THE NEW
HEALING
HERBS

THE NEW
HEALING
HERBS

THE **ESSENTIAL GUIDE** TO MORE THAN **130** OF NATURE'S MOST POTENT **HERBAL REMEDIES**

MICHAEL CASTLEMAN

RODALE.

This book is intended as a reference volume only, not as a medical manual. The information given here is designed
to help you make informed decisions about your health. It is not intended as a substitute for any treatment that may
have been prescribed by your doctor. If you suspect that you have a medical problem, we urge you to seek competent
medical help.

Mention of specific companies, organizations, or authorities in this book does not imply endorsement by the author
or publisher, nor does mention of specific companies, organizations, or authorities imply that they endorse this book,
its author, or the publisher.

Internet addresses and telephone numbers given in this book were accurate at the time it went to press.

A portion of this book was previously published in *The New Healing Herbs* in March 2010.

Rodale books may be purchased for business or promotional use or for special sales.
For information, please write to: Special Markets Department, Rodale, Inc.,
733 Third Avenue, New York, NY 10017

Printed in the United States of America

Rodale Inc. makes every effort to use acid-free ♾, recycled paper ♲.

Illustrations on pages 60, 69, 71, 74, 80, 91, 107, 110, 120, 122, 124, 176, 185, 196, 200,
224, 267, 292, 309, 312, 332, 340, 355, 357, 368, 373, 375, 377, 390, 393, 399, 408, 425, 435,
444, and 490 by Michael Gellatly; all others by Wayne Michaud

Book design by Christina Gaugler

Library of Congress Cataloging-in-Publication Data is on file with the publisher.

ISBN-13 978-1-62336-912-5 paperback

Distributed to the trade by Macmillan

2   4   6   8   10   9   7   5   3   1

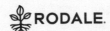

Contents

◇

PART I

◇

PART II

CHAPTER 6

Using the Healing Herbs:

Introduction

Twenty-seven years ago, when I wrote the first edition of *The Healing Herbs*, it was clear that herbal medicine was becoming increasingly popular. But no one involved with herbal healing in the late 1980s had any inkling of the explosion in popularity that herbal medicine would enjoy as the 20th century turned into the 21st. And in my wildest dreams, I could not imagine how popular *The Healing Herbs* would become—now more than 1 million copies have been sold in English, Spanish, French, Italian, and other languages.

Herbal medicine is currently a $6 billion a year industry, about five times the size it was when the original edition of this book appeared in 1991—not to mention another several billion dollars a year spent on cannabis alone. According to a national survey conducted for *Prevention* magazine, 49 percent of American adults—more than 100 million people—use an herbal medicine each year, and 24 percent—some 25 million people—call themselves regular users. And a study published in 2005 in *Archives of Internal Medicine* shows that 16 percent of men over 18 and 19 percent of women over 18 use a medicinal herb every week.

New herbs have been added to each edition of *The Healing Herbs,* from the 100 herbs in the first edition to 135 in this fourth edition. The newest herbs—cannabis, purslane, rooibos, saffron, stevia—are not "new" in the sense of newly discovered. These plants have been well-known for millennia. But only during the past decade have studies clearly shown how medicinally valuable they are.

Twenty-seven years ago, the medical profession was, at best, skeptical of herbal medicine. No longer. Today, it's not at all unusual for physicians to recommend:

- Echinacea for the common cold
- Ginger to prevent motion sickness and morning sickness
- Black cohosh for menopausal discomforts
- Cranberry to prevent urinary tract infections
- St. John's wort to treat depression
- Elderberry to treat flu
- Cannabis to treat nausea and pain

Doctors have become more open to herbal medicine in part because their friends and family members have reported success with them. In addition, mainstream American medical journals have changed their position on herbs. Twenty-seven years ago, major journals were quick to publish reports detailing the hazards of medicinal herbs (including several reports that turned out to be erroneous); rarely did they publish information about herbs' benefits. Today, these same journals publish studies that support herbal healing. A report in the *British Medical Journal* (now *BMJ*) was largely responsible for popularizing St. John's wort as an antidepressant. A review in the *Journal of Family Practice* concluded that echinacea is an effective cold treatment. Studies published in *Lancet* have demonstrated the effectiveness of feverfew for migraine prevention. A study in the *New England Journal of Medicine*, once openly hostile to herbs, showed that cranberry juice helps prevent urinary tract infections. And reports in the *Journal of the American Medical Association*, another traditional herb basher, have supported ginkgo as a treatment for Alzheimer's disease and saw palmetto for benign prostate enlargement. (This revised edition summarizes all these studies and many more.)

In other words, in the United States today, herbal medicine is more mainstream than it's been in 100 years. It's still not as medically accepted as it is in some other countries, notably Germany, nor is it as mainstream as it was in 19th century America before the pharmaceutical industry took medicine out of the herb garden and moved it into the laboratory. But herbal medicine is no longer the fringe practice that it was when the first edition of this book appeared in 1991.

Medicinal herb products have also come a long way in the last 27 years. There are many more of them and they are widely available, now stocked by many pharmacies and even some supermarkets. And they have become more reliable with the advent of "standardized extracts," preparations from plants bred to contain specific concentrations of pharmacologically active compounds, and then grown, harvested, stored, and prepared under controlled conditions to produce reliable dose uniformity. Standardized extracts are not quite as dose-controlled as laboratory-synthesized pharmaceuticals, but they're close, and considerably more dose-controlled than bulk herbs.

Unfortunately, since this book's original edition, we've also witnessed a few serious safety problems with herbs—two in particular. During the 1990s, an estimated 30 young adults died after taking mega overdoses of Chinese ephedra (*ma huang*). They were not using this herb medicinally, but rather to experience amphetamine-like intoxication. They took hundreds of times the dose that responsible herbalists would recommend. In addition, around the same time, 82 people worldwide suffered liver damage—and 9 died—while using kava, the South Pacific herbal tranquilizer. It turned out that kava's meteoric rise to popularity led to adulteration of the root with aerial parts of the plant that contain liver-toxic compounds. Because of the scandal, kava's popularity plummeted, adulteration ceased, and so did reports of liver damage.

But despite occasionally scary headlines, overall, herbal medicines have an admirable safety record. With more Americans using more medicinal herbs than at any time in a century, there have been few serious mishaps, especially when compared with the side effects—and deaths—from pharmaceuticals. (For more, see Chapter 2.)

Nonetheless, safety concerns seem destined to remain the most pressing issue in herbal medicine, largely because the Food and Drug Administration has, to date, refused to reopen its Review Process for over-the-counter drugs to include evaluation of herbs (see Chapter 1). But considerable numbers of FDA staff support the use of healing herbs. I'm cautiously optimistic that over the next decade, the FDA will adopt medicinal herb labeling regulations more appropriate to Americans' needs.

Meanwhile, *The New Healing Herbs*—completely revised, updated, and expanded—should help you use medicinal herbs confidently, effectively, and above all, safely.

Michael Castleman
San Francisco, September 2016

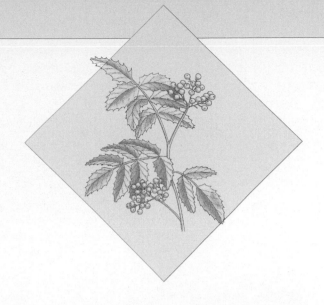

PART 1

There is nothing in the most advanced contemporary medicine whose embryo cannot be found in the medicine of the past.

—Maximilien E. P. Littré, French lexicographer

Chapter 1

FROM MAGIC TO MEDICINE

5,000 YEARS OF HERBAL HEALING

In 1991, glacial melting in the Italian Alps exposed a corpse preserved deep in the ice, the naturally mummified body of a prehistoric man who had frozen to death around 3300 BC.

Dubbed the Iceman, he wore straw-lined leather shoes, leather clothing, a thick coat made from woven grass, and a bearskin cap. He carried a wooden bow, a leather quiver filled with stone-tipped arrows, a flint-bladed knife, a wood-handled ax with a copper blade, and a food pouch that still contained dried deer meat and a prune.

The Iceman's pouch also contained two mysterious, walnut-sized cork-like lumps strung together on a leather thong, suggesting that they were of value. The lumps turned out to be bracket fungus (*Piptoporus betulinus*), mushrooms that grow in shelf-like plates on tree trunks. Bracket fungus contains agaric acid, a potent laxative, and an oily resin that is toxic to some bacteria and intestinal parasites.

Scientists studying the Iceman had no idea why he would have carried bracket fungus until, in 1998, a painstaking autopsy of his digestive tract turned up the eggs of an intestinal parasite (*Trichuris trichiura*).

It now appears that the Iceman knew he had a medical problem and was ingesting bracket fungus to treat his condition. Given its laxative and antiparasitic action, the fungus probably provided some benefit.

This discovery ranks as the world's oldest documented example of the practice of medicine, and it suggests that prehistoric humanity was more medically sophisticated than previously believed. After all, the Iceman or someone he knew had diagnosed his malady correctly and had recommended a reasonably appropriate treatment—an herbal treatment—5,000 years ago.

Animal Attractions

What exactly is a healing herb? "Herb" comes from the Latin for "grass." Technically, herbs are plants that wither each autumn, plants other than shrubs or trees. But many woody perennials are used in herbal healing: cinnamon, slippery elm, tea tree, and white willow, to name a few. To herbalists, "healing herbs" includes every plant with medicinal value.

Prehistoric sites show that Neanderthals

used yarrow, marshmallow, and other herbs as early as 60,000 years ago. What attracted them to these plants?

Animals played a key role. Prehistoric humans were keen observers of their world. No doubt our ancestors noticed that when animals appeared ill, they sometimes ate plants they ordinarily ignored. Humans sampled these plants and in many cases noticed curious effects, among them: wakefulness, sleepiness, laxative action, and increased urination. The herbs that caused these effects were incorporated into prehistoric shamanism, and later into medicine.

Animal-inspired herbalism is still with us. The controversial herbal cancer therapy marketed in the 1940s by Harry Hoxsey was reportedly inspired by a cancer-stricken horse that ate unusual herbs (more on this later).

Aromatic Magic

Early humans were also attracted to healing herbs' aromas. They rubbed strong-smelling herbs on their bodies to repel insects and to hide their scent from animals they feared or hunted. They also adorned themselves with sweet-smelling herbs to please their mates.

Fragrant herbs were eventually incorporated into perfumes and embalming mixtures. Demand for them spurred ancient trade. During the Middle Ages, when Europeans believed that bathing was unhealthy and farm animals often shared human living quarters, homemakers spread aromatic "strewing herbs" to freshen the air. Herbalists still prepare scent baskets (potpourris) today, and the perfume industry still creates most of its fragrances from herbal essences.

But foul odors, not fragrant ones, were key to the development of herbal healing. Early humans used plants such as rosemary, thyme, dill, and virtually all of today's culinary spices to mask the stench of rotting food, especially meats. Today, we use culinary herbs and spices only as flavor enhancers, but to prehistoric humanity, flavor enhancement was incidental to food preservation.

Prehistoric humanity had no refrigeration, and food spoiled quickly. Spoilage destroyed precious reserves, and early humans learned the hard way that eating rotten food caused illness and sometimes death. No doubt some prehistoric homemaker happened to lay some rotting food on a bed of mint, rosemary, sage, or some other aromatic herb, hoping the herb's fragrance would mask the item's stench. It did, and as a bonus, the food didn't spoil as quickly.

Our ancestors began wrapping food, especially meats, in aromatic herbs to preserve them, which led to other astonishing discoveries. Those who ate preservative herbs along with the food suffered less illness—and the food tasted better.

Surely, our ancestors thought, aromatic herbs were magical. As time passed and magic was incorporated into religion, ancient civilizations came to view aromatic herbs as gifts from the gods, which is why many herbs figure prominently in ancient myths and religions.

Thanks to modern science, we know that the oils that give aromatic herbs their fragrance and flavor contain potent antimicrobial compounds that kill many food-spoiling, disease-causing microorganisms. In fact, rosemary and sage have food-preservative action comparable to that of the commercial preservatives BHA and BHT.

Trial and Error

Our ancestors also most likely discovered many healing herbs by trial and error. They learned through experience that some plants healed, while others harmed. They had little control over their world. Average life expectancy was barely 30 years. Because their lives were so full of threatening, often fatal, surprises, anything that made life more predictable acquired an aura of magic and healing.

It's no coincidence that shamans from prehistoric times down to the present day have relied heavily on herbs, such as ipecac, buckthorn, and wormwood, that cause vomiting, purging, and hallucinations. Any predictable effect was better than none, and the ability to induce vomiting, purging, or visions made shaman/herbalists appear to possess magic powers.

The allure of predictable action remained central to medicine for thousands of years. Herbs that induced vomiting (emetics) or had powerful laxative action were used routinely in medicine until the late 19th century.

Major effects made big impressions, but early humans also recognized herbs' more subtle benefits. We'll never know what possessed some ancient Chinese peasant to brew a tea from the small, ungainly stalks of *ma huang* (Chinese ephedra), but several thousand years ago, someone did. In the process, that person stumbled upon one of the world's oldest medicines, a decongestant whose laboratory analog, pseudoephedrine, inspired the name of a popular cold/allergy product, Sudafed. (Over-the-counter Sudafed no longer contains pseudoephedrine.)

Similarly, we'll never know how many roots ancient Asians dug up before they discovered ginger. Or why Native Americans had a hunch that black cohosh might be useful in gynecology. However, around the world ancient peoples dug, dried, chewed, pounded, rubbed, and boiled the plants around them—and discovered the vast majority of medicinal herbs still used today.

Isolated Cultures, Similar Herbs

Botanical trial and error becomes even more remarkable considering that widely separated cultures independently arrived at similar uses for many healing herbs. There are four major herbal-medicine traditions: Chinese, Ayurvedic (India), European (including Egyptian), and Native American. The ancient spice trade introduced Asian herbs such as garlic, ginger, and cinnamon into Europe thousands of years ago. And a few ancient herbalists, notably the 1st-century Greek, Dioscorides, traveled extensively as a physician to Roman armies and absorbed the herbal wisdom of cultures throughout the ancient world.

Nonetheless, early Asian and European herbalists were largely isolated from one another. Until the 1st century AD, it took 2 years for spice traders to travel round-trip from Greece to India's black pepper farms.

Despite today's instant global communication, different healing systems still operate relatively independently. During the 1970s and early 1980s, ginkgo became an important medicine in France and Germany for aging-related ailments, with sales topping $500 million a year. Most U.S. medical school libraries stocked the German and French journals showing ginkgo's remarkable effectiveness, yet American physicians virtually ignored ginkgo well into the 1990s. How connected could the ancient herbalists have been?

Even granting a nearly impossible level of herbal mingling between Asia and Europe, the land bridge between Asia and North America became the Bering Sea about 10,000 years ago. Until the 15th century, Old World cultures were almost entirely isolated from the Americas. Nonetheless, Old and New World herbalists used many herbs similarly.

- Angelica and licorice. Asians, Europeans, and Native Americans relied on these herbs as treatments for respiratory ailments.

- Hop and the mints. All ancient herbal traditions used these herbs as stomach soothers.

- Blackberry and raspberry. Around the world, they were used to treat diarrhea.

- Uva-ursi. Asians, Europeans, and Native Americans all discovered its diuretic properties.

- White willow. All four herbal healing traditions used it to treat pain and inflammation.

During the 19th century, chemists used "herbal convergence" to point them to plants whose extracts became the first pharmaceuticals. According to a report in the journal *Science*, about 75 percent of the pharmaceuticals derived from plants came to drug companies' attention thanks to traditional herbal medicine.

Homage to the "Wise Women"

Most medical histories chronicle great achievements by great men: Hippocrates, the father of medicine; Galen, Rome's leading physician; William Harvey's explanation of blood circulation; Edward Jenner's inoculations against smallpox; Louis Pasteur's Germ Theory; Alexander Fleming's discovery of penicillin.

But from ancient times to the present day, a relatively small number of male physicians made the great discoveries and ministered to the rich and royal while an enormous number of unsung women herbalists took care of everyone else.

Women healers have gone by many names: midwives, wise women, green women, witches, old wives, and nurses. Most physicians have scoffed at women's folk healing, and scientists often dismiss folk wisdom as "old wives' tales." But medically untrained women still provide much of the world's primary care. Even in the United States, most people view physicians as the health care choice of last resort. The medical profession promotes the idea that family doctors are our primary providers, but studies show that before people call health professionals, about 90 percent consult a friend or family member. These informal heath advisers are overwhelmingly women.

Ancient physicians officially recognized women's leading role in obstetrics and gynecology more than 2,000 years ago in the Hippocratic Oath, still recited by many graduating medical students today: "I will prescribe no ... pessary [contraceptive device] to produce abortion." Anti-abortion activists have seized on this statement as a condemnation of abortion. In fact, this declaration withdrew male doctors from gynecology and gave the field—including abortion, which has been widely practiced since ancient times—to midwives.

Whatever your opinion of abortion, throughout history women have consistently sought to control their fertility. After all, until about 150 years ago, childbirth was a leading cause of female death.

Midwives completely dominated obstetrics and gynecology until the late 19th century. They used many herbs to calm the womb, trigger menstruation, induce abortion, promote or dry up mothers' milk, and treat infant colic and infectious diarrhea (still a leading cause of infant death in many nations). These were the daily concerns that female patients presented to their women healers.

Sometimes medically unschooled women herbalists introduced university-trained physicians to powerful medicines, for example, the heart drug digitalis from foxglove. But by and large, male physicians dismissed female folk healers as ignorant practitioners of medicine that was at best, inferior, and at worst, harmful.

Nonetheless, women herbalists have played a key—and largely undocumented—role in medical history. Just as herbs are the forgotten sources of many medicines, the "wise women" represent the forgotten healers whose thousands of years of collective experience taught us how to use herbs safely and effectively.

The wise women were particularly adept at contraception. Around 700 BC, an oracle sent Greek colonists to the coast of what is now Libya to found a colony, Cyrene. It was located in a dry, desolate, inhospitable place, but the colonists soon discovered a local plant that made them wealthy, silphion (in Latin, *silphium*), a species of fennel. Silphium was a remarkably effective contraceptive. When women ate it, they did not conceive. The herb quickly became the contraceptive of choice around the Mediterranean. Cyrenian coins depicted the plant, often held by a woman. Poets extolled its powers. Silphium became so popular that overharvesting eventually wiped it out.

Shen Nung and the Origins of Chinese Medicine

Legend has it that around 3400 BC (the Iceman's era) "the divine farmer," mythical emperor-sage Shen Nung, invented agriculture and discovered that many plants have medicinal value. He tested herbs on himself and recorded their effects—and died after ingesting one that was poisonous.

Chinese herbalists credit Shen Nung as the author of China's first great herb guide or "herbal," the *Pen Tsao Ching* (*Classic of Herbs*), which listed 237 botanical prescriptions using dozens of herbs, including cannabis, ephedra, rhubarb, and opium poppy. However, most authorities agree that the *Pen Tsao Ching* was passed down orally for millennia until published in book form during the Han dynasty, around AD 100.

Chinese herbalists discovered many medicinal plants, notably ginseng, tea, sesame, garlic, and cinnamon. Starting around AD 500, it became customary for Chinese emperors to commission updates of Shen Nung's herbal. Over the centuries, these became increasingly elaborate—and contradictory. By 1590, when Li Shih-Chen published his landmark 52-volume *Pen Tsao Kang Mu* (*Catalogue of Medicinal Herbs*), he included 1,094 medicinal plants and an astounding 11,000 herbal formulas.

Today, practitioners of Chinese herbalism still study Li's work, but they have simplified his art, employing some 300 herbs, 150 of which are considered indispensable, among them: Chinese angelica (*dang gui*), burdock, chrysanthemum, cinnamon, dandelion, garlic, ginger, ginseng, hawthorn, licorice, lotus, mint, rhubarb, scullcap, senna, and tea.

European colonialists introduced Western medicine into China, dismissing Chinese herbalism and acupuncture as nonsense. The Chinese felt the same way about the "foreign devils'" medicine, and the two systems seemed irreconcilable.

But shortly after the establishment of the People's Republic in 1949, the Chinese government decided that China's huge, medically underserved population could benefit from combining the two systems. Today, throughout China, Western-trained physicians practice alongside traditional herbalists and acupuncturists. Chinese and Western physicians examine the same patients, confer with each other, and often coordinate their recommendations.

A turning point in American acceptance of Chinese medicine occurred in 1972, when Richard Nixon became the first president to visit China. During his visit, American reporters visited a hospital and watched astonished as a woman had abdominal surgery while fully conscious, her only anesthesia being some acupuncture needles in her earlobes and feet.

On the trip, influential *New York Times* columnist James Reston developed appendicitis and had surgery. Afterward, he tried acupuncture for postsurgical pain control. He was so pleased with the results that he wrote a testimonial column that helped open the United States to acupuncture and Chinese herbalism.

Jivaka and the Vedas

According to legend, around 1200 BC a poor Indian boy named Jivaka studied medicine under the great Punarvasu Atreya, founder of India's first medical school at the University of Taxila in the Punjab. Having no money, the lad offered to become Atreya's servant in exchange for training.

Seven years later, Jivaka asked his teacher when his studies would be completed. Instead of answering, Atreya challenged him to scour the countryside and collect plants that were medi-

cally useless. Jivaka searched for a month, only to return sullen and empty-handed. He told his mentor that he was unable to find a single plant without healing power. Atreya replied, "Go! You now have the knowledge to be a physician."

Centered in the Indus Valley near the present India-Pakistan border, ancient Indian civilization was quite advanced. Excavations at Harappa and Mohenjo Daro dating to about 2500 BC have revealed municipal water and sewerage systems more advanced than the ones the Romans developed 2,000 years later.

Ancient Indians called their medicine Ayurveda, from two Sanskrit words: *ayur*, life, and *veda*, knowledge. Ayurvedic medicine developed from the *Vedas*, India's four books of classic wisdom.

The oldest, the 4,500-year-old *Rig Veda*, is a collection of 1,028 Hindu hymns, recited orally from 2500 BC and written 1,000 years later. The *Rig Veda* contains detailed descriptions of eye surgery, limb amputation, and medicinal formulas using 67 herbs, including ginger, cinnamon, and senna. The 3,200-year-old *Atharva Veda* also discusses many healing herbs.

Around 700 BC (400 years before Hippocrates), Charaka, a University of Taxila professor, wrote Ayurvedic medicine's first encyclopedia, the *Charaka Samhita*, listing 500 herbal formulas.

In 250 BC, India's King Asoka converted to Buddhism and launched a 1,000-year golden age of Ayurvedic medicine. Asoka sent Buddhist monk-physicians around the country to heal the sick and convert them to Buddhism. As the centuries passed, pilgrims came from as far away as China and Persia to receive Ayurvedic treatment.

One favorite Ayurvedic herb was *Rauwolfia serpentina*. It's the source of resperine, a drug used in Western medicine for much of the 20th century to manage high blood pressure.

Ayurvedic healing influenced Arab medicine, which combined Greco-Roman, Middle Eastern, and Asian therapies. Arab physicians in turn introduced some Ayurvedic practices into Europe.

During the 19th century, the British introduced Western medicine into India, but a majority of Indians and Pakistanis still rely on Ayurvedic medicine or homeopathy, both of which prefer medicinal herbs to drugs.

10,000 Healing Herbs

During ancient times, what we know today as Iraq was home to a succession of peoples: the Sumerians, Assyrians, Babylonians, and Persians. The early Sumerians had no physicians. Sick people congregated in public squares, and passersby gave them advice.

As Sumerian culture developed, so did its medicine. In late Sumerian mythology, the gods give Sumeria's original healer, Thrita, 10,000 healing herbs and the wisdom to use them. One of the world's oldest surviving prescriptions is a Sumerian clay tablet from around 2100 BC that mentions myrrh, cypress, and opium poppy.

By 1000 BC, Assyrians could consult three types of healers: herbalists (internists), knife wielders (surgeons), and counselors (psychiatrists). Herbalists were the most numerous and prominent, in part because Assyria was strategically placed along the ancient Spice Road (also known as the Silk Route) from Asia to Egypt. Archeologists have unearthed an Assyrian pharmacy that stocked 230 herbs, including almond, anise, caraway, coriander, juniper, saffron, sesame, turmeric, and willow.

The Assyrians, and later the Babylonians and Persians, were enthusiastic spice traders. Valued for taste, food preservation, and healing, spices were in great demand and generated huge profits. When properly dried and stored, spices could travel great distances without spoiling. They didn't have to be fed like cattle and slaves. And they took up little space, which meant they could be easily transported and hidden from thieves. No wonder that in Genesis 37:25, when Joseph's jealous brothers sold him into slavery, he was purchased by "a caravan . . . with camels bearing gum, balm, and myrrh on their way to Egypt."

Imhotep and the "Stinking Ones" of the Nile

In 1874, in the Valley of the Tombs near Luxor, the German Egyptologist Georg Ebers discovered the world's oldest surviving medical text, a 65-foot papyrus dating from 1500 BC. The Ebers Papyrus listed 876 herbal formulas from more than 500 plants: aloe, caraway, cardamom, chamomile, cinnamon, coriander, fennel, fenugreek, garlic, gentian, ginger, juniper, mint, myrrh, onion, opium poppy, saffron, sage, sesame, and thyme. The Ebers Papyrus shows that ancient Egyptians used around one-third of the herbs in today's Western herbal pharmacopoeia.

Some Ebers formulas strike the modern reader as bizarre, such as a shampoo made from a dog's paw, decayed palm leaves, and a donkey hoof, all boiled in oil. Others sound surprisingly prescient—the recommendation to bandage moldy bread over wounds to prevent infection. Penicillin was originally derived from a mold.

In Egyptian mythology, Thoth, god of knowledge, created medicine. He also invented writing, the arts, and science. The most notable Egyptian physician was Imhotep, who was also the architect to Pharaoh Zoser (3000 BC). Imhotep is credited with designing the first pyramid, but as time passed, he was revered mostly as a healer. He became deified, and around 700 BC, Egypt's medical school at Memphis and a nearby school for midwives were dedicated to him.

The Egyptians imported mountains of herbs for perfumes, embalming mixtures, and medicines. They also considered plants important spoils of war. In 1475 BC, when Pharaoh Thutmose III conquered what is now Syria, he demanded as tribute specimens of all Syrian plants not found in Egypt.

The Egyptians loved aromatic herbs. The ancient kingdom's access to both the Mediterranean and Arabian seas allowed them to import aromatics from as far away as Spain and the Spice Islands (Indonesia).

But the Egyptians also loved two herbs that many other ancients considered foul-smelling—garlic and onion. The Egyptians believed that they prevented disease (a view supported by modern science). They ate so much garlic and onion that the Greek historian Herodotus called them "the stinking ones." Both herbs were found in the tomb of King Tut.

The Egyptians also gave their slaves daily rations of garlic and onion to keep them strong and healthy. In 450 BC, Herodotus wrote of an inscription inside the Cheops Pyramid at Giza (built around 2900 BC) that said 1,600 talents of silver, enough to equip an army, had been spent on garlic and onions for its builders.

Once, a garlic shortage once forced the Egyptians to cut their slaves' rations. The slaves became so incensed that they refused to work. If this story is true, it would be the world's first documented strike.

Egyptian farmers could not satisfy the demand for garlic and onions, so the Egyptians turned to the Philistines, who lived in nearby Canaan (Israel). The Philistine city of Askelon, in Gaza, became a major garlic and onion trading center, for the Egyptians, Greeks, and Romans. The Romans favored the Philistines' small green onions, calling them *ascalonia* after Askelon. The word evolved into *escallon*, and finally into our "scallion."

Middle Eastern herbalists also used a great deal of opium to treat pain. Excavations of 3,000-year-old tombs in Israel have discovered pottery shaped like opium poppy pods and containing residues of opium, the narcotic still widely used today as codeine and morphine.

By about 500 BC, Egyptian herbalists were considered the finest in the Mediterranean, and rulers from Rome to Babylon recruited them as court physicians. Aspiring physicians—Rome's Galen among them—went to Egypt to study with the medical masters of the Nile.

From Aesculapius to Hippocrates

The early Greeks viewed illness as a divine curse and prayed to Apollo, god of medicine, for recovery. In Greek mythology, Apollo fathered a son, Aesculapius, a physician-god like Imhotep, who treated the sick helped by his daughters, Hygeia and Panacea. Hygeia, source of our word "hygiene," touted healthy living, while Panacea, whose name means cure-all, treated disease.

When ill, early Greeks visited temples dedicated to Aesculapius where physician-priests treated them with baths, exercise, massage, fasting, prayer, herbs, counseling, and animal sacrifices. The program was similar to the regimens at many contemporary health spas, except for the sacrifices.

Snakes were sacred to Aesculapius, and they slithered freely around his temple grounds. One omen of imminent recovery was to have a snake lick a patient's wounds. Snakes' tongues thus became symbols of healing, and they remained ingredients in medicinal potions well into the Middle Ages. Aesculapius was often pictured carrying a staff with a snake wrapped around it. The snake-staff combination became the caduceus, the symbol of medicine.

Sons of Aesculapian priest-doctors often followed their fathers into the healing temples. On the island of Kos, off Turkey, one Aesculapian family produced Hippocrates (460–377 BC), the father of Western medicine. Hippocrates rebelled against Aesculapius, however, by secularizing Greek medicine. He believed that diseases came not from the gods but from natural causes: the environment, climate, and diet.

In the *Iliad*, Homer claimed that Greek medicine came from Egypt. Kos is located only a short voyage from the land of Imhotep. But Hippocrates clearly elaborated on Egyptian practices. From his seat under a plane tree (a type of sycamore), he was the first physician known to examine patients closely and use case studies in medical training, a method still employed in medical education today.

Hippocrates never wrote a word, but his students compiled the 72-volume *Corpus Hippocraticum*. It mentions 350 medicinal plants, including anise, burdock, clove, cinnamon, mint, rosemary, and thyme.

Hippocrates taught that health depends on a balance among the body's four vital fluids, or "humors": blood, phlegm, yellow bile, and black bile. Hippocrates' Humoral Theory of illness remained a cornerstone of European medicine until the mid-19th century, when Pasteur's Germ Theory supplanted it.

The humors were said to have four qualities: hot, cold, dry, and wet. Hippocrates prescribed warming herbs such as ginger for diseases that he believed were caused by cold and cooling herbs such as mint for ailments produced by heat. All classic Western herbals assigned Hippocratic qualities to healing herbs—warming, cooling, and so on—and listed the "foul humors" they supposedly relieved.

Aesculapian priests and later Greek physicians grew and gathered many herbs. They also bought medicinal plants from herbalists known as root gatherers or rhizomists. (In botany, a rhizome is an underground stem.) The rhizomists were peasant foragers who gathered medicinal plants and sold them in market towns.

Hippocrates had no women students, but many midwives were also rhizomists. Homer mentions one named Agamede, who was famous for her knowledge of herbs.

Shortly before Hippocrates' death, the father of botany was born. Theophrastus (372–285 BC) was the author of *Historia Plantarum* (*An Inquiry into Plants*) and *De Causis Plantarum* (*The Growth of Plants*), which remained standard references for more than 1,000 years. Many of the 550 plants he discussed were used medicinally. Theophrastus operated a prominent herb shop in Athens. He and Aristotle were friends. When the seminal philosopher died, he bequeathed Theophrastus his garden.

Roman Herbalists: Dioscorides, Pliny, and Galen

The first medical botanist was the Turkish-born Greek Pedanius Dioscorides (AD 40–90), who served as a physician with Emperor Nero's Roman legions traveling from Germany to Arabia. In AD 78, he published *De Materia Medica* (*On Medicines*), Europe's first book on herbs. It discussed 600 plants, including aloe, anise, chamomile, cinnamon, dill, marjoram, poppy, rhubarb, and thyme.

As a military physician, Dioscorides focused on soldiers' needs, particularly wound treatment. But *De Materia Medica* also included a great deal of herbal folk wisdom, proving that he learned from many herbalists during his travels.

De Materia Medica remained a standard medical text for 1,500 years. Virtually every herbal published through the 17th century referred to it. After the invention of the printing press in 1440, *De Materia Medica* was one of the first books published. The oldest copy in the United States, from 1547, resides in the Lloyd Library in Cincinnati (more on the Lloyd Library later).

It's fitting that Rome's legions produced a great herbalist, because part of their mission was to protect the Roman spice trade with Asia from barbarian predation. By the 1st century AD, the herb and spice trade was a cornerstone of Roman commerce. Roman demand for medicinal, culinary, and perfume herbs was almost insatiable.

Shortly before the publication of *De Materia Medica*, Greek merchants discovered the secret of the Indian Ocean's shifting monsoon winds, which blew east toward India part of the year and west toward Egypt the rest. This insight allowed spice merchants to cut round-trips from Rome to India in half, from 2 years to 1. Faster transit meant cheaper herbs, such as the Roman favorite black pepper, whose price plummeted to the modern equivalent of around $100 per ounce. (I recently bought black peppercorns for $1 an ounce.)

While Dioscorides traveled the Empire, back in Rome, Caius Plinius Secundus, or Pliny the Elder (AD 23–79), was busy compiling ancient scientific knowledge into his 37-volume *Historia Naturalis* (*Natural History*). Volumes 12 through 19 dealt with botany, and 20 through 27 addressed herbal medicine. Pliny recommended some wild prescriptions—for colds, "kissing a mouse." But many of his herbal recommendations were more plausible and guided physicians for centuries.

In August AD 79, Pliny heard that Mount Vesuvius near Pompeii was rumbling. He had to see it and traveled there. When the volcano exploded on August 24, Pliny was perched on a nearby hill, taking notes. He died of asphyxiation.

Fifty years later, Claudius Galenus, better known as Galen (AD 131–200), became Rome's leading physician. Born into a wealthy family in Turkey, Galen studied medicine in Greece and Alexandria and then spent several years as a physician to gladiators. At age 30, he moved to Rome, and eventually he became the physician to Emperor Marcus Aurelius.

Galen was arrogant and dogmatic. He practiced a highly theoretical form of medicine that dominated European medical training for 1,500 years. At a time when midwife-herbalists relied on single herbs or formulas with a few ingredients, Galen practiced "polypharmacy," which used complex combination of herbs, animal parts, and minerals to create concoctions called "galenicals." Galen's wealthy patients liked galenicals because they were expensive and therefore exclusive. As the centuries passed, Europe's nobility came to favor costly galenicals, while the peasantry stuck with single herbs or simple formulas, which became known as "simples."

Roman rhizomists—*herbarii*, in Latin—congregated around Capitoline Hill. They were a motley crew. Physicians accused them of mislabeling and adulterating their herbs. Pliny and Galen boycotted them, provided tips on detecting adulteration (variations in color, taste, aroma), and urged physicians to grow and gather their own medicinal plants.

Roman Assassins: From Mithridates to Theriaca

Roman herbalists were as likely to be killers as healers. The Imperial court seethed with murderous intrigue. Among available assassination methods—knifing, "accidents," and poisoning among them—the herbal approach was most popular.

Political notables were typically surrounded by bodyguards, making knifings and accidents difficult to arrange. Physical assault also involved risk of capture. Poisoning could be accomplished from a safe distance. Death occurred sometime after the deed, allowing for escape or alibi. And in an age before autopsy, when apparently healthy people often sickened and died suddenly, wily poisoners might never be suspected.

As a result, rulers throughout the Roman Empire became obsessed with herbal poisons and the development of antidotes, known in Latin as *theriaca* (in English, "theriacs") from the Greek *theriakon*, meaning remedies for venom.

The ancient world's most poison-paranoid ruler was Mithridates Eupator (120–66 BC), king of Pontus, on the Black Sea. Mithridates governed by terror and feared being poisoned. As a result, he delved into botany, believing that familiarity with both poisonous and medicinal plants was his best defense. His botanical expertise is commemorated in the genus name of the herb boneset, *Eupatorium*.

In addition to formulating dozens of theriacs, Mithridates supposedly ordered his court physician to concoct the ultimate herbal poison. The ancient king took increasing doses to develop a tolerance and make himself immune.

Then, in 66 BC, the Romans attacked. Facing capture and certain execution, Mithridates tried to poison himself. But according to legend, he'd become so tolerant that no poison could kill him. He ordered a slave to stab him to death. To this day, the word *mithridatism* means an acquired tolerance to poisons.

Roman nobility offered to pay enormous sums for any antidotes attributed to Mithridates. Needless to say, Rome's unscrupulous *herbarii* were only too happy to peddle bogus mixtures as "Mithridates' Theriac."

A century after the unpoisonable king's death, Emperor Nero was driven nearly insane by fear of poisoning, in part because he'd gained the throne by poisoning his stepbrother. Nero ordered his physician, Andromachus of Crete, to improve on Mithridates' Theriac. Andromachus mixed 78 herbal, animal, and mineral ingredients—including opium, a lizard, and snake flesh (in homage to Aesculapius)—to create Andromachus' Theriac.

Slave midwife-herbalists were highly valued as poisoners. They could often be placed as concubines in the bedrooms of their intended victims, beyond the reach of bodyguards and tasters, who sampled rulers' food and drink before they ingested, just in case. A slave herbalist Locusta became famous for her poisoning skill. After one important murder, she received her freedom and a gift of land.

Not to be outdone by Andromachus, Galen wrote a book containing more than 100 theriac recipes. He also developed his own, Galene, a polypharmaceutical brew of 70 ingredients, including dozens of herbs, honey, wine, minerals, and animal parts that took 40 days to prepare.

When Rome fell, the barbarians seized not only Rome's lands and wealth but also its vast stores of herbs and spices. During one attack, the barbarians demanded horses, money—and 3,000 pounds of black pepper.

Theriaca eventually evolved into the Elizabethan English word "treacle." The Elizabethan peasantry used garlic as an all-purpose medicine and antidote, and it became known as "poor man's treacle."

Avicenna and the Invention of Pharmacy

As Rome collapsed, Arab civilization filled the intellectual vacuum. From AD 600 to 800, Islamic armies forged an empire stretching from Spain across Northern Africa to India. Unlike the barbarians who seized Roman Europe, the Arabs venerated Greco-Roman culture and learning. Along with the spoils of conquest, they sent tens of thousands of Greco-Roman books to Baghdad, for translation into Arabic.

Ibn-Sina, or Avicenna (AD 980–1037), was the era's leading Arab physician. While still quite young, he cured an Arab prince of a serious illness, triggering great demand for his services. A

follower of Galen, he wrote the *Canon of Medicine*, the West's medical bible for 600 years. Book Two discussed healing herbs, including cinnamon, clove, nutmeg, myrrh, rhubarb, and senna.

The Arabs revered Galen but were not ruled by polypharmacy. They simplified Galen's formulas and developed pharmacy as a field distinct from medicine. The first pharmacies appeared in Baghdad in the 9th century.

Arab pharmacists replaced galenicals with syrups, ointments, and tinctures (alcohol extracts). They were the first to distill pure alcohol, whose name derives from the Arabic *al-kohl*, or "quintessence." Arab medicine also gave us the terms alkalai, from *al-qali*, "ashes," and sugar, from *sukkar*, meaning "grain or pebble."

From AD 800 until Christians recaptured it in the 1400s, Spain rivaled Baghdad as a center of Arab herbalism. One influential herbalist was Abul-Kasim Khalef ibn Abbas, in Spanish, Abulcasis (AD 936–1013). He wrote *Liber Servitoris* (*The Book of Simples*), an important source for later European herbals.

The other prominent herbalist was Ibn al-Baitar (AD 1197–1248), a botanist who collected 1,500 plants from Spain to Syria. He also wrote the most complete Arab herbal, the *Corpus of Simples*. It introduced 200 new healing herbs (and poisons), including tamarind, aconite, and nux vomica (strychnine).

Monasteries and Liqueurs

After the fall of Rome, the Catholic Church dominated European medicine, reviving the pre-Hippocratic Greek belief that illness was a punishment from God and was treatable only by prayer and penance. But Catholic monks preserved Greco-Roman herbalism by copying their texts.

Among monastic orders, the Benedictines were the most avid herbalists. They adopted the Arab practice of making tinctures. They flavored wine with digestion-promoting herbs and created the forerunners of today's liqueurs. One is still called Benedictine.

Charlemagne (AD 742–814) was so impressed by the Benedictines' herb gardens that he ordered all of the monasteries in his vast realm to plant "physic gardens" to ensure an adequate supply of healing herbs. Charlemagne described herbs as "friends of the physician and cook."

Around AD 820, the Benedictines designed their ideal monastery, known as the Plan of St. Gall. In one corner was an infirmary that included rooms for bathing, examinations, and bloodletting. It also featured a 1,000-square-foot physic garden that contained two dozen herbs, including: cumin, fennel, fenugreek, mint, pennyroyal, rose, rosemary, rue, sage, savory, and watercress.

In another corner was a kitchen garden that also contained many herbs, including dill, which was commonly mixed with salt water to preserve vegetables, particularly cucumbers, forerunners of today's dill pickles.

The most notable Benedictine herbalist was Hildegard of Bingen (1098–1179), abbess of the Rupertsburg convent in the German Rhineland. Centuries before the Renaissance, Hildegard was a Renaissance woman, a nun, administrator, composer, writer, and herbalist. Her religious music is still performed today.

Hildegard claimed that visions of God commanded her to treat the sick and compile herbal formulas. Her book, *Hildegard's Medicine*, combined Catholic mystical, German folk medicine, and her own extensive herbal experience. Hilde-

gard's favorite herbs included aloe, apple, bay, blackberry, caraway, celery, clove, dill, fennel, garlic, hyssop, licorice, marjoram, myrrh, nettle, nutmeg, onion, oregano, parsley, raspberry, rosemary, rue, thyme, and watercress.

Hildegard's herbal is unique. At a time when the few literate Europeans, mostly monks, were content to copy the Greeks, Romans, and Avicenna, she composed an original medical text based on her own clinical experience. What's more, she was the only medieval woman who left any account of "wise woman" healing practices.

Today, much of Hildegard's advice sounds silly. For poor vision, she advocated rubbing the eyes with a topaz soaked in wine. However, many of her recommendations were quite sensible. She advocated eating a balanced diet and brushing teeth with aloe and myrrh—both of which have antibacterial, decay-preventive properties.

While Hildegard relied on simples, complex galenicals continued to be valued by the nobility, who had access to galenically inclined physicians and the wealth to afford all the ingredients that Galen's polypharmaceuticals required. The men who mixed medieval galenicals were the first alchemists.

Around the time that the Benedictines invented liqueur, Germanic Angles and Saxons were settling England. They brought European herbalism with them and learned how the native Celts and their priests, the Druids, used healing herbs.

Around AD 950, a nobleman named Bald persuaded England's King Alfred to commission the first British herbal. The book combined Anglo-Saxon and Celtic herbalism with Greco-Roman and Arab practices. It was called the *Leech Book of Bald*. (Leech comes from *laece*,

Anglo-Saxon for "doctor.") It discussed 500 plants, including vervain and mistletoe, both sacred to the Druids. A surviving copy is on display at the British Museum.

With the Renaissance, European medicine took a secular turn. After the invention of printing, monks stopped copying ancient herbals, but continued to tend their physic gardens. One Austrian monk-gardener was Gregor Mendel. In 1868, he published *Plant Hybridization*, an account of his experiments with peas. It launched the science of genetics.

Wise Women: From Healers to Witches

Hildegard of Bingen was lucky to have lived in the 12th century. Had she practiced herbalism from 1300 to 1650, she might have been burned as a witch.

It's not clear what led to Europe's 350 years of witch hunts. Feminists link the practice to the rise of secular medicine as a male-dominated profession. Others blame the hysteria on bubonic plague (the Black Death), which swept Europe in waves and killed much of its population.

Another theory holds that European rulers and the Catholic Church became alarmed by post–Black Plague population decline, which they blamed on contraceptive herbs touted by the wise women. The leading medieval contraceptive herbs were abortifacients, or in modern parlance "morning-after" plants. The most popular were pennyroyal, rue, and wormwood. Modern research shows that all three stimulate uterine contractions and abortion.

After 1300, witch hunts transformed folk herbalists' image from wise women to evil witches. The witch hunts started in Germany and eventually spread throughout Europe. Accusations of "sexual intercourse with the Devil" were typically accompanied by testimony that the alleged witch practiced herbal medicine and made healing mixtures, cosmetics, love potions, aphrodisiacs, abortifacients, and poisons.

Accusations of poisoning were particularly damning. It's possible that some women herbalists continued the Roman tradition of herbal assassination, but this was the era before the discovery of the dose-response relationship, the idea that the greater the dose, the greater the effect. Many so-called witches' plants, poisonous in large amounts, caused no harm in therapeutic or cosmetic amounts. Nonetheless, the witch hunters considered them poisons.

One plant associated with witchcraft was "devil's herb," which could be lethal if ingested. But applied topically, it was a cosmetic. Eventually, the plant was renamed "beautiful woman," or belladonna.

Another sorcerer's herb was witch's bells. Large amounts are poisonous, but small amounts stimulate the heart. After the witch-hunt era, the plant's name was changed to foxglove, source of the heart drug digitalis.

Conviction of witchcraft meant death. At the height of the witch hunts, as many as 600 women a year—about two a day—were executed in parts of Germany. At Toulouse, France, 400 were put to death in a single day.

North America did not escape the hysteria. The Salem witch trials in Massachusetts (1692) resulted in 20 executions of women. Records suggest that they were wise women herbalists.

After the witch hunts, the saintly Hildegard was forgotten, replaced by the witches of Shakespeare's *Macbeth*, whose bubbling cauldron contained mandrake, belladonna, and other herbs.

Witches were also vilified in the stories that became today's fairy tales. In *Snow White,* the evil queen-witch concocts an herbal poison, dips an apple into it, and slips it to Snow White, who falls into a coma, an echo of herbal poisoning dating back to the Romans.

The witch hunts failed to eradicate women's herbalism, but they succeeded in driving it underground. More than a century after the last witch hunts, the "old woman" who helped popularize foxglove said that it was a "secret family recipe." Her forebears had good reason to keep their use of witch's bells a secret.

A World Hungry for Spices

The fall of Rome devastated the spice trade. Arab merchants continued to import Asian herbs into Europe, but the commerce declined and prices soared. During the Middle Ages, a pound of ginger could buy a fat sheep. Black pepper was counted out corn by corn and used to pay rents, taxes, and dowries.

Then came the Crusades. From 1095 until 1291, European armies attempted to wrest the Holy Land from Islamic control. Militarily, they failed, but while in the Middle East, the Crusaders tasted Asian spices and returned home craving more.

The 1296 publication of Marco Polo's travelogue heightened European fascination with Asian herbs. Polo's father and uncle were merchants who set out from Venice to China in 1271, taking the 17-year-old Marco with them. The young Italian became a favorite of Kublai Kahn, and when he returned in 1295, his famous memoir was filled with mouthwatering accounts of Asia's tantalizing spices.

The ancient Spice Routes slowly reopened.

Around 1300, British spice dealers obtained a royal charter to become the Guild of Pepperers. They bought black pepper and other herbs from brokers in Venice, who traded with Arab importers. By 1400, Venice alone imported 2,500 tons of ginger and black pepper a year. European demand seemed limitless.

Then something terrible happened. During the 1400s, the Mongols, who supported trade with Europe, lost Western Asia to the Ottoman Turks, who closed the trade routes. In Venice and Genoa, cities enriched by the spice trade, Italian merchants grew desperate for new avenues to the East. If the world was round, as some claimed, it might be possible to sail west across the Atlantic to reach the Indies.

It was no coincidence that Christopher Columbus hailed from Genoa. He never reached the East Indies, but he returned from the New World with allspice and red pepper, known to Caribbean Indians as *kian*, or "cayenne."

In 1498, when the Portuguese explorer Vasco da Gama succeeded in sailing around Africa to India, he stepped ashore in Calcutta saying, "We come in search of Christians and spices."

The Portuguese and Dutch grabbed an early lead in exploration. They monopolized the sea route around Africa to India and the Spice Islands (Indonesia), as well as the trade in cinnamon, cloves, tea, and black pepper.

The Spanish concentrated on the New World and its gold. Sometimes they found the precious metal, sometimes other valuables. In 1519, Hernando Cortez watched as Mexico's Aztec ruler, Montezuma, toasted his arrival by sipping from a golden goblet. Cortez coveted the goblet—but the herbal beverage that it contained, *chocolatl* or "chocolate," eventually became more important than the Aztec's gold.

In addition to chocolate, Spanish conquistadors returned home with corn, tobacco, potatoes, carrots, strawberries, lima beans, tomatoes, sarsaparilla, passionflower, and the most important new healer of all, cinchona (Jesuit or Peruvian bark). Cinchona was the first effective treatment for malaria (also known as ague, intermittent fever, and swamp fever), which had plagued the Mediterranean area and Europe since ancient times. Centuries later, cinchona became the source of the antimalarial drug quinine.

The Spanish may also have returned from the New World with something else: syphilis. A doctor in Seville claimed he'd treated Columbus' crew in 1493. It's possible that they became infected in Haiti. Or perhaps increased trade spread a disease that had existed for ages in isolated pockets around the Mediterranean.

In any event, an epidemic of unusually virulent syphilis swept through Europe in 1494, killing thousands. Europeans considered the disease an import from the New World and looked across the Atlantic for a cure. They focused on sarsaparilla, which was widely used until well into the 19th century. (The herb turned out to be ineffective.)

Another syphilis treatment was mercury. It played a key role in the schism that developed in the early 19th century between promercury "regular" physicians and antimercury herbal "Eclectics."

Spain kept chocolate, cinchona, and other New World plants secret for years. Eventually, they were revealed in a book by Spanish physician-botanist Nicolas Monardes. The book became a huge bestseller. It was published in English in 1577, with the title *Joyful Newes Out of the Newe Founde Worlde.*

Twenty years after *Joyful Newes*, England played a minor role in world exploration. That changed in 1599, when the Dutch suddenly tripled the price of black pepper. England was outraged. Eighty London merchants pooled their capital and established the British East India Company, which began importing pepper and other herbs directly from India.

The English eventually took control of India and Ceylon (Sri Lanka). The East India Company also imported Chinese tea, which quickly became as English as the Union Jack.

The East India Company's tea was very popular in England's North American colonies. In 1773, when Parliament tried to tax it, New England tea lovers dumped several tons into Boston Harbor in protest. The Boston Tea Party helped ignite the American Revolution.

Paracelsus and the Doctrine of Signatures

Around 1500, Italian mathematician Giambattista della Porta conceived the first new medical philosophy since Galen. Called the Doctrine of Signatures, it claimed that a plant's physical appearance revealed its healing value. As British herbalist William Coles explained in his *Art of Simpling* (1656), God had not only "stamped upon plants . . . a distinct forme but also given them particular signatures whereby a Man may read the use of them."

According to Coles, "Wall-nuts [walnuts] have the perfect signature of the Head. The outer husk represents the cranium or outward skin of the skull, whereon the hair groweth, and therefore those husks are exceedingly good for wounds in the head. The inner woody shell hath the Signature of the Skull . . . and the

Kernel hath the very figure of the Brain. If the Kernel be bruised, moistened with wine, and laid upon the Head, it comforts the head and brain mightily." Some herbals still suggest walnuts for headache.

The most vocal champion of the Doctrine of Signatures was Phillippus Aureolus Theophrastus Bombastus von Hohenheim (1493–1541), the son of a Swiss alchemist/physician. A brilliant, arrogant student of medicine, he lived up to his name, Bombastus, then changed it to Paracelsus ("greater than Celsus"), convinced that he was more brilliant than the Roman physician Celsus (53 BC–AD 7), then considered on a par with Galen.

In the 1520s, Paracelsus taught at the University of Basel in Switzerland. At a time when medical students studied only Hippocrates, Galen, Celsus, and Avicenna, Paracelsus publicly burned their books to symbolize his rejection of Galenic dogma. He also rejected the ancient Humoral Theory of illness for the Doctrine of Signatures.

Strange as it sounds today, the doctrine was based on experience with healing herbs. For instance, the stems of dandelion are hollow, allowing air to pass through them. Based on this characteristic, the doctrine declared dandelion a respiratory remedy.

The Doctrine of Signatures quickly became the new medical dogma. Bile has a yellowish tinge, and jaundice, a liver problem, turns the skin yellow. Under the doctrine, any yellow flower or root was considered a liver medicine. Similarly, any plant with long, snaking roots was used to treat snakebite. Plants with heart-shaped leaves were considered heart remedies. Juicy plants were used as diuretics and lactation promoters.

In addition to promoting the insurgent medical philosophy, Paracelsus further offended medical professionals by rejecting Latin for the vernacular, opening medicine to those unschooled in the language of the universities. He correctly predicted the discovery of "active principles" in plants and pioneered the chemical extraction of plant oils.

Paracelsus also discovered the dose-response relationship. "Is it a poison or not?" he wrote. "It depends only on the dose." His insight came too late to save thousands of alleged witches executed in part for possession of alleged poisons, but it allowed Paracelsus to introduce small doses of many potentially toxic minerals into medicine: arsenic, sulphur, lead, antimony, and particularly mercury, not just to treat syphilis but also for other diseases. In time, physicians came to view mercury as a panacea.

The Age of Herbals

In the 1450s when printing arrived, herbals proliferated and England's university-trained physicians feared losing their medical monopoly. They lobbied their influential patients in the British Court to restrict the practice of medicine to them, outlawing it to "rogues, horse-gelders, rat catchers, idiots, and witches."

In a 1511 decree, Henry VIII limited doctoring to university-trained physicians and barber-surgeons who'd completed apprenticeships. Anyone else had to pass a test administered in Latin. Of course, few folk herbalists could even read English let alone Latin. Some stopped practicing. Many became "green men and women," latter-day rhizomists who supplied herbs to physicians and early pharmacists, or apothecaries, often while continuing to practice herbal healing on the sly.

In time, England's herbalists rebelled against the suppression of folk medicine by publishing two anonymous herbals. *Bancke's Herball* (1525), the first herbal printed in English, and *The Grete Herball* (1526), a combination of French and German references.

Henry VIII's edict eventually led to a major shortage of doctors. In 1543, he rescinded it with the Herbalists' Charter: "From henceforth, it shall be lawful for every . . . King's subject, having knowledge and experience of . . . Herbs and Roots . . . to practice, use, and minister to any Sore, Wound, Swelling, or Disease any Herbs, Ointments, Baths, Pulsters (poultices) and Emplaisters (plasters), according to their Cunning, Experience, and Knowledge . . . without Suit, Vexation, Trouble, Penalty, or Loss of their Goods."

The Herbalists' Charter came just one year after German botanist Leonhard Fuchs (1501–1566) published *De Historia Stirpium* (*On Plants*), the first original book of medical botany since Dioscorides' treatise 1,500 years earlier. Illustrated with woodcuts, it discussed 500 healing herbs, including 100 from the New World.

In 1546, the University of Padua in Italy planted the first academic botanical garden, which helped launch the science of botany. In time, most major universities and many physicians and apothecaries planted their own physic gardens.

William Turner, the father of British botany, published his *New Herball* in 1551. Subsequently, a London publisher commissioned Robert Priest to combine and translate French and German herbals into English, but Priest died before completing the project, and his translation disappeared.

Enter herbalist John Gerard (1545–1612), who established a noted physic garden in London's Fetter Lane that contained 1,000 species, including England's first potatoes. In 1586, Gerard was appointed curator of the College of Physicians' Physic Garden, and soon after, became herbalist to King James I.

In 1597, Gerard published his *Herball or Generall Historie of Plantes*, in which he displayed the College of Physicians' characteristic contempt for "overbold apothecaries, and foolish women." However, Gerard apparently had nothing against plagiarism. He obliquely acknowledged the late Robert Priest, leading to accusations that he'd obtained Priest's lost translation and published it as his own.

Gerard denied wrongdoing. His herbal contained considerable original material on herb gardening—but most authorities believe he stole Priest's work.

John Parkinson (1567–1650) was another pioneering British herbalist. In 1640, he published *Theatrum Botanicum* (*The Theater of Plants*), subtitled *The Universall and Complete Herball*, an 1,800-page book that discussed 3,800 plants, grouped into families such as Hot Plants, Venomous Plants, and Strange, Outlandish Plants.

Parkinson's classification system appears quaint today, but during the 17th century, herbalists struggled with organizing botanical medicines. Many scientists proposed systems, but none stuck until 1737 when Swedish naturalist Carl Linne, also known as Carolus Linnaeus (1707–1778), developed his Latin binomial genus-and-species system based on reproductive characteristics. After Darwin, scientists added evolutionary criteria, but to this day, plants and animals are still named using Linnaeus' binomial formula—genus and species in Latin, for example, garlic is *Allium sativum*.

As university medicine slowly became more

scientific, leading physicians stopped growing their own herbs. They turned instead to the increasing number of apothecaries, who used mortars and pestles to powder healing herbs. The mortar and pestle remain symbols of pharmacy today.

In 1673, London's apothecaries established Britain's finest medicinal herb garden, the 3.8-acre Chelsea Physic Garden, which still exists. Today, it contains 5,000 species of herbs from around the world. Located 2 miles west of Piccadilly Circus, it is open to the public.

Nicholas Culpeper: England's Herbal Robin Hood

Nicholas Culpeper was by far England's most influential herbalist. His *Complete Herbal and English Physician* (1652) has remained in print ever since in more than 100 editions, a record of longevity only a handful of books can claim. A century after Culpeper's death, literary lion Dr. Samuel Johnson wrote, "Culpeper . . . undoubtedly merits the gratitude of posterity."

Culpeper was—and still is—loathed as well as loved. His herbalist contemporary, William Coles, denounced him as "a man ignorant of simples." More than 250 years later, in *The Old English Herbals* (1922), Elinour Rohde wrote, "The infamous Nicholas Culpeper was a false prophet of herbalism . . . [author of] an absurd book." Today, scientists scoff at Culpeper's prescriptions and his devotion to astrology.

Egotistical and brash, Culpeper came of age during the English Civil War (1642–1648), which pitted King Charles I and the monarchist aristocracy against Oliver Cromwell and the Puritans. The Puritans won, abolished the monarchy, and executed Charles.

Culpeper came from an aristocratic family, but he fought for Cromwell. He took a musket ball in the chest, which left him in poor health for the rest of his life and spurred him to study medicine.

As an aristocrat, Culpeper attended Cambridge, where he fell in love and planned to elope. But on her way to meet him, Culpeper's fiancée was killed when lightning struck her carriage. Beside himself with grief, Culpeper left Cambridge and became an apothecary's apprentice, a trade considered far beneath anyone with a university education.

Culpeper was an anomaly. Trained at Cambridge, he could read Greek and Latin as well as Court physicians. But he resented the snobbery of former classmates who became doctors and disparaged apothecaries. Furthermore, as a Puritan, he was outraged that the monarchist College of Physicians ignored the medical needs of the largely Puritan lower classes. Culpeper's solution was to become England's medical Robin Hood.

In 1649, Culpeper translated the College of Physicians' Latin manual, the *Pharmacopoiea Londinensis*, into English, calling it *The London Dispensatory and Physical Directory*. It gave those illiterate in Latin their first look at the 1,600 simples and 1,100 other formulas that constituted the state of the art in 17th-century British medicine. Culpeper's audacity earned him physicians' undying hatred. However, apothecaries, midwives, and the common people lionized him for giving them access to professional medical information.

Culpeper's apothecary shop near London became wildly popular. He often treated the poor for free. The College of Physicians attacked him relentlessly, and in response, he became increasingly combative.

Culpeper wrote a series of essays in which he

accused the physicians of greed for their high fees and stupidity for their outdated devotion to Galen and Avicenna: "[We have] a company of proud, domineering doctors whose wits were born 500 years before themselves. . . . College, College, thou art Diseased, and I will tell thee the Cause. The Cause is Mammon [greed]. The Cure: Fear God. Be Studious. Hate Covetousness. Regard the Poor."

To make botanical medicine even more accessible, Culpeper published his own herbal in 1652. It gave equal weight to the official herbalism of the ancient masters and the homegrown folk wisdom of England's country people, who adored him all the more.

Today, critics dismiss Culpeper because of his devotion to astrology. In his herbal, Mars owned garlic, lavender was under Mercury, and the sun claimed rosemary under the celestial Ram. But in Culpeper's day, astrology was taught in all the universities, and the College of Physicians routinely factored it into diagnosis and treatment decisions. In fact, one reason the College hated Culpeper was that he accused them of making astrological errors.

Culpeper's real problem was that he rarely met an herb he didn't consider a panacea. He touted dozens of herbs "to heal all inward and outward hurts." He called about a third of the herbs in his herbal sure cures for "the bites and stings of venomous creatures." He also promoted scores of herbs to "bring down women's courses" (promote menstruation/abortion), many more than midwives of that era recommended.

But Culpeper can be forgiven his errors and exaggerations. In the 1650s, very little was known about the body, and statements that appear gross misrepresentations today were not far-fetched back then.

Physicians call most medical problems "self-limiting," that is, if you wait long enough, they go away. Take almost any herb for "inward or outward hurts," and most clear up, with or without all the herbs Culpeper recommended. The same goes for attacks by "venomous creatures." Few bites and stings are fatal. Left untreated, most eventually resolve.

Unfortunately, Culpeper's promotion of every herb for every ill has haunted herbalism ever since. Well into the 1970s, some herbals touted Culpeper-style hyperbole as truth, providing easy—and legitimate—targets for attacks by herb skeptics. Nicholas Culpeper was a seminal figure in botanical medicine, but his herbal should be viewed as history and nothing more.

Dr. Withering's Wise Woman

In 1767, 26-year-old William Withering had barely begun practicing medicine in Stafford, England, when he was called to treat 17-year-old Helena Cookes, who was bedridden with a lingering illness that prevented her favorite pastime, painting watercolors of wildflowers.

Like every other medical student, Withering had studied botany—and hated it. Still, he was taken with Miss Cookes. He gathered wildflowers for her to paint while in bed and 5 years later married her. Along the way, he developed a passion for medical botany.

"In 1775," he wrote, "my opinion was asked concerning a recipe for the cure of dropsy [congestive heart failure]. I was told it had been a family secret of an old woman in Shropshire, who sometimes made cures after regular practitioners had failed." The old woman's recipe contained 20 herbs, but Withering quickly decided that the heart stimulator was foxglove. Withering began using foxglove himself and gained a reputation for treating the heart problem.

In 1776, Dr. Erasmus Darwin (Charles' grandfather) asked Withering to treat a woman with dropsy. Withering gave her foxglove, and she improved. Darwin submitted a report to a British medical journal claiming that he himself had cured the woman with foxglove. He did not mention Withering.

Furious, Withering published his *Account of the Foxglove and Its Medical Uses*, summarizing his results in 163 cases. Foxglove was the original source of digitalis, a drug considered a state-of the-art treatment for congestive heart failure well into the 20th century.

Sickly Colonists, Robust Indians

Europeans considered Indians "ignorant savages"—except medically. Explorers and colonists were all too familiar with plagues and pestilence and marveled at the Indians' good health. Not surprisingly, many became eager students of Indian herbal medicine.

Each tribe had its own medical mythology, but this Cherokee tale is typical. Long ago, humanity grew too numerous. Hunters killed so much game that the animals feared for their survival and decided to afflict humans with diseases to reduce hunting. But the plants decided that the animals had acted unfairly. The trees, shrubs, grasses, and flowers showed humanity how they could cure the diseases the animals had unleashed.

An early European devotee of Indian medicine was Jacques Cartier, the French explorer who discovered Canada's St. Lawrence River. In 1536, he sailed to the site of present-day Quebec, where he and his crew dug in for the winter. Within a few months, 25 of his 100 men had died of "sailors' disease" (scurvy), and most of the rest were gravely ill.

During the Age of Exploration, scurvy was a scourge. On his first voyage around Africa, Vasco da Gama lost two-thirds of his crew to it. During the 16th and 17th centuries, sailors sometimes encountered unmanned "ghost ships" adrift on the high seas, their entire crews killed by scurvy.

Fortunately for Cartier, an Indian gave the sickly explorers a tea brewed from yellow cedar bark and leaves. Everyone recovered. Later, the tea was shown to contain vitamin C, which prevents and cures scurvy.

In Boston, Puritan minister Cotton Mather (1663–1728) wrote that Indian healers produced "many truly stupendous cures." And in the 1730s when John Wesley (1703–1791), founder of Methodism, visited America, he wrote that the Indians had "exceedingly few" diseases and that their medicines were "quick and generally infallible." Many early American physicians touted their apprenticeships to Indian herbalists. Later, even ardent Indian haters in the U.S. Army marveled at the effectiveness of Indian wound treatments.

Of course, Indian healers also had critics, mostly university-trained physicians. Philadelphia doctor Benjamin Rush (1745–1813), a signer of the Declaration of Independence, declared, "We have no discoveries in the materia medica . . . from the Indians. It would be a reproach to our schools of physic if modern physicians were not more successful than Indians."

Rush was mistaken. Indians introduced white settlers to many healing herbs: black cohosh, black haw, boneset, cascara sagrada, echinacea, chaparral, goldenseal, lobelia, Oregon grape, sarsaparilla, slippery elm, and witch hazel.

Healing Herbs in Early America

In their "kitchen gardens," American colonists grew both culinary and medicinal herbs, including: balm, basil, caraway, chamomile, comfrey, dill, fennel, garlic, lavender, licorice, marjoram, mints, mustard, parsley, rosemary, rue, savory, saffron, sage, tarragon, and thyme.

Thomas Jefferson was a typical herb grower. His 1,000-square-foot garden at Monticello contained 26 herbs. As president, while negotiating the Louisiana Purchase from France, he went to great lengths to obtain some French tarragon for his garden.

Nurse/midwives also grew medicinal herbs. One was Martha Ballard (1735–1812) of Maine, who kept a diary that included her practice of herbal medicine. She used 52 herbs grown in the area around her home on the Kennebec River, northeast of Portland, including anise, balm, buckthorn, burdock, chamomile, catnip, comfrey, feverfew, hop, mullein, mustard, onion, pennyroyal, rhubarb, rue, sage, shepherd's purse, and yarrow. She also purchased 24 imported herbs, among them aloe, licorice, myrrh, pepper, and senna.

Herbs were prized imports into colonial America. In addition to tea, black pepper was very popular. New England shipping magnate Elias Hasskett Derby, one of early America's first homegrown millionaires, made much of his money importing black pepper from Sumatra.

Herbs were also a major colonial export. Furs, tobacco, and cotton generated the most money, but pound for pound, nothing beat ginseng root, the herb prized in Asia as the ultimate whole-body strengthener (tonic).

French Jesuits began shipping Canadian ginseng to China in the early 1700s, where it brought the then-astounding price of $5 a pound. By the 1740s, news of the unassuming ground cover's value in the Orient spread south to the 13 colonies. Shipping agents bought roots for $1 a pound, more than the wholesale value of the rarest furs. Foragers scoured the countryside, and frontier scouts, surveyors, and trappers collected ginseng as a sideline to their other work.

By the 1770s, rapacious collection had wiped out ginseng east of the Appalachians, forcing collectors into the western wilderness. The search for ginseng played a key role in the exploration of western Pennsylvania, West Virginia, Kentucky, and Tennessee. One noted collector was Daniel Boone, who, according to one account, lost a cargo of ginseng when his boat capsized in the Ohio River.

The American Revolution gave the new nation not only its independence but also its first herbal, *Materia Medica Americana* (1787), by Johann David Schopf (1752–1800). Ironically, Dr. Schopf came to America to treat Hessian mercenaries who fought for the British. After the war, he stayed long enough to compile his book on medicinal plants.

America's first resident medical botanist was Constantine Rafinesque (1784–1841) who arrived as a young man and studied the herbs of the Mississippi Valley with Native American healers. In 1819, Rafinesque became a professor of botany at a Kentucky college where he wrote *Medical Flora* (1828).

Rafinesque coined the term "eclectic" to describe the kind of medicine he championed, a combination of European, Asian, Indian, and slave herbalism. Shortly after his death, 19th-century America's most scientific herbalists began calling themselves Eclectics.

The Shakers: America's Premier Healing Herb Growers

Today, most Americans associate "Shaker" with high-quality furniture. But throughout the 19th century, the Shakers were better known for the high quality of their medicinal herbs.

An English Quaker, Ann Lee, founded the sect in Manchester, England, in the early 1770s. She believed in worshiping God with singing and dancing called shaking, hence the name Shaking Quakers, then Shakers. Not surprisingly, Lee was briefly imprisoned as a witch.

In 1774, Lee and eight Shakers arrived in New York and founded a community near Albany. The Shakers practiced strict pacifism as well as gender equality and segregation. Marriage and sex were banned. Member families were broken up. Meals were eaten in devotional silence.

Eventually, the Shakers established 24 communities, from Maine to Indiana to Florida. Eight lasted through World War I. One survives—Sabbathday Lake in New Gloucester, Maine.

Ann Lee's motto was "Hands to work, hearts to God." Her industrious followers launched the American medicinal herb industry in 1799, first collecting healing herbs from the wild, then growing them. The herb business prospered, and in 1824, the Sabbathday Lake community built a large herb shed for drying and processing. It still stands.

The Shakers sold their herbs through a nationally distributed catalog. The first (1831) was headlined: "Why send to Europe's bloody shore for plants that grow by our own door?" It offered 142 herbs, roots, barks, and seeds, including angelica, basil, bayberry, belladonna, black and blue cohosh, boneset, cannabis (marijuana), catnip, chamomile, coltsfoot, comfrey, elecampane, gentian, hop, hyssop, jimson weed, juniper, lady's slipper, licorice, lobelia, marshmallow, mullein, motherwort, nux vomica, opium poppy, pennyroyal, peppermint, rosemary, saffron, senna, slippery elm, valerian, walnut, white oak, and wild cherry. The Shakers also sold a few culinary "sweet" herbs: sage, marjoram, savory, and thyme.

Unlike Rome's *herbarii*, the Shakers developed a reputation for honesty and herbal purity. In 1851, Rafinesque said that they had "the best medicinal gardens in the United States. They cultivate a great variety and sell them cheap, fresh, and genuine."

Pacifism did not prevent the Shakers from selling medicinal herbs to the Union Army during the Civil War. They supplied much of the Union's opium. After the war, the Shakers sold medicinal herbs directly to hospitals and the embryonic pharmaceutical industry.

The Shakers invented pills. Before pills, loose powdered herbs were packaged in envelopes, which were inconvenient to ship. Shaker craftsmen drilled holes in wood frames to create the first pill molds. The herbalists poured in measured amounts of powdered herbs, then hammered pegs into the holes to turn powders into the pellets we call pills.

When patent medicines became popular after the Civil War, the Shakers marketed several. Their top seller was Dr. Corbett's Shaker Sarsaparilla Syrup, with sarsaparilla, dandelion, black cohosh, yellow dock, juniper, and other herbs. The Shakers touted it for a dozen conditions. Two other popular items were Pain King, with opium, and Tamar Laxative, with dried prunes and senna.

The Shaker herb business died after World War II, but the Sabbathday Lake community revived it in the 1960s. The community's herb garden, herb shed, and museum are open to the public.

Thomson's Botanic Medicine

Early America's leading herbalist was Samuel Thomson (1760–1843). Born in Alstead, New Hampshire, he studied with midwives and Indian healers. Around 1800, Thomson's daughter became seriously ill. Unsure of his skills, he called a physician, who pronounced her incurable. Then, Thomson cured her with herbs and hot baths. Soon after, he declared himself a "doctor."

Thomson detested the regular physicians of his day, who relied on bloodletting, violent laxatives (cathartics), and mercury. These treatments were called "heroic medicine," but the heroism was entirely on the part of patients.

Consider George Washington. In 1799, the elderly but healthy father of our country developed a sore throat with a fever and chills. He probably had strep throat that likely would have cleared up with rest, hot liquids, and herbal antibiotics such as garlic and onion.

Instead, Washington's heroic physicians bled him of four pints of blood, leaving him anemic and weak. Then they gave him cathartics and mercury. He was dead a day later.

Inspired by European herbalism and mineral baths and Indian herbalism and sweat lodges, Thomson developed a medical system based on herbs and hot baths. His favorite herb was lobelia or Indian tobacco, which in large amounts causes vomiting, hence its common name "puke weed."

In 1809, Thomson was arrested for murder after allegedly administering a fatal dose of lobelia. But the prosecutor could not persuade jurors that lobelia was poisonous, and Thomson was acquitted.

Samuel Thomson may not have been the nation's greatest herbalist, but he was our first medical marketing genius. In 1813, he obtained a patent for Thomson's Improved System of Botanic Practice of Medicine, which allowed him to sell his Indian-inspired herbalism nationwide while still retaining ownership. Thomson sold "family rights" to his medical system for $20. Starting in 1822, he charged another $2 for his book, *The New Guide to Health, or the Botanic Family Physician.*

Thomson's motto was "Every man his own physician," but the vast majority of his "family rights" were purchased by women, many of whom welcomed the opportunity to add legitimacy to the word-of-mouth herbalism that they'd learned from their mothers and other women.

In 1839, at the height of his popularity, Thomson claimed 3 million adherents. This was an exaggeration, but Thomsonian herbalism was very popular. Thomson boasted that half of Ohio used his system. Detractors said it was only one-third.

Initially, Thomsonian herbalists used 65 herbs, all available from the Shakers. Then Thomson realized that he could boost his income by selling prepackaged herbal formulas. He organized his family members into Friendly Botanic Societies, cooperatives that bought his formulas and distributed them around the country. Because

Thomson's formulas were part of his patented medical system, they became known as "patent medicines."

As time passed, patent medicines became a major industry. Some were quality products, but many were worthless concoctions of alcohol, opium, and cocaine sold by hucksters whose outrageous claims eventually spurred Congress to create the Food and Drug Administration (FDA).

After Thomson's death in 1843, his medical system fell from fashion. But some practitioners preserved it. One was Dr. John Kellogg of Battle Creek, Michigan, who invented the nation's first health food, the cornflake, and founded Kellogg's cereal company. For the most part, though, Thomsonian medicine was replaced by homeopathy and Eclectic herbalism.

Homeopathy: Herbal Microdoses

From 1830 through World War I, the main competition for regular American physicians came from homeopathy, the herbally inclined medical system created by a disillusioned German physician, Dr. Samuel Hahnemann (1755–1843). Trained in heroic medicine, Hahnemann decided that bloodletting, cathartics, and mercury did more harm than good.

Hahnemann did not reject all heroic treatments. He was impressed with several, among them, cinchona bark, the antimalarial, and inoculation with cowpox to prevent smallpox. In healthy people, both of these treatments produce low-level symptoms of the diseases that they are used to prevent. Hahnemann called the phenomenon homeopathy, from the Greek for "treatment by similars."

Hahnemann tested hundreds of herbs and other substances on himself, carefully cataloging their effects. Eventually, he began using them to treat illnesses with similar symptoms. His approach was less drastic than heroic medicine's. He enjoyed considerable success and attracted a large following.

Homeopathy came to the United States in the 1830s, quickly winning many supporters fed up with heroic medicine, including Mark Twain, Daniel Webster, and John D. Rockefeller. Homeopaths popularized several drugs still used today, including ergot derivatives for migraines and nitroglycerin for angina.

By the early 20th century, however, homeopathy fell from U.S. medical fashion. One reason was the decline of heroic medicine. As regular physicians stopped opening veins and using mercury, their critics had less to criticize. Another reason was the unrelenting hostility of the American Medical Association (AMA). Around 1900, an estimated 25 percent of regular physicians also prescribed some homeopathic medicines. Then the AMA decreed that any physician caught using homeopathy would be expelled from the organization.

But the major reason for homeopathy's decline was its Law of Potentization, Hahnemann's assertion that his medicines grew *stronger* as they became more *dilute*. The Law of Potentization violated Paracelsus' dose-response relationship, a cornerstone of pharmacology. Critics charged that medicines homeopaths considered extremely powerful were so dilute that they did not contain even a single molecule of the active ingredient. As a result, American scientists dismissed homeopathy—and its largely herbal medicines—as nonsense. By the 1950s, American homeopathy was just about dead.

Homeopaths can't explain the Law of Potentization, but they insist that more than 150 years of clinical experience show that it works. They have a point. In recent years, rigorous scientific trials have found that homeopathic medicines, most of them herbal, effectively treat colds, flu, hay fever, asthma, fibromyalgia, rheumatoid arthritis, and infectious diarrhea.

In 1991, nonhomeopathic Dutch epidemiologists published an analysis of 105 homeopathy studies from 1966 to 1990. Of the 105, 81 (77 percent) showed significant benefit. Only 24 (23 percent) showed none.

However, few of these studies were double-blind, meaning that researcher bias might have contaminated the results. So the Dutch investigators spotlighted the results of the 21 most rigorous trials. Fifteen (71 percent) showed significant benefit. While questions remain about how homeopathy works, the researchers concluded that "the evidence presented in this review would probably be sufficient for establishing homeopathy as a regular treatment for certain conditions."

Since its founding, homeopathy has been popular in Europe. Today, the physician to the British royal family is a homeopath. Surveys show that many British, French, and German M.D.s prescribe some homeopathic medicines in their practices.

During the last 30 years, America has witnessed a modest homeopathic renaissance. Today, about 9 percent of U.S. doctors—some 5,000 M.D.s—incorporate homeopathic medicines into their practices. Several thousand other health professionals—dentists, podiatrists, veterinarians, nurses, and chiropractors—also use homeopathy.

A study by Harvard researchers suggested that more than 2.5 million Americans have tried homeopathy. Sales of homeopathic medicines now total more than $250 million a year, in part because major drugstore chains now carry them. What's more, in recent years, many celebrities have gone public with their use of homeopathy: singer Tina Turner, and actors Cher, Jane Fonda, and Angelica Huston.

The Eclectics: America's Scientific Herbalists

Despite the regular physicians' reliance on bloodletting, cathartics, and mercury, most 19th-century medicines were herbal. In 1820, two-thirds of the treatments in the *U.S. Pharmacopoeia*, the official list of the nation's drugs, were botanical. By 1880, the figure was almost three-quarters.

During the 1820s, a group of antiheroic practitioners—Thomsonians, Indian-trained herbalists, and disillusioned regulars—created the Reformed Medical Society to promote nonheroic, largely herbal healing. In 1830, the society met in New York to found a Reformed medical school. The reformers were mostly Easterners, but the East's cities were strongholds of regular medicine.

The Reformers decided to locate their school on the free-thinking western frontier, then located at the Mississippi River. Thomsonian medicine was very popular in Ohio, so the reformers established their school in Cincinnati. They adopted Rafinesque's term, eclectic, to describe their herb-based approach, which combined European, Asian, Indian, and slave herbalism. They called their school the Eclectic Medical Institute.

The institute was the nation's first medical

school to admit women, many of whom were Thomsonian herbalists interested in more training. In 1877, however, the Eclectics "yielded to prejudice," according to Eclectic historian Henry Felter, and barred women.

The Eclectics were scientific herbalists. They experimented with herbs, performing chemical analyses to identify active constituents. They published their findings in scientific journals and were prominent in the early pharmaceutical industry.

The two most distinguished Eclectics were John King and John Uri Lloyd, both professors at the Eclectic medical school. King (1813–1893) was a botanical pharmacologist who introduced physicians to podophyllin, a plant resin still used today to treat warts. In 1855, he published the first edition of his *King's American Dispensatory*, 19th-century America's most comprehensive scientific herbal. The 18th edition (1898) is still in print.

Lloyd (1849–1936) began his career at age 14 as a Cincinnati pharmacist's apprentice. He loved it and brought his brothers, Nelson Ashley Lloyd (1851–1925) and Curtis Gates Lloyd (1859–1926), into the field. Eventually, they established Lloyd Brothers Pharmacists, Inc.

John Lloyd specialized in plant chemistry and developed most of the company's products. He was also one of the first presidents of the American Pharmaceutical Association (1887–1888).

Nelson Lloyd managed the business side of Lloyd Brothers. His other love was baseball. He owned the Cincinnati team that eventually became the Reds, and later, he invested in the New York Giants.

Curtis Lloyd specialized in mushrooms. He also managed the brothers' large collection of botany books.

By 1864, the collection had outgrown the brothers' homes, so they established the Lloyd Library. Today, the library houses the world's largest private collection of botanical information: 300,000 books and pamphlets as well as 500 journals. For years, the Lloyd Library also published a botanical journal, *Lloydia*, now called the *Journal of Natural Products*. The Lloyd Library in Cincinnati is open to the public.

The years 1880 to 1900 marked the heyday of Eclectic medicine. But with the dawn of the 20th century, Eclectic medicine declined as herbal medicines were largely replaced by pharmaceuticals. The Eclectic Medical Institute graduated its last class in 1939, and American scientific herbalism faded and almost died.

But not quite. A handful of Eclectic-inspired physicians, who called themselves "naturopaths," hung on, particularly in the Pacific Northwest. Among them was John Bastyr, N.D. (1912–1995), of Seattle. He was affiliated with the National College of Naturopathic Medicine in Portland, Oregon, the sole surviving medical school of Eclectic herbalism.

In 1978, a group of Bastyr's former students founded the John Bastyr College of Naturopathic Medicine in Seattle, now Bastyr University in nearby Kenmore. In addition to the Portland and Washington schools, North America now boasts six other naturopathic medical schools:

- Bastyr University, San Diego, California
- Southwest College of Naturopathic Medicine, Scottsdale, Arizona
- Canadian College of Naturopathic Medicine, Etobicoke, Ontario

❧ Boucher Institute, Vancouver, British Columbia

❧ National University of Health Sciences, Chicago, Illinois

❧ College of Naturopathic Medicine, University of Bridgeport, Connecticut

Naturopaths are currently licensed to practice in 17 states: Alaska, Arizona, California, Colorado, Connecticut, Hawaii, Kansas, Maine, Maryland, Minnesota, Montana, New Hampshire, North Dakota, Oregon, Utah, Vermont, and Washington. The District of Columbia, Puerto Rico, and the U.S. Virgin Islands also license naturopaths as do five Canadian provinces: Alberta, British Columbia, Manitoba, Ontario, and Saskatchewan. Elsewhere, naturopaths practice under other medical credentials, typically as acupuncturists, chiropractors, or clinical nutritionists.

Naturopathic schools require standard college premedical courses for admission. The first 2 years at Bastyr combine a mainstream medical education—anatomy, physiology, biochemistry, pathology, microbiology, pharmacology, public health, and physical examination and diagnosis—with courses on naturopathic philosophy, clinical nutrition, homeopathy, and Western, Chinese, and Ayurvedic herbal medicine.

Third- and fourth-year students apprentice with mentor naturopaths, often at Bastyr's clinic in Seattle, which treats more than 25,000 patients a year. At first glance, the clinic looks like a mainstream medical facility. Closer examination reveals that its large in-house pharmacy stocks few pharmaceuticals, relying mostly on herbs, homeopathic medicines, and nutritional supplements.

The Collapse of Professional Herbal Medicine

Modern pharmacology dates from 1820, when a German chemist first synthesized an organic compound (urea) from inorganic chemicals. Early pharmacologists developed drugs largely by modifying compounds extracted from medicinal plants. They isolated morphine from opium poppy, aspirin from willow bark, caffeine from coffee, anesthetic menthol from peppermint, antimalarial quinine from cinchona, and decongestant ephedrine from Chinese ephedra, among many others.

After the Civil War, aspiring American doctors had two basic training choices: apprenticeship to practicing physicians or enrollment in medical schools in the United States or Germany. Compared with American programs, a German medical education was more extensive and scientifically rigorous, and the medical schools were affiliated with hospitals, allowing intensive clinical training.

German-trained American physicians scorned U.S. medical education and urged the nation's medical schools to adopt the German model. In 1870, Harvard was among the first to do so, after university president Charles Eliot wrote, "The ignorance and incompetence of the average graduate of American medical schools . . . is horrible to contemplate."

Three years later in 1873, a $7 million bequest led to the creation of a German-style medical school and hospital in Baltimore, Johns Hopkins University. When it opened in 1893, Hopkins took the unprecedented step of refusing to admit medical students without college degrees. Harvard quickly followed, making medical training a graduate program.

Other medical schools adopted the Harvard-Hopkins model, dropping botany in favor of pharmacology. Heroic treatment fell from fashion, but so did herbs, replaced by the drugs of the new pharmaceutical industry.

Laboratories and teaching hospitals were costly, so financing became critical. Well-endowed Harvard, Johns Hopkins, and other medical schools spent enormous sums on their facilities. More modestly endowed homeopathic and Eclectic schools could not keep up. As a result, doctors trained under the Harvard-Hopkins model were considered superior physicians, and state licensing boards began requiring the Harvard-Hopkins curriculum. Other medical schools saw enrollments shrink.

Then the influential Carnegie Foundation commissioned Abraham Flexner to survey the quality of the nation's medical training. His 1910 report endorsed the Harvard–Hopkins model and dismissed all others. Carnegie and other wealthy foundations supported only Harvard-Hopkins schools. By 1940, every surviving U.S. medical school offered only graduate training on the Harvard-Hopkins model, and none provided training in herbal healing.

Hoxsey's Controversial Herbal Cancer Treatment

For American herbal healing, the 1920s though the 1960s were lost decades. U.S. medical schools ignored herbal medicines as the nation's pharmacies replaced tinctures with pharmaceuticals.

But herbal healing didn't die. It reverted to what it had been throughout history, folk medicine practiced mostly by women who grew and gathered their own herbs and prescribed them as classic herbals recommended.

A few diehards continued to promote herbal healing. Dr. Benedict Lust (1869–1945), the father of modern naturopathy, came to the United States from Germany in 1895. He opened the nation's first health food store and established sanitariums in New Jersey and Florida that offered mineral baths and herbal medicines. His nephew, John Lust, penned an influential herbal, *The Herb Book* (1974), which is still in print.

In 1939, Jethro Kloss (1863–1946), a sanitarium manager and health food pioneer, published *Back to Eden*. Subtitled "A Story of the Restoration to Be Found in Herb, Root, and Bark," the book helped preserve herbal approaches to healing.

In England, C. F. (Hilda) Leyel (?–1957) almost single-handedly revived British herbalism when she opened the first of her Culpeper shops in 1927. In 1940, she successfully lobbied Parliament not to repeat Henry VIII's mistake of outlawing herbal medicine.

But the most flamboyant and controversial herbalist of the 20th century, was Harry Hoxsey (1901–1974), who loudly proclaimed that his herbal formula cured cancer. A former Appalachian coal miner, Hoxsey had no formal medical training. He attributed his Hoxsey Cancer Formula to his great-grandfather, who, he claimed, had witnessed a cancer-stricken horse recover after eating an odd combination of plants. Hoxsey started selling his family's formula in the 1930s. By the 1950s, his Dallas clinic was the world's largest privately owned cancer center, with branches in 17 states.

Hoxsey's claims outraged Texas medical authorities, and during the 1930s, a Dallas prosecutor arrested him for fraud more than 100 times. The Hoxsey formula didn't work for everyone, but the prosecutor could not find any patients who felt that they'd been defrauded. What's more, Hoxsey presented hundreds who swore that his formula had cured their cancers.

The Texas courts ruled in favor of the cancer maverick. Then the prosecutor's brother developed cancer and secretly took the Hoxsey formula. When he recovered, Hoxsey's former prosecutor became his defense attorney.

Hoxsey was also attacked by the AMA. He fought back in court. When AMA officials conceded that the Hoxsey Formula had merit for treating skin cancer, Hoxsey became the first person ever to win a libel suit against the AMA. The FDA eventually closed Hoxsey's clinics for violating federal drug-labeling regulations. His herbal ingredients were not FDA-approved cancer treatments.

Ironically, Hoxsey died of prostate cancer. He took his formula, but it didn't work for him.

The Hoxsey formula is available today at the Bio-Medical Center in Tijuana, Mexico. Studies show that nine of the formula's ingredients have antitumor action: barberry, buckthorn, burdock, cascara sagrada, red clover, licorice, poke, prickly ash, and bloodroot.

The Herbal Renaissance

Starting in the 1960s, many Americans began thinking differently about health and healing. They invested their energy in illness prevention rather than treatment.

One step involved a retreat from salt as the nation's main seasoning as research linked it to high blood pressure, heart disease, and stroke. Retiring their salt shakers, many Americans rediscovered culinary herbs and spices. Many also learned of herbs' medical benefits. In 2000, U.S. medicinal herb sales topped $4 billion and by 2014, $6.4 billion.

Several trends fueled the herbal renaissance:

- Growing interest in self-care. Mainstream medicine can produce miracles, but it has also become impersonal and often prohibitively expensive. To save time and money and limit dependence on doctors, many Americans have turned to prevention and self-care. Healing herbs fit neatly into lifestyles focused on a plant-based diet, fitness, and stress management.

- Enthusiasm for alternative healing arts. Once denigrated, homeopathy, naturopathy, and Chinese and Ayurvedic medicine have become increasingly popular. They all make extensive use of herbal medicines.

- Backlash against advanced technology. The very wizardry of high technology has spurred a yearning for more down-to-earth medicines. When there's a choice, many Americans prefer healing herbs to the drugs often derived from them.

- Environmental awareness. As climate change and rainforest destruction have become global issues, interest has grown in screening threatened plants for medicinal uses. The National Cancer Institute and governments around the world have launched testing programs, hoping to identify new therapeutic actions.

- Advocacy by the United Nations. A 1974 World Health Organization report concluded that adequate worldwide health care could not be achieved unless nonindustrialized nations were encouraged to nurture traditional herbal healing. Since then, the United Nations has encouraged the Chinese model of combining traditional and Western medicine.

✣ Increasing mainstream medical acceptance. From the 1960s through the 1980s, no mainstream medical schools taught courses on alternative medicine. Today, almost 100 do.

The FDA vs. Healing Herbs

Unfortunately, the Food and Drug Administration (FDA), the agency that regulates medicinal herbs, has been glacially slow to embrace the herbal renaissance. Herb critics are quick to cry "hucksterism" when herb marketers position their products as dietary supplements with vague labeling. But this sorry saga is a direct result of FDA policies.

During the 19th century, patent medicines laced with alcohol, cocaine, and even heroin raised cries for national drug regulation. But it took *The Jungle* (1906), Upton Sinclair's exposé of deplorable conditions in the meatpacking industry, to convince Congress to prohibit adulteration and mislabeling of foods and drugs.

Congress established the FDA in 1928, but the agency had more bark than bite. Then in 1937, a toxic ingredient in an antibiotic, elixir of sulfanilamide, killed 107 people. The following year, Congress passed the Food, Drug, and Cosmetic Act, which gave the FDA real regulatory power.

But the agency remained weak on enforcement until 1959, when 8,000 European babies were born with terrible birth defects because, when pregnant, their mothers had taken Thalidomide, an over-the-counter sedative. After the

Thalidomide scandal, the FDA got tough on drug safety.

The agency declared that, before new drugs could be approved, their makers had to demonstrate safety and effectiveness in rigorous studies. These trials were very expensive—millions of dollars per drug in the 1960s and, by some estimates, $100 million today.

Those who marketed over-the-counter (OTC) pharmaceuticals screamed that the FDA had no right to require costly testing of drugs that had been used safely in many cases for centuries. So the agency appointed panels of physicians, pharmacists, and pharmacologists to review the safety and effectiveness of OTC ingredients. The panels wrote reports, monographs, that served as the basis for grandfathering approval of drugs judged safe and effective. The OTC Review Panel process ran from 1972 to 1985.

When the reviews began, more than 100 herbal medicines were listed as safe and effective in the *U.S. Pharmacopoeia*, the nation's official drug reference, and deserved grandfathered approved as OTC medicines. Unfortunately, the OTC Review Panels did not review the medical literature. They only considered information submitted in support of ingredients the OTC manufacturers hoped to retain on pharmacy shelves.

By the end of the review process, hundreds of ingredients had been analyzed in monographs, including two dozen herbs, for example, the active constituents in most OTC laxatives (senna, psyllium seed, and cascara sagrada), and decongestants (peppermint oil, eucalyptus oil, and two compounds in Chinese ephedra).

But the approved herbs represented only a tiny fraction of the hundreds of botanical medicines known to be safe and effective. For example, before World War II, all U.S. pharmacies stocked valerian-based sleep aids. By the time of the OTC review process, drug companies had dropped valerian in favor of sedative antihistamines (diphenhydramine, Benadryl). As a result, no valerian products were presented to the OTC Review Panel, and none were approved. As a result, the panels ignored dozens of herbs.

Why didn't medicinal herb companies present their products to the OTC Review Panels? Several reasons:

- During the review process, the 1970s and early 1980s, botanical medicine was just beginning to recover from its lowest ebb in U.S. history. The few surviving botanical medicine companies were, by and large, mom-and-pop enterprises run by herbalists whose marketing efforts consisted mainly of brewing medicinal teas for friends and selling them at local health food stores. Most had no idea that the OTC review process was even taking place, let alone how to participate. When they found out, it was too late.

- At the time, many herbalists rejected the word "drug." Most saw their products as foods, not drugs, despite the fact that their teas and tinctures were used for pharmacological, not nutritive, purposes. A few herbalists tried to organize participation in the OTC review process, but their efforts largely fell on deaf ears.

- Finally, the OTC Review Panels appeared unsympathetic to herbs. They were composed of mainstream health professionals who were largely unfamiliar with botanicals. Except for the few herbs that were approved, the OTC Review Panels basically ignored medicinal plants.

In 1985, when the OTC review process ended, it was closed. Any drug or herb that was not already approved had to undergo the expensive and time-consuming tests that the FDA required of new drugs—even if the herbal drugs had been widely used for millennia.

Furthermore when a new drug wins FDA approval, its owner gets a patent, the exclusive right to market it for many years. But who would spend millions to prove that valerian is an effective sleep aid? It is, and many studies have confirmed its effectiveness and safety, but since no one can patent valerian, there's no way to recoup the huge investment in approval trials.

FDA regulations have left healing herbs in limbo. Even if they've been used for thousands of years, to be approved as drugs they must be tested as brand-new compounds, which makes no sense economically because they can't be patented. Thus, the vast majority of medicinal herbs are sold as dietary supplements, a designation several rungs down the regulatory ladder.

The catch is that dietary supplements cannot make medicinal claims, which is why product labels are vague about the herbs' effects.

In 1994, Congress passed the Dietary Supplement Health and Education Act (DSHEA), which directed the FDA to consider petitions that would allow herbs (and vitamin and mineral supplements) to make medicinal claims. To date, a few claims have been approved, notably that soy protein lowers cholesterol. But the FDA has declined entreaties by the herb industry to reopen the OTC review process.

Germany treats medicinal herbs more rationally. Like the FDA, the German government requires pre-approval safety and efficacy testing for all newly synthesized pharmaceuticals. However, it does not hold herbs, which the Germans call traditional medicines, to quite so high a standard.

In 1978, drug regulators in the former West Germany convened an expert panel, Commission E, to study the extensive scientific literature on 650 herbs. In a process similar to the FDA's OTC review, the Commission E published monographs that declared hundreds of herbs safe and effective for dozens of ailments. The commission also recommended dosages and warned of possible side effects.

German herb companies are allowed to make medicinal claims supported by Commission E monographs as long as they market unadulterated, properly labeled herbs and adhere to the commission's dose recommendations. Currently, Commission E monographs represent the world's most authoritative government-sponsored, expert information on medicinal herbs' benefits, dosages, and side effects.

In this country, the National Institutes of Health's Office of Complementary and Alternative Medicine (OCAM) has sponsored meetings of FDA officials and herbal medicine advocates. The dialogue has focused on the possibility of reopening the OTC review process along the lines of Commission E. Some FDA officials support the idea, but as this book goes to press, the agency has taken no action.

It would clearly serve the public interest for the FDA to embrace an herbal medicine regulatory model similar to Commission E. According to a national survey conducted for *Prevention* magazine, 49 percent of American adults have used at least one herbal medicine. Another 24 percent consider themselves regular users.

Without clear labeling to specify benefits, side effects, and dosage—labeling that the FDA currently prohibits for all but a few medicinal herbs—many Americans remain confused about how best to use herbal medicines.

Increasingly Popular—But Still a Long Way to Go

A 2002 survey in the *Journal of the American Medical Association* showed that during a typical week, 14 percent of American adults used at least one medicinal herb (other than coffee or tea). Today, it's 20 percent—some 50 million people—and 10 percent of American adults have had herbs suggested by health professionals. In addition, pet owners increasingly treat their animals with herbs, notably chlorella.

However, the news media continue to be biased against herbs. In 2008, Canadian researchers compared newspaper coverage of clinical trials involving pharmaceuticals and herbal medicines. "Compared with pharmaceuticals, newspaper coverage of herbal clinical trials was more negative. Media coverage is not providing the public with the information necessary to make informed medical decisions."

But that's slowly changing, at least in medical journals. Until the 1990s, mainstream medical journals usually vilified herbs. Today, leading journals—including the *Journal of the American Medical Association (JAMA)* and *the New England Journal of Medicine*—are still quick to knock them, but now they also tout herbs' benefits, in part because the families and friends of medical researchers and journal editors use herbs, and in part because herbal medicine research has exploded. In 1977, English-language medical journals published 739 studies of medicinal herbs. By 2007, journal articles totaled 6,364, almost nine times as many.

Compared with American physicians, English doctors are more supportive of herbal medicine. But in a 2010 survey of 1,157 British doctors:

* 47 percent admitted feeling poorly informed about medicinal herbs.

* 63 percent did not ask patients if they used herbs.

* 72 percent said the public has too much faith in botanical medicines.

* 76 percent said their colleagues knew little about herbs.

Compared with American physicians, Scandinavian doctors are more supportive of herbs. But in a 2013 survey of 1,642 Norwegian adults, 80 percent said they used botanical medicines, but only 20 percent mentioned it to their doctors. The top reason why? *My doctor didn't ask.*

That's why it's so important for herbal medicine users to say so during doctor visits. Discussing your use of herbs helps reduce risk of possibly harmful herb-drug interactions, and it coaxes doctors to take herbal medicines more seriously, learn more about them, and—let's hope—recommend them.

Chapter 2

TEMPEST IN A TEAPOT

Are Healing Herbs Safe?

Before you take anyone's advice about using medicinal herbs, ask, "Are herbs safe?" If the answer is a blanket "yes," consult someone else.

The fact is, some of the world's most potent poisons are herbal, for example, poison hemlock or wild parsley. *Never* pick parsley in the wild. Another example is the *Amanita* mushroom, aptly called "death cap." *Never* forage for mushrooms in the wild unless you're *certain* you can identify them correctly.

So are herbal medicines safe? Most popular medicinal herbs, including those discussed in this book, are reasonably safe for most people most of the time when taken in recommended amounts. But medicinal plants contain pharmacologically active compounds that have drug effects on the body, and while drugs can heal, they also have the potential to harm: allergic reactions, side effects, possible fetal injury, and interactions with other herbs and drugs.

Overall, herbs are safer than pharmaceuticals, but they can still cause problems, and anyone who uses them should do so cautiously and responsibly.

Herb Safety in the Headlines

In recent years, headlines have called many herbs hazardous:

- Potentially serious surgery-related bleeding complications have developed in people taking herbs with anticoagulant action, among them: garlic, ginkgo, and ginseng. (Turns out ginkgo has been falsely accused.)

- Kava has been blamed for serious liver failure, including several deaths.

- Chinese ephedra (*ma huang*) has been abused by people seeking amphetamine-like intoxication. At very high doses, it can cause death.

- Herbal laxatives (buckthorn, cascara sagrada, rhubarb, and senna) have also caused problems: abdominal cramps, bloody stool, and even potentially serious electrolyte imbalances from regular use of unusually high doses.

No question, herbal medicines can cause problems. That's why this book contains extensive information on safety and side effects for every herb discussed. However, herbs are much safer than drugs.

❦ In 2014, Americans contacted the nation's poison control centers more than 1 million times. Pharmaceuticals prompted 991,307 calls, herbs, 42,535. So drugs accounted for 96 percent of suspected poisonings, herbs just 4 percent. Some of these exposures caused deaths. In 2014, accidental nonsuicidal poisonings with drugs killed 1,888 Americans, herbs none. *Zero.* Clearly herbs are much safer than drugs.

❦ University of Toronto researchers analyzed 30 years of the American medical literature for reports of drug side effects among hospital patients. They estimated that drug side effects kill an astonishing 106,000 U.S. hospital patients a year and cause 2.2 million serious but nonfatal medical problems. In other words, adverse reactions to pharmaceuticals rank as this country's fourth leading cause of death, accounting for more fatalities than AIDS, suicide, and homicide *combined.* These side effects did not result from medical errors. They occurred when drugs were administered in accordance with FDA dosage guidelines (*Journal of the American Medical Association*, April 15, 1998).

Clearly, pharmaceuticals may be hazardous. But which are more dangerous, drugs or herbal medicines? Drugs by a mile. Even the regrettable death tolls from all potentially hazardous herbs combined are dwarfed by the problems caused by pharmaceuticals.

Of course, many more Americans use drugs than herbs. From a cost-benefit perspective, it's reasonable to prescribe potentially hazardous drugs to treat life-threatening conditions. The point here is not to condemn pharmaceuticals but rather to point out that despite occasional problems, herbal medicines do not pose any significant public health hazard.

A Double Standard

Herbal medicines are victims of a double standard. Doctors and the public generally trust pharmaceuticals more than herbs because they are more tightly regulated. (See Chapter 1 for regulatory issues.) In many cases, though, the FDA's supposedly tight regulations deliver little more than the illusion of safety—as evidenced by the fact that use of prescription pharmaceuticals within FDA prescribing guidelines is responsible for more than 100,000 U.S. deaths a year and more than 2 million serious adverse reactions.

The FDA requires pharmaceutical companies to conduct clinical trials to demonstrate new drugs' safety and effectiveness, but most of these trials involve at most only a few thousand people. What about side effects that affect only 1 person in 10,000 or 50,000 or 1 million? They don't show up until the drug has become widely used. Within 5 years of approval, an estimated 50 percent of pharmaceuticals have their labels revised to include side effects—some potentially serious—that were discovered after the drugs were released.

Herbal medicines may not be as tightly regulated as pharmaceuticals, but they usually have much longer histories of use: decades, centuries, millennia. They have withstood the test of time. Every now and then, an age-old herb turns out to pose a new hazard, for example, potentially liver-damaging pyrrolizidine alkaloids in comfrey. But such discoveries are rare compared with postapproval side effects of recently approved pharmaceuticals.

The herb-safety double standard extends to the mass media. Media health experts tend to be much less familiar and comfortable with herbs than pharmaceuticals. Media experts tend to question herb safety and overstate herb hazards. Meanwhile, familiarity breeds acceptance. These same experts tend to understate drug hazards.

That's why reports of relatively minor herb hazards tend to generate big headlines and persist in the media. By comparison, reports of drug hazards—for example, the fact that pharmaceuticals are the nation's fourth leading cause of death—make headlines for a day and then are largely forgotten.

Of course, as more people with a greater variety of medical conditions begin using healing herbs, especially in combination with pharmaceuticals, some new problems are bound to turn up. The interactions between St. John's wort and several drugs are good examples. Herbs should always be used cautiously, especially by those taking other medications. By and large, however, herbal medicines are gentler and safer than pharmaceuticals.

The Issue of Dose Control

Some critics of herbal medicine contend that herbs are hazardous because typical preparation directions—1 to 2 teaspoons of dried herb per cup of boiling water, steeped for 10 minutes—yield infusions with highly variable doses of the medicinally active compounds. In contrast, when people take pharmaceuticals, they know precisely how much of the active ingredients they're getting.

The critics have a point. Herb potency depends on plant genetics, growing conditions, maturity at harvest, time in storage, the possibility of adulteration, preparation method, and dose. On the other hand, suicide statistics show that precise dose control is no guarantee that pharmaceuticals will be used safely. In addition, drug effects depend on body weight. A standard dose of a pharmaceutical taken by a person who weighs 120 pounds has a greater effect than the same dose ingested by someone who weighs 200 pounds. Finally, individuals vary. Different people often have very different reactions to the same drugs.

How do you react to drugs? For headache, the standard adult aspirin dose is two tablets every 4 hours. Through experience, some people learn that one tablet provides sufficient relief, while others must take three.

In general, healing herbs cause fewer side effects than pharmaceuticals. Pharmaceuticals tend to be highly concentrated, and pills and capsules have little taste, factors that make taking an overdose easy. The active constituents in herbs are typically less concentrated, and most herbs taste bitter, both of which help discourage overdose. Nonetheless, anyone who uses healing herbs must strive for good dose control.

The doses recommended in this book represent a consensus of the opinions found in both traditional herbals and scientific references. In the few cases where sources disagreed significantly, this book recommends the smaller amount—better to err on the side of caution.

These days, an increasing number of herbal medicines are available in pills and capsules as standardized extracts. This means that the plants were grown from seeds or clones known to produce a certain concentration of the pharmacologically active compounds. Then the plants were harvested, stored, and prepared under controlled conditions to produce reasonable dose uniformity.

Standardized extracts are not quite as dose-controlled as laboratory-synthesized pharmaceuticals, but they're considerably more dose-controlled than bulk herbs. When you buy commercial preparations, look for standardized extracts.

How to Use Herbs Safely

To use healing herbs safely, you don't need to be a doctor or master herbalist. All that's required is a little information:

- Before taking any herb, read up on it. Don't just listen to family and friends. Each herb profiled in this book contains extensive information on safety and side effects. Take warnings seriously. When in doubt about using any herb for any reason, don't use it until you've consulted a health professional.

- Don't take herb identity for granted. Look for products that identify herbs by their Latin binomials—genus and species. For example, garlic's binomial is *Allium sativum*. Latin binomial identification is no guarantee that the herb is labeled properly. But it suggests that the marketer understands the importance of proper identification and has taken steps to do that.

- Don't exceed recommended dosage. Some people assume that if a little is good, more must be better. Wrong. Don't put yourself at risk by taking overdoses. Whenever using commercial preparations—teas, tincture, pills, or capsules—follow the label directions carefully.

- Respect your individuality. Individuals vary. You may be allergic to one or more herbs or develop other unusual reactions. When you take herbal medicines, stay alert for adverse reactions such as abdominal upset, diarrhea, headache, itching, rash—anything out of the ordinary. If you notice unusual symptoms soon after taking a medicinal herb, stop and discuss your reaction(s) with your doctor.

- Who is most sensitive to healing herbs? Generally, those who suffer allergies (hay fever, hives), those with illnesses often linked to allergies (asthma, eczema), and those who have experienced serious, potentially fatal allergic reactions (anaphylaxis).

- Anaphylaxis triggered by medicinal herbs is extremely unlikely but always possible. The main symptom is difficulty breathing. If you develop any trouble breathing, call your emergency medical number immediately and tell the operator that you're experiencing suspected anaphylaxis. Then give your address and phone number and follow the operator's directions.

- Track your reactions. Even if you're not allergic, you may still be unusually sensitive to one or more medicinal herbs, in doctor-speak an "idiopathic" reaction, meaning "for unknown reasons"—just one of those things. Out of the blue, you may react badly to an herb that's generally considered safe. It happens.

- Pay attention to your body. If things go awry and you suspect that an herb is to blame, stop taking it and consult your physician.

- If you're over 65, start with a low dose. As people grow older, they often become more sensitive to drug effects, so a low dose might suffice. In addition, older people often take other medications. Starting with a low dose of medicinal herbs reduces the risk of adverse herb-drug interactions. You can always increase the dose later.

✤ If you're pregnant or nursing, use herbs with extreme caution. With a few exceptions, such as raspberry or ginger, women who are pregnant or nursing should not take medicinal amounts of healing herbs. Herbs that cause no problems for adults may still harm the unborn and newborns. Moms-to-be and nursing moms who wish to try herbal medicines should do so only in consultation with their health care providers.

✤ With few exceptions, don't give healing herbs to children under age 2. While some herbalists contend that herbal medicines are okay for children 6 months and older, this book takes a more conservative position. As gentle as most herbs are, they're usually not appropriate for the very young. The few exceptions include cinnamon, chamomile, cranberry, dill water, and ginger—and even these should be given cautiously.

✤ When administering any herb to a child, dilute the remedy in accordance with the child's weight. Standard herb doses are appropriate for a 150-pound person. A child who weighs 50 pounds should get one-third of the adult dose.

✤ Beware of herb-drug interactions. Exercise caution when using herbs if you already take pharmaceuticals or other herbs. Do not duplicate a drug's effects with herbs. If you're already taking an antidepressant drug, don't use the herbal antidepressant St. John's wort without consulting your doctor. If you're taking a pharmaceutical blood thinner (antico-agulant) such as aspirin, don't add anticoagulant garlic or white willow to your treatment plan. If you're already taking a tranquilizer or an anti-anxiety medication, steer clear of herbal tranquilizers: kava, passionflower, skullcap. Or switch from tranquilizers to calming herbs.

✤ Think twice before jumping on any new herb's bandwagon. Be extra careful when taking any newly popular herb or any old herb with a new use. In the mid-1990s, when the age-old herb St. John's wort was shown to have antidepressant action, it flew off the shelves. As the number of users jumped into the millions, rare side effects that strike only one person in a million suddenly began showing up. That's how doctors identified St. John's wort's interactions with several pharmaceuticals. Until the herb became popular, too few people took it for these problems to be noticed.

✤ Be prudent when using herb oils. Aromatic herbs' essential or volatile oils are highly concentrated, and small amounts may cause serious harm. For example, as little as a teaspoon of pennyroyal oil can cause death. Many herbal oils are available commercially. They are best used topically. If you ingest any, take only a drop or two at a time. Keep herbal oils well out of the reach of children.

✤ Pay attention to symptoms of toxicity. If you develop stomach upset, nausea, diarrhea, headache, or dizziness within a few hours of taking any healing herb, stop taking it and see if your symptoms subside. When in doubt, call your local Poison Control Center or your physician or pharmacist. If you experience a severe reaction, call your local emergency number immediately.

❦ Keep your physician informed. In any medical consultation, tell the doctor which herbs you take and why. Forthrightness helps prevent potentially harmful herb-drug interactions. (It also helps educate doctors about herbs.)

❦ Discontinue anticoagulant herbs at least 2 weeks before surgery. Anticoagulant herbs include: evening primrose oil, garlic, ginger, turmeric (curcumin), and white willow.

Potentially Problematic Herbs

Become familiar with the following herbs and exercise extra caution when taking them:

❦ Stimulants. These are the herbs most likely to cause trouble. Large doses of Chinese ephedra (*ma huang*) may cause amphetamine-like effects and potentially fatal heart problems. Unusually large doses of other herbal stimulants can also cause problems. Herbal stimulants include ginseng and those that contain caffeine: coffee, tea, cocoa (chocolate), maté, and kola. Don't exceed recommended doses. With herbs that contain caffeine, don't take more than what you're used to. In addition, don't take two or more stimulant herbs simultaneously. The effects are additive.

❦ Laxatives. Aloe, buckthorn, cascara sagrada, and senna all contain potent laxative compounds (anthraquinones). Even in recommended doses, they may cause violent purging and abdominal distress. In larger doses, they cause bloody diarrhea and other problems. Chemical laxatives—both herbal and pharmaceutical—should be last-resort treatments for constipation. Before taking them, drink more fluids, particularly prune juice, eat more plant foods to boost dietary fiber (bran cereal for breakfast), and get more exercise. If that doesn't work, try a fiber supplement, for example, Metamucil, whose active ingredient is the medicinal herb psyllium. If that doesn't provide sufficient relief, try a chemical laxative such as senna—but if you need to use it more than once a week, consult your doctor.

❦ Tranquilizers and sedatives. Herbal tranquilizers-sedatives include catnip, chamomile, hop, kava, lavender, lemon balm, passionflower, and valerian. Beware of combining these herbs. Don't take these herbs with alcohol, and don't combine them with pharmaceutical tranquilizers or sedatives.

Undoubtedly, the future holds more herbs-are-hazardous headlines as more people use herbal medicines more frequently, for more ailments, and in combinations with more drugs. And unfortunately, some people are likely to suffer harm. But by following the advice in this chapter and in the discussions of individual herb, you should be able to avoid most problems.

Chapter 3

STORING AND PREPARING HEALING HERBS

Getting the Most from Nature's Medicine

These days, most medicinal herbs are available in pills and/or capsules. It's as easy to take them as it is to take Tylenol.

Some herbs come in tinctures (alcohol extracts). Typically, the bottle includes an eyedropper cap, so it's easy to add the recommended number of drops to a glass of water, juice, or herbal beverage tea.

But you may enjoy growing and preparing your own herbs. Or you may choose to use some herbs available only as dried bulk plant material. That can feel daunting. Don't let it intimidate you.

Directions for Drying

Culinary herbs that also have medicinal applications—peppermint, rosemary, ginger— can be used fresh. But the convention among herbalists is to start with dried plant material, which is easier to store and resists spoiling.

Traditionally, herb growers simply tied their harvests in bunches and hung them in a warm, dry, shady place until they crumbled easily. With roots, they washed, split, and spread them in a single layer on a clean tray. These drying methods are still used today. In fact, some herb shops sell herbs in dried bunches.

However, traditional drying has two disadvantages. It often requires more room than people have, and it takes time—days to weeks for many leaves, stems, and flowers, and sometimes months for barks or roots. To preserve the volatile aromatic oils in many herbs, the faster the drying, the better. That's why most commercial herb producers use special equipment for drying their herbs.

An easy way to dry herbs at home is to place them on a baking sheet or a piece of clean window screen in an oven on the lowest temperature setting. Oven drying is convenient and inexpensive, but it has two drawbacks. If you harvest in heat of summer, you may not want to turn on your oven. And some ovens don't heat evenly, so some plant material may char while some doesn't dry.

Another approach is to purchase a small produce dryer, a tabletop appliance that blows hot-air to dry not only herbs but also other produce. Ask a local nursery, check garden catalogs or Web sites, or search the Internet for "herb dryers."

Powdering Made Easy

Once herbs are dry, for convenience, herbalists usually reduce them to powders. Traditional herbalists powdered herbs with mortars and pestles, a method that still works well for those processing only small amounts. Or try a small electric coffee grinder. For gardeners who produce bushels of herbs, larger grinders are available.

Setup for Storing

This may surprise those who store kitchen spices in clear glass jars, but light is one of the two biggest destroyers of herb flavor and medicinal potency. The other is oxygen.

To best preserve herbs' medicinal constituents, store them in opaque glass or ceramic containers. Fill containers to the top to limit the amount of oxygen in them. As you use your herbs, add cotton wadding to limit oxygen in containers.

When stored carefully, aromatic herbs—sage, rosemary, thyme—can remain potent for a year or more. Nonaromatic herbs—alfalfa, uva-ursi—last considerably longer.

Moisture is another herb killer. If your herbs get wet, re-dry them quickly to prevent mold growth.

Insects may also take a toll. Drying kills many pests, but watch for signs of infestation. When not using your herbs, keep containers closed tight.

Procedures for Preparation

Healing herbs may be used as infusions, decoctions, tinctures, capsules, ointments, and compresses. They may also be added to baths.

Making Infusions

Infusions are hot-water extracts. Some herbalists use the terms infusion and tea interchangeably, but the two are quite different. Infusions are prepared like teas, but they are steeped longer and become considerably stronger.

The standard traditional infusion recipe calls for $1/2$ to 1 ounce of dried herb steeped in a pint of boiling water for 10 to 20 minutes, then strained. But infusions do not have long shelf lives and should be made as needed. So modern herbalists generally recommend 1 to 2 rounded teaspoons of dried herb per cup of boiling water, steeped for 10 to 20 minutes.

Of course, after 20 minutes, infusions are no longer hot. Drink them at room temperature or reheat.

To use fresh herbs instead of dried, double the amount of herb—2 to 4 rounded teaspoons. Compared with dried herbs, fresh ones contain more water. They're bulkier, so you need more.

Making infusions can be as therapeutic as drinking them. While your infusion is steeping, inhale the warm, steamy vapors. For colds, flu, cough, bronchitis, and allergies, the vapors act as a nasal decongestant. As you inhale the vapors, close your eyes and visualize your immune system attacking your illness and making you well. Studies show that such meditative visualizations stimulate the immune system, marshalling the body to better fight the illness.

Some herbal infusions—chamomile, ginger, peppermint—are quite tasty. Others are horribly bitter. This is nature's way of discouraging overdose, but if you can't get your medicine down, it can't do any good. To make bitter infusions more palatable, add sugar, honey, or lemon, or mix them with herbal beverage blends or fruit juice. If you still can't stomach an infusion, try a different preparation.

Preparing Decoctions

Similar to infusions, decoctions are hot water extracts of roots and barks. Compared with flowers, leaves, and stems, it's more difficult to coax medicinal constituents out of roots and barks. Instead of steeping, bring the water to a boil, reduce the heat and gently simmer the dried herb material for 10 to 20 minutes, then strain.

Making Tinctures

Tinctures are alcohol extracts. They're highly concentrated, so they're more portable than infusions or decoctions. They also remain potent longer—up to several years.

To make tinctures, commercial manufacturers typically use pure grain alcohol, which is 198 proof. But most home tincture makers use 100 proof vodka.

The standard tincture recipe calls for 1 ounce of powdered dried herb steeped in 5 ounces of distilled spirits for 6 weeks. Some tips:

- Seal tincture containers tightly.
- Despite sealing, some containers may ooze. Don't store developing tinctures on valuable furniture.
- Label each tincture with the herb used and the date you put it up to steep. That way, you'll know when 6 weeks have passed.
- Shake each mixture every few days to encourage alcohol uptake of the herb's medicinal constituents.
- Keep tinctures out of direct sunlight.
- If possible, use brown glass containers to minimize light damage.
- Don't be surprised if tincture change color as they develop.
- If the liquid level in developing tinctures fall, top off with more distilled spirits.
- After 6 weeks, most herbalists strain out the plant material, but this is not necessary.
- Store tinctures in a cool place.
- Keep tinctures away from children. Tinctures are quite potent, and a small amount might cause harm.

People who abstain from alcohol can make tinctures using warm (but not boiled) vinegar. Herbalists recommend wine or apple cider vinegar, not white vinegar. The directions are the same as for alcohol tinctures.

Using Capsules

Powdered herbs can also be packed inside standard pharmaceutical gelatin capsules. Capsules are a convenient way to carry healing herbs when traveling or taking herbs that taste unpleasant. Many herb supply catalogs offer empty capsules and capsule-packing devices.

Capsules come in different sizes. The "00" size is standard. If you make capsules, measure how much powdered herb fits into the capsules you're using so you won't exceed the dosage recommended in this book.

Store capsules away from light and away from children.

External Preparations: Ointments, Compresses, and Baths

To make herbal ointments, add 1 to 2 teaspoons of tincture per ounce of commercial skin lotion.

For compresses to treat cuts, burns, and other skin problems, dip a clean cloth in a cool infusion or decoction and drape it over the affected area for 20 minutes. Repeat as needed.

To make baths more relaxing, fill a cloth bag with a few handfuls of aromatic herbs, then allow water to run over it. For additional aroma, leave the herb bag in the water as you bathe.

Chapter 4

HOW TO OBTAIN HEALING HERBS

The Best Sources Are Close at Hand

Healing herbs may be obtained by gathering, growing, or buying them.

Gathering

If you enjoy long walks in meadows and forests, gathering herbs can be great fun. Of course, not all healing herbs grow in the United States, but many do.

To go "herbing," you need a good field guide. The best ones are *A Field Guide to Medicinal Plants: Eastern and Central North America* by noted herbalists Steven Foster and James A. Duke, Ph.D., and *A Field Guide to Western Medicinal Plants and Herbs* by Steven Foster and another distinguished herbalist, Christopher Hobbs. Both books are part of the Peterson Field Guides series. Each book discusses more than 500 healing herbs. The Eastern book includes 500 pen-and-ink drawings and 200 color photos. The Western book features more than 600 color photos. Both are excellent.

Some herbs, such as dandelion, are easy to recognize and safe to pick. In fact, with dandelions, your neighbors will probably thank you for pulling plants out of their lawns. But other herbs, particularly ginseng, are more difficult to find.

Some healing herbs—including blackberry, raspberry, nettle, and rose—have thorns. Wear gloves, long pants, and long sleeves to gather these favorites.

Other herbs—angelica root and cascara sagrada bark—are safe to ingest when dried but hazardous when fresh.

Sometimes, the medicinal parts are safe but other parts cause problems, for instance, blue cohosh. Its medicinal root is safe when used properly, but its berries are poisonous. Likewise, rhubarb's medicinal root can be used safely, but its leaf blades are poisonous.

Finally, a few poisonous plants resemble healing herbs. Three poisonous species of hemlock look like parsley. Some herb gatherers have died because they mistook poison hemlock—also known as fool's parsley—for the familiar garnish. Never ingest any wild parsley.

If you stalk the wild healers, dress appropriately, read up on the herbs in Chapter 5 to see if they're safe or problematic, and use a good field guide. Most important, when in doubt about any plant's identity, don't ingest it.

Growing

The herb entries in Chapter 5 contain directions for cultivating the healing herbs that grow in the United States. To get started, you'll still need cuttings, seeds, or root divisions.

Cuttings can be difficult to obtain. You have to know an herb gardener. But cuttings are rarely necessary. Most nurseries and seed catalogs carry culinary herb seeds. Most nurseries also carry herb seedlings. If you don't see the herbs you want, ask if your nursery can obtain them.

For the committed herb gardener, nothing compares with the specialty catalogs published by many of the nation's hundreds of commercial herb growers. Most charge a small fee for the catalog.

❦ Companion Plants features more than 300 varieties of plants and 100 varieties of seeds. CompanionPlants.com. (740) 592-4643. 7247 North Coolville Ridge Road, Athens, OH 45701.

❦ The Rosemary House offers more than 100 varieties of plants and 200 varieties of seeds. TheRosemaryHouse.com. (717) 697-5111. 120 South Market Street, Mechanicsburg, PA 17055.

❦ Mountain Rose Herbs sells more than 100 varieties of herbs, seeds, herbalist supplies, and other herbal products. MountainRoseHerbs.com. (800) 879-3337. PO Box 50220, Eugene, OR 97405.

❦ Sandy Mush Herb Nursery features more than 1,000 herbs and other plants. SandyMushHerbs.com. (828) 683-2014. 316 Surrett Cove Road, Leicester, NC 28748.

❦ The International Herb Association (IHA) provides an enormous number of services to herb growers. It publishes a member directory and newsletter and sponsors conferences. Iherb.org. PO Box 5667, Jacksonville, FL 32247.

Buying

Supermarkets now carry many herbal beverage teas, some of which can be brewed into medicinal infusions. For a better selection, try a health food store. Most carry dozens of bulk herbs, medicinal herb blends, tinctures, oils, and tablets.

Bulk herbs, tinctures, oils, and tablets can also be purchased by mail. Many of the gardeners' resources listed above sell dried herbs and herb preparations. In addition, these companies and the companies below offer large selections:

❦ Jean's Greens features more than 200 varieties of organic and wildcrafted herbs, and other herbal products. JeansGreens.com. (518) 479-0471. 1545 Columbia Turnpike, Castleton, NY 12033.

❦ Monterey Bay Spice Company sells more than 500 herbs and spices. Herbco.com. (800) 500-6148. 241 Walker Street, Watsonville, CA 95076.

❦ HerbPharm features more than 250 herb products. Herb-Pharm.com. 800-348-4372. PO Box 116, Williams, OR 97544.

Noteworthy Herb Publications

Another way to find herbs—and to learn more about them—is to read the herb press. Recommended publications include:

❧ *HerbalGram*, the magazine of the American Botanical Council and the Herb Research Foundation. It's an excellent, authoritative source of the latest herb research, with an emphasis on herbal healing. HerbalGram .org. (512) 926-4900. 6200 Manor Road, Austin, TX 78723.

❧ *The Herb Quarterly* is a wonderful magazine with a broad scope, including herb gardening, cookery, crafts, history, and herbal medicine. HerbQuarterly.com. (510) 668-0268. 4075 Papazian Way #208, Fremont, CA 94538.

❧ Consumer Lab. This independent laboratory tests supplements and herbal products to see if they stand up to their label claims. Results are available to members. $39.00/year. ConsumerLab.com. (914) 722-9149. 333 Mamaroneck Avenue, White Plains, NY 10605.

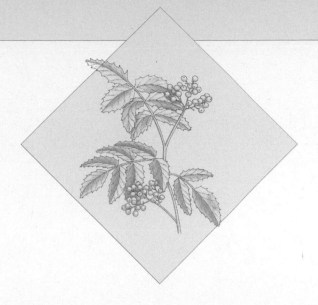

PART II

He causeth the grass to grow for the cattle

and herbs for the service of humanity.

—Psalms 104:14

Chapter 5

135 HEALING HERBS

The Cream of the Herbal Crop

This chapter profiles the history, folklore, and science of 135 medicinal plants. Why these 135?

❧ They're available. The selected herbs are generally Western in origin, from the Middle Eastern, European, and Native American healing traditions. Some Asian herbs have also been included. However, plants unique to Chinese herbalism have been omitted, despite their medical effectiveness, because they're not widely available in the United States.

❧ They're useful. All of the selected herbs have practical applications for everyday health concerns.

❧ They're reasonably safe. The selected herbs rarely cause serious side effects when used as recommended. Each profile provides detailed information on dosage, precautions, and potential hazards. (See Chapter 2 for a general discussion of herb safety.)

❧ They're often found in kitchen spice racks. Centuries ago, all of the herbs and spices used in cooking today were prized mainly for their use in food preservation and healing. Few people realize that they have valuable pharmacies in their kitchens.

❧ They're fascinating. The Pied Piper was as much an herbalist as a musician (page 473). The makers of Bayer were originally skeptical of aspirin (page 320). A 19th-century battle over abortion popularized a modern remedy for menstrual cramps (page 103). And cowboys who drank sarsaparilla were less interested in refreshment than in preventing venereal diseases (page 420).

❧ They're popular. Every year, the American Botanical Council, the leading medicinal herb organization, ranks medicinal herbs by popularity based on sales. This book includes all bestselling herbs.

ALFALFA

Hope for the Heart

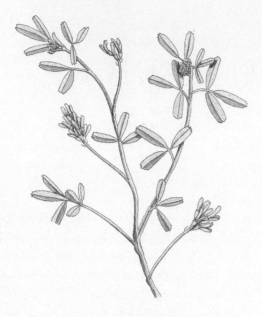

Family: Leguminosae; other members include beans and peas

Genus and species: *Medicago sativa*

Also known as: Chilean clover, buffalo grass, and lucerne (in Britain)

Parts used: Seeds, sprouts, and leaves

Alfalfa is the world's oldest forage crop. Farmers have prized it since before the dawn of history. Since the 1970s, alfalfa sprouts have become a popular salad vegetable. But the seeds contain the real healing power. They reduce cholesterol, which helps prevent heart disease and most strokes.

Healing History

What's good for cattle is also good for people, or so the ancient Chinese thought. Their animals ate alfalfa so enthusiastically that the Chinese began cooking the herb's tender young leaves as a vegetable. Soon, traditional Chinese physicians were using the plant to stimulate appetite and treat digestive problems, particularly ulcers.

Ancient India's traditional Ayurvedic physicians also used alfalfa to treat ulcers, and also prescribed it for arthritis and fluid retention (edema).

The ancient Arabs fed their horses alfalfa, believing that it made the animals swift and strong. They called it al-fac-facah, or "father of all foods," which the Spanish changed to alfalfa.

Spain introduced alfalfa into the Americas, where it became a popular forage crop, particularly in the Great Plains. Like the ancient Chinese, the pioneers believed that what was good for their cattle was good for them. They used alfalfa to treat arthritis, boils, cancer, scurvy, and urinary and bowel problems. Pioneer women used it to produce menstruation.

After the Civil War, alfalfa fell out of favor as a healing herb. It wasn't until the 1970s that it returned to popularity via the salad bowl.

Therapeutic Uses

Most of alfalfa's traditional therapeutic uses have long been disproved. But scientists have discovered an alfalfa benefit our ancestors never dreamed of. This herb helps prevent heart disease, stroke, and cancer, the nation's top three killers.

HEART DISEASE AND STROKE. Animal studies show that alfalfa leaves and seeds reduce blood cholesterol levels. High cholesterol raises risk for heart attack and most strokes. (Alfalfa sprouts produce a similar, but less pronounced benefit.) Scandinavian researchers gave alfalfa seeds (1.5 ounces three times a day) to 15 people with high cholesterol. After 8 weeks, their cholesterol level fell significantly.

CANCER. One study suggests that alfalfa helps neutralize cancer-causing substances in the intestine. Another, published in the *Journal of the National Cancer Institute*, shows that the herb binds carcinogens in the colon and helps speed their elimination.

WOMEN'S HEALTH. Alfalfa seeds contain two compounds, stachydrine and homostachydrine, that promote menstruation. They may also trigger miscarriage. Pregnant women should not eat alfalfa seeds. But women should not consider this herb a reliable contraceptive.

BAD BREATH. Alfalfa is rich in the green plant pigment chlorophyll, the active ingredient in most commercial breath fresheners. Sip an alfalfa infusion if you're concerned about bad breath.

Intriguing Possibility

In laboratory studies, alfalfa helps fight disease-causing fungi. One day, it may be used to treat fungal infections.

Medicinal Myths

Some herbalists still espouse the age-old view that alfalfa treats ulcers, but scientific research has found no support for this.

Herbalists also recommend alfalfa for bowel problems and as a diuretic to treat fluid retention. Unfortunately, these traditional uses have not held up under scientific scrutiny either.

Although some supplement manufacturers promote alfalfa tablets as a treatment for asthma and hay fever, a study published in the *Journal of the American Medical Association* shows that these claims have no merit. Alfalfa contains neither bronchodilators, which arrest an asthma attack, nor antihistamines, which relieve hay fever.

Rx Recommendations

While alfalfa sprouts dress up salads, it's the leaves and seeds that are used in herbal healing. Alfalfa leaf and seed tablets and capsules are available in most health food stores and supplements shops. Take them according to package directions.

When using the bulk herb, prepare medicinal infusions with 1 to 2 teaspoons of dried leaves and/or bruised seeds per cup of boiling water and steep for 10 to 20 minutes. Enjoy up to 3 cups a day to help reduce cholesterol in addition to cholesterol-lowering drugs your doctor prescribes. Alfalfa has a hay-like aroma and tastes like chamomile, with a slightly bitter aftertaste.

Safety

Wash alfalfa sprouts carefully. They may become contaminated with *E. coli* or *Salmonella* bacteria and cause food poisoning.

Do not consume more than recommended amounts of alfalfa seeds. They contain the potentially toxic amino acid canavanine. According to a report in *Lancet*, over time, eating large quantities of seeds may cause the reversible blood disorder pancytopenia. This condition impairs infection-fighting white blood cells and platelets, necessary for clotting.

The canavanine in alfalfa seeds has also been linked to systemic lupus erythematosus, a potentially serious auto-immune disease. Alfalfa seeds have reactivated the disease in people who were in remission, according to the *New*

England Journal of Medicine. Another study shows that the seeds induce lupus in monkeys. If you have lupus or have ever had pancytopenia, do not use alfalfa.

Pregnant and nursing women should not use alfalfa, except sprouts in salads.

Do not give alfalfa to children under 2. In older children, adjust the recommended dose based on the child's weight. Give a 50-pound child one-third of the dose a 150-pound adult would take.

If you're over 65, start with a low dose, and increase only if necessary.

Inform health professionals of the herbs you use. Problematic herb-drug interactions are possible.

Alfalfa may cause allergic reactions or other unexpected side effects. If any develop, reduce your dose or stop taking it. For more on herb safety, see Chapter 2.

If symptoms get worse or persist longer than 2 weeks, consult a health professional.

Gardening

Alfalfa grows throughout most of the United States. The plant is a deep-rooting, bushy perennial that grows to 3 feet, resembling tall clover. The leaves are divided into three leaflets. Depending on location, the herb's lavender, blue, or yellow flowers bloom from May through October.

Alfalfa grows best in loamy soil. It tolerates clay but not sand, which lacks sufficient nutrients. Prepare the soil with manure and rock phosphate. Sow seeds in autumn in rows 18 inches apart. Young plants require regular watering, but once established, they become fairly drought tolerant.

Harvest when plants bloom by cutting them back to within 3 inches of the ground, then hang them to dry. When dry, pick off the leaves.

ALOE
The Herbal Wound Soother

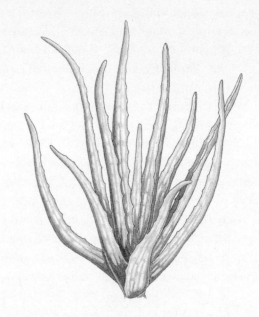

Family: Liliaceae; other members include lily, tulip, garlic, and onion

Genus and species: *Aloe vera* and an estimated 500 other species

Also known as: Cape, Barbados, Socotrine, and Zanzibar aloe

Parts used: Leaf gel, juice, or latex

Every kitchen windowsill should house a potted aloe. That's where minor burns, scalds, and cuts occur. It's easy to snip one of the plant's thick, fleshy leaves and scoop the inner gel onto the injury. Aloe gel dries into a natural bandage. It also promotes wound healing and helps prevent infection.

In addition, aloe latex, extracted from cells on the leaf's inner skin, is a powerful laxative— so potent that many authorities discourage ingesting it.

Healing History

Our word aloe comes from the Arabic *alloeh*, meaning "bitter and shiny," an apt description of the plant's wound-healing leaf gel. Drawings of aloe have been found in Egyptian temples dating to 3000 BC. The Bible mentions aloe several times, for example, "I have perfumed my bed with myrrh, aloes, and cinnamon" (Proverbs 7:17).

Egyptian prescriptions from 1500 BC recommend aloe for infections and skin problems and as a laxative, uses supported by modern science.

Aloe is one of the few non-narcotic plants to cause a war. When Alexander the Great conquered Egypt in 332 BC, he heard of a plant with amazing wound-healing powers on an island off Somalia. Intent on healing his soldiers' wounds—and on denying this healer to his enemies—Alexander sent an army to seize the island and the plant, which turned out to be aloe.

The Greek physician Dioscorides recommended aloe externally for wounds, hemorrhoids, ulcers, and hair loss. The Roman naturalist Pliny prescribed it for internal use as a laxative.

Arab traders carried aloe from Spain to Asia around the 6th century, introducing it to India's traditional Ayurvedic physicians, who used it to treat skin problems, intestinal worms, and menstrual discomforts. Chinese healers used it similarly.

More recently, American pioneers relied on aloe gel to treat wounds, burns, and hemorrhoids.

Therapeutic Uses

Contemporary herbalists—and scientists— agree with Dioscorides' 2,000-year-old observation that applied topically, aloe treats wounds.

WOUNDS (burns, scalds, scrapes, and sunburn). Aloe contains compounds—bradykinase, salicylic acid, and magnesium lactate—that reduce the pain, inflammation, swelling, and redness of wounds. Scientific evidence of aloe's wound-healing power was first documented in 1935, when an American medical journal reported accelerated healing of X-ray burns with aloe gel scooped from the plant's cut leaves. Since then, dozens of studies have supported the herb's ability to stimulate healing of first- and second-degree burns. Asian researchers analyzed many studies of aloe for wound healing. Compared with standard care, the wounds of those using aloe healed significantly faster—up to 8 days faster.

Aloe works best for superficial wounds. In a study published in the *Journal of Dermatology and Surgical Oncology*, the herb sped the healing of pimples by 3 days compared with standard medical treatment. For deep wounds, however, aloe *slows* healing. That's what researchers found in a study of aloe treatment of cesarean section incisions. Their study, published in *Obstetrics and Gynecology*, showed that incisions not treated with aloe gel healed in 53 days, but those treated with aloe took 83 days. Use aloe gel on superficial wounds, but don't use it on deep wounds requiring stitches.

INFECTIONS. In addition to wound healing, aloe gel also helps prevent wound infections. Several studies have shown aloe to kill many different bacteria and fungi that can infect wounds, including *E. coli*, *Staphylococcus*, *Streptococcus*, *Salmonella*, *Shigella*, and *Candida*. It also boosts the immune system, which helps the body fight infection.

ACNE AND POISON PLANTS. Beyond wounds, aloe also helps heal other minor skin afflictions, including acne and rashes caused by poison ivy, oak, and sumac.

PSORIASIS. Affecting some 7 million Americans, this autoimmune skin condition causes eruptions of red, raised skin patches usually topped with scaly tissue. At Malmo University Hospital in Sweden, researchers gave 60 people with psoriasis either a medically inactive placebo cream or one containing 0.5 percent aloe gel. The participants applied the creams three times a day, 5 days a week, for 16 weeks. Among those using the placebo cream, 7 percent experienced substantial clearing of their skin patches. But in the aloe group, that figure was 83 percent.

GENERAL SKIN CARE. To make her more alluring, Cleopatra's servants massaged aloe gel into her skin. The herb remains a popular ingredient in skin-care products. But if you're after beautiful skin, do what the legendary beauty did: Use the fresh leaf gel. The "stabilized" (preserved) gel found in commercial skin-care products and shampoos may not provide the fresh herb's benefits. If you enjoy aloe fragrance in shampoos and skin lotions, that's fine. Just don't expect them to turn you into Cleopatra.

DIABETES. Several animal studies show that aloe juice reduces blood sugar (glucose) levels in experimental animals. Thai researchers gave 72 diabetics either a placebo or aloe juice (1 teaspoon twice daily). After 6 weeks, the aloe group's blood sugar fell significantly.

GUM DISEASE. Indian researchers gave 345 young adults with gum disease (gingivitis) either a placebo, a drug used to treat it (chlorhexidine), or a mouthwash containing aloe vera juice. After a month the drug and herb worked significantly better than the placebo, and aloe was as effective as the drug.

Intriguing Possibilities

Aloe juice and aloe-based beverages are widely available in health food stores. Their labels claim that they soothe the digestive tract. Anecdotal reports suggest possible benefits for inflammatory bowel disease (colitis and Crohn's disease), but there is no rigorous research to support this.

Laboratory studies show that aloe kills the fungus that causes vaginal yeast infections (*Candida albicans*), and some herbalists recommend using it to treat the infection itself. But just because it kills the fungus in test tubes doesn't mean that it treats the infection in the body. No scientific studies support this use, and an FDA advisory panel found insufficient evidence to recommend aloe as a yeast treatment.

In laboratory tests, a compound in aloe called aloe-emodin has shown promise against leukemia. But National Cancer Institute scientists say that experimental preparations are still too toxic to give to people with leukemia.

Finally, folk herbalists have recommended topical aloe to treat skin cancer. This has never been studied scientifically.

Rx Recommendations

To help soothe and heal burns, scalds, scrapes, and sunburn and to help prevent superficial wound infections, first clean the wound with soap and water. Then select a lower (older) aloe leaf and cut off several inches. Slice it lengthwise, scoop the gel onto the wound, and let it dry. As for the injured leaf, it quickly closes its own wound. Its remaining gel can be used another time.

To enjoy the cosmetic benefits of aloe, apply

the leaf gel to freshly washed skin. Stop if it causes irritation.

Safety

Aloe gel is safe for external use by anyone who does not develop an allergic reaction.

If a wound treated with aloe does not heal significantly within two weeks or if it gets worse, consult a doctor.

Commercial aloe juice may have a mild laxative effect, but stay away from laxatives containing aloe latex. The latex contains laxative compounds (anthraquinones) with powerful purgative action that may cause cramping, diarrhea, and severe intestinal cramps. Other laxative herbs—senna, rhubarb, buckthorn, and cascara sagrada—also contain anthraquinones, but work more gently.

Despite recommendations not to use aloe as a laxative, some supplement companies sell aloe laxative tablets on the strength of approval by Commission E, the expert panel that evaluates herbal medicines for the German counterpart of the FDA. If you try aloe as a laxative, never exceed the dose on the label, and if you develop intestinal cramps, reduce your dose or stop taking it. If you're looking for a natural laxative, start with an effective but gentler herb, psyllium (page 370).

Women who are pregnant or trying to conceive should not take aloe latex, as its cathartic nature may stimulate uterine contractions and trigger miscarriage. Nor should the latex be used by nursing mothers. It enters mother's milk and may cause stomach cramps and violent catharsis in infants.

Aloe latex's cathartic power may also aggravate ulcers, hemorrhoids, diverticulosis, diverticulitis, colitis, Crohn's disease, or irritable bowel syndrome. Anyone with a gastrointestinal illness should not use aloe latex as a laxative.

In general, aloe latex is not recommended for internal use in children or adults.

Inform health professionals of the herbs you use. Problematic herb-drug interactions are possible.

Aloe may cause allergic reactions or other unexpected side effects. If any develop, reduce your dose or stop taking it. For more on herb safety, see Chapter 2.

If symptoms get worse or persist longer than 2 weeks, consult a health professional promptly.

Gardening

Got a brown thumb? Then aloe is your perfect houseplant. All it requires is a little water. Aloe prefers sun, but it tolerates shade and doesn't mind poor soil. The only conditions this hardy succulent cannot tolerate are poor drainage and cold. Bring potted aloe indoors before the temperature falls below 40°F.

Aloe periodically produces offshoots, which you may remove and replant when they are a few inches tall. Simply uproot or unpot the plant, work the soil gently to separate the offshoot, and return the mother plant to its bed or pot.

ANDROGRAPHIS

The "King of the Bitters" Fights
Colds—and More

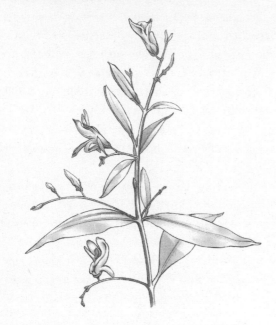

Family: Acanthaceae; other members include
acanthus

Genus and species: *Andrographis paniculata*

Also known as: Kalmegh, Kan Jang

Parts used: Mostly leaves, sometimes root

Many healing herbs taste bitter. But andrographis, an annual native to India, is so bitter that centuries ago, Indians named it *kalmegh*, Bengali for "king of the bitters."

Healing History

Like many bitter herbs, India's traditional Ayurvedic physicians prescribed andrographis to promote digestion, increase appetite, and treat stomach distress. In addition, they recom-mended the herb to treat fever, snakebites, and jaundice (liver disease). Traditional Chinese physicians considered andrographis a "cold" herb and used it to treat conditions involving excessive heat, for example, fever.

Therapeutic Uses

IMMUNE STIMULATION. Andrographis boosts the ability of white blood cells to gobble up invading germs, including *E. coli*, the bacteria that cause urinary tract infections, and *Shigella*, which causes infectious diarrhea (dysentery).

COLDS, FLU, AND SINUS INFECTION. Andrographis also improves the body's ability to fight the viruses that cause colds and flu. Swedish researchers gave either a placebo or the herb to 179 adults with cold symptoms: sore throat, nasal congestion, runny nose, watery eyes, and cough. After 3 days, the andrographis group showed highly significant benefit, especially in relief of sore throat. A dozen other studies around the world agree that treatment with andrographis results in shorter, milder colds in both adults and children, without significant side effects.

Russian researchers gave a placebo or andrographis to 540 people with flu symptoms (cold symptoms plus fever and muscle aches). Their conclusion: The herb "contributes to quicker recovery and reduces risk of post-influenza complications," for example, bronchitis. Andrographis caused no significant side effects.

Finally, Thai researchers analyzed many cold and flu studies of andrographis. They concluded that the research "supports the usefulness of andrographis in reducing the severity of upper respiratory tract infections."

FEVER, PAIN, AND INFLAMMATION.

At a dose of 6 grams, the herb reduces fever, validating this use by traditional Chinese physicians. In one Chinese study, the herb reduced fevers in 70 of 84 subjects within 48 hours. In another, Thai researchers gave either a placebo or andrographis (6 grams/day) to 152 people with fever and sore throat caused by tonsillitis. After one week, the herb group reported significantly greater relief, results similar to that produced by acetaminophen (Tylenol).

URINARY TRACT INFECTION. Thai researchers gave either andrographis (1,000 milligrams/day) or antibiotics to women with UTI. The herb was as effective as the pharmaceuticals.

LIVER PROTECTION. When people ingest liver-toxic chemicals or develop hepatitis, the organ overproduces several enzymes. In animal studies, andrographis helps return liver enzyme to normal, especially when the cause of the damage was alcohol, certain carcinogens, or parasites. Andrographis protects the liver as well as the milk thistle extract, silymarin (page 323).

Intriguing Possibilities

An Armenian study showed andrographis beneficial for sinus infection.

One animal study shows that pretreatment with andrographis reduced deaths from cobra venom, possibly validating the traditional Indian practice of using the herb to treat snakebite.

Animal studies suggest that andrographis lowers blood sugar, which might help control diabetes.

Pilot studies suggest that andrographis might combat malaria.

The herb also appears to reduce blood clotting, including the internal blood clots that cause heart attack and most strokes. If con-

firmed, someday andrographis might help prevent these conditions.

Rx Recommendations

For immune stimulation in adults, try 2 to 3 grams/day of liquid extract (1 to 2 teaspoons). To treat colds and flu, the dose is 6 grams/day (4 teaspoons). But liquid extracts are too bitter to be palatable. Most andrographis products are sold as capsules. Follow package directions.

Safety

Andrographis is considered nontoxic, however, at doses several times higher than recommended, stomach distress, loss of appetite, nausea, and vomiting are possible.

Andrographis impairs blood clotting. If you have a clotting disorder or are taking anticoagulant medication (including aspirin), talk to your doctor before using andrographis. Stop using it 2 weeks before elective surgery.

At high doses, andrographis suppresses the fertility of both male and female laboratory animals. The one human trial showed sperm suppression. Couples hoping to conceive should avoid it.

Pregnant and nursing women should not use andrographis.

Do not give andrographis to children under 2. In older children, adjust the recommended dose based on the child's weight. Give a 50-pound child one-third of the dose a 150-pound adult dose.

If you're over 65, start with a low dose, and increase only if necessary.

If you use this herb, inform your health professionals. Problematic herb-drug interactions are possible.

Andrographis may cause allergic reactions or other unexpected side effects. If unusual symptoms develop, reduce your dose or stop taking it. For more on herb safety, see Chapter 2.

If symptoms get worse or persist longer than 2 weeks, consult a health professional promptly.

Gardening

Andrographis is not grown in the United States.

ANGELICA
An Herbal Angel

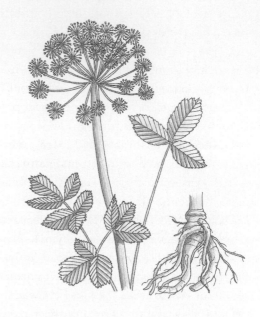

Family: Umbelliferae (carrot, parsley, celery, fennel, dill)

Genus and species: *Angelica archangelica* (European), *A. atropurpurea* (American), *A. sinensis* (Chinese), and other species

Also known as: Wild celery and masterwort; in China, *dang gui* or *dong quai*

Parts used: Roots, leaves, and seeds

Tall, striking, and attractive, angelica has played a role in magic and medicine for thousands of years. But the species used in Western and Chinese herbal medicine differ. So, too, are the opinions of the herb's medicinal value.

In the West, European angelica has always been a minor healing herb. But in Asia, Chinese angelica, usually called *dang gui*, has long been considered a major boon for gynecological complaints. This claim is controversial, but Western researchers may have been too quick to dismiss Chinese angelica as worthless.

Healing History

In Asia, Chinese angelica has been used since the dawn of history. It has always been considered the premier tonic for menstrual problems, menopausal complaints, and other women's health concerns. Traditional Chinese practitioners and Indian Ayurvedic physicians continue to prescribe it for gynecological conditions, arthritis, abdominal pain, colds, and flu.

During the Middle Ages, European peasants considered European angelica magical. They fashioned angelica leaves into necklaces to protect their children from illness and witchcraft. Angelica was reputed to be the only herb witches never used. Its presence in women's gardens or cupboards was considered a persuasive defense against charges of witchcraft.

During the 16th and 17th centuries, the juice from crushed angelica roots was combined with other herbs to make "Carmelite water." This medieval drink was said to cure headache, promote relaxation and long life, and protect against poisons and witches' spells.

In 1665, Europe was decimated by bubonic plague. Legend has it that a monk dreamed he met an angel, who gave him an herb to cure the scourge. The monk named the herb angelica, in honor of the messenger in his dream. The name stuck, and the Royal College of Physicians in London incorporated angelica water into England's official plague remedy, the King's Excellent Plague Recipe.

History provides no clear verdict on the effectiveness of the "excellent recipe," but the old monk's dream may have been prophetic. Bubonic plague is a bacterial disease, and modern science has discovered that compounds in angelica have antibacterial action.

European angelica has hollow stems. Air can pass through them. Under the Doctrine of Signatures—the medieval belief that an herb's physical appearance reveals its healing benefits—hollow-stemmed plants were considered beneficial for respiratory problems, and during the 17th century, angelica was a popular treatment for colds, flu, and asthma.

When European colonists arrived in North America, they found Native Americans using American angelica as they did—to treat respiratory ailments, particularly tuberculosis. Eventually, the colonists began using large doses to induce abortion.

Nineteenth-century American Eclectic physicians, forerunners of today's naturopaths, recommended angelica for heartburn, indigestion, bronchitis, malaria, and typhoid.

Therapeutic Uses

Contrary to legend, angelica does not deliver humanity from epidemic disease, but the Chinese herb has caused a good deal of controversy. Some studies show benefit for menopausal discomforts, while others do not. Meanwhile, most traditional uses for European angelica look iffy.

Contemporary herbalists recommend angelica mostly for digestive problems and to help clear mucus. These uses may have some validity.

MENOPAUSAL COMPLAINTS. Israeli researchers gave 55 women complaining of hot flashes either a placebo or a combination of *dang gui* and chamomile (75 milligrams *dang gui* and 30 milligrams chamomile, five times a day).

After 12 weeks, the herb group reported significantly greater relief.

Researchers at the National College of Naturopathic Medicine in Portland, Oregon, and Bastyr University, the naturopathic medical school in Kenmore, Washington, gave thirteen menopausal women either medically inactive placebos or a Chinese herbal formula containing *dang gui*, licorice root, hawthorn leaf, burdock root, and wild yam root. After 3 months, the women who took the herbal formula reported significantly greater relief.

However, Kaiser Permanente researchers in Oakland, California, gave *dang gui* to 71 menopausal women for 3 months. They reported no benefit. Experts in Chinese herbal medicine have criticized the Kaiser Permanente study because it used only *dang gui*. In Chinese herbal medicine, the herb is never used alone.

While the jury is still out on *dang gui* for menopausal complaints, formulas containing the herb appear to soothe hot flashes.

HEART DISEASE AND STROKE. Angelica species contain compounds, coumarins, with anticoagulant (blood-thinning) action. Blood thinners are used to prevent the internal blood clots that trigger heart attacks and most strokes. Chinese studies show that *dang gui* extract administered by injection helps dissolve the clots that cause stroke.

RESPIRATORY AILMENTS. Score one for the Doctrine of Signatures. German researchers have determined that angelica relaxes the windpipe, suggesting that it may have some value in treating colds, flu, bronchitis, and asthma.

DIGESTIVE COMPLAINTS. The same German investigators found that angelica relaxes the intestines. This lends some cre-

dence to the herb's traditional use in treating digestive complaints.

ARTHRITIS. Japanese researchers report that angelica has anti-inflammatory effects, so there may be something to its traditional Asian use for treating joint pain.

Intriguing Possibilities

A Chinese pilot study suggests that *dang gui* may increase red blood cell production, hinting that it may someday prove beneficial in treating anemia.

The Chinese have also found that *dang gui* improves liver function in people with cirrhosis or chronic hepatitis. Their research is preliminary, however, and no specific recommendations can be made at this time about using angelica for liver problems.

A Chinese pilot study suggest that *dang gui* may help treat ulcerative colitis.

Rx Recommendations

If you'd like to use Chinese angelica to treat gynecological problems, consult a practitioner of Chinese herbal medicine for a multi-herb formula.

Commission E, the expert panel that evaluates herbal medicines for the German counterpart of the FDA, endorses European angelica as a treatment for appetite loss, abdominal distress, and flatulence.

For an infusion, use 1 teaspoon of powdered seeds or leaves per cup of boiling water. Steep for 10 to 20 minutes and strain if you wish.

For a decoction, use 1 teaspoon of powdered root per cup of water. Bring to a boil and simmer for 2 minutes. Remove from the heat, let stand for 15 minutes, and strain if you wish. Drink up to 2 cups a day. Angelica decoctions taste bitter. Add sweetener.

With a homemade tincture, use ½ to 1 teaspoon up to twice a day.

When using commercial preparations, follow the package directions.

Safety

Angelica has never been shown to stimulate uterine contractions, but given its traditional use to induce menstruation and abortions, women who are pregnant or trying to conceive should avoid it.

Angelica contains compounds known as psoralens. Exposure to sunlight may cause a rash in those who ingest psoralens (photosensitivity). Psoralens may also promote tumor growth, leading the authors of a report in the journal *Science* to advise against taking angelica internally.

On the other hand, an animal study showed that the angelica constituent alpha-angelica lactone has an anticancer effect. Angelica's role in human cancer, if any, remains unclear. People with cancer histories probably should not use it until the controversy has been settled.

Fresh angelica roots are poisonous. Drying eliminates the hazard. Dry roots thoroughly before using them.

Unless you are a confident field botanist, do not collect angelica in the wild. It's easy to confuse with water hemlock (*Cicuta maculata*), which is extremely poisonous.

For adults who are not pregnant or nursing and have no history of cancer, heart attack, or photosensitivity, angelica is considered reasonably safe in amounts typically recommended.

Do not give angelica to children under 2. In older children, adjust the recommended dose based on the child's weight. Give a 50-pound child one-third of the dose a 150-pound adult would take.

If you're over 65, start with a low dose, and increase only if necessary.

Inform health professionals of the herbs you use. Problematic herb-drug interactions are possible.

Angelica may cause allergic reactions or other unexpected side effects. If any develop, reduce your dose or stop taking it. For more on herb safety, see Chapter 2.

If symptoms get worse or persist longer than 2 weeks, consult a health professional promptly.

Gardening

Angelica often blooms around May 8, the feast day of St. Michael the Archangel, which is the source of European angelica's species name, *archangelica*. The plant grows to 8 feet and resembles celery—hence its common name, wild celery. It's a biennial that dies after producing seeds.

Angelica grows from seeds or root divisions. Seed viability is relatively brief, only about 6 months, but refrigeration extends it up to a year. Germination may take a month. Sow angelica in the fall or spring ½ inch deep in well-prepared beds. Space plants 2 feet apart in all directions.

Angelica thrives in rich, moist, well-drained, slightly acidic soil. It prefers partial shade. Leaves may be harvested in the fall of the first year and roots during the spring or fall of the second year.

Angelica is not usually considered a culinary herb, but fresh leaves provide a zesty accent to soups and salads. Leaves have a fragrant aroma and a warm, vaguely sweet taste reminiscent of juniper, followed by a bitter aftertaste. You can eat steamed stems with butter. Chopped stems add flavor to roast pork.

APPLE

The Sweet, Juicy, Crunchy Healer

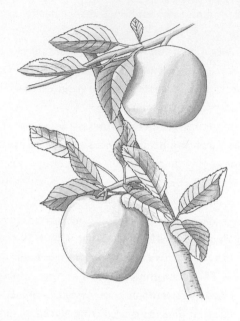

Family: Rosaceae; other members include rose, peach, almond, and strawberry

Genus and species: *Malus sylvestris* or *Pyrus malus*

Also known as: No other common names

Parts used: Fruits

An apple a day keeps the doctor away. The old rhyme is truer than ever, particularly if the doctor is a gastroenterologist, oncologist, or cardiologist. Apples help prevent and treat both diarrhea and constipation and may also help prevent America's top three killers: cancer, heart disease, and stroke.

Few herbalists consider the apple an herb, but the tasty fruit has a long tradition as a healer. So much of what ancient herbalists believed about this delectable fruit has been scientifically supported that it's time to return the apple to the herbal-medicine roster.

Healing History

The Bible never identifies the Garden of Eden's "forbidden fruit," but since ancient times, people have believed that it was an apple. Legend has it that a piece got stuck in Adam's throat, hence our "Adam's apple."

The "apple of discord" started the Trojan War. A poisoned apple induced Snow White's coma. William Tell shot an apple off his young son's head. And let's salute early America's apple eccentric, John Chapman, Johnny Appleseed. This pioneer spent most of his life wandering around Pennsylvania, Ohio, and Indiana sowing apple seeds—and becoming legendary.

The ancient Egyptians, Greeks, and Romans loved apples and developed dozens of varieties, but it was ancient India's Ayurvedic physicians who first prescribed them to relieve diarrhea. Applesauce is still a popular home remedy for diarrhea.

Traditional Chinese physicians have used apple bark for centuries to treat diabetes, another use that's supported by modern science.

The medieval German abbess/herbalist Hildegard of Bingen prescribed raw apples as a tonic for healthy people and cooked apples as the first treatment for any sickness.

In medieval England, people said, "Eating an apple before going to bed/Makes the doctor beg his bread." You know what this evolved into.

Seventeenth-century English herbalist Nicholas Culpeper recommended apples "for hot and bilious stomachs . . . inflammations of the breast and lungs . . . [and] asthma." He also suggested boiled apples in milk as a treatment for gunpowder burns.

The Americas had no native apples, but the Pilgrims brought seeds, and the fruit quickly became, well, as American as apple pie. Apples, apple bark, and apple cider soon became mainstays of American folk medicine.

Speaking of apple pie, when the poor baked pies, they used only a bottom crust. Richer bakers could afford to add a top crust—hence our description of the wealthy as "upper crust."

A century ago, American Eclectic physicians, forerunners of today's naturopaths, had several recommendations for apples: raw for constipation, baked or stewed for minor fevers, a bark decoction for intermittent fever (malaria), and apple cider for fever.

Therapeutic Uses

Modern science has discovered that Johnny Appleseed's favorite fruit has tremendous value in healing thanks to its pulp, which is high in pectin, a soluble fiber.

DIARRHEA. Pectin helps relieve diarrhea because intestinal bacteria transform it into a soothing, protective coating for the irritated intestinal lining. In addition, pectin adds bulk to the stool, which helps resolve diarrhea.

Infectious diarrhea is caused by bacteria. One study found that apple pectin is effective against several types of bacteria that cause diarrhea: *Salmonella*, *Staphylococcus*, and *E. coli*. In fact, pectin is the "pectate" in the over-the-counter diarrhea preparation Kaopectate.

CONSTIPATION. Physicians recommend diets high in fiber to add bulk to stool. Pectin is a type of fiber that helps resolve constipation by adding bulk and stimulating bowel contractions.

HEART DISEASE AND STROKE. A high-fiber diet helps reduce cholesterol, a key risk factor for heart disease and most strokes. With fiber in the gut, the cholesterol we eat remains in the intestine until elimination. If you have a pectin-rich, high-fiber baked apple for dessert after eating meat and dairy, you enjoy some protection from their cholesterol.

In a long-term study of 805 Dutch men, those who ate the most apples experienced the fewest heart attacks. The scientists concluded that in addition to pectin, compounds in apples called flavonoids played an important protective role. Flavonoids are antioxidants that help prevent the cell damage at the root of the arterial narrowing that triggers heart attack.

CANCER. The American Cancer Society recommends a high-fiber diet to help prevent several cancers, particularly colon cancer. A study published in the *Journal of the National Cancer Institute* shows that pectin binds cancer-causing compounds in the colon, speeding their elimination.

The antioxidant flavonoids in apples also help prevent the cell damage that causes many cancers.

DIABETES. Physicians also recommend a high-fiber diet to control diabetes. A report in *Annals of Internal Medicine* showed that apple pectin helps reduce blood sugar (glucose) in diabetics.

HEAVY METAL EXPOSURE. European studies suggest that apple pectin helps eliminate lead, mercury, and other toxic heavy metals from the body.

WOUNDS. Although pectin is the apple's major medicinal component, the fruit's leaves contain an antibiotic called phloretin. If you cut yourself out in the orchard, press apple leaves against the wound as you seek soap and water.

Intriguing Possibility

A few studies, including one published in the *Journal of the National Cancer Institute*, hint that pectin may help prevent cancer from spreading (metastasizing).

Rx Recommendations

For first-aid for minor wounds, crush some apple leaves and apply them to the cut or scrape until you can wash and bandage it.

Eat the whole fresh fruit to enjoy a wide range of healthful benefits. Green apples tend to be tart, but they usually have more "snap." Red apples are usually sweeter but may have a mealy texture. Wash apples with soap and water before eating to eliminate any pesticide residue.

Safety

James A. Duke, Ph.D., retired USDA herbal medicine authority (and poet), sums up apple safety this way:

An apple a day keeps the doctor away,
Or at least that's what some people say.
But one man, we read,
Ate a cupful of seed,
And this man died.
Poisoned by cyanide.

Strange but true: Apple seeds contain cyanide, the powerful poison. About ½ cup of seeds can be deadly for the average adult, but considerably less is fatal for children and the elderly. Many parents are familiar with the stomachaches that young children develop when they eat apple cores. The few seeds in the typical core pose little risk of serious poisoning. But to be prudent, teach children not to eat apple seeds.

Gardening

Archeological evidence shows that humans have enjoyed apples since 6500 BC. Prehistoric apples resembled today's crab apples—small, dry, and mealy. But as agriculture developed, apples became one of the world's first hybridized orchard fruits.

Today, about 300 apple varieties grow in the 50 states. Special varieties have been developed for just about all growing conditions in North America. Consult a nursery for the varieties best suited to your locale.

Full-size apple trees grow to about 40 feet and spread over 1,600 square feet (40 by 40). Genetic dwarf apple varieties produce delicious, full-size fruits but grow to only 6 to 12 feet and spread over less than 150 square feet (12 by 12).

Plant the rootstock in a sunny location and water regularly. Prune at planting, then annually. Different apple varieties have different fertilizer requirements and different pest problems. Consult a nursery.

ARNICA

The Controversial Homeopathic Wound Treatment

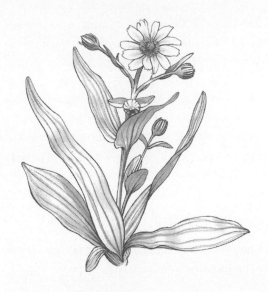

Family: Asteraceae; other members include daisy

Genus and species: *Arnica montana*

Also known as: Mountain daisy, wolf's bane, leopard's bane

Parts used: Dried flower heads

Arnica is homeopathic first-aid for wounds, injuries, and muscle soreness. But mainstream physicians scoff at homeopathy in general and homeopathic arnica in particular. The studies go both ways, some showing benefit, others showing none. But the weight of the evidence tilts in favor of this mountain flower.

Healing History

For centuries, European herbalists used arnica in salves and ointments as a topical treatment for injuries, bruising, and pain. They also prescribed teas and tinctures for a variety of conditions, including paralysis, menstrual problems, and typhoid.

The German philosopher Johann Wolfgang von Geothe drank arnica tea to ease his chest pain (from angina). But he used a very low dose because he knew that large doses could be toxic. Even modest amounts cause nausea, vomiting, and diarrhea. Larger amounts suppress respiration, causing coma and death. As a result, America's 19th century Eclectic physicians limited this herb to external uses to treat wounds, bruising, pain, and inflammation.

Arnica is most widely prescribed by homeopaths. Homeopathy, developed in the 1830s by the German physician Samuel Hahnemann (1755–1843), is controversial because its microdose medicines are so dilute that pharmacologists insist they could not possibly have any effect. Nonetheless, for reasons science cannot currently explain, many homeopathic herbal treatments, including arnica, have shown benefits in rigorous studies.

Therapeutic Uses

Recent studies of arnica are confusing. Some show benefit. Others do not. And results showing benefit are often barely statistically significant. Meanwhile, results showing no benefit often barely miss statistical significance of benefit. So the scientific cases for and against arnica are not very compelling. Nonetheless, the majority of studies show benefit, and in homeopathic doses, this herb is safe and inexpensive.

SURGICAL PAIN AND BRUISING. Homeopaths typically prescribe arnica for pain caused by injuries. As a result, most arnica research has focused on pain, with the herb ingested in homeopathic micro-doses or applied topically in ointments.

German researchers gave 88 people having bunion surgery either a standard drug for pain and inflammation (diclofenac, Voltaren) or homeopathic arnica (10 tiny pills three times a day). Four days after surgery, the two treatments were equally effective for bruising, swelling, and wound tenderness. Diclofenac was more effective for pain. But those taking arnica got back on their feet more quickly and comfortably. The researchers concluded: "After foot operations, arnica can be used instead of diclofenac."

Welsh scientists gave 190 adults having tonsillectomies either a placebo or homeopathic arnica (two tiny pills six times the day after surgery, then two tiny pills a day for the next week). The arnica group reported significantly less pain.

German researchers gave 60 people having surgery to remove varicose veins either a placebo or arnica (5 tiny pills three times a day for 2 weeks). The arnica group reported significantly less bruising and pain.

Plastic surgeons in Farmington, Connecticut, gave 29 people having face-lifts either a placebo or arnica for 10 days after surgery. The arnica group experienced less bruising.

Swiss researchers gave 204 people with osteoarthritis of the hands either a standard ointment containing ibuprofen (Motrin, Advil) or an arnica ointment. After 21 days, both groups reported the same relief.

MUSCLE SORENESS. Norwegian researchers tested arnica in runners in two Oslo Marathons (1990 and 1995). A total of 82 runners were given either a placebo or arnica (five tiny pills starting the evening before the races then morning and evening of race day and for 3 days after). The arnica group reported less muscle soreness.

An Australian study of 20 runners concurred, showing that arnica ointment reduced delayed-onset muscle soreness.

OSTEOARTHRITIS. Swiss researchers gave 204 people with arthritis of the fingers either ibuprofen gel or arnica tincture mixed with skin lotion. Three weeks later, both participants and their doctors rated the herb as slightly more effective with fewer side effects.

Commission E, the German counterpart of the FDA, approves arnica ointments for muscle aches, inflammation, and insect bites and stings.

Intriguing Possibilities

Animal studies suggest that arnica may stimulate the immune system.

Rx Recommendations

When using arnica ointments or homeopathic pills, follow package directions. Or consult a homeopath.

Safety

Do not ingest arnica plant material. It's poisonous, causing nausea, vomiting, gastrointestinal distress, and in high doses, coma, cardiac arrest, and death. If you grow arnica, keep the plant away from young children, and warn older children not to ingest it.

Ingest this herb *only* in homeopathic doses, which are too low to cause problems. Consult a homeopath for appropriate dosages for children and those over 65.

Pregnant and nursing women should not

ingest arnica. Use of topical ointments is fine.

If you use this herb, inform your health professionals. Problematic herb-drug interactions are possible.

Arnica may cause allergic reactions or other unexpected side effects. If unusual symptoms develop, reduce your dose or stop taking it. For more on herb safety, see Chapter 2.

If symptoms get worse or persist longer than 2 weeks, consult a health professional promptly.

Gardening

Arnica is native to cool mountainous regions of Europe and Russia. It also grows at higher elevations in the northwest United States. Arnica is a perennial that grows to 12 inches and produces bright yellow, daisy-like flowers, hence its common name, mountain daisy. Sow seed in the spring in a mix of loam, peat moss, and sand. Arnica likes acid pH, full sun, moisture, and high altitude. The flowers smell unpleasant, but the odor subsides as they dry. Pulverize dried flowers and make a tincture. Mix some tincture with hand lotion or skin cream for a topical ointment.

ARTICHOKE

The Delicious Vegetable with Surprising Healing Benefits

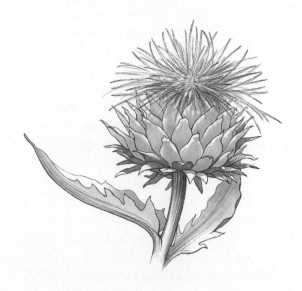

Family: Compositae or Asteraceae; other members include thistle

Genus and species: *Cynarae scolymus*

Also known as: Garden artichoke, globe artichoke

Parts used: The flower and lower portions of the barbed scales that enclose it

What's the best herb for preventing and treating liver problems? If you're familiar with herbal medicine, you know it's milk thistle (page 323). But artichoke, a close botanical relative of milk thistle, is almost as beneficial. Its species name, *scolymus*, derives from the Greek for thistle. In traditional European herbal medicine, the two plants were used almost interchangeably. In addition, artichoke also soothes the stomach, lowers cholesterol, and treats irritable bowel syndrome.

Healing History

Around 300 B.C, the ancient Greek naturalist, Theophrastus, described a plant native to Sicily. He called it scolymus, now artichoke's species name: "The head [flower bud] is most pleasant, being boiled." Theophrastus' scolymus was wild artichoke, or cardoon (*Cynara cardunculus*). Ancient farmers cultivated it and bred it, selecting for larger flower buds. By the Middle Ages, they had produced today's globe artichokes— which continued to be called cardoons (or cardone, cardoni, carduni or cardi) until the 19th century.

Around the ancient Mediterranean, herbalists used artichoke/cardoon as both a food and medicine. As a food, it was considered a delicacy. As a medicine, the flower and the plant's juice were used to promote digestion and treat upset stomach and liver problems (jaundice).

One type of artichoke, blessed thistle, was so popular in 17th-century England that in his *Complete Herbal* (1652), the noted English herbalist, Nicholas Culpeper, wrote: "I shall spare the labour of writing a description as almost everyone may describe them from their own knowledge." Culpeper called blessed thistle "an excellent remedy" for jaundice and gallbladder problems and recommended it for plague, boils, and "the bites of mad dogs and venomous beasts." He also said it "cures the French pox," that is, syphilis.

In France, for centuries artichoke juice has been a traditional liver tonic.

America's 19th century Eclectic physicians recommended artichoke for liver disease, gout,

and muscle aches (rheumatism). They also considered artichoke juice an aphrodisiac.

Therapeutic Uses

LIVER PROBLEMS. Like milk thistle, artichoke has considerable antioxidant action that spurs regeneration of liver cells. Several studies show that in animals treated with liver-toxic chemicals, artichoke minimizes liver damage and increases survival.

INDIGESTION. German researchers gave 244 adults with chronic indigestion either a placebo or artichoke extract (640 mg twice a day). After 6 weeks, the artichoke group reported significantly greater relief and improved quality of life. In a similar study, British scientist reported the same findings.

IRRITABLE BOWEL SYNDROME (IBS). This common condition causes chronic digestive problems: abdominal pain, cramping, bloating, and diarrhea or constipation. Because artichoke helps treat indigestion, British researchers thought it might also alleviate IBS. They gave 208 adult IBS sufferers either a placebo or artichoke extract (320 or 640 milligrams/day). Two months later, the artichoke group reported 41 percent greater relief.

CHOLESTEROL. Several studies show that artichoke lowers cholesterol. In one trial, German researchers gave people with high cholesterol either a placebo or artichoke extract (450 milligrams/day). After 6 weeks, the placebo group's total cholesterol fell 9 percent, but in the artichoke group, it dropped twice as much, 19 percent. For every 1 percent decrease in total cholesterol, heart attack risk drops 2 percent. So thanks to artichoke, participants' risk of heart attack decreased 38 percent. The researchers called their findings "clear evidence for recommending artichoke" as a treatment for high cholesterol.

Italian scientists gave 92 adults with high cholesterol either a placebo or artichoke leaf extract (250 milligrams/day). After 8 weeks, the placebo group showed no increase in HDL (good cholesterol), but among the artichoke takers, HDL increased significantly.

ATHEROSCLEROSIS. Often called hardening of the arteries, atherosclerosis involves the development of cholesterol-rich deposits on artery walls that limit blood circulation and raise risk of heart disease and stroke. An Italian study shows that artichoke juice (1 cup a day) helps prevent atherosclerosis.

ANTIMICROBIAL. Artichoke inhibits the activity of several bacteria and fungi.

DIGESTIVE SUPPORT. Commission E, the German counterpart of the FDA, notes that artichoke increases bile flow, which helps digest fats. The Commission approves fresh artichoke, its leaf extract, and juice for indigestion.

Intriguing Possibilities

Pilot studies suggest that artichoke may have some pain-relieving and anti-inflammatory action.

The herb may also reduce blood sugar and help manage diabetes.

And one study shows that when male laboratory animals are exposed to chemicals that damage testicular tissue, artichoke treatment minimizes the damage.

Medical Myth

Some folk medical traditions recommend artichokes for hangover. British researchers gave 15 adults either artichoke extract (three standard capsules) or a placebo immediately after drinking sufficient alcohol to cause intoxication and hangover. One week later, the treatments were switched (a cross-over trial). The artichoke group took the placebo and vice versa. There were no differences in hangover duration or discomfort between the artichoke and placebo groups. Artichoke does not reduce hangover.

Rx Recommendations

Artichoke extract is available at health food stores or on the Internet. But why buy extract when artichokes themselves are cheaper? Steam the delicious vegetable for 30 to 45 minutes. Pull off the outer scales. Dip the inner scales in butter, yogurt, or mustard and eat the fleshy base. When you get down to the flower, remove the immature scales and central hairs, and eat the heart.

Safety

Frequent contact with artichoke may cause allergic reactions, notably skin irritation or hives.

Commission E warns that people with gallstones or obstructed bile ducts should consult a physician before using artichoke medicinally.

Gardening

Don't confuse this plant with Jerusalem artichoke (*Helianthis tuberosus*), a species of sunflower.

Artichoke is a perennial that grows to 6 feet and 4 feet wide. Flower buds (heads) appear in July in the Southern United States, or in August in the Northern United States and Canada.

Growing requires 100 frost-free days a year. Soil should be rich with compost and manure and well drained. Artichokes like slightly acid soil (pH 6.0). Seeds can be started indoors in early spring and transplanted after the last frost. Watering encourages large artichokes.

Replace some older plants each year. Take suckers or side roots from your healthiest plants to propagate.

ASHWAGANDHA

India's Potent Adaptogen

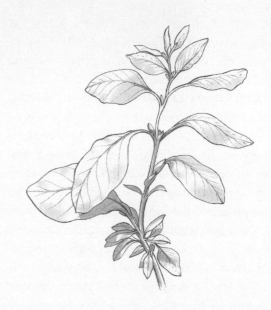

Family: Solanaceae; other members include tomato, potato, and bell peppers

Genus and species: *Withania somnifera*

Also known as: Withania, Indian ginseng, winter cherry, dunal

Parts used: Root

Ashwagandha (ash-wah-GAHN-da) derives from two Sanskrit words—*ashwa* meaning horse, and *gandha* for essence, that is, the herb makes users as strong as horses. That's an exaggeration, but recent studies show that it does improve muscle strength.

Ashwagandha is not related to ginseng but it's often called "Indian ginseng" because its effects are similar to the Chinese herb. It's an "adaptogen" that strengthens the whole body, treating fatigue, weakness, debility, and many age-related conditions.

Healing History

Ashwagandha is a small evergreen shrub native to India. It also grows in the Middle East and East Africa. Its small, smooth, round, fleshy fruit contains many seeds and turns reddish-orange when ripe, hence the name winter cherry.

Ashwagandha has been revered in India's traditional Ayurvedic medicine for 3,000 years. It's discussed in several ancient Ayurvedic medical texts, including the *Charaka,* which recommends it as a whole-body tonic, particularly for those suffering from debility and for enhancing reproductive function and longevity. Ayurvedic physicians prescribe it to treat arthritis, muscle aches, inflammations, conditions associated with aging, and insomnia, hence its species name *somnifera.*

Therapeutic Uses

Like ginseng and rhodiola, Chinese and Ayurvedic physicians consider ashwagandha a "tonic" or *adaptogen,* meaning whole body strengthener. The term *adaptogen* was coined in 1947 by Russian scientist, N. V. Lazarev, who was interested in drugs that helped the body overcome physical and emotional stress. His student Israel I. Brekhman popularized the term and showed that the most powerful adaptogens are not drugs, but herbs. Lazarev and Brekhman believed that adaptogens should:

❧ Counteract the adverse effects of stress.

❧ Increase energy.

❧ Increase the body's resistance to a broad range of adverse influences.

❧ Have a normalizing effect, improving many conditions while aggravating none.

❧ Cause minimal side effects.

Since Brekhman's death in 1994, the term adaptogen has been generalized to include herbs that don't necessarily boost energy or counteract stress, but have a number of benefits including enhanced immune function, antioxidant action, and physiological normalization.

Unfortunately, in America, "tonics" are suspect. Many 19th century patent medicines sold as "rejuvenating tonics" contained mostly alcohol and/or opium. In addition, most Americans believe that individual drugs treat just one problem, maybe two. We're not used to the idea that one drug—or herb—can produce a broad range of physical and mental health benefits. But animal studies show that ashwagandha produces several: immune stimulation, heart protection, improved stamina, and greater resistance to the physiological damage caused by stress.

Human trials agree.

STRESS AND ANXIETY PROTECTION. Indian scientists gave 130 adults either a placebo or ashwagandha (500 milligrams/day). After a year, the herb group showed significantly less anxiety and improved well-being.

Researchers at SUNY Upstate Medical Center in New York analyzed five studies of ashwagandha as a treatment for stress/anxiety. In all five, a total of 400 participants showed significant benefit, reduced stress and anxiety. And ashwagandha caused fewer side effects than pharmaceutical tranquilizers.

BLOOD PRESSURE. Indian scientists

gave 20 young adult men either a placebo or ash-wagandha (1,000 milligrams/day). After 2 weeks, the groups switched treatments. When taking the herb, participants' blood pressure declined significantly. Blood levels of the stress hormone, cortisol, also fell.

CHOLESTEROL. Indian researchers gave ashwagandha daily to diabetics with high cholesterol. After a month, their cholesterol levels dropped significantly.

DIABETES. In the cholesterol study just mentioned, the diabetics' blood sugar levels also declined. The decrease "was comparable to that produced by oral diabetes medication."

FATIGUE. Malaysian researchers gave either a placebo or ashwagandha (2,000 milli-grams four times a day) to 100 women suffering fatigue from cancer chemotherapy. After 6 months, the placebo group reported slightly less fatigue, but those taking ashwagandha reported much less—plus better appetite, less insomnia, pain, and constipation and greater well-being and quality of life.

REACTION TIME. Indian researchers gave 20 men, age 20 to 35, either a placebo or ashwa-gandha (1,000 milligrams/day). After 2 weeks, they registered significantly speedier reaction times.

STRENGTH. Indian scientists gave ashwa-gandha (750 to 1,250 milligrams root extract/day) to 18 young adults. After a month, their handgrip strength and stamina increased sig-nificantly. Other Indian researchers conducted a similar study in children (2,000 milligrams/day). Two months later, they also registered signifi-cantly increased grip strength.

INFERTILITY. Indian researchers gave ashwagandha (5 grams of powdered root/day) to 180 infertile men and 50 with normal fertil-ity. After 3 months, the control group showed no fertility changes, but those taking the herb showed improvements: higher sperm counts and improved sperm motility with fewer deformed sperm.

ADAPTOGEN. After taking ashwagandha for a year, Indian men showed reduced choles-terol, more red blood cells, and enhanced sexual function.

Intriguing Possibilities

Ashwagandha appears to have some antide-pressant action. It may also protect against sei-zures and loss of cognitive function due to toxic chemicals.

Rx Recommendations

The recommended dose is 1 to 6 grams/day (2 to 12 teaspoons) in capsules or tea. In tincture or liquid extract, use 2 to 4 milliliters 3 times/day.

Safety

Very high doses of ashwagandha may cause stomach upset, diarrhea, nausea, vomiting, drowsiness, dulling of reflexes, and loss of motor abilities.

Large doses may trigger abortion. Pregnant and nursing women should not use ashwagandha.

Do not give ashwagandha to children under 2. In older children, adjust the recommended dose based on the child's weight. Give a 50-pound child one-third of the dose a 150-pound adult would take.

If you're over 65, start with a low dose, and increase only if necessary.

If you use this herb, inform your health professionals. Problematic herb-drug interactions are possible.

Ashwagandha may cause allergic reactions or other unexpected side effects. If unusual symptoms develop, reduce your dose or stop taking it. For more on herb safety, see Chapter 2.

If symptoms get worse or persist longer than 2 weeks, consult a health professional promptly.

Gardening

Ashwagandha grows primarily in dry, subtropical areas of India to an elevation of about 5,000 feet. It also grows from Pakistan to Egypt, and in Spain, Morocco, the Canary Islands, and South Africa. In the United States, it can be grown in the South and Southwest. The plant is an erect shrub that in the wild grows to 3 feet, but cultivated plants grow larger.

Keep seeds moist but not too wet. They germinate within 2 weeks at 70°F. This herb prefers full sun and sandy soil. Harvest the fruit in the fall. Dry the bright yellow seeds for planting the following spring. Harvest the medicinal root in the fall after the first frost. Roots are either dried whole or cut into pieces and dried.

ASTRAGALUS
An Asian Immunity Booster

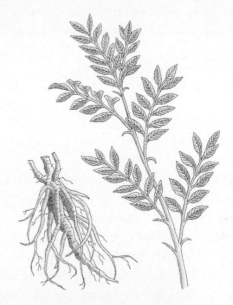

Family: Leguminosae; other members include beans and peas

Genus and species: *Astragalus membranaceus*

Also known as: Huang qi, yellow leader, and milk vetch

Parts used: Roots

The Chinese refer to astragalus as *huang qi*, meaning "strengthener of *qi*." *Qi* (or *chi*) is the Chinese term for life force, vitality, stamina, disease resistance, and the ability to cope with stress. As a strengthener of *qi*, astragalus is powerful medicine.

Healing History

Chinese herbalists have prescribed astragalus for 2,000 years. Today practitioners of Chinese medicine believe the herb strengthens all body systems and is particularly effective for treating illnesses that cause fatigue. They consider it similar to ginseng, and they prescribe it for diabetes, heart disease, and high blood pressure.

Therapeutic Uses

Western scientists have begun to study astragalus only recently, so there are still more questions than answers about the herb's effects. However, research to date confirms traditional Chinese claims.

ENHANCED IMMUNITY. The first Western study of astragalus took place in 1983 at the University of Texas M. D. Anderson Cancer Center in Houston. The herb improved immune function in 19 cancer patients who were being treated with immune-suppressing chemotherapy drugs.

Since then, several studies—animal and human—have shown that astragalus, administered either orally or by injection, improves immune function. In one animal study, astragalus improved the germ-devouring ability of macrophages, infection-fighting white blood cells. In another, astragalus boosted the infection-fighting ability of T-cells, another type of white blood cell.

In a Chinese study, doctors administered astragalus extract (injections of 8 grams/day) to 10 people with viral heart infections and depressed immune systems. Their immune function improved significantly.

In another Chinese study, 235 women with various chronic viral infections, among them herpes, were treated with immune-boosting interferon and/or astragalus. The herb by itself did not provide much benefit. But astragalus plus interferon produced the greatest antiviral benefit.

HEART DISEASE. Chinese researchers gave astragalus to 92 people with angina, a form of heart disease. The herb reduced chest pain in 83 percent. In another Chinese study, compared with heart attack sufferers who did not take the herb, those treated with astragalus showed significantly improved heart function.

LIVER DAMAGE. Chinese researchers gave 208 people with chronic hepatitis B, average age 38, either a placebo or an herbal formula that was primarily astragalus (dose not specified, three times a day). After 2 months, the herb users showed significantly improved liver function.

CHRONIC FATIGUE. Korean scientists gave a placebo or a combination of astragalus and Chinese sage (3 to 6 grams/day). A month later, the placebo group showed scant change but the herb takers showed significantly less fatigue.

HAY FEVER. Croatian researchers catalogued the allergy symptoms of 41 hay fever sufferers, then gave them either a placebo or astragalus (160 milligrams twice daily). After six weeks the herb group showed significantly less sneezing, itchy eyes, and runny nose—with no side effects.

Intriguing Possibilities

Chinese studies suggest that astragalus improves sperm motility, reduces blood pressure, and enhances immune function in people infected with HIV, the virus that causes AIDS.

Rx Recommendations

In China, growers peel and dry carrot-like astragalus roots. They cut roots into long slices that resemble popsicle sticks. When using dried roots, finely chop four or five and simmer them in 4 cups of boiling water for 1 hour. Drink 1 cup in the morning and 1 cup in the evening. Astragalus tastes mildly sweet, but you may prefer it blended with other beverage herbs.

Astragalus is also available in a variety of commercial preparations, including tinctures, capsules, and tablets. Follow package directions.

Safety

When used as recommended, astragalus is generally considered safe. One laboratory test, however, found that a strong decoction caused chromosome mutations, a hint that the herb might be carcinogenic. Traditional Chinese herbalists recommend using astragalus for only a few weeks during an illness, and not routinely. This would be prudent advice if mutagenicity is confirmed.

Chinese practitioners advise against taking astragalus for acute infections; instead, they recommend reserving it to strengthen the body after it has begun to heal.

Pregnant and nursing women should not use astragalus.

Do not give astragalus to children under 2. In older children, adjust the recommended dose based on the child's weight. Give a 50-pound child one-third of the dose a 150-pound adult would take.

If you're over 65, start with a low dose, and increase only if necessary.

Inform health professionals of the herbs you use. Problematic herb-drug interactions are possible.

Astragalus may cause allergic reactions or other unexpected side effects. If any develop, reduce your dose or stop taking it. For more on herb safety, see Chapter 2.

If symptoms get worse or persist longer than 2 weeks, consult a health professional promptly.

Gardening

Astragalus is a perennial plant native to northern China and Mongolia that produces small yellow flowers. Its thick root has a tough fibrous skin with a yellowish interior, which is the medicinal part. The root has a sweetish, licorice-like taste. Astragalus is not grown in the United States.

BACOPA

This Herb Can Make You Smarter

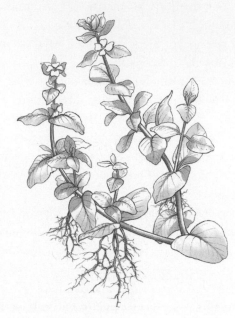

Family: Scrophulariaceae; other members include snapdragon

Genus and species: *Bacopa monnieri*

Also known as: Brahmi, water hyssop

Parts used: Whole plant

Bacopa is an age-old Ayurvedic remedy for the nervous system. Another Ayurvedic herb, gotu kola (page 260) has been used similarly. As a result, both of these herbs share the Sanskrit name, *brahmi*, meaning "expands consciousness." To avoid mixing up the two plants, most herbalists have stopped using the term, brahmi, and refer to these herbs as bacopa and gotu kola.

Healing History

Over the centuries, India's traditional Ayurvedic physicians have prescribed bacopa to aid learn-ing, memory, and concentration. It was also recommended to treat anxiety, seizures, and mental illness. Modern research has shown that bacopa offers so many health benefits that Indian researchers consider it an "adaptogen" like ginseng, ashwagandha, or rhodiola—an herb that enhances total well-being.

Therapeutic Uses

LEARNING, MEMORY, CONCENTRA-TION. Contemporary research has confirmed bacopa's brain-boosting power. The herb contains compounds, bacosides, that improve nerve impulse transmission. As early as 1966, a study showed that bacopa increases learning-related neurotransmitter levels in the brain. Since then many animal studies and clinical trials have shown that it's a brain booster.

In several studies, Australian and Indian researchers gave middle-aged adults standard cognitive function tests, and then either a placebo or bacopa (300 milligrams/day). In one study, after 5 weeks, the herb improved learning and other measures of mental acuity. In another, after 12 weeks, the bacopa group showed significant improvement in learning and memory consolidation.

Australian scientists analyzed six rigorous studies of bacopa for memory enhancement. Bacopa did not produce miracles, but it aided recall.

Researchers at Oregon Health Sciences University in Portland gave standard tests of memory and learning to 48 elderly men, average age 74. Then participants took either a placebo or bacopa (300 milligrams/day). Three months later, retesting showed no change in the placebo group, but significantly improved results in those who used bacopa.

Another Indian report shows that 3 to 9 months of daily bacopa improve children's IQs.

To improve cognitive function, herbalists generally say it takes several weeks of daily bacopa use. But in good news for students cramming for exams, an Australian report suggests that even one dose may help. Researchers gave 24 adults, ages 18 to 56, cognitive function tests and then a placebo or one dose of bacopa (320 milligrams). Re-testing showed that bacopa improved ability to do math in one's head. So, students, one dose of bacopa doesn't guarantee an A, but it may help.

ATTENTION DEFICIT/HYPERACTIVITY DISORDER (ADHD). Indian psychiatrists gave 36 children with ADHD either a placebo or bacopa (50 milligrams twice a day). After 12 weeks, the herb group showed improvement in memory and learning.

ANXIETY. In one Indian study, 35 people suffering severe anxiety took large doses of bacopa (12 grams/day). After 2 weeks, they were significantly less anxious.

Oregon and Australian scientists gave 48 elderly folks a placebo or bacopa (300 milligrams). After 12 weeks, the placebo takers showed increased anxiety, but the bacopa group showed less.

ANTIOXIDANT. How do the bacosides in bacopa boost brain power? They have antioxidant action. Antioxidants prevent or reverse the cell damage caused by highly reactive oxygen ions (free radicals). Antioxidants usually reduce risk of heart disease and cancer without affecting mental acuity. But for reasons that remain unclear, bacosides appear to focus their antioxidant action on the parts of the brain involved in reasoning and memory, the frontal cortex and hippocampus.

LIVER PROTECTION. The antioxidants in bacopa protect the liver from drug-induced damage.

HYPOTHYROIDISM. Bacopa also stimulates production of thyroid hormone, suggesting value in treating hypothyroidism.

INFLAMMATION. Bacopa has anti-inflammatory action. One study suggests it's as effective as the standard nonsteroidal anti-inflammatory drug (NSAID), indomethacin (Indocin), but without the stomach upset common with NSAIDs.

Intriguing Possibilities

Traditional Ayurvedic physicians used bacopa to treat epileptic seizures. Animal studies show it has anticonvulsant action—but only at very high doses.

In animal studies, bacopa opens the airway into the lungs (bronchodilator). As a result it may help treat bronchitis and asthma.

Pilot studies suggest that bacopa relaxes the digestive tract and may prove beneficial for indigestion and irritable bowel syndrome. Bacopa also appears to suppress *Helicobacter pylori*, the bacteria that causes ulcers.

Finally, in laboratory studies, the herb has been shown to inhibit growth of some cancers.

Rx Recommendations

The traditional adult dose is 5 to 10 grams of powdered herb/day in divided doses; or 5 to 12 milliliters/day of fluid extract; or 200 to 400 milligrams/day of bacopa extracts standardized to 20 percent bacosides. Follow package directions.

Safety

At recommended doses, bacopa causes no known side effects. But at unusually high doses, it becomes a sedative.

Pregnant and nursing women should not use bacopa.

Do not give bacopa to children under 2. In older children, adjust the recommended dose based on the child's weight. Give a 50-pound child one-third of the dose a 150-pound adult would take.

If you're over 65, start with a low dose, and increase only if necessary.

Inform health professionals of the herbs you use. Problematic herb-drug interactions are possible.

Bacopa may cause allergic reactions or other unexpected side effects. If any develop, reduce your dose or stop taking it. For more on herb safety, see Chapter 2.

If symptoms get worse or persist longer than 2 weeks, consult a health professional promptly.

Gardening

Bacopa is a hardy, creeping, succulent-like, perennial ground cover with small oblong leaves and white or purple flowers. It likes marshy soil and can be grown in temperate or warmer areas at elevations to 4,500 feet with adequate water. Water frequently.

BARBERRY
A Powerful Infection Fighter

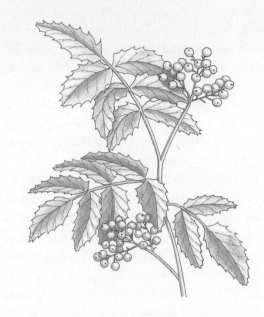

Family: Berbericlaceae; other members include May apple, mandrake, and blue cohosh

Genus and species: *Berberis vulgaris;* Oregon grape: *B. aquifolium* or *Mahonia aquifolium*

Also known as: Berberry, berberis, and jaundice berry

Part used: Root

Who says herbs can't compete with pharmaceutical drugs? In one study, berberine, the active constituent in barberry, proved more potent against bacteria than chloramphenicol, a powerful pharmaceutical antibiotic.

But there's a lot more to this herb than infection treatment. Barberry, and its close relative, Oregon grape, may also stimulate the immune system, reduce blood pressure, and even shrink some tumors.

Healing History

Barberry has been a prominent herbal healer for more than 2,500 years. The ancient Egyptians used it to prevent plague, probably effectively considering the herb's antibiotic action. India's traditional Ayurvedic healers prescribed barberry for dysentery, another use that's been scientifically confirmed.

During the early Middle Ages, European herbalists were guided by the Doctrine of Signatures, the belief that a plant's physical appearance revealed its therapeutic benefits. Barberry has yellow flowers, and its roots produce a yellow dye. These features were linked to the yellowing of the skin and eyes of jaundice, a symptom of liver disease. As a result, barberry was widely used to treat liver and gallbladder ailments, earning the name jaundice berry.

Traditional Russian healers recommended it for skin inflammations, high blood pressure, and abnormal uterine bleeding.

When colonists introduced barberry into North America, the Native Americans recognized it as a relative of the native Oregon grape, a holly-like plant that they considered a powerful healer. Many tribes adopted barberry and used it to treat dysentery, mouth ulcers, sore throat, wound infections, and intestinal complaints.

The 19th-century American Eclectic physicians, forerunners of today's naturopaths, prescribed barberry as a purgative and treatment for jaundice, dysentery, eye infections, cholera, fevers, and "impurities of the blood," a euphemism for syphilis.

Barberry was also an ingredient in the popular but highly controversial Hoxsey Cancer Formula, an alternative cancer therapy marketed from the 1930s to the 1950s by ex-coal miner Harry Hoxsey (page 31).

Therapeutic Uses

Most contemporary herbalists limit their recommendations to gargling barberry decoction for a sore throat and drinking infusions for diarrhea and constipation. Actually, it's useful for much more.

INFECTIONS. The berberine in barberry has remarkable infection-fighting properties. Studies around the world show that it kills microorganisms that cause wound infections (*Staphylococcus* and *Streptococcus*), diarrhea (*Salmonella* and *Shigella*), dysentery (*Entamoeba histolytica*), cholera (*Vibrio cholerae*), giardiasis (*Giardia lamblia*), urinary tract infections (*Escherichia coli*), and vaginal yeast infections (*Candida albicans*).

ENHANCED IMMUNITY. In addition to antibiotic action, berberine also stimulates the immune system. It activates macrophages (literally, "big eaters"), the white blood cells that devour harmful microorganisms.

LIVER DAMAGE. Score one for the Doctrine of Signatures and "jaundice berry." Pakistani researchers gave laboratory animals large doses of acetaminophen to produce liver damage, signified by increased blood levels of liver enzymes. Then some animals were treated with barberry. Their enzymes declined, showing significant normalization of liver function. The researchers concluded, "This study provides a scientific basis for the traditional use of barberry in liver disorders."

HIGH BLOOD PRESSURE. Barberry contains compounds that enlarge (dilate) blood vessels. This lends support to the herb's traditional Russian use as a treatment for high blood pressure.

CHOLESTEROL. A Chinese analysis of 11 studies involving 874 participants showed that berberine (1 to 1.5 grams/day for 8 to 16 weeks) significantly reduced cholesterol.

DIABETES. Chinese scientists in Shanghai gave diabetics either a standard medication (metformin) or berberine (500 milligrams three times a day). After 3 months, the herb lowered blood sugar as much as the drug.

HEART DISEASE. High cholesterol, high blood sugar, and high blood pressure are all major risk factors for heart disease. Because berberine diminishes them all, it also reduces risk of heart disease.

PSORIASIS. German researchers confirmed barberry's traditional use in treating skin problems in a 4-week study involving 82 people with psoriasis, which produces red, raised, scaly skin eruptions. Each participant was given two ointments marked "left" and "right," one with barberry extract, the other without. Participants applied each ointment to one side of their bodies. The barberry ointment produced significantly greater shrinkage of skin eruptions.

PINKEYE (CONJUNCTIVITIS). In Germany, doctors prescribe a berberine preparation, Ophthiole, to treat sensitive eyes, inflamed lids, and pinkeye. Unfortunately, the product is not available in the United States. To try it, apply a compress of barberry infusion.

Intriguing Possibilities

Perhaps Harry Hoxsey was right. Animal studies suggest that barberry helps shrink some tumors. Pilot studies also hint that the herb has anti-inflammatory activity, suggesting possible value in treating arthritis.

Rx Recommendations

To prepare a decoction, boil ½ teaspoon of powdered root bark in 1 cup of water for 15 to 30 minutes, then strain if you wish. Let it cool, and drink up to 1 cup a day. The taste is quite bitter, but you can mask it with honey or an herbal beverage blend.

When using commercial preparations, follow the package directions.

To make a compress to treat pinkeye, soak a clean cloth in a barberry infusion.

Safety

In large doses, barberry may cause nausea, vomiting, convulsions, hazardous drops in blood pressure, and depression of heart rate and breathing. People with heart disease or chronic respiratory problems should stick to recommended dosage and take this herb only in consultation with their physicians.

Berberine may stimulate uterine contractions. Women who are pregnant, nursing, or trying to conceive should not use it.

If barberry causes diarrhea, dizziness, stomach upset or light-headedness, decrease dosage or stop using it. Tell your doctor if you experience any unpleasant effects or if your symptoms do not improve significantly after 2 weeks on this herb.

Do not give barberry to children under 2. In older children, adjust the recommended dose based on the child's weight. Give a 50-pound child one-third of the dose a 150-pound adult would take.

If you're over 65, start with a low dose, and increase only if necessary.

Inform health professionals of the herbs you use. Problematic herb-drug interactions are possible.

Barberry may cause allergic reactions or other unexpected side effects. If any develop, reduce your dose or stop taking it. For more on herb safety, see Chapter 2.

If symptoms get worse or persist longer than 2 weeks, consult a health professional promptly.

Gardening

Barberry is a perennial shrub that reaches 10 feet. It has smooth gray bark, long spines, and hanging clusters of bright yellow flowers that bloom in spring.

Barberry grows easily in the Northeast and Midwest. Plant seeds in the fall in fertile, moist, well-drained soil. Germination occurs the following spring. The shrub can also be propagated from cuttings.

Barberry prefers sun but tolerates shade. Prune in spring after the shrub flowers. Neglected shrubs become overgrown and unhealthy, but they can be rejuvenated by fertilizing and cutting back to within a foot of the ground in late winter. In areas with very cold winters, shelter the plant from the wind. Harvest the root bark in spring or fall, and dry it.

The herb's edible berries make tasty jams and jellies. The berry juice may be substituted for lemon juice.

BAYBERRY
All-American Fever Treatment

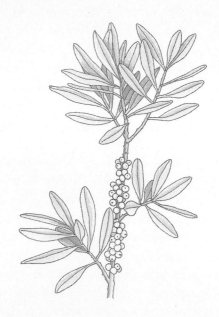

Family: Myricaceae; other members include myrtle

Genus and species: *Myrica* various species

Also known as: Wax myrtle, candleberry, and tallow shrub

Part used: Root bark

Before electric lights, bayberry was prized as the source of a fragrant candlewax that produced considerably less smoke than tallow. Today, bayberry candles are still with us, largely used around Christmas.

Healing History

Bayberry trees grow up and down the East coast. But its medicinal use was largely confined to the South, where the Choctaw boiled the leaves and drank the decoction to treat fever. An account from 1722 says white settlers adopted the plant and drank bayberry wax in hot water "as a certain cure for violent dysentery."

During the early 19th century, Samuel Thomson, an Indian-trained New England herbalist and creator of some of the first patent medicines, popularized bayberry, touted it as second only to red pepper for producing "heat" in the body. Thomson recommended bayberry for colds, flu, and other infectious diseases as well as for diarrhea and fever.

After the Civil War, the more scientific Eclectic physicians, forerunners of today's naturopaths, prescribed bayberry topically for bleeding gums and internally for diarrhea, dysentery, sore throat, scarlet fever, menstrual difficulties, and typhoid.

Since then, bayberry's popularity has waned, but some contemporary herbalists recommend it externally for varicose veins and internally for diarrhea, dysentery, colds, flu, bleeding gums, and sore throat. One modern herbal goes so far as to advocate treating uterine bleeding by packing the vagina with cotton soaked in bayberry tea. (Do not try this. Consult a physician promptly for unusual uterine bleeding.)

Therapeutic Uses

Two hundred years ago, bayberry was widely used medicinally. It's a shame that this native American herb has been largely forgotten, because science has shown that bayberry may have some real benefits in treating fever and diarrhea.

DIARRHEA. Bayberry root bark contains myricitrin, an antibiotic that fights a broad range of bacteria and protozoa. Myricitrin's antibiotic action supports bayberry's traditional use against diarrhea and dysentery. Bayberry also contains astringent tannins, which add to its value in treating diarrhea.

FEVER. Myricitrin also reduces fever, lending credence to bayberry's traditional use among the Choctaws.

Intriguing Possibilities

An Indian animal study suggests that bayberry may open the bronchi and help relieve asthma.

Myricitrin promotes the flow of bile, so bayberry may potentially help treat liver and gallbladder ailments.

Rx Recommendations

To prepare a decoction, boil 1 teaspoon of powdered root bark in 1 pint of water for 10 to 15 minutes, then strain if you wish. Add a bit of milk and drink up to 2 cups a day of the cooled beverage. You'll find the taste bitter and astringent.

A tincture might go down more easily. If you use a homemade tincture, take ½ teaspoon up to twice a day. When using commercial preparations, follow package directions.

Safety

Bayberry's high tannin content makes it iffy for anyone with a history of cancer. In various studies, tannins show both pro- and anticancer actions. Their cancer-promoting action has received more publicity, notably from a study published in the *Journal of the National Cancer Institute*, which showed that tannins produce malignant tumors in laboratory animals. But tannins have also been found to have an anticancer effect on some animal tumors.

Tannins' impact on human cancers remains unclear. Small quantities have never been implicated in human tumors, but Asians who drink large quantities of tea, which contains tannins, show unusually high rates of stomach cancer. The British also love tea, but their rates of stomach cancer remain low—probably because they add milk, which neutralizes tannins.

People with a history of cancer, particularly stomach or colon cancer, should avoid bayberry. Others should consume no more than the recommended amounts.

In large doses, bayberry root bark may cause stomach distress, nausea, and vomiting. People with chronic gastrointestinal conditions, such as colitis, should use it cautiously.

Bayberry changes the way the body uses sodium and potassium, so people who must watch their sodium/potassium balance—those with kidney disease, high blood pressure, or congestive heart failure—should consult their physicians before using it.

Pregnant and nursing women should not use bayberry.

Do not give bayberry to children under 2. In older children, adjust the recommended dose based on the child's weight. Give a 50-pound child one-third of the dose a 150-pound adult would take.

If you're over 65, start with a low dose, and increase only if necessary.

Inform health professionals of the herbs you use. Problematic herb-drug interactions are possible.

Bayberry may cause allergic reactions or other unexpected side effects. If any develop, reduce your dose or stop taking it. For more on herb safety, see Chapter 2.

If symptoms get worse or persist longer than 2 weeks, consult a health professional promptly.

Gardening

Bayberry is an evergreen tree native to the United States east of the Mississippi. Around the Great Lakes, mature plants rarely grow taller than 3 feet. But in the South it grows to 35 feet.

Bayberry has grayish bark, waxy branches, and dense, narrow, delicately toothed leaves dotted with resin glands that produce a fragrant aroma when crushed. Yellow flowers appear in spring and produce nutlike fruits thickly covered with the wax once so highly valued in candle making.

Bayberry grows from seeds planted in spring or early fall. It prefers peaty soil under full sun but tolerates poorer, sandy soil along streams and in swampy areas. Plants require little care other than pruning. Harvest the root bark after a few years.

BILBERRY

Sharpen Your Vision

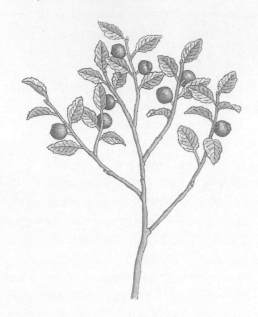

Family: Ericaceae; other members include azalea, blueberry, cranberry, and uva-ursi

Genus and species: *Vaccinium myrtillus*

Also known as: European blueberry, bogberry, and whortleberry

Parts used: Fruits

Bilberries are small and blue, hence the name European blueberry. The little blue fruits have been used in herbal medicine for centuries. But it wasn't until World War II that the herb's real value was discovered—not by scientists, but by aviators.

Healing History

No one knows when herbalists first recommended bilberries. The first written prescription dates from the 12th century, when abbess/herbalist/composer Hildegard of Bingen endorsed the berries for a variety of complaints, including respiratory problems.

Bilberries are astringent, meaning that they draw tissue together. Bilberry and other astringent herbs, such as tea, have been used for thousands of years to treat wounds, mouth sores, and diarrhea.

In Elizabethan England, a combination of bilberries and honey, called "rob," was a popular remedy for diarrhea. Later, bilberries became popular as jam. Over time, those who ate berries or jam reported clearer vision, and folk herbalists began touting bilberries for sharper vision. Herbalists also recommended them to treat diabetes.

During World War II, British fliers ate bilberry jam before nighttime bombing missions, swearing that the berries sharpened their vision. After the war, researchers began studying the herb and discovered that it does, indeed, improve night vision and help the eyes adjust to glare.

Therapeutic Uses

Bilberries owe their blue color to potent antioxidant pigments called anthocyanosides. Antioxidants help prevent and reverse the cell damage inflicted by highly reactive oxygen molecules called free radicals. Scientists now agree that the damage produced by free radicals (oxidative damage) is an underlying cause of heart disease, many cancers, and other degenerative illnesses.

GENERAL HEALTH. Antioxidants—including vitamins C and E, the mineral selenium, carotenoids (including beta-carotene), and anthocyanosides—are found in plant foods.

They help prevent and even reverse the cell damage at the root of heart disease, most cancers, and other illnesses. At the Jean Mayer USDA Human Nutrition Research Center on Aging at Tufts University, researchers analyzed the antioxidant content of dozens of common plant foods. Those richest in antioxidants turned out to be the dark-colored fruits and berries that contain generous amounts of anthocyanosides: blueberries, blackberries, raspberries, cherries, cranberries, red grapes, plums, raisins, and prunes.

The study ignored bilberries because they are uncommon in the United States, but they're about as rich in anthocyanosides as blueberries, which ranked near the top in terms of antioxidant content.

CATARACTS. Cataracts are a major cause of vision impairment and blindness among older adults. The condition results from oxidative damage to the normally clear lens of the eye, which leads to the development of cloudy spots that impair vision.

For reasons that remain unclear, the anthocyanosides in bilberry have unusually powerful effects on the eyes. In one Italian study, 50 people with early-stage cataracts were given bilberry extracts three times a day in combination with another antioxidant, vitamin E. The treatment stopped the progression of cataracts in 97 percent of study participants.

GLAUCOMA. Italian researchers gave bilberry (120 milligrams/day) to 20 adults with elevated intra-ocular fluid pressure (IOP), the main risk factor for glaucoma. Nineteen others remained untreated. Baseline IOP was comparable in both groups. After 6 months 1 of the 19 in the control group had significantly lower IOP. But in the bilberry group, 19 of 20.

MACULAR DEGENERATION. The nerve-rich retina in the back of the eye is essential to good vision. Macular degeneration involves deterioration of the macula, the central retina responsible for seeing what's directly in front of you.

European researchers gave bilberry extract to 31 people with various retinal problems. Those with macular degeneration experienced significant vision improvement.

For another study, a South Dakota researcher gave lists of antioxidant-rich fruits and vegetables to 10 adults, age 61 to 77, suffering macular degeneration and asked them to eat two daily servings of the fruits and three servings of the vegetables. He also instructed the participants to take supplements containing antioxidant vitamins and minerals plus extracts of bilberry and ginkgo (like bilberry, ginkgo is an antioxidant). One year later, all 10 people showed significant vision improvement.

DIABETIC RETINOPATHY. Diabetes damages the blood vessels, including the tiny capillaries in the eye that nourish the retina. When these capillaries develop diabetes-related damage, they leak blood into the eye, causing the blurred vision of diabetic retinopathy.

Bilberry's powerful antioxidants help strengthen retinal blood vessels, reducing blood leakage from the capillaries. In the European study mentioned above, bilberry significantly improved diabetic retinopathy.

VARICOSE VEINS. Varicose veins result from weakening of the biological "glue" that cements the veins' cell structure. Weakened veins stretch abnormally, allowing blood to pool. Varicose veins usually occur in the legs. When they affect the anal-rectal area, they're called hemorrhoids.

Bilberry strengthens the veins and helps treat varicosities. When Italian researchers gave bilberry extract to 47 people with this varicose veins, their symptoms improved significantly.

DIARRHEA AND MOUTH SORES. Commission E, the expert panel that evaluates herbal medicines for the German counterpart of the FDA, endorses bilberry as a treatment for diarrhea and mouth sores—the herb's primary traditional uses.

Intriguing Possibilities

A Japanese pilot study suggests that bilberry might counteract myopia.

Some studies suggest that bilberry lowers blood sugar levels in people with diabetes, a finding that supports another of the herb's traditional uses. In addition, animal studies suggest that it helps prevent and treat ulcers.

Rx Recommendations

European herbalists have bred a variety of bilberry that is processed into a standardized extract containing 25 percent anthocyanosides. Check the labels of commercial preparations. In most studies, participants took one or two 80- to 160-milligram capsules of standardized bilberry extract three times a day. Follow package directions.

Safety

Bilberry is a food. Pregnant and nursing women may use it in consultation with their health care providers.

Inform health professionals of the herbs you use. Problematic herb-drug interactions are possible.

Bilberry may cause allergic reactions or other unexpected side effects. If any develop, reduce your dose or stop taking it. For more on herb safety, see Chapter 2.

If symptoms get worse or persist longer than 2 weeks, consult a health professional promptly.

Gardening

Bilberry is a shrubby perennial that grows to about 18 inches in forested areas of Northern and Central Europe. The leaves are oval, bright green, and about an inch long. Red or pink bell-shaped flowers appear in spring, with blue-black or blue-purple berries forming in late summer and fall. Bilberry does not grow well in the United States and is rarely cultivated here.

BITTER MELON

Diabetes? Obesity? Try This Herb

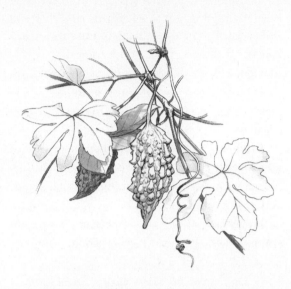

Family: Cucurbitaceae; other members include melons, gourds, cucumber, pumpkin, squash

Genus and species: *Momordica charantia*

Also known as: Bitter cucumber, bitter gourd, balsam pear

Parts used: Fruit, leaves, seed, and seed oil

Bitter melon is an annual vine that grows to 6 feet in Asia, Africa, South America, and the Southeastern United States. It produces an edible but bitter orange-yellow fruit shaped like a cucumber, gourd, or small melon—hence its common names.

Healing History

Bitter melon has a long folk medical history on several continents. Externally applied to the skin, it has been used to treat wounds and abscesses. Internally, traditional herbalists recommended it for asthma, constipation, diabetes, intestinal parasites, kidney stones, psoriasis, stomach upset, and some tumors.

Therapeutic Uses

DIABETES. All parts of bitter melon, but especially the fruit, contain compounds chemically similar to the hormone insulin. Several animal studies show that these compounds reduce blood sugar and help manage diabetes. Researchers at India's University of Mumbai (Bombay) gave an extract of bitter melon fruit to diabetic rats. It reduced their blood sugar by 48 percent, an effect comparable to that of the widely prescribed diabetes drug, glibenclamide (Glyburide, Micronase).

Several clinical trials have shown that bitter melon reduces blood sugar levels in Type 2 diabetics. If you have diabetes, talk to your doctor about supplementing your diet and medication regimen with this herb.

OBESITY. Being overweight raises risk for diabetes. Several animal studies show that animal diets supplemented with bitter melon reduce weight gain and fat accumulation. University of Hong Kong researchers placed rats on a high-fat diet with or without supplemental bitter melon extract. The animals in the herb group gained less weight and accumulated less body fat. The researchers concluded that the herb "strongly counteracts the [harmful] effects of a high-fat diet."

IMMUNE STIMULATION. Bitter melon boosts production of interferon, a component of the immune system that prevents infection.

Intriguing Possibilities

One protein in bitter melon fruit and seed inhibits the replication of several viruses: polio, herpes, and HIV, the virus that causes AIDS.

Animal studies suggest that bitter melon reduces cholesterol. Japanese researchers fed rats an extract and documented a "marked reduction in cholesterol."

Bitter melon also increases blood levels of key antioxidants, notably glutathione and superoxide dismutase. Antioxidants help prevent cancer. Japanese researchers added bitter melon extract to rats' drinking water. A known percentage of rats spontaneously develop breast cancer. But among those ingesting the herb, the rate of breast cancer was significantly less than expected. Indian researchers have found that bitter melon also reduces risk of animal stomach cancer.

It's still too early to call the herb a treatment for herpes, HIV, high cholesterol, and cancer, but in the future, that's a possibility.

Rx Recommendations

Some herbalists recommend bitter melon juice for diabetes—$\frac{1}{2}$ to 1 cup a day. When using the fruit, the typical dose is 900 milligrams three times a day (2,700 milligrams total) with meals.

Several supplements are available. Most are capsules containing 250 to 500 milligrams of fruit extract. Follow package directions.

Safety

No published reports document serious side effects in adults taking recommended doses of bitter melon.

However, large amounts of juice have sickened children, causing vomiting. In some animal studies, bitter melon has suppressed fertility and raised liver enzyme levels, an indication of liver damage. Couples trying to conceive and people with liver disease should not use bitter melon.

Diabetics who try bitter melon should inform their physicians, monitor their blood sugar closely, and be prepared to reduce their dose of insulin and other medications.

Pregnant and nursing women should not use bitter melon.

Do not give this herb to children under 2. In older children, adjust the recommended dose based on the child's weight. Give a 50-pound child one-third of the dose a 150-pound adult would take.

If you're over 65, start with a low dose, and increase only if necessary.

Inform health professionals of the herbs you use. Problematic herb-drug interactions are possible.

Bitter melon may cause allergic reactions or other unexpected side effects. If any develop, reduce your dose or stop taking it. For more on herb safety, see Chapter 2.

If symptoms get worse or persist longer than 2 weeks, consult a health professional promptly.

Gardening

Bitter melon can be cultivated along the Gulf Coast, particularly in Florida. It's a climbing annual vine with long-stalked leaves and yellow flowers. The fruits look like small warty cucumbers.

BLACKBERRY

Beyond Jam, Jelly, and Pie

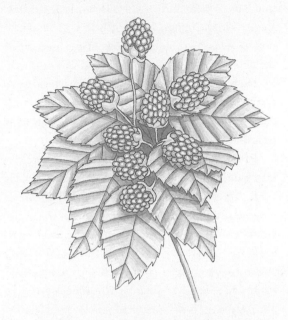

Family: Rosaceae; other members include rose, peach, almond, apple, and strawberry

Genus and species: *Rubus fruticosus* (European), *R. villosus* (American), and other species

Also known as: Bramble, dewberry, goutberry

Parts used: Leaves, bark, roots, and fruits

Yes, of course, blackberry jams, jellies, and pies are delicious. But the blackberry bush was once as highly prized for its medicinal leaves, bark, and roots as for its sweet, juicy fruit.

Blackberry spent most of the 20th century as a minor medicinal herb. Today that's changed based on research showing that the pigment that gives blackberries their color is a potent antioxidant with remarkable healing benefits.

Healing History

The ancient Greeks used blackberry to treat gout. Greek medicine was so influential in Europe that well into the 18th century, the herb was called goutberry.

The Romans chewed the leaves and bark for bleeding gums and drank a decoction for diarrhea.

The ancient Chinese used the unripe berries to treat kidney problems, urinary incontinence, and impotence.

Arab physicians in the 10th century considered the fruit an aphrodisiac. (It isn't).

During the Middle Ages, blackberry leaves were applied to the skin to soothe burns and scalds.

In his influential *Herbal*, 17th-century English herbalist Nicholas Culpeper described blackberry as "very binding" and good for "fevers, ulcers, putrid sores of the mouth and secret parts [genitals], spitting blood [tuberculosis], piles [hemorrhoids], stones of the kidney, too much flowing of women's courses [menstruation], and hot distempers of the head, eyes, and body."

Nineteenth-century American Eclectic physicians, forerunners of today's naturopaths, recommended a preparation made from blackberry fruit as "an excellent syrup which is of much service in dysentery, being pleasant to the taste, mitigating the sufferings of the patient, and ultimately effecting a cure." They also recommended blackberry leaves for gonorrhea, vaginal discharges, recovery from childbirth, and "cholera infantum," an archaic term for infectious diarrhea, which, in the days before antibiotics, was often fatal (and in many parts of the world still is).

Few contemporary herbalists recommended blackberry for anything beyond treating diarrhea until the mid-1990s, when scientists discovered the value of the pigment that gives the berries their dark color.

Therapeutic Uses

Contrary to Culpeper's claims, blackberry doesn't do much for the genitals. But the fruit and leaves of this herb help prevent and treat quite a few common ills.

Blackberries owe their healing power to high levels of anthocyanosides, compounds in the fruit's dark pigment. Anthocyanosides are potent antioxidants that help prevent and reverse the cell damage produced by highly reactive oxygen molecules called free radicals (oxidative damage). Scientists now agree that oxidative damage is the underlying cause of heart disease, many cancers, and other degenerative illnesses.

GENERAL WELLNESS. Antioxidants including vitamins C and E, the mineral selenium, carotenoids (including beta-carotene), and anthocyanosides are found only in plant foods. In a study conducted at the Jean Mayer USDA Human Nutrition Research Center on Aging at Tufts University, researchers assessed the antioxidant content of dozens of common plant foods. The scientists determined that the most concentrated sources of antioxidants are the dark-colored fruits that contain generous amounts of anthocyanosides: blackberries, blueberries, cherries, red grapes, plums, raisins, and prunes.

CATARACTS. Cataracts are a major cause of older adult vision impairment and blindness. The condition occurs when oxidative damage to the normally clear lens of the eye develops cloudy spots.

For reasons that remain unclear, anthocyanosides have unusually powerful effects on the eyes. Most of the research demonstrating this has been conducted in Europe using a similar, distinctly European fruit, bilberry, that's similar to American blueberries. But medicinal herb experts, including James A. Duke, Ph.D., formerly the U.S. Department of Agriculture's top herbal medicine authority, agree that all fruits rich in anthocyanosides produce similar benefits.

In one Italian study, 50 people with early-stage cataracts were given bilberry extracts three times a day, along with vitamin E, which is also an antioxidant. In 97 percent of the study participants, cataract progression stopped.

MACULAR DEGENERATION. The back of the eye contains a nerve-rich area, the retina, which is crucial to vision. The most sensitive part of the retina, the macula, is responsible for discerning what's directly in front of you (central vision) as well as fine detail. Macular degeneration involves deterioration of the macula, which can lead to the loss of central vision.

In a European study, 31 people with macular degeneration and various other types of retinal problems were treated with anthocyanosides in the form of bilberry extract. Those with macular degeneration showed significant vision improvement.

On this side of the Atlantic, a South Dakota researcher conducted a study involving 10 men and women, age 61 to 77, who all had macular degeneration. The researcher instructed his volunteers to eat five daily servings of high-anthocyanoside plant foods—two servings of fruit and three servings of vegetables. He also asked each person to take supplements containing antioxidant vitamins and minerals, plus bilberry (with its antioxidant anthocyanosides) and ginkgo (also an antioxidant). One year later, all 10 people showed significant vision improvement in at least one eye.

DIABETIC RETINOPATHY. Diabetes damages blood vessels throughout the body, including the tiny capillaries that nourish the retina. When injured, these capillaries leak blood into the eye, causing the blurred vision of diabetic retinopathy.

With their powerful antioxidant action, anthocyanosides help strengthen retinal blood vessels, thus reducing blood leakage into the eye. In the European study mentioned above, diabetics treated with bilberry anthocyanosides showed significantly improved vision.

VARICOSE VEINS. Varicose veins occur when the biological "glue" that cements the veins' cell structure weakens. This weakening stretches the veins abnormally, causing blood to pool. The condition can affect veins in the legs or anal area (hemorrhoids).

Anthocyanosides help treat varicose veins by strengthening their structure. In an Italian study, when 47 people received anthocyanosides (as bilberry extract) for their varicose veins, they experienced significant improvement in their symptoms.

HEMORRHOIDS. The herb's astringent nature explains its traditional use as a hemorrhoid remedy.

DIARRHEA. Blackberry leaves contain large amounts of astringent tannins. In the digestive tract, tannins helps control diarrhea and dysentery, confirming a traditional use for the herb. Commission E, the expert panel that evaluates herbal medicines for the German counterpart of the FDA, endorses blackberry leaf as a treatment for diarrhea.

WOUNDS. Tannins' astringent action also constricts blood vessels and minimizes minor bleeding, explaining blackberry's traditional use as a topical wound treatment. Blackberry thorns often cause minor cuts, so it's nice to know that first-aid is close at hand.

MOUTH SORES AND SORE THROAT. Tasty, astringent blackberry leaf tea may help soothe mouth sores and sore throat.

Intriguing Possibilities

One study showed that a strong infusion of blackberry leaves reduces blood sugar levels in rabbits with diabetes, hinting at possible value in diabetes management.

Research has shown that blackberry's close relative, raspberry, relaxes the uterus. Women might try blackberry leaf tea for painful menstrual cramps.

Rx Recommendations

To reduce risk of heart disease, cancer, cataracts, and macular degeneration, eat lots of blackberries. It doesn't matter how you eat them—fresh, frozen, canned, or in preserves, jams, jellies, or pies. In any form, blackberries contain generous amounts of healing anthocyanosides.

To treat diarrhea or soothe a sore throat, try an infusion, decoction, or tincture. To prepare an infusion, use 2 to 3 teaspoons of dried leaves per cup of boiling water. Or instead of dried leaves, use a handful of dried or crushed berries or 1 to 2 teaspoons of dried powdered bark. Steep for 10 to 20 minutes, strain, and add a bit of milk. Drink up to 3 cups a day.

For a decoction, use 1 teaspoon of powdered root per cup of water. Boil for 30 minutes and strain if you wish. Drink up to 1 cup a day with a bit of milk.

When using homemade tinctures, take up to 1 teaspoon up to twice a day.

To treat wounds or hemorrhoids, soak a clean cloth in a tincture or strong infusion and apply.

When using commercial preparations, follow the package directions.

Safety

Blackberries are considered safe for anyone who is not allergic, but questions have been raised about the tannins in medicinal preparations of blackberry leaf. In various studies, tannins show both pro- and anticancer action. Their cancer-promoting action has attracted a lot more attention, primarily because of a study published in the *Journal of the National Cancer Institute*, which showed that tannins produce malignant tumors in laboratory animals. But in some animal trials, tannins also appear to have antitumor effects.

The relationship between tannins and human cancers remains unclear. In small quantities—the amount found in blackberry fruits—the compounds have never been shown to cause human tumors. Asians who drink large quantities of high-tannin tea show unusually high rates of stomach cancer. The British also love tea, but their rates of stomach cancer remain low. One reason may be that they add milk, which neutralizes tannins.

People with a history of cancer, particularly stomach or colon cancer, should avoid blackberry leaf tea. Others should take no more than the recommended amount of infusion or decoction and, for extra safety, add a bit of milk.

In large amounts, tannins may cause stomach distress, nausea, and vomiting. Blackberry root bark contains the most tannins, followed by the leaves and, in distant third, the fruits. People with chronic gastrointestinal conditions, such as colitis, probably should not use the roots.

Pregnant and nursing women should not use blackberry leaf tea. However, anyone may eat sweet, juicy blackberries.

Do not give blackberry leaf tea to children under 2. In older children, adjust the recommended dose based on the child's weight. Give a 50-pound child one-third of the dose a 150-pound adult would take.

If you're over 65, start with a low dose, and increase only if necessary.

Inform health professionals of the herbs you use. Problematic herb-drug interactions are possible.

Blackberry leaf may cause allergic reactions or other unexpected side effects. If any develop, reduce your dose or stop taking it. For more on herb safety, see Chapter 2.

If symptoms get worse or persist longer than 2 weeks, consult a health professional promptly.

Gardening

Blackberry bushes grow wild throughout most of North America. They have long, tangled, thorny stems; lush foliage; and a profusion of berries that turn red as they ripen and become a juicy, purplish blue-black by midsummer.

Blackberry bushes can become thick, thorny, and impenetrable. Rooting them out is almost impossible—just ask any gardener who has tried. Even after bushes have been removed, root fragments often continue to send up new shoots. To minimize problems, plant this shrub in containers or surround its roots with sheet metal.

Blackberries grow easily from ½-inch root cuttings taken in autumn and stored through the winter in cool sand (around 50°F). Plant cuttings vertically 1 to 3 feet apart in 3 to 4 inches of soil.

Blackberries adapt to many conditions but grow best in loose, moist, rich soil amended with manure or finished compost. The plants flower in spring and bear fruit throughout the summer.

Harvest leaves and roots anytime. For ease of harvesting berries, train the branches along supports and prune them mercilessly.

BLACK COHOSH
The Women's Herb

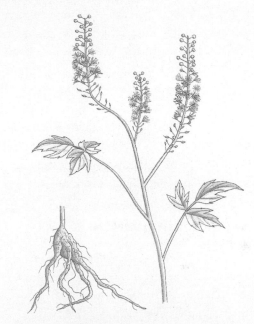

Family: Ranunculaceae; other members include buttercup, larkspur, and peony

Genus and species: *Actea racemosa* (formerly *Cimicifuga racemosa*) or *Macrotys actaeoides*

Also known as: Squawroot, snakeroot, cimicifuga

Parts used: Rhizomes and roots

Among the 19th century's most popular patent medicines was Lydia E. Pinkham's Vegetable Compound, introduced in 1876 to treat "female weakness," that is, premenstrual syndrome, menstrual cramps, and menopausal complaints. Pinkham's compound—developed by its namesake, a Lynn, Massachusetts, homemaker and herbalist—contained several medicinal herbs, chief among them, black cohosh, an age-old Algonquin treatment for gynecological complaints.

Pinkham's Compound also contained an enormous amount of alcohol. During the 19th century, respectable ladies did not drink liquor, but often satisfied a thirst for alcohol with the Vegetable Compound. However, its black cohosh helped treat menstrual and menopausal symptoms.

After World War II, Pinkham's Vegetable Compound was reformulated to contain very little alcohol. Ironically, the revamped recipe also omitted the active ingredient, black cohosh.

Healing History

The "black" in black cohosh refers to the plant's dark medicinal root. "Cohosh" is Algonquin for "rough," another reference to the roots.

Native Americans boiled black cohosh's gnarled roots in water and drank the decoction for fatigue, sore throat, arthritis, and rattlesnake bite—hence another of the plant's popular names, snakeroot. But it was most popular among Native American women who used it for gynecological problems and recovery after childbirth.

Wild black cohosh grew most profusely in the Ohio River valley, which seems fitting. After all, the herb was championed by 19th-century American Eclectic physicians, forerunners of today's naturopaths, whose medical school was located on the banks of the Ohio in Cincinnati. The Eclectics called the herb by a different name, macrotys, and recommended it for fever, rashes, insomnia, malaria, yellow fever, and all "hysterical" (gynecological) ailments. The Eclectic medical text *King's American Dispensatory* (1898) stated, "In dysmenorrhea [menstrual cramps], it is of greatest utility, being surpassed by no other drug."

Non-Eclectic ("regular") physicians remained unimpressed by black cohosh. But Lydia Pinkham sided with the Eclectics and included the herb in her compound.

Black cohosh does not grow in China, but Chinese physicians use several related plants to treat headache, measles, diarrhea, bleeding gums, and some gynecological problems. Homeopaths recommend microdoses of black cohosh for menstrual problems and childbirth recovery.

Contemporary herbalists recommend the herb primarily for premenstrual syndrome (PMS), menstrual cramps, and menopausal symptoms. Since the 1990s, many herb companies have marketed black cohosh for women's reproductive health concerns.

Therapeutic Uses

Black cohosh root contains several medicinal compounds: acetein, formononetin, and triterpenes. In the 1940s, German scientists discovered that these compounds are "estrogenic," meaning that they mimic the effects of the female sex hormone estrogen. Herbal medicine is much more mainstream in Germany than in the United States, and by the 1950s, German women were using a commercial standardized extract, Remifemin, to treat PMS, menstrual cramps, and menopausal hot flashes. Remifemin is now widely available in the United States.

Most contemporary herbalists consider black cohosh estrogenic. It is, but indirectly. The herb suppresses secretion of luteinizing hormone (LH), which in turn leads to estrogenic action.

MENOPAUSAL COMPLAINTS. Most black cohosh studies have focused on its alleviation of hot flashes and other menopausal discomforts. Occasionally a study shows no benefit. But the great weight of the evidence supports the herb as a treatment for hot flashes.

From 1982 through 1991, German researchers conducted eight clinical trials involving a total of 1,170 women. The studies differed in design, but all tested the black cohosh extract, Remifemin (40 drops twice a day or two 40-milligram tablets daily for 6 to 12 weeks). All of these trials produced the same results: fewer, briefer hot flashes, improved mood, relief from fatigue, and less vaginal dryness. In the largest of these reports, involving 629 women, within a month, 80 percent reported significant improvement of menopausal discomforts. Many experienced complete relief within 6 to 8 weeks. The herb caused no significant side effects. Commission E endorses black cohosh as a treatment for menopausal discomforts.

Since this report, various studies have supported or rejected black cohosh for hot flashes, but the weight of the evidence tilts toward its effectiveness in relieving menopausal complaints.

- German researchers asked 6,141 women to rate their menopausal symptoms using a standard scale and then gave them black cohosh (Remifemin, label dosage). A year later, their menopausal discomforts had diminished significantly. (For emotional upsets, a combination of Remifemin and St. John's wort was effective.)

- Canadian scientists analyzed nine rigorous trials. Two showed no benefit, but seven showed significant relief of hot flashes.

- Spanish researchers surveyed 122 menopausal women and then instructed them to take Remifemin (label dose). Three months later, the women reported fewer menopausal complaints and better mental health.

PREMENSTRUAL SYNDROME. Germany's Commission E, the expert panel that evaluates herbal medicines for the German counterpart of the FDA, endorses black cohosh as a treatment for PMS. The panel's position is based on more than 50 years of German clinical experience with Remifemin.

MENSTRUAL CRAMPS. Commission E also endorses black cohosh as a treatment for menstrual cramps.

HORMONE REPLACEMENT ALTERNATIVE. The ovaries synthesize most of women's estrogen. During menopause, production of the hormone slowly declines. Among women of any age who have their ovaries removed, estrogen production suddenly plummets.

To make up for lost estrogen, mainstream physicians may recommend hormone replacement therapy. German researchers compared pharmaceutical hormone replacement with black cohosh (two Remifemin tablets twice a day) in 60 women who had their ovaries removed before age 40. After 6 months, both groups reported similar satisfaction with their treatment, but the black cohosh group experienced fewer significant side effects—none.

STRESS AND ANXIETY. Black cohosh is not on the list of stress-relieving herbs but Japanese researchers surveyed the stress loads of 36 mentally healthy women and then gave them either a placebo or black cohosh (200 milligrams/day). After a week, the groups switched treatments (a cross-over trial). While taking the herb, participants showed significantly lower blood levels of stress hormones.

Stress reduction may explain black cohosh's mechanism of action for menopausal complaints. As mentioned, the herb is not directly estrogenic, so how could it relieve hot flashes?

Possibly because of its antianxiety effect.

BREAST CANCER PREVENTION. Estrogen spurs the growth of breast tumors, and anything with estrogenic effects can be presumed to do the same. For a while, scientists warned breast cancer survivors and women at high risk for the disease not to use black cohosh because of its estrogenic effect. However, as mentioned, the herb is only indirectly estrogenic. University of Missouri researchers gave it to menopausal women and measured both its effect on hot flashes and biomarkers for estrogenic effects. After 12 weeks, the women reported significant relief from hot flashes—but showed no increase in estrogenic markers. In other words, black cohosh does not have typical estrogenic action and should not stimulate the growth of breast tumors.

In fact, black cohosh may *reduce* risk of breast cancer. In laboratory studies, German scientists have shown that it inhibits the growth of breast cancer cells. University of Pennsylvania researchers surveyed 2,473 older women about their use of black cohosh. Some were breast cancer survivors. Others had never had the disease. "Use of black cohosh had a significant breast-cancer–protective effect."

UTERINE FIBROIDS. Fibroids are noncancerous growths that many women develop during the decade or so before menopause. Large ones can cause unusually heavy menstrual flow and other symptoms. Fibroids are a frequent reason for hysterectomy. But surgery is controversial because fibroids typically disappear on their own as women become menopausal. So women with large fibroids face an uncomfortable choice—endure them until menopause or cut them out. Now there's a third option: Remifemin.

Chinese researchers gave 62 women with fibroids either tibolone, a drug sometimes used to treat them, or Remifemin (40 milligrams/day). After 3 months, the tribolone group's fibroids increased in volume by 5 percent, but among those who used Remifemin, volume decreased up to 30 percent.

HIGH BLOOD PRESSURE. A study in *Nature* revealed that black cohosh reduces blood pressure by opening blood vessels in the limbs (peripheral vasodilation). Consult your physician before using it for this purpose.

Intriguing Possibilities

Pilot studies suggest that black cohosh may relieve pain and inflammation, possibly explaining its traditional use for arthritis. Another report hints that it helps preserve bone, promoting its potential use in osteoporosis prevention. Other research involving the herb showed cholesterol and blood pressure reduction, antiulcer effects, and blood sugar regulation, pointing toward possible value in controlling diabetes. Black cohosh also appears to inhibit the growth of prostate cancer cells. Finally, animal studies hint that the herb may have antibiotic, sedative, and stomach-soothing properties.

Rx Recommendations

For a decoction, use ½ teaspoon of powdered root per cup of water and boil for 30 minutes, then strain if you wish. Let cool before drinking. Black cohosh has an unpleasant aroma and a sharp, bitter taste. Add lemon and honey and/or mix the herb with a beverage herb. Take 2 tablespoons every few hours, up to 1 cup a day.

With a homemade tincture, take 2 to 4 teaspoons twice a day.

When using commercial preparations, follow the package directions.

Safety

First, double-check the label to be sure that you have black cohosh, not *blue* cohosh. The latter should not be used by most women. Or simply buy Remifemin, which is black cohosh.

Nineteenth-century researchers gave laboratory animals doses of black cohosh 90 times the recommended human equivalent. It caused dizziness, diarrhea, vomiting, tremors, depressed heart rate, miscarriage, and other side effects. These studies continue to be cited today. On the other hand, in the eight studies that examined black cohosh as a treatment for menopausal discomforts, no significant side effects turned up. In fact, the only side effect was stomach upset in 7 percent of participants. The consensus of the modern scientific research is that black cohosh is safe when used as recommended.

Since 2000, a few case reports have documented liver damage in women taking black cohosh, raising the possibility that the herb might be liver-toxic. On closer examination, all these women were taking drugs known to increase risk of liver damage.

In 2007, the European Medicines Agency investigated 42 case reports of liver damage in women taking black cohosh, typically Remifemin. No cases were conclusively linked to the herb. Black cohosh "probably" caused two cases, and "possibly" contributed to two more. But even if all four cases of liver damage caused by the herb, black cohosh was unrelated to 90 percent of liver toxicity cases.

Italian researchers analyzed 16 clinical trials involving several thousand participants. They found no evidence of liver damage.

There is currently no compelling evidence that recommended doses of black cohosh harm the liver. But women with liver disease should discuss use of this herb with their doctors and probably avoid it.

Women who are pregnant or nursing or whose physicians have advised them not to take birth control pills should not use black cohosh.

There is no reason to give black cohosh to children.

If you're over 65, start with a low dose, and increase only if necessary.

Inform health professionals of the herbs you use. Problematic herb-drug interactions are possible.

Black cohosh may cause allergic reactions or other unexpected side effects. If any develop, reduce your dose or stop taking it. For more on herb safety, see Chapter 2.

If symptoms get worse or persist longer than 2 weeks, consult a health professional promptly.

If you are taking postmenopausal hormone replacement therapy, consult your physician before taking black cohosh.

Let your doctor know if you experience any unpleasant effects or if the symptoms for which you are using the herb do not improve significantly within 4 weeks.

Gardening

Black cohosh is native to the area from Ontario south to Tennessee and west to Missouri. It's a leafy perennial that reaches 9 feet. Its white flowers bloom throughout summer. Black cohosh has knotty black roots and a smooth stem with large, toothed, compound leaves and small, multiple white flowers that develop on long projections (racemes).

Black cohosh grows from seeds sown in spring or root divisions taken in spring or fall. Harvest the roots in fall after the fruits have ripened and cut them lengthwise to dry.

BLACK HAW

An Herb with Southern Roots

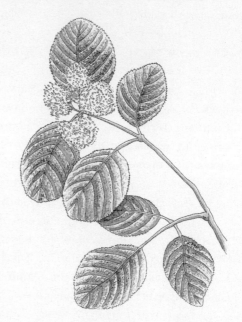

Family: Caprifoliaceae; other members include honeysuckle and elder

Genus and species: *Viburnum prunifolium*

Also known as: Viburnum

Part used: Bark

Indiana poet James Whitcomb Riley wrote, "What is sweeter, after all / Than black haws in early fall?" He was referring to the shrub's olive-sized blue-black fruits.

But it's the reddish brown bark of this native American shrub that boasts centuries of folk use as a remedy for gynecological complaints—a history confirmed by modern science. Native American women drank a decoction of black haw bark for menstrual cramps, childbirth recovery, and menopausal discomforts, but especially to prevent miscarriage.

Healing History

Before the Civil War, black haw's miscarriage-preventing action played a small but uncompromising role in relations between slave women and their owners. Slaveholders wanted the women to bear as many children as possible and often "bred" them by rape. Many slaves quietly protested this abuse by taking abortifacient herbs to terminate resulting pregnancies. In reaction, many slave owners forced slave women to ingest black haw to prevent abortion.

A popular abortion-inducing herb was cotton root, readily available on most plantations. As explained in *King's American Dispensatory* (1898), the textbook of the 19th-century American Eclectic physicians, forerunners of today's naturopaths, "It was customary for planters to compel female slaves to drink an infusion of black haw daily whilst pregnant to prevent abortion from taking cotton root."

An Eclectic physician from Mississippi introduced black haw to the North, where it quickly became an herbal mainstay for gynecological complaints. The Eclectics valued it highly: "As a uterine tonic, it is unquestionably of great utility . . . for menstrual pains . . . and a good remedy for menopause. . . . But the condition for which black haw is most valued is threatened abortion. By its quieting effect upon the irritable womb, women who have been previously unable to go to term have been aided to pass through pregnancy without mishaps."

Today, black haw is a minor medicinal herb. But it's still recommended for menstrual cramps and threatened abortion. Some herbals encourage women to drink black haw tea throughout pregnancy, but this turns out to be a bad idea.

Therapeutic Uses

Scientists have confirmed that black haw may be a good treatment for gynecological complaints.

MENSTRUAL CRAMPS. A study published in *Nature* showed that black haw contains a uterine relaxant called scopoletin, thus supporting the herb's value in treating menstrual cramps. In Germany, where herbal medicine is more mainstream than in the United States, black haw preparations are widely recommended for cramps. These products are not available in the United States, but the herb itself is fairly easy to obtain.

THREATENED MISCARRIAGE. Black haw has been used for centuries to prevent miscarriage. As a uterine relaxant, it may indeed do the job. Unfortunately, it also contains salicin, a close chemical relative of aspirin. Because aspirin has been linked to birth defects, pregnant women should not take black haw, except possibly under a physician's supervision to prevent premature delivery.

FEVER AND PAIN (INCLUDING HEADACHE AND ARTHRITIS). The aspirin-like compound in black haw may reduce fever and relieve pain.

Rx Recommendations

For relief of menstrual cramps, fever, headache, and general aches and pains, prepare a decoction using 2 teaspoons of dried black haw bark per cup of water. Boil for 10 minutes, then strain and cool. Drink up to 3 cups a day. The herb has an extremely bitter taste. Add lemon and honey or sugar, or mix with a beverage tea.

As a homemade tincture, take up to 2 teaspoons three times a day.

When using commercial preparations, follow package directions.

The plant's aspirin-like action may cause a rare but potentially fatal condition, Reye syndrome.

Safety

Like aspirin, the salicin in black haw is a pain reliever (analgesic), which may contribute to the herb's ability to relieve menstrual cramping. But aspirin has been implicated as a cause of birth defects in the children of women who take it while pregnant. Aspirin is most hazardous to the unborn early in pregnancy. Recognizing this, the classic British herbal, *Potter's New Cyclopaedia of Botanical Drugs and Preparations,* advises black haw use only during the final 5 weeks of pregnancy to prevent premature delivery.

Any woman facing a possible premature birth should discuss her situation with her obstetrician. Drugs (including herbs) are a last resort and should be used only with the consent of a doctor.

Do not give black haw to children under age 2 or to children under age 16 who have colds, flu, or chickenpox. There is no reason for postmenopausal women to use it.

For adults over age 65, start with low-strength preparations and increase the strength if necessary.

Inform health professionals of the herbs you use. Problematic herb-drug interactions are possible.

Black haw may cause allergic reactions or other unexpected side effects. If any develop, reduce your dose or stop taking it. For more on herb safety, see Chapter 2.

If symptoms get worse or persist longer than 2 weeks, consult a health professional promptly.

Gardening

In the North, black haw is a deciduous spreading shrub with reddish brown bark. In the South, it becomes a small tree. The leaves are pointed, serrated ovals resembling plum leaves. They turn red in the fall.

Depending on location, black haw blooms from early spring to summer. The flowers are large, clustered, white, and showy.

Black haw grows best in rich, moist, well-drained soil under full sun. It tolerates poorer soil and partial shade as long as it gets adequate water.

The branch bark may be collected in summer; the trunk bark should be collected in fall. Dry it in the shade.

BONESET

A Traditional Remedy for Colds and Flu

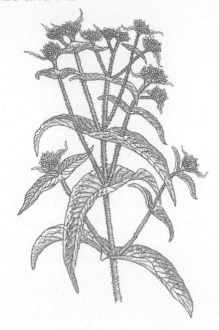

Family: Compositae; other members include daisy, dandelion, and marigold

Genus and species: *Eupatorium perfoliaturn*

Also known as: Feverwort, agueweed, and sweat plant

Parts used: Leaves and flowers

Boneset has nothing to do with mending broken bones. The name comes from its traditional use as a treatment for breakbone fever, a 19th-century term for dengue fever (pronounced DENG-ee). Dengue is a mosquito-borne viral infection that causes muscle pain so intense that people fear their bones are breaking, hence the condition's traditional name. Today, dengue is rare in the United States, except near the Gulf Coast from Florida to Texas, and among overseas travelers, who sometimes return from the tropics with it.

Ironically, boneset has never been shown to provide significant relief from dengue fever. But it may help treat minor viral and bacterial illnesses by revving up the immune system's response to infection.

Healing History

Native Americans introduced boneset to early colonists as a sweat inducer, an old treatment for fever. They used it for all fever-producing illnesses, including influenza, cholera, dengue, malaria, and typhoid, hence the herb's popular names: feverwort, sweat plant, and agueweed ("ague" is an archaic term for fever).

Native Americans also used boneset to relieve arthritis and to treat colds, indigestion, constipation, and loss of appetite.

Colonists adopted boneset so enthusiastically that it became one of early America's most popular healing herbs. During the Civil War, soldiers used it not only to treat fever but also as a tonic to keep them healthy. (This is a bad idea—see "Safety" page 106.)

In his classic 19th-century text, *American Medicinal Plants*, Dr. C. F. Millspaugh had this to say about boneset: "There is probably no plant more extensively or frequently used than this. The attic or woodshed of almost every farm house has bunches hanging from the rafters, ready for immediate use should some family member or neighbor be taken with a cold."

Dr. Millspaugh also considered boneset excellent against malaria, a major health problem during his day. He wrote that he'd seen the herb cure cases of malaria that didn't respond to Peruvian cinchona bark, source of the antimalarial drug, quinine.

Boneset was listed as a treatment for fever in the *U.S. Pharmacopoeia*, a standard drug reference, from 1820 through 1916 and in the *National Formulary*, the pharmacists' reference, from 1926 through 1950. But during the 20th century, it fell from favor, replaced by another fever fighter, aspirin, introduced by Bayer in 1899.

Some contemporary herbalists continue to recommend boneset for fever.

Therapeutic Uses

Contemporary herb critics ridicule boneset as passionately as physicians a century ago praised it. One claims, "It simply doesn't work." Another sniffs, "Boneset lacks therapeutic merit." A third writes, "In view of [boneset's] singular lack of effectiveness, it seems incredible that the plant held official status from 1820 to 1950."

The critics have a point: Boneset has never been shown to suppress fever as well as aspirin. But several studies suggest that it has some therapeutic value after all.

COLDS AND FLU. European studies show that boneset helps treat minor viral and bacterial infections thanks to immune-stimulating compounds that spur white blood cells to devour more germs. In Germany, where herbal medicine is more mainstream than in the United States, physicians use boneset to treat colds and flu.

ARTHRITIS. One study suggests that boneset is anti-inflammatory, lending some support to its traditional use in treating arthritis.

Intriguing Possibility

Some studies suggest that the herb's immune-stimulating compounds may have anticancer action.

Medicinal Myth

Despite its traditional use, boneset has never been shown to be effective against dengue fever or malaria.

Rx Recommendations

To prepare an infusion, use 1 to 2 teaspoons of dried leaves per cup of boiling water and steep for 10 to 20 minutes. Drink up to 3 cups a day. This herb tastes very bitter and astringent. Add sugar or honey or lemon or mix with an herbal beverage tea.

As a homemade tincture, take $\frac{1}{2}$ to 1 teaspoon up to three times a day.

When using commercial preparations, follow the package directions.

Safety

In large amounts, boneset may cause nausea, vomiting, and diarrhea. In addition, the herb contains pyrrolizidine alkaloids (PAs), chemicals that, in large amounts, cause liver damage. Boneset's effect on human cancer, if any, is unclear, because the plant also contains anticancer compounds.

The PAs in some healing herbs, notably comfrey (see page 174), have caused liver damage when people have taken more than the recommended dose for long periods. If you use boneset, use it sparingly.

Do not eat fresh boneset. It contains tremerol, a toxic chemical that causes nausea, vomiting, weakness, muscle tremors, and at high doses, possibly coma and death. Drying the herb eliminates the tremerol and the possibility of poisoning.

Pregnant and nursing women should not use boneset.

Do not give boneset to children under 2. In older children, adjust the recommended dose based on the child's weight. Give a 50-pound child one-third of the dose a 150-pound adult would take.

If you're over 65, start with a low dose, and increase only if necessary.

Inform health professionals of the herbs you use. Problematic herb-drug interactions are possible.

Boneset may cause allergic reactions or other unexpected side effects. If any develop, reduce your dose or stop taking it. For more on herb safety, see Chapter 2.

If symptoms get worse or persist longer than 2 weeks, consult a health professional promptly.

Gardening

Boneset is easy to identify because its long, narrow, pointed leaf pairs are indistinct—connected and pierced by the stem. The herb has round, erect, hairy, hollow stems that grow to 5 feet, then split into three branches, each of which produces tiny, densely clustered white to bluish florets from midsummer through fall.

A hardy perennial, boneset grows easily from seeds planted in spring or root divisions planted in spring or fall. It prefers rich, moist, well-drained soil under full sun but tolerates poorer soil and partial shade.

Harvest as the plant flowers by cutting the entire plant a few inches above the ground.

BORAGE
"Essential" to Healing

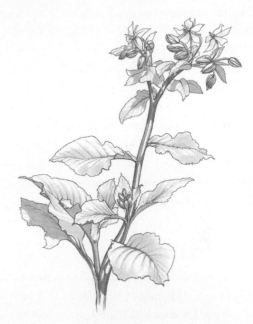

Family: Boraginaceae; other members include comfrey and forget-me-not

Genus and species: *Borago officinalis*

Also known as: star flower, bee bread, bee fodder, cool tankard

Parts used: Seed oil

Borage is an annual native to Syria that grows to 2 feet. The stem and leaves are covered with prickly hairs. It produces large star-shaped flowers, hence the common name star flower. The flowers are magnets for bees, hence the names bee bread and bee fodder. When steeped in water or wine, fresh borage imparts a cool, vaguely cucumber flavor. For centuries, it was mixed in wine, producing a beverage known as cool tankard, which became another of the plant's common names.

Healing History

The ancient Greek naturalist Dioscorides described the earliest documented use of borage— as a Mickey Finn, a drug added to wine or liquor that made drinkers pass out.

The early English herbalist John Parkinson recommended borage to revive hypochondriacs and "expell melancholie."

From ancient times until the early 19th century, borage infusion was also used as a diuretic, as a treatment for colds and bronchitis, and to increase milk production in lactating women.

Therapeutic Uses

Borage seeds yield an oil that is the richest plant source of the essential fatty acid (EFA) gamma-linolenic acid (GLA), about twice the GLA content of a more popular medicinal herb, evening primrose oil (page 210). Essential fatty acids play many important roles in the body. The brain is about 20 percent EFAs. Some EFAs have inflammatory effects that can harm the body. But others, notably GLA, have potent anti-inflammatory action. Essential fatty acids cannot be synthesized by the body and must be obtained from food. Cold water fish such as salmon contain EFAs, notably omega-3s, but many Americans who eat a meat-centered diet are deficient in EFAs, especially GLA.

When experimental animals are placed on GLA-deficient diets, they develop health problems: infertility, immune suppression, cardiovascular disease, liver abnormalities, poor wound healing, and eczema-like skin eruptions. This led researchers to try GLA supplementation in people with these conditions. The results have been remarkably positive.

Borage seed oil has not been studied as extensively as evening primrose oil. But considerable research has been conducted. Studies show that borage oil offers all the benefits of evening primrose oil—possibly greater benefits— because it contains more GLA.

DRY SKIN. GLA helps moisturize the skin. Older adults often develop dry skin. German researchers wondered if borage oil might help. They instructed 20 dry skin sufferers, average age 69, to apply some (360 or 720 milligrams) daily. After 2 months, their skin retained significantly more water. A common symptom of dry skin is itching. Before borage oil treatment, 34 percent of the participants reported frequent itching. After applying the oil, zero.

ECZEMA. This condition, known medically as atopic dermatitis, causes itchy red patches on the skin. A few studies discredit borage oil for eczema, but several show that its anti-inflammatory action provides significant benefit. German researchers gave a dozen eczema sufferers either a placebo or borage seed oil. In the placebo group, 20 percent showed benefit, but in the borage oil group, the figure was 71 percent.

Japanese researchers gave new undershirts to 32 children with eczema. Half of the shirts had been coated with borage oil. After 2 weeks, the children wearing the borage oil-coated shirts showed significantly normalized skin.

ASTHMA. Asthma involves inflammation of the bronchial tubes. Canadian researchers gave 35 asthma sufferers either a placebo or a combination of GLA and another essential fatty acid with anti-inflammatory action. After 4 weeks, the GLA group reported fewer asthma symptoms and less use of inhalers.

ACUTE RESPIRATORY DISTRESS SYNDROME. Often caused by serious infections, ARDS involves airway inflammation and potentially fatal breathing impairment. Ohio State University researchers fed 146 ARDS sufferers either a standard hospital diet or that diet with added borage oil and another essential fatty acid with anti-inflammatory action. After a week, the borage oil group showed significantly less airway inflammation and better oxygenation of their blood.

Mayo Clinic physicians gave 150 people with ARDS either standard treatment or that plus borage seed oil. The herb group has 35 percent fewer fatalities.

PRETERM INFANTS. Preemies are prone to health problems that retard normal development. British researchers gave 238 preemies either a standard diet or one supplemented with borage oil and fish oil, another source of GLA. Compared with untreated infants, the preemies given GLA showed greater growth and weight gain.

RHEUMATOID ARTHRITIS. GLA has anti-inflammatory action. Rheumatoid arthritis involves painful joint inflammation. University of Pennsylvania researchers gave 37 people with rheumatoid arthritis either cotton seed oil, which contains no GLA, or borage oil (1.4 grams/day of GLA). After 6 months, "treatment with GLA resulted in clinically important reduction in signs and symptoms of the disease." GLA reduced the number of tender joints by 36 percent, and the number of swollen joints by 28 percent. GLA reduced join pain, tenderness, and swelling by 40 percent.

University of Maryland researchers analyzed 13 studies of GLA treatment of rheumatoid arthritis. Results varied, but overall, GLA was beneficial.

BREAST CANCER. British researchers gave 38 women with breast cancer the drug tamoxifen or tamoxifen plus GLA (8 capsules/day totaling 2.8 grams). Biopsies before and after assessed changes in estrogen receptors. Those receiving the drug and herb oil showed a significant decrease in estrogen receptors, a sign of desired clinical response.

Intriguing Possibilities

Pilot studies suggest that borage oil improves bone mineral density.

Rx Recommendations

In most studies, researchers have used 1 to 3 grams/day.

Safety

Borage seed oil is considered safe in recommended doses. However, it should be used cautiously, if at all, by those with liver disease. Borage leaves, flowers, and seeds contain liver-toxic compounds (pyrrolizidine alkaloids). Concentrations of these chemicals are low, and there are no reports of borage causing liver damage. But people with liver disease should err on the side of caution and use evening primrose oil.

Pregnant women who would like to use borage oil should discuss it with their physicians.

Breast milk is rich in GLA, so nursing women may use borage seed oil in consultation with their physicians.

Do not give borage oil to children under 2. In older children, adjust the recommended dose based on the child's weight. Give a 50-pound child one-third of the dose a 150-pound adult would take.

If you're over 65, start with a low dose and increase only if necessary.

Inform health professionals of the herbs you use. Problematic herb-drug interactions are possible.

Borage oil may cause allergic reactions or other unexpected side effects. If any develop, reduce your dose or stop taking it. For more on herb safety, see Chapter 2.

If symptoms get worse or persist longer than 2 weeks, consult a health professional promptly.

Gardening

Borage grows in most warm and temperate climes. It prefers sandy, well drained soil. Plant seeds, cuttings, or root divisions in spring. Thin seedlings to space plants about every 15 inches. Borage self-seeds and grows year after year.

BOSWELLIA (INDIAN FRANKINCENSE)

Hello Boswellia, Goodbye Arthritis

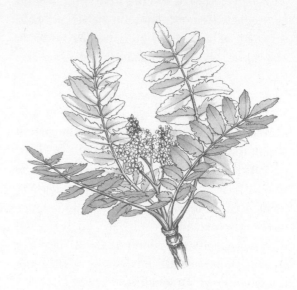

Family: Burseraceae; other members include myrrh and frankincense

Genus and species: *Boswellia serrata*

Also known as: Indian frankincense, Indian Olibanium

Parts used: gum resin

Christians believe that the three wise men who visited baby Jesus presented him with frankincense. In Leviticus (24:5–7), frankincense was offered in sacrifices to God. And in Isaiah (60:6), the prophet imagined pilgrims arriving in Jerusalem bearing gifts of gold and frankincense.

Frankincense, like its botanical relative, myrrh, is an aromatic resin exuded from the bark of tropical *Boswellia* trees that grow from North Africa to India and in tropical regions of the Western Hemisphere. In the Bible, frankincense was burned on sacrificial altars, imparting a distinctive fragrance to the proceedings. Scholars believe that Biblical frankincense was *Boswellia carterii*, found in Arabia. Indian frankincense is very similar. In herbal medicine, the terms boswellia and Indian frankincense are used interchangeably.

Healing History

India's traditional Ayurvedic healers have used boswellia resin for thousands of years. They recommended it topically for acne, boils, wounds, scars, and wrinkles. Internally they suggested it for dysentery, ulcers, muscle aches (rheumatism), and respiratory and menstrual problems. It was also widely used as a perfume on hair and clothing, as an indoor air freshener, and in Indian weddings and religious ceremonies.

Therapeutic Uses

Boswellia resin contains anti-inflammatory compounds (boswellic acids) that counteract other compounds in the body, leukotrienes, which maintain inflammation.

OSTEOARTHRITIS (OA). OA is the most common cause of chronic joint pain and inflammation. Several studies show reduced pain with boswellia. Indian researchers gave 66 people with OA of the knee either a standard pharmaceutical or boswellia (333 milligrams three times/day). After 6 months, both treatments produced similar benefit. The drug provided faster relief. The herb had no effect for the first month. But after terminating treatment, the boswellia group reported greater residual benefit.

Another Indian research team gave 30 osteoarthritis sufferers either a placebo or boswellia. After 8 weeks, the groups switched treatments. While taking the herb, every participant reported less pain. Other Indian studies using multiherb formulas containing boswellia (with turmeric, myrrh, and ashwagandha) have produced similar benefits.

Other Indian scientists gave 70 people with OA either a placebo or boswellia (100 or 250 milligrams/day). After 3 months, both doses of the herb provided significantly greater relief from pain and stiffness.

A German researcher analyzed seven clinical trials of boswellia for OA. All showed benefit.

RHEUMATOID ARTHRITIS (RA). Often more painful than osteoarthritis, RA causes joint inflammation, redness, and tenderness and possibly other symptoms. Indian researchers gave boswellia to 175 people with RA, and 122 reported benefit. A boswellia-based RA medication, Sallaki, have been approved in India since 1982.

ULCERATIVE COLITIS. The intestinal inflammation that causes colitis results, in part, from leukotrienes. Boswellia suppresses leukotrienes. Indian scientists gave colitis sufferers either a standard pharmaceutical (sulfasalazine) or boswellia (350 milligrams three times a day). After 6 weeks, 75 percent of the drug group went into remission; in the herb group, 82 percent. The researchers repeated this study and results were even better—40 percent remission in the drug group versus 90 percent among those taking boswellia.

ASTHMA. Inflammation plays a key role in asthmatic airway constriction. German researchers gave 40 asthmatics either a placebo or boswellia (300 milligrams three times a day). Six weeks later, 27 percent of the placebo group showed improvement; in the herb group, 70 percent.

Intriguing Possibilities

Indian pilot studies suggest that boswellia reduces cholesterol and triglycerides (blood fats), suggesting that it may help prevent and treat heart disease.

A pilot study in Texas suggests that boswellia may help treat chronic kidney disease.

In laboratory studies, the herb also suppresses replication of DNA in leukemia, hinting that it might have potential as a cancer treatment.

Rx Recommendations

For asthma, osteoarthritis, and colitis, take 300 milligrams of powdered resin three times a day. For osteoarthritis, take 400 milligrams three times a day. When using commercial products, follow package directions.

Safety

At recommended doses, boswellia is considered safe, but stomach distress, nausea, diarrhea, and heartburn have been reported.

Boswellia may stimulate menstruation. Pregnant and nursing women should not use it.

Do not give boswellia to children under 2. In older children, adjust the recommended dose based on the child's weight. Give a 50-pound child one-third of the dose a 150-pound adult would take.

If you're over 65, start with a low dose, and increase only if necessary.

Inform health professionals of the herbs you use. Problematic herb-drug interactions are possible.

Boswellia may cause allergic reactions or other unexpected side effects. If any develop, reduce your dose or stop taking it. For more on herb safety, see Chapter 2.

If symptoms get worse or persist longer than 2 weeks, consult a health professional promptly.

Gardening

Boswellia serrata is a moderate-size deciduous tree that grows in the hot arid mountains of central India. It requires limestone-rich soil. It is not grown commercially in the United States, but might grow in places like the mountains of the Southwest. Resin harvesters cut a thin strip of bark near the base of the tree and tap the tree in a manner similar to harvesting maple sap for syrup. Tapping takes place from November to May.

BUCHU

The South African Diuretic

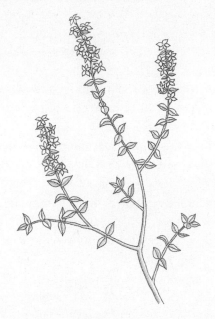

Family: Rutaceae; other members include orange, lemon, and rue

Genus and species: *Barosma betulina* or *Agathosma betulina, B. crenulata,* and *B. serratifolia*

Also known as: Bookoo, buku, bucku, and bucco

Parts used: Leaves

This 5-foot southern African shrub has finely toothed opposite or alternate leaves containing an oil that increases urination.

Healing History

Long before contact with Europeans, the indigenous people of what is now Namibia and South Africa used buchu for urinary problems. When Dutch (Afrikaner) colonists settled the region, they adopted the herb as a treatment for urinary tract infections, kidney stones, arthritis, cholera, and muscle aches.

Later, English settlers adopted buchu and used it to treat so many illnesses that some considered it a panacea.

In 1847, New York patent medicine entrepreneur Henry T. Helmbold introduced Helmbold's Compound Extract of Buchu as a remedy for urinary problems, kidney stones, and "diseases arising from imprudence [sexually transmitted infections]." Buchu made Helmbold rich. He called himself the Buchu King and deserves credit for introducing Americans to this healer.

Therapeutic Uses

PREMENSTRUAL SYNDROME (PMS). Many women complain of bloating from water retention before their periods. Buchu is an ingredient in several herb teas marketed to relieve the bloating of PMS.

URINARY TRACT INFECTIONS. Many herbals continue to recommend buchu for urinary tract infections. One study of the herb's effects on the bacteria that cause this infection showed no benefit. Still, many herbalists endorse buchu as an infection fighter.

HIGH BLOOD PRESSURE AND CONGESTIVE HEART FAILURE. Physicians often prescribe diuretics to treat these conditions. If you have either conditions, consult your physician about including buchu in your treatment plan.

Medicinal Myth

For years, buchu was a common ingredient in herbal weight-loss products. Diuretics can cause temporary loss of excess water weight, but no science-based weight-loss program endorses the use of diuretics for permanent weight control.

Rx Recommendations

For relief of premenstrual bloating, try an infusion or tincture of buchu. To prepare an infusion, use 1 to 2 teaspoons of dried, crumbled leaves per cup of boiling water and steep for 10 to 20 minutes. Drink up to 3 cups a day. Buchu has a minty aroma and a pleasant, minty taste.

If using a homemade tincture, take ½ to 1 teaspoon up to three times a day.

When using commercial preparations, follow package directions.

Safety

There are no reports of significant harm from using recommended amounts of buchu.

Diuretics deplete body stores of potassium. If you take buchu, increase your consumption of potassium-rich foods—bananas and fresh vegetables.

Pregnant and nursing women should not use buchu.

Do not give buchu to children under 2. In older children, adjust the recommended dose based on the child's weight. Give a 50-pound child one-third of the dose a 150-pound adult would take.

If you're over 65, start with a low dose, and increase only if necessary.

Inform health professionals of the herbs you use. Problematic herb-drug interactions are possible.

Buchu may cause allergic reactions or other unexpected side effects. If any develop, reduce your dose or stop taking it. For more on herb safety, see Chapter 2.

If symptoms get worse or persist longer than 2 weeks, consult a health professional promptly.

Gardening

Buchu is not grown in the United States.

BUCKTHORN

An Old-Time Constipation Cure

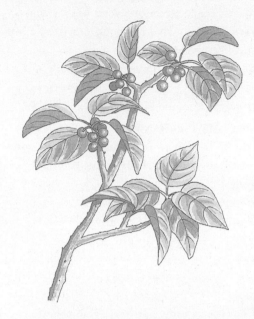

Family: Rhamnaceae; other members include cascara sagrada

Genus and species: *Rhamnus cathartica* and *R. frangula*

Also known as: Purging buckthorn, frangula, and alder buckthorn

Parts used: Berries and bark

The species name for buckthorn, *cathartica*, is no joke. This herb is a potent laxative—so powerful, in fact, that it should be used only as a last resort, after other, gentler laxatives have failed.

Healing History

European herbalists popularized buckthorn around the 13th century. At the time, physicians believed that the key to curing disease lay in purging "foul humors." With such a focus on purging, powerful laxatives were widely prescribed. Buckthorn was a favorite because it produced quick, reliable results—while often leaving users with intestinal cramps.

Over the centuries, herbalists have also recommended buckthorn for jaundice, hemorrhoids, gout, arthritis, and menstruation promotion. In addition, this herb has a long history as a cancer treatment. In America, it was an ingredient in the popular but controversial Hoxsey Cancer Formula (see page 31).

Therapeutic Uses

Buckthorn doesn't treat jaundice or arthritis, and it's more likely to aggravate hemorrhoids than to relieve them. But its laxative action is reliable—and powerful to a fault.

CONSTIPATION. No one disputes buckthorn's laxative action. It has been an ingredient in many pharmaceutical and herbal laxatives. Commission E, the expert panel that evaluates herbal medicines for the German counterpart of the FDA, approves it as a laxative.

Buckthorn contains chemicals called anthraquinones. They're dramatic purgatives—too powerful for most people. That's why buckthorn should be considered a last-resort treatment for constipation.

Intriguing Possibility

Harry Hoxsey may have been on the right track. Buckthorn has an antitumor effect, according to research published in the *Journal of the National Cancer Institute*. But one study does not establish efficacy as a cancer treatment.

This herb is many years away from cancer care—if it's ever used that way.

Rx Recommendations

In Germany, physicians prescribe an infusion containing ½ teaspoon each of dried buckthorn bark, fennel seeds, and chamomile flowers (which soothe the stomach). Steep the blend in 1 cup of boiling water for 10 minutes, then strain. Drink it before going to bed. You'll find the taste initially sweet, then bitter.

If you prefer a decoction, boil 1 teaspoon of dried buckthorn in 3 cups of water. Steep for 30 minutes, then strain. Drink it cool, 1 or 2 table-spoons before bed.

As a homemade tincture, take ½ teaspoon before going to bed.

When using commercial preparations, follow the package directions.

Safety

Because of buckthorn's powerful purgative action, people with chronic gastrointestinal problems—ulcers, colitis, Crohn's disease, diverticulitis, hemorrhoids, and irritable bowel syndrome—should not use it.

Don't take buckthorn for more than 2 weeks at a time. If you use it for too long, it causes lazy bowel syndrome, an inability to have bowel movements without chemical stimulation.

If you use bulk buckthorn, be sure that it has been dried thoroughly. Otherwise, it causes vomiting, severe abdominal pain, and violent diarrhea. Most herbalists recommend drying the berries or bark for at least a year—some say 2 years—before using them. Commercial preparations use aged bark.

You can dry fresh buckthorn quickly by bak-ing it at 250°F for several hours. If you experi-ence nausea and abdominal distress after taking the herb, seek professional medical attention immediately.

Pregnant and nursing women should not use buckthorn.

Do not give buckthorn to children.

If you're over 65, start with a low dose, and increase only if necessary.

Inform health professionals of the herbs you use. Problematic herb-drug interactions are possible.

Buckthorn may cause allergic reactions or other unexpected side effects. If any develop, reduce your dose or stop taking it. For more on herb safety, see Chapter 2.

If symptoms get worse or persist longer than 2 weeks, consult a health professional promptly.

Gardening

Buckthorn is a shrub or small tree that can reach 20 feet. It has shiny, dark green leaves and produces black, pea-size berries. It is not a garden plant.

BURDOCK

Likely to Stick Around

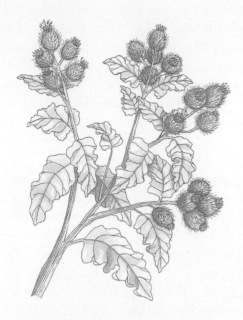

Family: Compositae; other members include daisy, dandelion, and marigold

Genus and species: *Arctium lappa*

Also known as: Great burdock and burr

Parts used: Primarily roots, also leaves and seeds

"Burdock" is a combination of "bur," meaning tenacious burrs, and "dock," Old English for "plant." The name is apt. Burdock burrs seem to reach out and grab anything near them. The same could be said for its place in modern herbal healing. While many scientists have dismissed burdock as useless, it seems destined to hang on as a healing herb, particularly as a potential treatment for cancer.

Healing History

Burdock has had its ups and downs. When it wasn't reviled as a weed, it was recommended as a treatment for a surprising variety of conditions.

Ancient Chinese physicians considered it a remedy for colds, flu, throat infections, and pneumonia. India's traditional Ayurvedic healers used it similarly.

The medieval German abbess/herbalist Hildegard of Bingen prescribed burdock to treat cancerous tumors.

During the 14th century in Europe, the herb's leaves were used to make wine and treat leprosy.

England's overly imaginative 17th-century herbalist Nicholas Culpeper recommended burdock for uterine prolapse, a condition in which the ligaments supporting the uterus weaken and cause it to fall into the vagina. Culpeper's bizarre prescription: Place burdock on the crown of the head to draw the womb back up.

Later European herbalists prescribed burdock root for fever, cancer, eczema, psoriasis, acne, gout, ringworm, skin infections, syphilis, gonorrhea, and problems associated with childbirth.

America's 19th-century Eclectic physicians, forerunners of today's naturopaths, considered the herb an excellent diuretic. They prescribed it for painful urination, urinary tract infections, and kidney problems, in addition to skin infections and arthritis.

Centuries after Hildegard recommended burdock for cancer, the herb's reputation as a tumor treatment spread to Russia, China, India, and the Americas. From the 1930s to the 1950s, burdock was an ingredient in the alternative cancer treatment marketed by ex–coal miner Harry Hoxsey (see page 31).

Contemporary herbalists have abandoned burdock as a cancer treatment (perhaps prematurely). But they continue to recommend it for skin problems, wound healing, urinary tract infections, arthritis, sciatica, ulcers, and even anorexia nervosa.

Therapeutic Uses

Many modern herb experts give a thumbs-down to burdock as a healing herb. *In Natural Product Medicine*, Ara Der Marderosian, Ph.D., and Lawrence Liberti write, "There is little evidence to suggest burdock is useful in treatment of any human disease." And in *Tyler's Honest Herbal*, the late Varro E. Tyler, Ph.D., writes, "Despite its long folkloric use, no solid evidence exists that burdock exhibits any useful therapeutic activity."

Most traditional claims for burdock have not withstood scientific scrutiny. The herb does not treat leprosy, arthritis, uterine prolapse, or congestive heart failure. Still, several studies suggest that it may prove to be therapeutic after all.

INFECTIONS. Burdock's traditional use against the fungal and bacterial infections has been experimentally confirmed. German researchers have discovered that fresh burdock root contains compounds (polyacetylenes), that kill disease-causing bacteria and fungi. Brazilian researchers have shown that the herb inhibits the growth of *Candida albicans*, the fungus that causes yeast infections, and several types of bacteria: *Staphylococcus, Pseudomonas,* and *Enterococcus.*

Intriguing Possibilities

Burdock has been used extensively around the world as a cancer treatment. Several studies show that compounds in the herb have antitumor activity. An article published in *Chemotherapy* identified one, arctigenin, as an "inhibitor of tumor growth." And a study in *Mutation Research* determined that burdock decreases mutations in cells exposed to mutation-causing chemicals. (Most substances that cause genetic mutations also cause cancer.)

Researchers in Slovakia induced coughs in laboratory animals and then gave them a variety of herbs. Marshmallow, an herbal cough suppressant with a long history of effectiveness, worked best (page 314). But burdock also worked quite well.

In animal studies, German researchers have discovered that burdock, applied topically, interferes to some extent with the type of allergic swelling that causes hives.

Finally, burdock has an as-yet-unexplained antipoisoning effect. Experimental animals fed the herb were somehow protected against several toxic chemicals.

In view of these tantalizing findings, let's hope scientists cling to burdock research as tenaciously as the plant's burrs cling to just about anything.

Rx Recommendations

Use burdock as a decoction or tincture. To prepare a decoction, boil 1 teaspoon of root in 3 cups of water for 30 minutes, then let cool. Drink up to 3 cups a day. Burdock has a sweet taste similar to celery root.

When using a homemade tincture, take ½ to 1 teaspoon up to three times a day.

When using commercial preparations, follow package directions.

Safety

No one questioned the safety of burdock until the *Journal of the American Medical Association* linked the herb to one case of serious poisoning. A woman who drank a strong decoction experienced blurred vision, dry mouth, and hallucinations, all classic symptoms of atropine poisoning. Burdock does not contain atropine, but belladonna, a plant that looks similar, does. Presumably, some belladonna accidentally adulterated the woman's burdock.

One case of adulteration is not cause for alarm. Still, if you use burdock and develop any symptoms of atropine poisoning, seek emergency medical treatment immediately.

Pregnant and nursing women should not use burdock.

Do not give burdock to children under 2. In older children, adjust the recommended dose based on the child's weight. Give a 50-pound child one-third of the dose a 150-pound adult would take.

If you're over 65, start with a low dose, and increase only if necessary.

Inform health professionals of the herbs you use. Problematic herb-drug interactions are possible.

Burdock may cause allergic reactions or other unexpected side effects. If any develop, reduce your dose or stop taking it. For more on herb safety, see Chapter 2.

If symptoms get worse or persist longer than 2 weeks, consult a health professional promptly.

Gardening

Burdock's medicinal root has brown bark and a white, spongy, fibrous interior that becomes hard when dried. Its stem is multibranched, with long, egg-shaped leaves. A bristled flower—actually a clump of many purplish flowerlettes—tops each branch. The flowers produce its infamous burrs.

Burdock grows easily from seeds planted in spring. Thin seedlings to 6-inch spacing. Burdock prefers moist, rich, deeply cultivated soil and full sun, but tolerates poorer soils. Mix wood chips and sawdust into burdock beds to keep the soil loose so roots are easier to harvest.

Burdock roots deeply, so it's not advisable to transplant it once established. Harvest roots during the fall of the first year or the spring of the second.

BUTCHER'S BROOM

Sweep Away Varicose Veins and Hemorrhoids

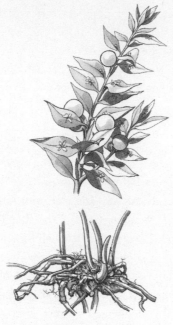

Family: Liliaceae; other members include lilies, tulips, and onions

Genus and species: *Ruscus aculeatus*

Also known as: Ruscus, box holly, knee holly, sweet broom

Parts used: Rhizome and root

For centuries, European butchers bound the stiff twigs of this plant into bundles and used the small brooms to keep their cutting boards clean. However, many plants were used to make brooms and acquired the name "broom." If you want butcher's broom, confirm that the herb you're buying is *Ruscus aculeatus.*

Butcher's broom is native to the Mediterranean and Middle East but grows throughout much of Europe. Its leaves resemble holly leaves, hence some of its common names and its generic name, ruscus, which is derived from the Anglo-Saxon term for holly.

Healing History

In ancient times, butcher's broom was used as a laxative and diuretic. A root decoction in wine was used to treat kidney stones.

Seventeenth-century English herbalist Nicholas Culpeper recommended a root decoction and a poultice of the berries for broken bones.

Then the plant fell into disuse. In the 1950s, scientists discovered that butcher's broom's underground stems (rhizomes) made veins less likely to leak fluid (reduced venous permeability, or venous insufficiency) and might be useful in treating varicose veins including hemorrhoids.

Therapeutic Uses

Most published studies have used a French proprietary formula, Cyclo 3 Fort. It contains butcher's broom (150 milligrams/capsule) extract plus vitamin C (100 milligrams) and hesperidin methyl chalcone (150 milligrams), a compound from citrus fruits that also helps reduce venous permeability.

VARICOSE VEINS/CHRONIC VENOUS INSUFFICIENCY. Chronic venous insufficiency means that the veins, particularly the leg veins, don't properly return blood to the heart. Blood pools in the legs, eventually causing varicosities. An estimated 80 million Americans, about 40 percent of the adult population, have varicose veins. While not life-threatening, they can be painful, unsightly, and costly to treat.

Italian researchers analyzed 20 studies of Cyclo 3 Fort for chronic venous insufficiency. Compared with placebo treatment, the herb product "significantly reduced" swelling and the severity of pain, heaviness, cramping, and tingling. The researchers called their analysis "a strong demonstration of the efficacy of Cyclo 3 Fort in treating chronic venous insufficiency."

Several studies also show that Cyclo 3 Fort relieves pregnancy-related varicose veins. The research to date has not established the absolute safety of butcher's broom during pregnancy, but an article in *Alternative and Complementary Therapies* says, "Both animal and human studies indicate a high degree of safety during pregnancy."

Commission E, the German counterpart of the FDA, approves butcher's broom for varicose veins.

LYMPHEDEMA. Lymph is a fluid that circulates throughout the body and contains infection-fighting white blood cells. When lymph vessels become damaged, lymph drainage becomes blocked, and excess fluid accumulates, causing swelling and discomfort. When lymph nodes are removed from the underarm as part of breast cancer surgery, lymphedema is a common side effect. French researchers gave fluid-draining arm massage, a standard therapy, to 57 women who had developed lymphedema after breast cancer surgery. The women also took either a placebo or Cyclo 3 Fort daily. After 3 months, the herb group showed significantly less arm swelling.

HEMORRHOIDS. Hemorrhoids are varicose veins around or near the anus. French researchers gave Cyclo 3 Fort to 124 hemorrhoid sufferers (six capsules daily for 3 days, then four capsules daily for 4 days). Using standard measures of hemorrhoid pain, the herb product provided significant relief. Commission E approves butcher's broom for hemorrhoids.

Intriguing Possibilities

Pilot studies suggest that Cyclo 3 Fort may relieve some women's premenstrual bloating.

Rx Recommendations

Take two to four capsules of Cyclo 3 Fort a day. Or follow package directions. Cyclo 3 Fort is available in the United States. Check where you buy medicinal herbs or the Internet.

Safety

Butcher's broom is considered safe in recommended doses, but stomach upset and diarrhea have been reported.

Pregnant women interested in trying Cyclo 3 Fort for varicose veins should discuss this with their physicians.

Do not give butcher's boom to children under 2. In older children, adjust the recommended dose based on the child's weight. Give a 50-pound child one-third of the dose a 150-pound adult would take.

If you're over 65, start with a low dose, and increase only if necessary.

Inform health professionals of the herbs you use. Problematic herb-drug interactions are possible.

Butcher's broom may cause allergic reactions or other unexpected side effects. If any develop, reduce your dose or stop taking it. For more on herb safety, see Chapter 2.

If symptoms get worse or persist longer than 2 weeks, consult a health professional promptly.

Gardening

Butcher's broom is a prickly, low-growing evergreen shrub that thrives throughout much of the southern United States. Its shoots look like asparagus and are edible. But the berries are toxic. This plant grows best in moist, chalky soil. It can grow in many parts of the United States, but most of the herb used medicinally is imported.

BUTTERBUR

For Hay Fever and Migraine Relief

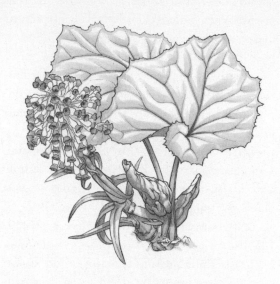

Family: Asteraceae; other members include daisy

Genus and species: *Petasites hybridus*

Also known as: Pestilence wort, bog rhubarb, butter dock, butterfly dock

Parts used: Leaf and root extract

Butterbur is a perennial shrub native to Europe. Its leaves are large and downy, hence its generic name, *Petasites*, from the Greek *petasos* for the broad-brimmed felt hats worn by shepherds. During the Middle Ages, the leaves were used to wrap butter in warm weather, hence butterbur. This herb also has a long history of use in healing. But from the late-19th to late-20th centuries, it was largely forgotten. Then studies in the 1990s showed that it deserves a place in herbal medicine.

Healing History

The ancient Greeks used butterbur to treat asthma. This use continued through the Middle Ages when butterbur was also used to treat fevers, cough, headache, ulcers, and plague, hence one of its names, pestilence wort.

Therapeutic Uses

The medicinally active constituent in butterbur is petasin.

MIGRAINE PREVENTION. Mention herbs for migraines, and herbalists immediately say feverfew (page 220). It works, but so does butterbur, validating one of the herb's folk uses.

German researchers gave 60 migraine sufferers either a placebo or butterbur (pyrrolizidine-free, 50 milligrams twice a day). After 12 weeks, the herb group suffered 60 percent fewer migraines. In a 4-month study at Albert Einstein College of Medicine in the Bronx, New York, butterbur extract (pyrrolizidine-free, 75 milligrams twice a day) reduced migraine frequency 48 percent. Another German group found that among 33 migraine sufferers, the herb (pyrrolizidine-free, 50 milligrams twice a day) reduced migraine frequency by at least half in 45 percent of them. A third German team treated 108 children, age 6 to 17, with the herb (pyrrolizidine-free, 50 to 150 milligrams/day, depending on age). After 4 months, 77 percent reported attack frequency reduced by at least 50 percent.

HAY FEVER. Swiss scientists gave 125 allergy sufferers either a popular antihistamine (Zyrtec) or butterbur (pyrrolizidine-free, 50 milligrams four times a day). The herb worked as well as the drug. But the drug caused drowsiness in 75 percent of users. The herb did not.

Other studies—but not all—support butterbur's antiallergy action. To settle the matter, British researchers conducted a meta-analysis, a statistically sophisticated review. They included all published studies that met standard criteria for scientific rigor—subjects were randomly assigned to either herb or placebo groups (or a popular antihistamine), and neither the subjects nor the researchers knew who was in which group. The researchers found six rigorous butterbur trials. Five showed that the herb was effective. It worked better than the placebo and as well as standard antihistamines.

Intriguing Possibilities

One study suggests that butterbur (pyrrolizidine-free, 50 milligrams three times a day) reduces the number, duration, and severity of asthma attacks. Another suggests that the herb may help relieve psychosomatic anxiety and depression.

Rx Recommendations

Look for tablets containing 50 milligrams of a standardized carbon dioxide extract containing 8 milligrams of petasin per tablet. Take one tablet two or three times a day. Or follow package directions.

Safety

Butterbur contains pyrrolizidine alkaloids toxic to the liver. The root contains more than the leaves. Commission E, the German counterpart of the FDA, says intake of pyrrolizidine alkaloids should be limited to no more than 1 microgram/day. Butterbur roots contain as much as 100 micrograms/gram. However, commercial preparations use carbon dioxide to remove these compounds. Look for butterbur products that specify no pyrrolizidines or a CO_2 extract.

Headache, itchy eyes, stomach upset, constipation, and diarrhea have been reported.

Pregnant and nursing women should not use butterbur.

Do not give butterbur to children under 2. In older children, adjust the recommended dose based on the child's weight. Give a 50-pound child one-third of the dose a 150-pound adult would take.

If you're over 65, start with a low dose, and increase only if necessary.

Inform health professionals of the herbs you use. Problematic herb-drug interactions are possible.

Butterbur may cause allergic reactions especially in those with ragweed allergies, or other unexpected side effects. If any develop, reduce your dose or stop taking it. For more on herb safety, see Chapter 2.

If symptoms get worse or persist longer than 2 weeks, consult a health professional promptly.

Gardening

Butterbur grows in temperate climates, including North America. It prefers wet, marshy soil adjacent to streams. Once established, it spreads aggressively. Snip flowers before they open to stop spreading. Stems were once cooked as a vegetable, hence the name bog rhubarb. Do not eat the stems. They contain pyrrolizidine alkaloids.

CANNABIS (MARIJUANA)

From Prohibition to Growing Acceptance of Its Healing Value

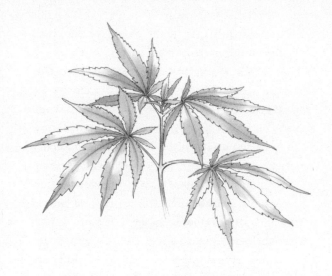

Family: Cannabaceae; other members include hemp and hop

Genus and species: *Cannabis sativa* and *C. indica*

Also known as: marijuana, weed, pot, reefer, dope, grass, hemp, sinsemilla, hash, hashish, bud, maryjane, bhang, kif, wacky tobaccy, ganja (Jamaica), Acapulco gold (Mexico), Panama red (Panama), Durban poison (South Africa), Thai stick (Asia), and a vast array of American strains, including Mowie wowie (Hawaii), Train Wreck, AK-47, Sour Diesel, Green Crack, Pineapple Express, and God's Gift

Parts used: Flower buds, leaves

NOTE: As this book goes to press, possession, cultivation, and sale of cannabis (marijuana) is illegal under federal law. Possession of any amount can bring 1 to 3 years in prison and fines up to $5,000. Cultivation and/or sale, depending on amount, carry federal penalties of 5 years to life with fines up to $1 million. In addition, most states laws also prohibit cannabis possession, cultivation, and sale with violators facing similar state penalties.

However, since 1996, 28 states and the District of Columbia have legalized cannabis for medicinal use: Alaska, Arizona, Arkansas, California, Colorado, Connecticut, Delaware, Florida, Hawaii, Illinois, Maine, Maryland, Massachusetts, Michigan, Minnesota, Montana, Nevada, New Hampshire, New Jersey, New Mexico, New York, North Dakota, Ohio, Oregon, Pennsylvania, Rhode Island, Vermont, and Washington.

In addition, seven states have legalized cannabis for recreational use: Alaska, California, Colorado, Massachusetts, Nevada, Oregon, and Washington, and the District of Columbia has decriminalized adult possessions of up to 2 ounces.

This book's publisher believes in obeying the law—but cannabis law is rapidly evolving. Currently, cannabis is among the nation's most widely used medicinal herbs. Unfortunately, it is also the subject of a great deal of misinformation. This chapter presents what's currently known about cannabis, both its benefits and risks.

Healing History

Currently, most people use the terms "marijuana" and "cannabis" interchangeably. But as the herb passes from illicit indulgence to legiti-mate medicine, "marijuana" is fading and "cannabis" is ascendant.

Cannabis comes in two varieties—tall, thin-leafed *C. sativa* from central Asia and shrubbier, broader-leafed *C. indica* from India. Humans have used cannabis for 10,000 years. The oldest remains have been discovered at Asian archeological sites dating from as early as 8,000 BC. It remains unclear how prehistoric humans used the plant—medicinally, for fiber, as a food, as an intoxicant, or some combination.

Cannabis and hemp started out as the same plant. During prehistoric times, cannabis/hemp contained varying amounts of psychoactive compounds. Over the millennia, growers bred cannabis for intoxication and hemp for its soft, strong, durable fiber. Thomas Jefferson wrote the Declaration of Independence on hemp paper, and Betsy Ross sewed the first American flag using hemp cloth. Today, industrial hemp is used to make rope and textiles and contains negligible amounts of psychoactive compounds.

The first written reference to medicinal cannabis appeared around 3400 BC, in China's first great herbal, the *Pen Tsao Ching* (*Classic of Herbs*) by mythological emperor Shen Nung. By the first century AD, Chinese herbals included cannabis in more than 100 herbal prescriptions.

Cannabis reached the Mediterranean about 1500 BC. The Greek historian Herodotus (484 BC–c. 425 BC) was the first to document its intoxicating effects. He described how the Scythians of central Asia heated stones upon which revelers threw cannabis flowers and seeds. They inhaled the vapor and became euphoric.

The ancient Greek herbalist Dioscorides and Galen, Rome's leading physician, both recommended cannabis medicinally, particularly for gastrointestinal complaints. India's Ayurvedic physicians also prescribed it for gastrointestinal distress and for pain, particularly migraines.

The ancient Persians of present-day Iraq considered cannabis an indispensible medicine. Noted Persian physician Mohammad-e Zakariaya Razi (865–925 AD) cited a broad range of therapeutic uses.

During the Age of Exploration (1400–1600), European nations vastly expanded their navies. Their ships required a great deal of rope and cloth for sails. Both came from hemp, and along with the fibrous variety, medicinal cannabis also arrived in Europe and England. In his *Anatomy of Melancholy* (1621), one of the first medical discussions of depression, English physician Robert Burton recommended hemp, "which puts [sufferers] for a time into a kind of Extasis [ecstasy] and makes them gently to laugh."

Irish physician Sir William O'Shaughnessy, M.D., (1809–1889) was the first Westerner to study cannabis as medicine. During his life, England ruled India so he focused on *C. indica*, recommending it enthusiastically for pain and anxiety. In 1894, the report of England's India Hemp Drugs Commission called *C. indica* "medicinal in character" and concluded "occasional use of hemp in moderate doses may be beneficial."

In 1860, cannabis was incorporated into the *U.S. Pharmacopeia*, the compendium of the nation's formulary, for pain and stomach distress. By the early 20th century, most U.S. drug makers offered cannabis preparations for pain, anxiety, sleep problems, gastrointestinal problems, and "hysteria," that era's term for premenstrual, menstrual, and menopausal discomforts.

In an 1890 report in the medical journal *Lancet*, J. R. Reynolds, M.D., personal physician to Queen Victoria, wrote, "In almost all painful maladies, I have found Indian hemp by far the most useful of drugs."

In 1915, Sir William Osler, a founder of Johns Hopkins Medical School, called cannabis "probably the most satisfactory remedy" for migraine.

In her 1931 *A Modern Herbal*, noted English herbalist Maude Grieve wrote that *C. indica* produced "exhilarating intoxication" and recommended it for "easing pain and inducing sleep."

In 1964, Israeli researcher Raphael Mechoulam identified the main psychoactive constituent of cannabis, delta-9-tetrahydrocannabinol (THC).

Cannabis prohibition dates from the early 20th century, when, shortly after the Mexican revolution (1910), large numbers of Mexicans decamped to the American Southwest. Many Americans objected to the influx and sought to rid the country of Mexicans—and their social intoxicant, marijuana. The U.S. Department of Treasury agreed and, despite all evidence to the contrary, called marijuana addictive and linked it to insanity, criminality, and use of harder drugs such as heroin. In 1937, Congress passed the Marijuana Tax Act, which effectively outlawed cannabis in the United States. In 1942, the *U.S. Pharmacopeia* dropped cannabis.

But many Americans objected to marijuana prohibition, among them, the American Medical Association and New York City Mayor Fiorello LaGuardia (after whom the airport is named). LaGuardia asked the New York Academy of Sciences to evaluate marijuana's effects. In 1944 the LaGuardia Committee released its findings, concluding that cannabis was not addictive, played no role in insanity or criminality, was not a gateway to harder drugs, and had legitimate medical uses. But pro-cannabis sentiments had no effect on U.S. government policies. Marijuana remained illegal with federal officials considering it as dangerous as heroin.

That's pretty much where things stood for 50 years—government agencies demonizing cannabis, while, starting in the 1960s, millions of otherwise law-abiding Americans embraced it as a social intoxicant more benign than alcohol and as a medicine.

Cannabis prohibition limited research, but during the 1970s, small pilot studies published in journals including the *Journal of Clinical Pharmacology* showed that, just as the ancients believed, cannabis was a useful treatment for pain, with 10 milligrams of oral THC as effective as 60 milligrams of codeine.

In 1986, the journal *Pharmacological Reviews* devoted an entire issue to cannabis. The articles affirmed its pain-relieving action, refuted allegations that it contributed to criminality, aggression, brain damage, and loss of motivation, and documented its ability to reduce risk of glaucoma by lowering intraocular pressure.

In 1996, the American Public Health Association called for an end to prohibition of medical cannabis research. That same year, California became the first state to legalize medical marijuana. Today, more than half the states have legalized it as medicine. Approximately two-thirds of Americans live in states with legal medical marijuana.

For a 1997 report in the *American Journal Public Health*, researchers reviewed the medical records of 65,000 HMO patients who admitted using marijuana. Compared with nonusers, they showed no greater risk of illness, drug addiction, mental health problems, or death.

Legal or not, the U.S. Department of Health and Human Services' Substance Abuse and Mental Health Administration estimates that 10 percent of Americans over age 12 have used cannabis during the past year (25 million people), 6 percent have used it in the past month (15 million), and 1 percent use it daily (2.5 million). Sources including *Forbes*, CNBC, the National Organization for Reform of Marijuana Laws, and Jeffrey Miron, Ph.D., a Harvard authority on cannabis, estimate annual U.S. production at some 65 million plants (10,000 tons) with a value exceeding $10 billion a year, making cannabis one of the nation's largest cash crops and among America's most widely used herbal medicines.

Therapeutic Uses

Cannabis contains dozens of compounds with potential medicinal value, but the two most studied are tetrahydrocannabinol (THC) and cannabidiol (CBD). THC causes intoxication. CBD does not. THC can be used to treat a broad range of conditions including anxiety, nausea, pain, gastrointestinal distress, and insomnia. CBD treats pain. Today, growers breed cannabis to be high in THC, high in CBD, or both. Some studies have used herbal cannabis, while others have employed dose-standardized extracts—Sativex nasal spray or oral nabilone or dronabinol (Marinol).

In 2017, the National Academies of Science, Engineering, and Medicine, an arm of the federal government, issued the most comprehensive review to date of the medical uses of cannabis. It strongly recommended that the federal government remove cannabis from the list of Schedule 1 drugs, those that have no medical value and a high risk of abuse, for example, heroin, and reclassify it as therapeutic. The National Academies report documents many medical uses.

Decades of prohibition have limited cannabis research, but here's a summary of recent findings.

NAUSEA OF CHEMOTHERAPY. Cancer chemotherapy often causes nausea and vomiting. Swiss and British researchers reviewed 30 studies involving 1,366 people that compared pharmaceutical antiemetics with cannabis (ingested extracts, various doses). Cannabis worked best.

GASTROINTESTINAL DISTRESS. Many studies show that the GI tract is rich in cannabinoid receptors, which presumably explains why cannabis is so effective for nausea. The herb also treats other forms of GI distress, for example, stomach cramping, irritable bowel syndrome, and gastritis. Surveys of people with inflammatory bowel disease (Crohn's) show that one-third to one-half use cannabis for symptomatic relief.

MULTIPLE SCLEROSIS. English researchers gave 667 MS sufferers either a placebo or cannabis (10 to 25 milligrams THC depending on weight) twice a day. After 15 weeks, the cannabis group reported less pain, fewer jerky movements (spasticity), and improved walking ability.

German researchers assessed spasticity in 276 people with MS and then gave them Sativex (52 percent THC, 48 percent CBD, 7 sprays a day). After 4 weeks, spasticity declined a highly significant 40 percent.

RHEUMATOID ARTHRITIS. English researchers gave 58 RA sufferers either a placebo or Sativex. The Sativex group reported significantly less joint pain and better sleep.

FIBROMYALGIA. University of Manitoba investigators gave 40 fibromyalgia sufferers either a placebo or synthetic cannabis (nabilone). After 4 weeks, the nabilone group reported significantly less pain.

Researchers in Barcelona, Spain, surveyed 58 middle-aged women with fibromyalgia who smoked cannabis an average of three times a day. All reported improvement in one or more symptoms: insomnia, pain, stiffness, and ability to relax.

NERVE (NEUROPATHIC) PAIN. Nerve pain, for example, sciatica, can feel unbearable. University of California, San Francisco, researchers gave 50 people with AIDS-related neuropathy either a placebo or cannabis (3.6 percent THC, a low dose) three times a day. After the first treatment, the placebo group experienced a 15 percent reduction in neuropathic pain, the cannabis group, 72 percent less. After 5 days, the cannabis group continued to experience significantly greater relief from nerve pain.

English scientists gave 125 neuropathy sufferers either a placebo or Sativex (up to 48 sprays a day). After 5 weeks, the placebo group reported 8 percent less pain, the Sativex group 22 percent less. The Sativex group also reported better sleep.

OPIOID OVERDOSE DEATHS. Drugs derived from opium (codeine, morphine, and synthetic opioids) are effective for pain, but carry a high risk of addiction and death from overdose. In a 2014 report, Johns Hopkins researchers compared opioid deaths from 1999 to 2010 in states with or without legalized medical cannabis. During those 12 years, in states that prohibited the drug, opioid deaths increased. But in states with legal medical cannabis, opioid deaths fell 25 percent.

Medical Myths

LOSS OF MOTIVATION? Ever since it became clear that cannabis is not an addictive gateway to harder drugs, critics have raised a new objection—that it saps motivation, especially among teens. This may be the case for some, but the National Assessment of Educational Progress reports that from 1970 to 2004, a period when cannabis availability and potency increased substantially, U.S. students' achievement scores in reading, writing, math, and science remained about the same. And according to the National Bureau of Economic Research American labor productivity has increased 15 percent since 2007. There is no evidence to suggest that cannabis has reduced Americans' overall motivation or achievement.

BLOODSHOT EYES? Many believe that smoking cannabis makes the eyes bloodshot, advertising that people have used it. Facial exposure to large amounts of any kind of smoke may cause red, bloodshot eyes, but today's high-potency cannabis is unlikely to produce a significant amount of smoke. Users need only a pinch of today's herb to achieve their desired effect. In addition, increasing numbers of users ingest cannabis-laced edibles rather than smoking it.

MORE—OR LESS—SEXUAL PLEASURE? Some people say that cannabis enhances lovemaking and don't have sex without it. Others say the herb ruins sex and never use it before lovemaking. In the one survey to address this issue, respondents were split. Sixty percent said cannabis enhances sex. Thirty percent said it ruins lovemaking. And 10 percent said the herb's sexual impact depends on their mood, their partner, and the cannabis strain.

Intriguing Possibilities

Laboratory studies suggest that CBD may reduce the aggressiveness of breast cancer. Animal studies hint that cannabis may slow the progression of dementia.

Rx Recommendations

When smoked, it takes 6 to 10 minutes to produce maximum blood levels of THC and CBD. When eaten, it takes an hour or two. When possible, use high-potency cannabis (15 percent THC or greater). This minimizes lung exposure to combustion products. If you use edibles, experiment to determine your therapeutic dose.

Safety

The most common side effect is dry mouth. Dizziness, lightheadedness, eye irritation, and cough are also possible. Long-term heavy use may impair memory and reduce male fertility.

Smoking cannabis may cause bronchial irritation, and heavy long-term use is associated with an increased risk of bronchitis. However, today's high-potency strains and increasing use of vapor inhalation devices have greatly reduced the amount of smoke most users inhale, which limits this problem. As part of the long-term Coronary Artery Risk Development in Young Adults study, University of California, San Francisco, researchers followed 5,115 adults from their 20s into their 40s. They found no association between smoking cannabis up to three times a month and lung impairment.

Those suffering schizophrenia, bipolar disorder, or severe depression should not use cannabis unless a doctor says they may.

Those with asthma, chronic obstructive pulmonary disease (COPD), or other chronic lung conditions should not smoke cannabis, but they may use edibles.

While cannabis is usually calming, anxiety attacks are possible. If you experience anxiety, panic, or paranoia, stop using it.

Pregnant and nursing women should not use cannabis.

Do not give cannabis to children.

In states with legal cannabis, edibles account for almost 100 percent of emergency room visits—cannabis cookies, brownies, cakes, and candies. Dose control is difficult with edibles, and many inexperienced users eat too much. If you use edibles, begin with a small amount, wait 2 hours, and eat more only if necessary.

Compared with alcohol, cannabis causes much less driving impairment, but most authorities recommend against driving while using it. There is some evidence that cannabis use increases risk of automobile fatalities. However, marijuana markers remain in the blood for days, so it remains unclear if exposed drivers involved in fatal crashes were high at the time or if they'd used the drug previously but were not intoxicated when they crashed. The effects of cannabis on driving are sure to be the subject of continuing research as the drug becomes increasingly legal.

There is no evidence that smoking cannabis increases risk of lung cancer. French researchers compared the cannabis histories of 1,212 people with lung cancer and 1,040 cancer-free controls. After controlling for tobacco use, they found no association between smoking cannabis and lung cancer. UCLA researchers conducted a similar study using 601 lung cancer cases and 1,040 controls and also found no reason to believe that cannabis causes lung cancer. Finally, Case Western Reserve researchers analyzed 19 studies of cannabis and lung damage. They found that smoking the herb damages lung tissue, but that even long-term use is not associated with lung cancer.

The following medications *increase* cannabis intoxication:

- Alcohol
- Erythromycin (Robimycin, Ilosone, Acnasol) antibiotic
- Clarithromycin (Biaxin) antibiotic
- Miconazole (Moniastat) antifungal
- Ketoconazole antifungal
- Itraconozole (Sporanox) antifungal
- Fluconazole (Diflucan, Trican) antifungal
- Diltiazem (Cardizem, Tiazac, Dilacor) angina, high blood pressure
- Verapamil (Calan, Veralan, Isoptin) cardiac arrhythmias
- Amiodorone (Cordarone) cardiac arrhythmias
- Isoniazid (Nydrazid, Rifamate) tuberculosis
- Ritonavir (Norvir) HIV

Cannabis is much less likely to cause dependence than opiates, tobacco, or alcohol. Nonetheless, dependence is possible. For suspected dependence, consult your physician.

Gardening

C. sativa grows to 20 feet, *C. indica* to 6 feet. Few pure-strain plants are available in the

United States. The vast majority are hybrids with one of the two strains dominant.

Cannabis is dioecious—some plants are male, others female. The female flowers produce more resin containing THC and CBD. Most growers use cuttings (clones) from female plants. Cannabis grows easily from seeds, hence its common name, weed, but seeds often produce less desirable males.

Cannabis tolerates many conditions, but prefers rich, well-watered soil. However, outdoor cultivation invites theft and arrest, so many growers have moved indoors using high-tech hydroponic systems. To grow cannabis indoors, buy one of the many books on the subject.

CARAWAY

The Ancient Egyptian Digestive Aid

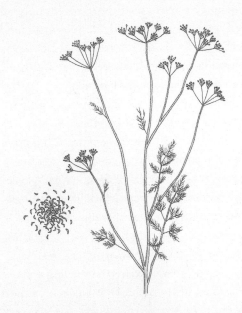

Family: Umbelliferae; other members include carrot, celery, parsley, fennel, and dill

Genus and species: *Carum carvi*

Also known as: Carum

Parts used: Fruits (seeds)

Caraway is best known as the seed that flavors rye bread. The reason it's in bread and other foods is that its seeds have been used since ancient times to calm the digestive tract and expel gas.

Caraway seeds have been found in prehistoric food remains from 3500 BC. The ancient Egyptians loved the seeds. The Ebers Papyrus, among the world's oldest surviving medical documents (1500 BC) recommended them for digestive upsets.

Healing History

Caraway is a rarity, an herb whose major medicinal uses have remained unchanged throughout history. The Greek physician Dioscorides mentioned the seeds to aid digestion, and herbals down through the ages have recommended them for indigestion, gas, and infant colic.

In Shakespeare's day, baked apples with caraway seeds were considered a stomach-soothing dessert. In *Henry IV*, a meal ends with "a pippin and a dish of caraway."

Seventeenth-century English herbalist Nicholas Culpeper noted that caraway "helpeth digestion . . . and easeth the pains of the wind colic."

America's 19th-century Eclectic physicians, forerunners of today's naturopaths, believed that the seeds "gently excite the digestive powers . . . [and can be] used in flatulent colic, especially of children."

Throughout history, in Europe, the Middle East, and early America, caraway was a favorite addition to laxative herbs because it tempered their frequently violent effects.

Caraway's only other traditional uses relate to women's health—for relieving menstrual cramps, promoting menstruation, and aiding milk production in nursing mothers.

Therapeutic Uses

The Egyptians were right about caraway. It's an effective digestive soother.

DIGESTIVE PROBLEMS. Modern researchers have discovered that two compounds in caraway seeds, carvol and carvene, soothe the smooth muscle tissue of the digestive tract and help expel gas.

In Germany, where herbal medicine is more mainstream than in the United States, a popular over-the-counter digestive product, Enteroplant, contains two active ingredients: peppermint oil (90 milligrams) and caraway oil (50 milligrams). German researchers gave 45 people with chronic indigestion either a placebo or Enteroplant (one capsule three times a day with meals). After 4 weeks, the placebo group reported no change in abdominal distress, but among those taking Enteroplant, 94.5 percent reported significant improvement, with 63 percent declaring themselves pain-free.

In another German study, after 2 weeks of daily use, a formula containing oils of peppermint, caraway, fennel, and wormwood produced similar relief. No wonder Commission E, the expert panel that evaluates herbal medicines for the German counterpart of the FDA, endorses caraway as a treatment for indigestion and abdominal distress.

IRRITABLE BOWEL SYNDROME. IBS causes an array of chronic, distressing symptoms: bloating, flatulence, abdominal pain and cramping, and diarrhea or constipation. German scientists gave 100 IBS sufferers either a placebo or Enteroplant (one capsule three times a day). A month later, 25 percent of the placebo group reported improvement, but in the herb group, 63 percent.

MENSTRUAL CRAMPS. The antispasmodics in caraway soothe not only the digestive tract but also other smooth muscles, such as those of the uterus. Thus, caraway may relax the uterus, not stimulate it. Women might try this herb for relief of menstrual cramps.

Rx Recommendations

Chew fresh caraway seeds a teaspoon at a time or mix them into food. To soften them, mix with water. They're often used in breads, soups, salads, stews, cheeses, sauerkraut, pickling brines, and meat dishes. Add them to just about any recipe.

Caraway oil is also used to flavor two digestive liqueurs: German Kummel and Scandinavian Aquavit.

For a pleasant-tasting infusion to aid digestion or relieve gas or menstrual cramping, use 2 to 3 teaspoons of crushed seeds per cup of boiling water. Steep for 10 to 20 minutes, then strain. Drink up to 3 cups a day.

If you prefer a homemade tincture, take $\frac{1}{2}$ to 1 teaspoon up to three times a day.

When using commercial preparations, follow the package directions.

For colic and gas, infants may be given low-strength caraway infusions.

Safety

There have been no reports of caraway causing harm. However, herbal oils are highly concentrated and small amounts—a teaspoon or two—may be toxic. Follow package directions.

Although the herb has antispasmodic properties, meaning that it may relax the uterus, it has been used historically to promote menstru-ation. Pregnant women should exercise caution.

Caraway may cause allergic reactions or other unexpected side effects. If any develop, reduce your dose or stop taking it. For more on herb safety, see Chapter 2.

If symptoms get worse or persist longer than 2 weeks, consult a health professional promptly.

Gardening

Caraway is an attractive biennial that reaches 2 feet. It has feathery leaves and umbrella-like clusters of tiny white flowers that bloom in early summer.

Caraway grows easily from seeds planted in spring $\frac{1}{2}$ inch deep and 8 inches apart. The plants like rich, well-drained soil and full sun. Keep them moist but not wet.

The first year, caraway produces a small rosette of leaves and a long taproot. Don't transplant it once it has become established. During the second year, caraway sends up its stem, reveals its feathery leaves, and produces its seeds.

Seeds appear in midsummer. Harvest them when they ripen. Leave some seeds behind, and the plants self-sow.

CASCARA SAGRADA

Goodbye Constipation

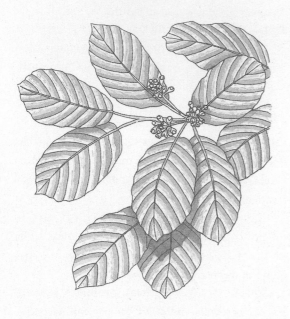

Family: Rhamnaceae; other members include buckthorn

Genus and species: *Rhamnus purshiana* or *Frangula purshiana*

Also known as: Cascara, sacred bark, and chittem bark

Part used: Bark

The 16th-century Spanish explorers who first visited northern California had a problem—constipation. Local Native Americans offered a solution, a tea made from the bark of a tree they held sacred. The herb worked, and the Spanish named it cascara sagrada, "sacred bark." It has been the answer to millions of prayers ever since. But the FDA calls it too hazardous to use.

Healing History

The Spanish recognized cascara sagrada as a relative of buckthorn, the powerful European herbal laxative. But cascara was gentler. The explorers sent some back to Spain, where its comparatively mild action was hailed as a wonder of the New World.

But Spanish explorers were more interested in finding gold than laxatives. For a long time, cascara remained a West Coast folk remedy, known as chittem bark, a polite variant of the Gold Rush '49ers' more vulgar name, sh—tin' bark.

Nineteenth-century Eclectic physicians, forerunners of today's naturopaths, touted cascara sagrada for "restoring bowel tone." In an 1877 home medical guide, one Eclectic extolled the herb's mildness, prompting Parke, Davis, the pharmaceutical firm, to market a commercial preparation. Cascara sagrada has been popular ever since. It entered the *U.S. Pharmacopoeia,* a standard drug reference, in 1890 and remains there today.

In Appalachian folk medicine, cascara sagrada has also been used to treat cancer. It was an ingredient in the popular but controversial Hoxsey Cancer Formula, an alternative therapy marketed from the 1930s to the 1950s by ex–coal miner Harry Hoxsey (see page 31).

Therapeutic Uses

Cascara sagrada contains anthraquinone laxative compounds.

CONSTIPATION. Commission E, the expert panel that evaluates herbal medicines for the German counterpart of the FDA, endorses cascara sagrada as a safe, effective laxative. Many European laxative products contain it.

In 19th- and 20th-century America, cascara sagrada was an ingredient in many over-the-counter laxatives. Today senna (see page 430) has largely replaced it. In 2002, the FDA banned cascara sagrada from over-the-counter laxatives, saying that it's too powerful and cathartic. However, it continues to be the active ingredient in a few prescription laxatives, among them: Cascara Aromatic and Aromatic Cascara Fluid Extract.

Intriguing Possibility

Harry Hoxsey may have been on the right track. Cascara sagrada contains aloe-emodin. In laboratory animals, this compound demonstrates antileukemia action, lending credence to the herb's use in treating cancer. Unfortunately, aloe-emodin is also toxic.

Rx Recommendations

Over-the-counter laxatives in the United States no longer contain cascara sagrada. If you'd like to use it, buy dried, year-old bark and prepare a decoction or ask your doctor for a prescription.

To prepare a decoction, boil 1 teaspoon of well-dried bark in 3 cups of water for 30 minutes, then strain and let cool to room temperature. Drink 1 to 2 cups a day. The taste is quite bitter. You may find that a tincture is more palatable; take $\frac{1}{2}$ teaspoon at bedtime.

When using a prescription product, follow the pharmacist's directions.

Safety

Anthraquinone laxatives are last resorts for constipation. First, increase your fiber intake (more fruits, vegetables, and whole grains), drink more fluids, and get more exercise. If that doesn't work, try a bulk-forming laxative, such as psyllium (page 370). And if that doesn't provide relief, try cascara sagrada.

Do not use cascara for more than 2 weeks. Over time, it causes lazy bowel syndrome, an inability to have bowel movements without chemical stimulation. If constipation persists, consult a physician.

Cascara bark must be stored for at least a year before use. The fresh herb contains compounds that can cause violent diarrhea and severe intestinal cramps. Drying results in milder action. Fresh bark may also be artificially dried by baking it at 250°F for several hours.

Cascara sagrada should not be used by anyone with ulcers, ulcerative colitis, Crohn's disease, irritable bowel syndrome, hemorrhoids, or other gastrointestinal conditions.

Pregnant and nursing women should not use cascara sagrada.

Do not give this herb to children.

If you're over 65, start with a low dose, and increase only if necessary.

Inform health professionals of the herbs you use. Problematic herb-drug interactions are possible.

Cascara sagrada may cause allergic reactions or other unexpected side effects. If any develop, reduce your dose or stop taking it. For more on herb safety, see Chapter 2.

If symptoms get worse or persist longer than 2 weeks, consult a health professional promptly.

Gardening

Cascara sagrada is an unassuming, 20-foot tree with reddish brown bark and thin, finely serrated leaves. It grows in the northwestern United States. It's not a garden herb.

CATNIP

Enjoy It with Kitty

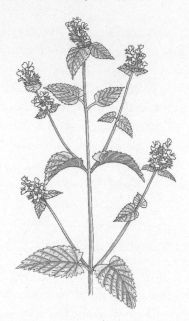

Family: Labiatae; other members include mints

Genus and species: *Nepeta cataria*

Also known as: Catmint, catnep, catswort, and field balm

Parts used: Flowers and leaves

Catnip makes most cats act drunk. But here's a case where one species' intoxicant is another's calmer. In people, catnip helps soothe the nerves and digestive tract. It offers gardeners handy first-aid and may also soothe menstrual cramps.

Healing History

From Europe to China, catnip has been used medicinally for at least 2,000 years. In teas, its lemon-minty vapors were considered a cold and cough remedy, relieving chest congestion and loosening phlegm. Old herbals praised its ability to promote sweating, a traditional treatment for fever.

Catnip has a long history of use as a tranquilizer, sedative, digestive aid, menstruation promoter, and treatment for menstrual cramps, flatulence, and infant colic. Centuries ago, people hung small bags of it around their necks to inhale its soothing vapors.

A blend of equal parts of catnip and saffron (page 408) was once recommended as a remedy for smallpox and scarlet fever. Catnip leaves were chewed to relieve toothache and, as crazy as this sounds today, smoked to treat bronchitis and asthma.

In pre-Elizabethan England, catnip was a popular beverage tea. During the Age of Exploration, a more stimulating Chinese herb, tea (*Camellia sinensis,* page 449) replaced it. But some English catnip lovers regretted this change. In her book *The Herb Garden*, a certain Miss Bardswell clucked, "Catmint Tea was . . . a good deal more wholesome."

Colonists introduced catnip into North America. The plant quickly went wild and now grows across the continent. Native Americans adopted it and used it as colonists did, as a beverage and to treat indigestion and colic.

Early Americans believed that catnip roots made even the kindest person mean. Hangmen consumed roots before executions to prepare for their work.

Catnip was listed as a stomach soother in the *U.S. Pharmacopoeia*, a standard drug reference, from 1842 to 1882 and in the *National Formulary*, the pharmacists' reference, from 1916 to 1950.

A 1969 report in the *Journal of the American Medical Association* claimed that when smoked, catnip produces marijuana-like intoxication. Newspapers ran screaming headlines, and bewildered pet shop owners reported a sudden run on cat toys.

The report was quickly discredited. Botanists flooded the medical journal with mail pointing out that the article's "catnip" photos were actually marijuana. Catnip has no history as a human intoxicant, and authorities quickly dismissed the notion that smoking it causes anything but sore throat.

Unfortunately, the same cannot be said for the popular press. As the late Varro E. Tyler, Ph.D., wrote in *Tyler's Honest Herbal*, "Once an erroneous statement appears in print, it is almost impossible to eradicate. Catnip is now listed in many books devoted to drugs of abuse as a mild intoxicant." For the record: It isn't.

Cat intoxication is another matter. A report in *Economic Botany* affirms that all cats are attracted to catnip, but only about two-thirds exhibit strong "feline catnip euphoria." Kitty euphoria is an inherited trait, and not all cats have the necessary gene.

Contemporary herbalists continue to embrace catnip. One writes, "Surely a plant with such a powerful impact on our feline friends . . . could not be destitute of medicinal value in humans." Modern herbals recommend catnip as a tranquilizer, sedative, digestive aid, and treatment for colds, colic, diarrhea, flatulence, and fever.

Therapeutic Uses

Modern herbalists tend to overstate this herb's value, but scientists have confirmed several of its traditional uses.

DIGESTIVE PROBLEMS. Like other

mints, catnip has antispasmodic action. It soothes the smooth muscles of the digestive tract. If you're prone to indigestion or heartburn, try a cup of catnip tea after meals.

INSOMNIA AND ANXIETY. German researchers report that the catnip compounds responsible for feline intoxication (nepetalactone isomers) are similar to the natural sedatives in valerian (valepotriates, page 473). This supports catnip's traditional use as a mild tranquilizer and sedative. If you feel tense or have trouble falling asleep, try a cup of catnip infusion.

INFECTIONS. Catnip has some antibiotic action, which lends credence to the herb's traditional use in some cases of diarrhea and fever. But it's not a particularly powerful antibiotic, so don't rely on it to prevent infection.

MENSTRUAL CRAMPS. Antispasmodics calm not only the digestive tract but also other smooth muscles, such as the uterus. Catnip's antispasmodic effect supports the traditional recommendation that it minimizes menstrual cramps.

Intriguing Possibility

Research at Iowa State University suggests that compounds in catnip oil are "highly effective" mosquito repellents—more effective than DEET. If you grow it, you can see for yourself. In late afternoon when mosquitoes come out, crush a few leaves, rub them on your skin, and see if you get bitten.

Rx Recommendations

Enjoy a pleasant, minty infusion as a digestive aid or mild tranquilizer or to soothe menstrual cramps.

For an infusion, use 2 teaspoons of dried herb per cup of boiling water. Steep for 10 to 20 minutes, then strain. (Do not boil catnip; boiling dissipates its healing oil.) Drink up to 3 cups a day.

If you prefer a homemade tincture, take ½ to 1 teaspoon up to three times a day.

When using commercial preparations, follow package directions.

For infant colic, you may give weak, cool catnip infusions cautiously in consultation with the child's doctor.

If you grow catnip, press some crushed leaves on minor garden cuts and scrapes to prevent infection until you can wash and bandage them.

Safety

Traditional herbalists recommended catnip as a menstruation promoter. There's no reason to believe this, but pregnant women should exercise caution and not take medicinal amounts.

Catnip is considered nontoxic, but some people may experience upset stomach or allergic reactions.

In children over 2, adjust the recommended dose based on the child's weight. Give a 50-pound child one-third of the dose a 150-pound adult would take.

If you're over 65, start with a low dose, and increase only if necessary.

Inform health professionals of the herbs you use. Problematic herb-drug interactions are possible.

Catnip may cause allergic reactions or other unexpected side effects. If any develop, reduce your dose or stop taking it. For more on herb safety, see Chapter 2.

If symptoms get worse or persist longer than 2 weeks, consult a health professional promptly.

Gardening

Catnip is a gray-green aromatic perennial that grows to 3 feet and bears all the hallmarks of the mint family: a square stem, fuzzy leaves, and twin-lipped flowers.

The herb grows easily from seeds or root divisions planted in spring or fall. It thrives in almost any well-drained soil with full sun or partial shade. Some growers say that keeping the soil on the dry side produces more aromatic plants. Thin seedlings to 18-inch spacing.

Harvest leaves and flowers in late summer when the plants are in bloom. Dry and store them in opaque, tightly sealed containers to preserve the volatile oil.

Gardeners' mythology holds that cats are not attracted to catnip in the ground. An old rhyme goes, "If you set it / Cats will get it. / But if you sow it / Cats won't know it." Don't believe it. Euphoric cats often roll all over sown plants.

The current consensus is that sowing, per se, does not keep cats away. The key is to prevent leaf bruising. Unbruised plants reportedly hold little attraction for cats. Any bruising, however, releases the aromatic oil, and cats come running.

CAT'S CLAW
The Peruvian "Life-Giver"

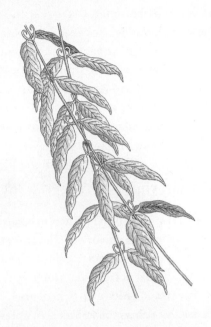

Family: Rubiaceae; other members include coffee and gardenia

Genus and species: *Uncaria tomentosa, U. guianensis*

Also known as: *Una de gato,* life-giving vine of Peru

Parts used: Inner bark

Cat's claw—in Spanish, *una de gato*—is a climbing, woody South American vine whose strands can grow longer than 1,000 feet. It climbs trees with the help of curved spines that resemble—guess what. It first attracted American herbalists' attention in the early 1990s. It's still a minor medicinal herb. But that may change as its benefits become more widely known.

Healing History

Indigenous South Americans have used cat's claw's inner root bark for centuries to spur wound healing and treat intestinal distress. In Peru, where cat's claw is particularly popular, herbalists recommend it for dysentery, gonorrhea, and cancers. Some Amazon Indian tribes believe that cat's claw has "life-giving" powers. They drink a cup of decoction weekly to prevent all manner of disease.

Therapeutic Uses

OSTEOARTHRITIS (OA). When people complain of arthritis, they mean OA. Several studies confirm that cat's claw has anti-inflammatory and pain-relieving action. At the Peruvian National University Medical School in Lima, researchers gave either a placebo or cat's claw to 45 people with OA of the knee. After 4 weeks, both groups reported less pain, but the herb group significantly less. The researchers concluded: "Cat's claw is an effective treatment for osteoarthritis."

RHEUMATOID ARTHRITIS (RA). Compared with OA, RA is not as common—2.5 million Americans have it—but it's more severe and may cause joint deformity and impairment. At Innsbruck University Hospital, Austrian scientists gave 40 RA sufferers standard drugs plus a placebo or cat's claw. After 6 months, the herb group reported significantly fewer painful, swollen joints.

IMMUNE ENHANCEMENT. Life-giving is a stretch, but cat's claw boosts immune function. It increases the number of germ-fighting white blood cells. It stimulates them to gobble up more germs. And it increases levels of the key immune proteins, interleukin-1 and -6. Writing in the *Journal of Ethnopharmacology*, Canadian researchers confirm what Amazonian Indians believe, that this herb is a "strong immunostimulant," make it useful in preventing and treating all manner of infections.

ANTIOXIDANT. Cat's claw also has antioxidant action. Antioxidants help prevent the DNA damage at the root of heart disease, cancer, and many other conditions. The herb has been shown to prevent cell mutations that can lead to cancer. Swedish researchers gave a dozen people a drug known to damage DNA. Subsequently, four of them took a placebo while the eight others took cat's claw (250 milligrams/day or 350 milligrams/day). After 8 weeks, the herb groups showed significantly greater DNA repair and less DNA damage. It's still too early to call cat's claw a cancer treatment, but when Italian researchers exposed rapidly dividing human breast cancer cells to an extract of the herb, it reduced cancer-spreading cell division 90 percent.

Intriguing Possibilities

Animal studies suggest that cat's claw lowers cholesterol and relaxes the arteries, lowering blood pressure. If it has the same effects in humans, it might be used to prevent and treat heart disease and stroke.

Rx Recommendations

To make a decoction, boil 1 teaspoon of powdered bark per cup of water for 1 minutes. Drink 1 to 3 cups a day.

If using tincture, the recommended dose is

1 to 2 teaspoons two to three times a day.

When using a standardized extract, the recommended dose ranges from 350 to 700 milligrams/day. Follow label directions.

Safety

Cat's claw is nontoxic and rarely causes side effects, but in rare cases, headache, dizziness, and stomach upset have been reported.

Because it stimulates the immune system, cat's claw should not be used by those suffering autoimmune conditions (lupus, multiple sclerosis) or taking immune-suppressing medications (organ transplant or skin graft recipients).

Pregnant and nursing women should not use cat's claw.

Do not give cat's claw to children under 2. In older children, adjust the recommended dose based on the child's weight. Give a 50-pound child one-third of the dose a 150-pound adult would take.

If you're over 65, start with a low dose, and increase only if necessary.

Inform health professionals of the herbs you use. Problematic herb-drug interactions are possible.

Cat's claw may cause allergic reactions or other unexpected side effects. If any develop, reduce your dose or stop taking it. For more on herb safety, see Chapter 2.

If symptoms get worse or persist longer than 2 weeks, consult a health professional promptly.

Gardening

Not grown in the United States.

CELERY

Good for Gout and High Blood Pressure

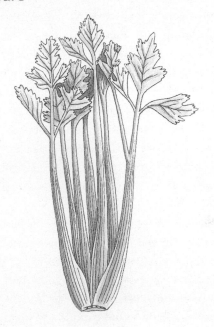

Family: Umbelliferae; other members include carrot and parsley

Genus and species: *Apium graveolens*

Also known as: Marsh parsley and wild celery

Parts used: Stalks and fruits (seeds)

Dieters often eat celery stalks, believing that chewing the stringy vegetable burns more calories than it contains. Most experts dismiss this as a myth.

However, celery does more than add crunch to salads. Scientists have discovered a surprising number of healing benefits in its stalks and especially its seeds. This herb may help relieve gout, insomnia, high blood pressure, and high cholesterol.

Healing History

The ancient Greeks gave celery wine to winning athletes. Celery drinks have been used medicinally throughout history. A contemporary echo of this, minus any medicinal claims, is the celery seed soft drink, Dr. Brown's Cel-Ray Soda, available in New York City, Philadelphia, and South Florida, but hard to obtain elsewhere.

For centuries, India's traditional Ayurvedic physicians have prescribed celery seed as a diuretic to treat water retention (edema). They also recommend it as a treatment for colds, flu, indigestion, arthritis, and diseases of the liver and spleen.

The medieval German abbess/herbalist Hildegard of Bingen wrote, "Whoever is plagued by gout . . . should powder celery seeds . . . because this is the best remedy." English herbalist John Gerard claimed celery "provoketh urine" as an aid to weight loss and expelled "phlegm out of the head." And 17th-century England's Nicholas Culpeper recommended celery seed as a diuretic for dropsy (congestive heart failure).

Later herbalists suggested celery to treat insomnia, obesity, nervousness, and several cancers, to promote menstruation, and to induce abortion. It has even been recommended as an aphrodisiac.

Oddly, for America's 19th-century botanical physicians, celery did not impress the Eclectics, forerunners of today's naturopaths. They considered the herb a footnote to its close relative, parsley. If parsley was unavailable, the Eclectics grudgingly recommended celery as "a nerve tonic" and remedy for arthritis and chest congestion.

Contemporary herbalists recommend celery as a diuretic, tranquilizer, sedative, and menstruation promoter and as a treatment for gout, arthritis, obesity, anxiety, and lack of appetite (gustatory, not sexual).

Therapeutic Uses

Few studies have investigated the medicinal benefits of celery, but research to date validates several of the herb's traditional uses.

GOUT. Eight hundred years after Hildegard of Bingen endorsed celery as "best" for gout, science has endorsed her claim. Gout is caused by a buildup of uric acid that forms crystals in the joints, notably the big toe.

In the 1990s, James A. Duke, Ph.D., the U.S. Department of Agriculture's herbal medicine authority (retired), developed gout. "My doctor urged me to take the drug allopurinol. I did, until I read a study showing that celery seed extract speeds elimination of uric acid. It seemed as though four daily 800-milligram tablets of celery seed extract would provide protection equivalent to allopurinol. Now, I'm a believer. My uric acid level has stayed below the level that triggers gout. I haven't had any gout attacks since I began using celery seed."

Of course, one testimonial does not prove that celery seed extract works. If you'd like to try it, consult your doctor.

HIGH BLOOD PRESSURE. Chinese medical practitioners recommend celery for high blood pressure. To mainstream physicians, this seemed ludicrous. Celery stalks contains considerable salt (sodium), which often raises blood pressure.

Then in 1992, Minh Le, father of a University of Chicago medical student, was diagnosed with high blood pressure. His doctor prescribed standard medication. Le ignored his doctor and began eating a quarter-pound of celery a day (about four stalks). Before long, his blood pressure dropped from 158/96 to 118/82.

Le's son, Quang Le, and University of Chicago pharmacologist William Elliot, Ph.D., isolated the active compound (3-n-butyl phthalide) and injected rats with an amount equal to four stalks of celery. The animals' blood pressure dropped 13 percent, and their cholesterol declined 7 percent.

If you want to add celery to your high blood pressure treatment regimen, consult your doctor. It might help. But if you're especially salt-sensitive, it may do more harm than good.

HIGH CHOLESTEROL. In addition to the 3-n-butyl phthalide it contains, celery is high in fiber, which helps reduce cholesterol.

CONGESTIVE HEART FAILURE. Doctors prescribe diuretics to treat both high blood pressure and congestive heart failure, which involves serious fluid buildup in the body. Celery seed has been shown to have diuretic action, which supports its traditional role as a treatment for congestive heart failure. If you'd like to try celery seed for this purpose, consult your doctor.

DIABETES. Several studies have indicated that celery seed reduces blood sugar (glucose), which is key to managing diabetes. Diabetes requires professional treatment. If you'd like to use celery seed as part of your treatment plan, ask your physician.

ANXIETY AND INSOMNIA. Celery seed oil contains phthalides, compounds that sedate animals. Of course, findings in animals don't always apply to humans, but if you're anxious, nervous, or wakeful, the herb can't hurt.

WOMEN'S HEALTH. Celery seed stimulates uterine contractions in animals, lending support to its traditional uses in promoting menstruation and inducing abortion. For this reason, pregnant women should not consume the seeds or their oil. The stalks may be eaten safely.

Other women may want to try celery seed to bring on their periods. But don't use the herb to try to induce abortion.

Diuretics help relieve the bloated feeling caused by premenstrual fluid retention. Women who are bothered by premenstrual syndrome might try some celery seed during the uncomfortable days before their periods.

Intriguing Possibilities

Celery contains psoralens, compounds used to treat psoriasis and, more recently, one form of cancer, cutaneous T-cell lymphoma. Might celery help? Currently we don't know, but it's possible.

Medicinal Myth

Celery seed's diuretic action lends some credence to its traditional use in treating obesity. However, lost water weight usually returns. Celery may aid weight loss in the short term, but the key to permanent weight control is a low-calorie, low-fat, plant-based diet and daily exercise.

Rx Recommendations

To treat gout, ask your doctor about adding four 800-milligram tablets of celery seed extract a day to your treatment program.

To treat high blood pressure, high cholesterol, or congestive heart failure, eat four stalks of celery a day, in consultation with your doctor.

For a pleasant-tasting, relaxing infusion that might help treat diabetes, use 1 to 2 teaspoons of freshly crushed seeds per cup of boiling water. Steep for 10 to 20 minutes, then strain. Drink up to 3 cups a day.

When using a tincture, take ½ to 1 teaspoon up to three times a day or follow package directions.

Safety

Diuretics should be used in consultation with a physician. They can deplete body stores of potassium, an essential nutrient. People who use them should also eat foods high in potassium to replace lost electrolytes—bananas and fresh vegetables.

High blood pressure, elevated cholesterol, congestive heart failure, and diabetes are potentially serious conditions. Celery seed may help manage them, but it should be used in consultation with your physician as part of an overall treatment plan.

Do not give celery seed extract to children under 2. In older children, adjust the recommended dose based on the child's weight. Give a 50-pound child one-third of the dose a 150-pound adult would take.

If you're over 65, start with a low dose, and increase only if necessary.

Inform health professionals of the herbs you use. Problematic herb-drug interactions are possible.

If symptoms get worse or persist longer than 2 weeks, consult a health professional promptly.

Gardening

Celery thrives in well-watered, richly organic soil. Less ideal conditions produce tougher, stringier, more bitter stalks.

In mild climates, celery grows virtually year-round. Elsewhere, start seeds indoors in January and plant seedlings in early spring after the danger of frost has passed. Soak the seeds before planting.

Germination takes about 10 days. Transplant at approximately 3 months, when the seedlings are about 3 inches high. Space the plants about 6 inches apart, and water copiously. The juiciness of the stalks depends on how much water the plants receive. Harvest seeds when they mature.

The psoralens in celery sometimes cause rashes in agricultural workers. Gardeners, take note: Wearing sunscreen prevents this.

CHAMOMILE

Pretty, Fragrant Flowers,
Potent Medicine

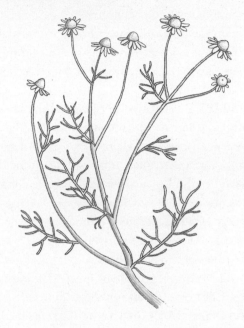

Family: Compositae; other members include daisy, dandelion, and marigold

Genus and species: *Matricaria chamomilla* (German or Hungarian) and *Anthemis nobilis* (Roman or English)

Also known as: Camomile, matricaria, anthemis, and ground apple

Parts used: Flowers

In "The Tale of Peter Rabbit," the young bunny eats himself sick in Mr. McGregor's garden, then gets chased out at the wrong end of the angry farmer's hoe. When Peter gets home, his mother gives him chamomile tea.

Peter's mother was a wise herbalist. Chamomile helps treat indigestion and soothes jangled nerves. Perhaps Peter's mother feared that his ordeal might give him an ulcer. Chamomile helps prevent them. Or maybe Mr. McGregor's hoe grazed Peter's tender skin. Chamomile compresses help heal superficial wounds.

Unfortunately, few people who sip tasty, apple-flavored chamomile tea realize what a healer they hold in their paws . . . sorry, hands.

Healing History

Chamomile is not one herb but two: German (or Hungarian) chamomile and Roman (or English) chamomile. The two plants are botanically unrelated, but oddly, both produce the same light blue oil that's been used medicinally since ancient times.

Chamomile's daisy-like flowers reminded the ancient Egyptians of the sun. They used the herb to treat fever, particularly the recurring fevers of malaria.

The Greek physician Dioscorides, the Roman naturalist Pliny, and India's ancient Ayurvedic physicians prescribed chamomile to treat headaches and kidney, liver, and bladder problems.

Germans have used chamomile since the dawn of history to ease digestive upsets, promote menstruation, and relieve menstrual cramps.

The 17th-century English herbalist Nicholas Culpeper recommended chamomile for fevers, digestive problems, aches, pains, jaundice, kidney stones, and dropsy (congestive heart failure) and "to bring down women's courses" (promote menstruation).

British and German immigrants introduced both chamomiles into North America. Today, most American-grown chamomile is the German variety.

America's 19th-century Eclectic physicians,

forerunners of today's naturopaths, recommended chamomile poultices to speed wound healing and prevent gangrene. They prescribed infusions for digestive problems, malaria, typhus, menstrual cramps, and menstruation promotion and for all birth-related difficulties: to quiet fetal kicking, arrest premature labor, relieve sore breasts and nipples, suppress milk production, and treat infant colic.

Today, chamomile is one of the nation's bestselling herbs, not as a medicine, but as a beverage tea, by itself or in blends. Its apple aroma gives many herbal skin care products their fragrance, and it has been used in shampoos since the Vikings because it adds luster to blond hair.

Medicinally, contemporary herbalists recommend chamomile as an external treatment for wounds and inflammation and as an internal treatment for fever, digestive upsets, anxiety, and insomnia.

Therapeutic Uses

In Germany, where herbal medicine is more mainstream than in the United States, one pharmaceutical company markets a popular chamomile product called Kamillosan. The Germans use it externally for wounds and inflammations and internally for indigestion and ulcers. Kamillosan is available in the United States—search it on the Internet.

Chamomile is so popular among Germans that many call the herb *alles zutraut*, or "capable of anything." That's an exaggeration, but not by much.

DIGESTIVE PROBLEMS. Dozens of studies support chamomile's traditional use as a digestive aid. Several compounds in chamomile oil—primarily bisabolol—relax the smooth muscle tissues that lines the digestive tract (antispasmodic). In fact, one study showed that chamomile relaxes the digestive tract as well as the opium-based drug papaverine.

Commission E, the expert panel that evaluates herbal medicines for the German counterpart of the FDA, endorses chamomile for gastrointestinal conditions.

ANXIETY. Chamomile's long history as a tranquilizer has a scientific basis. Argentinian researchers discovered that a compound in the oil, apigenin, binds to the same cell receptors as diazepam (Valium), suggesting that chamomile has similar effects. Japanese researchers induced stress in laboratory animals, and when they treated the animals with chamomile, stress hormone levels fell significantly.

Philadelphia researchers gave 57 anxiety sufferers either a placebo or chamomile extract (220 milligrams/day to 1,100 milligrams/day). After 8 weeks, the chamomile group showed significantly less anxiety.

In another British report, chronic anxiety sufferers received massages using one of two lotions—a placebo or a lotion containing chamomile oil. Both treatments reduced anxiety, but "the addition of chamomile oil seems to enhance the effect and to improve physical and psychological symptoms, as well as quality of life."

INSOMNIA. A British study has shown that chamomile is a mild sedative, which confirms its tranquilizing action. University of Michigan researchers gave 34 longtime insomniacs either a placebo or chamomile (270 milligrams twice a day). Before and after survyes showed that the chamomile group fell asleep faster, woke up less, and slept longer.

WOUND HEALING. Iranian researchers

treated 72 people's surgical wounds with either the topical steroid (hydrocortisone) or chamomile (compresses of a strong infusion twice a day). After 28 days, the herb-treated wounds healed faster.

DIARRHEA. German researchers gave either a placebo or chamomile tea to 79 children with diarrhea. The kids ranged from 6 months to 6 years. After 3 days, more of those in the chamomile group were cured.

DEPRESSION. British researchers used standard psychological tests to assess mood in 200 people and then gave them chamomile. Their mood improved. Chamomile's mood-elevating effects are mild. It's unlikely to have any impact on those with serious depression. But for minor everyday blues, a cup of chamomile tea might help.

OSTEOARTHRITIS. Ninety-nine adults with arthritis of the knee participated in an Iranian study, using one of three treatments: a placebo ointment, a salve containing a standard pharmaceutical (diclofenac), or one with chamomile (a concentrated infusion mixed with sesame oil). In addition they were allowed to take Tylenol and recorded its use. After 3 weeks, the chamomile group took the least Tylenol.

INFECTIONS. The Eclectic physicians were onto something when they suggested using chamomile compresses to prevent wound infections. Some studies show that chamomile oil applied to the skin speeds the healing of burns. The herb also has anti-inflammatory action, thanks to the azulene it contains. Commission E endorses chamomile topically as a wound treatment.

Other studies show that the herb impairs replication of polio virus and kills *Staphylococcus* bacteria and *Candida albicans*, the yeast fungus that cause vaginal infections.

IMMUNE STIMULATION. No one knew why chamomile prevented infections until British researchers discovered that it stimulates the immune system's infection-fighting white blood cells (macrophages and B-lymphocytes).

MENSTRUAL CRAMPS. Antispasmodics relax not only the digestive tract but also other smooth muscles, such as the uterus. Chamomile's antispasmodic properties support its age-old use to soothe menstrual cramps and reduce the risk of premature labor.

Oddly, however, chamomile was also used to stimulate menstruation. The apparent contradiction remains unresolved, but European researchers have isolated a substance in chamomile that stimulates uterine contractions. It's not clear which effect predominates.

ARTHRITIS. In animal studies, chamomile has relieved joint inflammation. Animal findings don't necessarily apply to people, but traditional herbalists recommended chamomile to treat arthritis. See if it works for you.

Intriguing Possibility

Japanese animal studies suggest that chamomile may help heal gastrointestinal ulcers and control blood sugar levels.

Rx Recommendations

For a pleasant, refreshing, apple-flavored infusion, use 2 to 3 heaping teaspoons of flowers per cup of boiling water. Steep for 10 to 20 minutes, then strain. Drink up to 3 cups a day.

As a homemade tincture, take 1/2 to 1 teaspoon up to three times a day.

When using commercial preparations, follow package directions.

Feel free to give weak infusions of chamomile cautiously to children under age two for colic. For older children and adults over age 65, start with low-strength preparations and increase the strength if necessary.

Try a chamomile infusion when you feel anxious, or add chamomile flowers to a hot bath. Just tie a handful of chamomile flowers into a cloth and run the bath water over it, inhaling the vapors.

For cuts, scrapes, and burns, brew a strong infusion, then soak a clean cloth in the liquid and apply it as a compress.

Safety

Controversy about chamomile erupted in the 1970s, when a report in the *Journal of Allergy and Clinical Immunology* claimed that it might cause a potentially fatal allergic reaction (anaphylaxis) in those allergic to its botanical cousin, ragweed. Herb critics immediately warned the millions of people with ragweed allergy to shun the herb. Herb advocates insisted that chamomile had been vilified unfairly.

To settle the issue, researchers compiled all world-wide reports of chamomile-induced allergic reactions from the 95-year period from 1887 to 1982. The grand total: no deaths and 50 allergic reactions—45 involving Roman chamomile and just 5 involving German, the type typically grown in the United States.

Chamomile poses no significant health hazard. The only people who should think twice about using it (and its close botanical relative, yarrow, page 487) are those with histories of previous anaplylaxis from ragweed.

Of course, adverse reactions are possible. Large amounts of highly concentrated chamomile preparations—much more concentrated than the typical infusion—have caused nausea and vomiting.

Women should feel free to try chamomile both to soothe menstrual cramps and to promote the onset of menstruation, but women who are pregnant or trying to conceive should steer clear of medicinal amounts.

Inform health professionals of the herbs you use. Problematic herb-drug interactions are possible.

Chamomile may cause unexpected side effects. If any develop, reduce your dose or stop taking it. For more on herb safety, see Chapter 2.

If symptoms get worse or persist longer than 2 weeks, consult a health professional promptly.

Gardening

German chamomile is an annual that reaches 3 feet. The Roman herb is a perennial groundcover that rarely exceeds 9 inches. Both have downy stems, feathery leaves, and daisy-like flowers with yellow centers and white rays.

The German variety grows easily when sown in spring after frost danger has passed. Scatter the tiny seeds on well-prepared beds, then gently tamp them down. Seedlings up to 2 inches tall transplant well; taller plants do not.

German chamomile prefers sandy, well-drained soil in partially shaded gardens. It shrivels under full sun. The plant flowers at about 6 weeks, producing lush flowers even in the short summers of northern climes. Flowering lasts several weeks, and if some are left unharvested, the plant self-sows. Don't leave too many, though, as this herb may become a pest.

Perennial Roman chamomile comes in two subtypes: single-flower and double-flower. Herbalists prefer the double-flower variety, which adapts to almost any soil but favors moist, well-manured loam. Seeds may be sown, but most gardeners prefer to propagate from off-shoots. Plant them about 18 inches apart in early spring. Roman chamomile is quite hardy, but if your winters are particularly severe, protect the plants with mulch.

Oddly enough, Roman chamomile grows best when it's stepped on. In Britain, it is often used as a ground cover on garden paths. Walking on it releases the herb's lovely apple fragrance and does not hurt the plant. After harvesting, dry the flowers and store them in sealed containers to preserve their volatile oil.

CHAPARRAL

A Cavity-Preventive Mouthwash

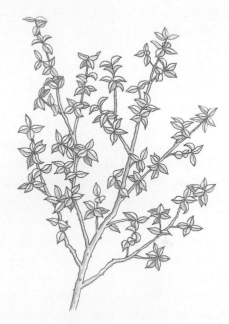

Family: Zygophyllaceae; other members include caltrop, star thistle, and bean caper

Genus and species: *Larrea divaricata* and *L. tridentata*

Also known as: Stinkweed, greasewood, and creosote bush

Parts used: Twigs and leaflets

Chaparral smells nasty and tastes horrible. Nonetheless, it's most widely used in mouthwashes.

We're not talking minty fresh here. You wouldn't want to reach for chaparral mouthwash before puckering up for a kiss. But the unassuming shrub, native to the American Southwest, contains a compound, nordihydroguaiaretic acid (NDGA) that kills some of the germs that cause tooth decay. NDGA also kills other microorganisms that turn fats and oils rancid.

Healing History

If, as many believe, effective medicines smell foul and taste terrible, chaparral should be a wonderful healer. Its leaves exude a waxy resin that smells like creosote, hence its popular names: stinkweed, greasewood, and creosote bush (though the plant contains no actual creosote).

Native Americans of the Southwest rubbed chaparral resin on burns. They used its tea to treat colds, bronchitis, chickenpox, snakebite, and arthritis. And they heated the tips of chapparal twigs and applied the hot resin to painful teeth.

White settlers adopted the plant, using it externally for bruises, rashes, dandruff, and wounds and internally for diarrhea, upset stomach, menstrual problems, venereal diseases, and several cancers.

Chaparral was listed as an expectorant (to clear mucus from the respiratory system) and bronchial antiseptic in the *U.S. Pharmacopoeia,* a standard drug reference, from 1842 to 1942. Today, few herbalists mention it, though some suggest it externally to prevent wound infections and internally to treat intestinal parasites and bacterial and viral infections.

Therapeutic Uses

Chaparral is both intriguing and controversial.

TOOTH DECAY AND GUM DISEASE. Chaparral's traditional use as a toothache treatment spurred scientists to test it against the bacteria that cause tooth decay and gum disease. A study in the *Journal of Dental Research* showed that chaparral mouthwash reduced cavities 75 percent.

Oral microorganisms also cause gum disease, the leading cause of adult tooth loss. Chaparral mouthwash is no substitute for regular brushing and flossing, but it may provide added protection.

WOUNDS. The NGDA in chaparral is a potent antiseptic with antibacterial and antifungal action, lending credence to the herb's traditional use as a wound treatment.

DEGENERATIVE ILLNESS PREVENTION. NGDA is a powerful antioxidant that helps prevent the cell damage at the root of many degenerative conditions: heart disease, cataracts, and many cancers.

Intriguing Possibilities

Life-extension advocates say that antioxidants like NGDA help slow the aging process and may even extend the human life span. One French study found that NGDA significantly lengthens the average life span of laboratory animals. Other scientists claim that the chemical almost doubles the average life span of laboratory insects. While science has not yet found a way to extend the human life span, these results are certainly intriguing.

Animal studies suggest that chaparral has anti-inflammatory action, lending support to its traditional use in treating arthritis.

Rx Recommendations

To prepare a mouthwash or an infusion, use 1 tablespoon of dried leaves and stems per quart of boiling water. Steep for 1 hour, then strain. Gargle or drink up to 3 cups a day. To mask its unpleasant taste, add honey and lemon or mix it with a beverage tea.

Safety

Chaparral is safe for use as a mouthwash—assuming you spit it out.

Since 1990, there have been 18 reports of liver damage in people taking chaparral. Most used tablets or capsules, not the tea traditionally preferred in herbal medicine. One person developed liver damage after only 3 weeks, but most took chaparral for several months. Most were also using other liver-damaging substances, such as alcohol and over-the-counter and/or prescription drugs. In all cases, the liver abnormalities cleared up after they stopped using chaparral.

In 1992, after reports of a half-dozen cases of liver damage, the American Herbal Products Association (AHPA) asked members to voluntarily suspend chaparral sales pending the outcome of an investigation. Scientists at the University of Texas Health Sciences Center reviewed case reports supplied by the FDA. They found no pattern clear enough to warrant action against chaparral. So, in 1995, the AHPA rescinded its voluntary suspension request. The FDA has taken no action against sale of the herb.

Still, in light of the possibility of liver damage, no one with liver disease or a history of it should ingest chaparral. Nor should it be used by anyone who is alcoholic or taking any medication regularly—including over-the-counter drugs.

Others who wish to try chaparral should use an infusion, not tablets or capsules, and should not take it for longer than a few months. Stop using chaparral if you develop any signs of liver trouble, such as nausea, fatigue, fever, or jaundice (dark-colored urine or yellowing of the eyes).

Pregnant or nursing women should not take chaparral.

Do not give chaparral to children.

If you're over 65, start with a low dose, and increase only if necessary.

Inform health professionals of the herbs you use. Problematic herb-drug interactions are possible.

Chaparral may cause allergic reactions or other unexpected side effects. If any develop, reduce your dose or stop taking it. For more on herb safety, see Chapter 2.

If symptoms get worse or persist longer than 2 weeks, consult a health professional promptly.

Gardening

Chaparral is a woody, olive green or yellow shrub that dominates the arid Southwest. It grows to about 10 feet and resembles dwarf oak. Its roots radiate far beyond its above-ground parts and release compounds that kill other plants. Chaparral is not a garden herb.

CHASTE TREE

Balancing Hormones Naturally

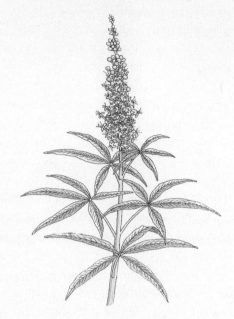

Family: Verbenaceae; other members include verbenas and many tropical trees and shrubs

Genus and species: *Vitex agnus-castus*

Also known as: Vitex, monk's pepper, and wild pepper

Parts used: Fruits (berries)

Chaste tree produces small, dark fruits resembling peppercorns. Since ancient times, Europeans believed that they suppressed women's libido. Vowing chastity, nuns used the fruits to suppress sexual urges, hence the name chaste tree. The plant's species name, *agnus-castus*, means "chaste lamb."

This herb has no documented effect on libido, but it changes the balance of female sex hormones, making it useful for several women's health conditions.

Healing History

Native to the Mediterranean, chaste tree was well-known to ancient Greek physicians. Hippocrates, the father of mainstream Western medicine, recommended it as a treatment for injuries and inflammations.

Dioscorides, author of the West's first herbal, *De Materia Medica (On Medicines)*, recognized chaste tree's effect on the female reproductive system, especially its ability to increase nursing mothers' milk production. He recommended the leaves and berries to treat lactation problems and to expel the placenta and control post-delivery bleeding. "If blood flows from the womb," Dioscorides wrote, "let the woman drink dark red wine in which the leaves of the chaste tree have been steeped."

In the *Iliad*, Homer calls the herb a symbol of virginity. In ancient Rome, the vestal virgins carried chaste tree twigs as symbols of their chastity. Oddly, however, during the 1st century AD, the Roman naturalist Pliny cited chaste tree as an aphrodisiac.

During the Middle Ages, chaste tree flowers were strewn on the ground before the feet of novitiates as they entered convents and monasteries, symbolically preparing them for lifelong chastity. Monks ate the fruits to suppress sexual urges, hence one of the plant's common names, monk's pepper.

During times of war or social upheaval, when Asian black pepper was difficult to obtain, Europeans used peppery chaste tree fruits as a substitute, hence another of the plant's common names, wild pepper.

Nineteenth-century American Eclectic physicians, forerunners of today's naturopaths, prescribed chaste tree berries to increase milk production in nursing mothers.

Therapeutic Uses

Modern research has shown that chaste tree targets the pituitary gland, increasing production of luteinizing hormone and decreasing secretion of follicle-stimulating hormone. These changes influence the balance of female sex hormones, reducing levels of estrogen and increasing levels of progesterone.

PREMENSTRUAL SYNDROME (PMS). Shifting the estrogen-progesterone balance helps relieve the irritability, breast tenderness, fluid retention, and other symptoms of PMS. In Germany, where herbal medicine is more mainstream than in the United States, an over-the-counter tincture of chaste tree (Agnolyt) has been marketed since the 1950s as a treatment for PMS. German women consider the herb particularly helpful for relieving PMS-related bloating and breast tenderness.

Several studies support the use of chaste tree for PMS symptoms. In one German trial, 1,542 women took 50 drops of chaste tree tincture daily for 6 months. Ninety percent reported substantial or complete relief of PMS symptoms.

In another German trial, 175 women with PMS took either chaste tree (50 drops) or vitamin B_6 (200 milligrams/day), a treatment with demonstrated effectiveness for premenstrual complaints. After 3 months, 61 percent called B_6 helpful, but chaste tree relieved PMS in 77 percent.

British researchers gave a placebo or chaste tree to 600 women. After 3 months, the herb showed significant benefit for relieving premenstrual discomfort.

Australian scientists analyzed six rigorous clinical trials. Five showed chaste tree effective for PMS. Commission E, the German counter-part of the FDA, approves chaste tree for prevention and treatment of premenstrual discomforts.

MENSTRUAL PROBLEMS. Chaste tree's hormonal effects also help relieve menstrual problems, notably scant or heavy flow and midcycle spotting. In one German study, 126 reproductive-age women took 40 drops of chaste tree tincture every day for several months. The women experienced significant normalization of their menstrual cycles.

Women with erratic cycles, scant or unusually heavy menstrual flow, midcycle spotting, nonovulatory periods, or menstrual cramps might try chaste tree in consultation with a physician. Commission E approves chaste tree for menstrual irregularity.

MENSTRUAL-RELATED BREAST PAIN. Czech studies show that chaste tree relieves cyclic breast pain (mastalgia). In one, 97 women with breast pain took either a placebo or the herb (30 drops of tincture twice a day). After three cycles, those using chaste tree reported significantly greater relief. Commission E, the German counterpart of the FDA for herbal medicines, approves chaste tree for cyclic mastalgia.

LACTATION PROBLEMS. The ancients were right: A German study shows that after taking the herb for several weeks, nursing mothers' milk production increased.

LIBIDO REDUCTION. In men, chaste tree reduces levels of the male sex hormone, testosterone. Most men produce more testosterone than necessary to fuel normal libido, so suppressing it has little effect. But in the small proportion of men with low testosterone, the herb might reduce libido, suggesting that some of the monks who prayed for it to inhibit their libido might have had their prayers answered.

Intriguing Possibility

German researchers gave a placebo or chaste tree to 96 women suffering infertility. After 3 months, in the placebo group, 36 percent became pregnant. In the herb group, the figure was 57 percent. However, these results did not quite reach statistical significance, so they might have occurred by chance. Nonetheless, chaste tree may help treat infertility.

In laboratory studies, chaste tree has suppressed the growth of cervical, uterine, ovarian, and breast cancer cells. It's too early to call it a treatment for these diseases, but in the future, that's possible.

Rx Recommendations

Most studies with chaste tree have used standardized tinctures—100 milliliters contains the equivalent of 9 grams of dried berries. The standard dose is 40 drops daily for at least 12 weeks.

Chaste tree capsules are also available. Recommended doses vary from 30 to 175-milligrams/day. Follow package directions.

Chaste tree may increase lactation in a few weeks, but for other indications, allow a few months.

Safety

Chaste tree has never been linked to any significant side effects, but minor problems are possible. In the 6-month German study of PMS, 17 women dropped out because of stomach upset. A few cases of itching, rash, fatigue, and hair loss have also been reported.

Pregnant women should not use this herb.

Do not give chaste tree to girls who have not reached puberty.

Inform health professionals of the herbs you use. Problematic herb-drug interactions are possible.

Chaste tree may cause allergic reactions or other unexpected side effects. If any develop, reduce your dose or stop taking it. For more on herb safety, see Chapter 2.

If symptoms get worse or persist longer than 2 weeks, consult a health professional promptly.

Gardening

Chaste *tree* is a misnomer. The plant is more of a shrub, generally growing to about 10 feet, although in favorable conditions, it may reach 20. It likes moist riverbanks in the southern European Mediterranean.

Chaste tree has finger-shaped leaves, slender violet flowers that bloom in summer, and dark brown or black berrylike fruits the size of peppercorns that appear in fall.

European colonists introduced chaste tree into the United States. Today, it grows along the eastern seaboard from Maryland to Florida and throughout the South as far west as Arkansas, Oklahoma, and Texas.

CINNAMON

Spice with a Punch

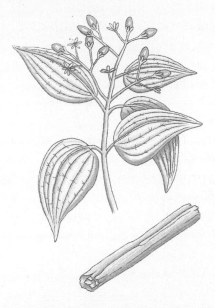

Family: Lauraceae; other members include bay, avocado, nutmeg, and sassafras

Genus and species: *Cinnamomum zeylanicum*, *C. cassia*, and *C. saigonicum*

Also known as: Cassia, Ceylon cinnamon, and Saigon cinnamon

Part used: Inner bark

We sprinkle it on toast, add it to cookie dough, stir it into hot apple cider, and find it in candies. But cinnamon is more than a sweet treat. It's one of the world's oldest healers. Modern science has confirmed its value for preventing infection and indigestion—plus it helps manage diabetes.

Healing History

Cinnamon originally grew in southern Asia. Chinese herbals from as early as 2700 BC mention the aromatic herb as a treatment for fever, diarrhea, and menstrual problems. India's ancient Ayurvedic healers used it similarly.

Ancient travelers introduced the herb to the Egyptians, who added it enthusiastically to embalming mixtures. Egyptian demand for cinnamon (and other Asian spices) played a major role in ancient trade.

The Biblical Hebrews, Greeks, and Romans adopted cinnamon as a spice, perfume, and treatment for indigestion. After the fall of Rome, trade with Asia came to a virtual halt, but somehow, cinnamon still found its way to Europe. The 12th-century German abbess/herbalist Hildegard of Bingen recommended it as "the universal spice for sinuses" and as a treatment for colds, flu, cancer, and "inner decay and slime."

By the 17th century, Europeans considered cinnamon primarily a kitchen spice. Medicinally, they used it only to mask the bitterness of other herbs.

As time passed, however, cinnamon regained its former prominence as a healer. America's 19th-century Eclectic physicians, forerunners of today's naturopaths, prescribed it for stomach cramps, flatulence, nausea, vomiting, diarrhea, and infant colic. The Eclectic medical text *King's American Dispensatory* (1898) also endorsed it for uterine problems: "[Cinnamon's] most direct action is on the uterine muscle fibers, causing contraction and arresting bleeding. For postpartum and other uterine hemorrhages, it is one of the most prompt and efficient remedies."

Modern herbalists recommend cinnamon to relieve nausea, vomiting, diarrhea, and indigestion and as a flavoring agent for bitter-tasting herbal preparations. But they disagree about its effects on the uterus. Some say it stimulates uterine contractions. Others insist it calms the organ.

Therapeutic Uses

Cinnamon delights the taste buds, but it also benefits other parts of the body.

INFECTIONS. Cinnamon oil is included in toothpastes and dental floss for more than just flavor. Like all culinary spices, it's a powerful antiseptic. It kills many decay- and disease-causing bacteria, fungi, and viruses. Try sprinkling some on minor cuts and scrapes after they've been thoroughly washed.

Perhaps toilet paper should be permeated with cinnamon. One German study showed that it "suppresses completely" the bacteria that cause most urinary tract infections (*Escherichia coli*) and the fungus responsible for vaginal yeast infections (*Candida albicans*). Cinnamon also suppresses *Salmonella* bacteria, a cause of food poisoning.

FOOD SPOILAGE. Spanish researchers impregnated food-wrapping paper with cinnamon oil. It extended the mold-free shelf life of fruits, vegetables, breads, and meats.

PAIN. Beyond antimicrobial action, cinnamon contains eugenol, a natural anesthetic oil that may help relieve the pain of cuts and scrapes.

DIGESTIVE UPSETS. Along with lending flavor to foods, cinnamon assists the body in digesting ice cream and other high-fat treats. A study in the British journal *Nature* shows that cinnamon helps the digestive system break down fats, apparently by boosting the activity of the digestive enzyme trypsin.

Commission E, the expert panel that evaluates herbal medicines for the German counterpart of the FDA, endorses cinnamon for indigestion, abdominal distress, bloating, and flatulence.

CHOLESTEROL. Pakistani researchers gave cinnamon (1 gram/day, a heaping teaspoon) to 60 people with high cholesterol and Type 2 diabetes. After 40 days, their cholesterol dropped 12 to 26 percent, significantly reducing their risk of heart disease. If you have high cholesterol, it can't hurt to sprinkle a teaspoon a day on your food.

DIABETES. Animal studies have shown that cinnamon reduces blood sugar. The Pakistani study just mentioned above showed that cinnamon reduced human blood sugar about 20 percent. Since then, dozens of studies around the world agree that cinnamon reduces blood sugar. Researchers at the University of California, Davis, analyzed eight clinical trials. "Cinnamon significantly lowers blood glucose in Type 2 diabetics."

MUSCLE SORENESS. Cinnamon contains anti-inflammatory compounds. Iranian researchers asked 60 women who exercised regularly to add one of three supplements to their meals: placebo, ginger (3 grams/day), or cinnamon (3 grams/day). After 8 weeks, the women exercised beyond their conditioning level, a workout designed to produce sore muscles. Compared with the placebo group, both herb groups showed lower levels of inflammation markers and reported less soreness.

Intriguing Possibility

Japanese researchers report that cinnamon helps reduce blood pressure. If yours is high, it can't hurt to use more of this tasty spice.

Rx Recommendations

For a warm, sweet, spicy infusion, use ½ to ¾ teaspoon of powdered herb per cup of boiling water, steep for 10 to 20 minutes, and strain if you wish. Drink up to 3 cups a day.

To treat minor cuts and scrapes, wash the affected area thoroughly, then sprinkle on a little powdered cinnamon.

Safety

Culinary amounts of cinnamon are nontoxic. However, cinnamon oil is a different story. On the skin, it may cause redness and burning. Used internally, it can cause nausea, vomiting, and kidney damage. Do not ingest the oil.

Despite some modern herbalists' contention that cinnamon helps calm the uterus, the weight of historical evidence suggests the opposite. For this reason, pregnant women should limit their use of cinnamon to culinary amounts.

Inform health professionals of the herbs you use. Problematic herb-drug interactions are possible.

Cinnamon may cause allergic reactions or other unexpected side effects. If any develop, reduce your dose or stop taking it. For more on herb safety, see Chapter 2.

If symptoms get worse or persist longer than 2 weeks, consult a health professional promptly.

Gardening

Cinnamon does not grow in the United States. Our supply comes from Asia and the West Indies. The trees reach a height of 30 feet. Collectors strip the aromatic bark from young branches no more than 3 years old.

CLOVE
Your Dentist Loves It

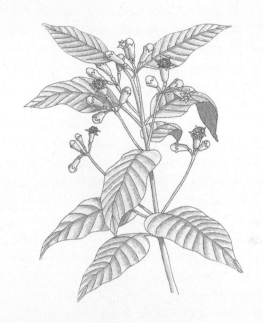

Family: Myrtaceae; other members include myrtle, tea tree, and eucalyptus

Genus and species: *Eugenia caryophyllata* or *Syzygiurn aromaticum*

Also known as: Clavos and caryophyllus

Parts used: Flower buds

Step into any spice shop, take a deep breath, and enjoy the rich, warm aroma that fills the air. Chances are the dominant fragrance is clove, one of the world's most aromatic healing herbs.

Step into your dentist's supply room and, although things smell quite different, chances are that clove oil is one of the items on the shelf. It's a dental anesthetic—and more.

Healing History

Clove is the bud of a fragrant Asian tropical evergreen tree. During the Han dynasty (20 BC to AD 220), those who addressed the Chinese emperor were required to hold cloves in their mouths to mask bad breath.

For millennia, traditional Chinese physicians have prescribed clove to treat indigestion, diarrhea, hernia, and ringworm, along with athlete's foot and other fungal infections. India's traditional Ayurvedic healers used clove to treat respiratory and digestive ailments.

A highly coveted luxury clove arrived in Europe around the 4th century AD. The medieval German abbess/herbalist Hildegard of Bingen recommended the rare herb in her antigout herb formula.

Demand for clove and other Asian spices helped launch the Age of Exploration. In 1512, the remnants of Magellan's world-circling flotilla carried some back to Spain.

Once the herb became widely available in Europe, herbalists prized it as a treatment for indigestion, flatulence, nausea, vomiting, and diarrhea. It was also used to treat cough, infertility, warts, worms, wounds, and toothache.

America's 19th-century Eclectic physicians, forerunners of today's naturopaths, recommended clove to treat digestive complaints and added it to bitter herbal medicine preparations to make them more palatable. The Eclectics were also the first to extract clove oil from the buds. They used it on the gums to relieve toothache, a practice adopted by modern dentists.

Contemporary herbalists recommend clove for digestive complaints and its oil for toothache.

Therapeutic Uses

Clove oil is 60 to 90 percent eugenol, which is the source of its anesthetic and antiseptic properties.

TOOTHACHE AND ORAL HYGIENE. Dentists use clove oil as an anesthetic and to disinfect root canals. It's an ingredient in some over-the-counter toothache remedies, for example, Dentapaine. The topical anesthetic, benzocaine, is more popular, but that might change if a Kuwaiti study get publicized. The researchers gave 73 toothache-suffering adults one of four treatments: clove oil, a placebo resembling clove oil, benzocaine, or a placebo resembling the drug. Both clove oil and benzocaine provided significantly greater pain relief than the placebos—with "no significant difference" between them. Commission E, the expert panel that evaluates herbal medicines for the German counterpart of the FDA, endorses clove oil as an oral anesthetic.

Toothaches require professional care. Clove oil may provide temporary relief, but see a dentist promptly.

DIGESTIVE PROBLEMS. Like all culinary spices, clove helps relax the smooth muscle lining the digestive tract, supporting the herb's age-old use as a digestive aid.

PARASITES AND INFECTIONS. Clove oil kills intestinal parasites and "exhibits broad antimicrobial properties against fungi and bacteria," according to one of many reports supporting the herb's traditional use as a treatment for diarrhea, intestinal worms, other digestive ailments, and ringworm.

HAY FEVER. Clove has some antihistamine action. If you have hay fever, clove probably won't replace pharmaceutical antihistamines, but it may provide additional relief.

Rx Recommendations

For temporary relief of toothache prior to professional care, dip a cotton swab in clove oil and apply it to the affected tooth and surrounding gum. When using commercial clove oil or eugenol preparations, follow the package directions.

To make a warm, pleasant-tasting infusion, use 1 teaspoon of powdered herb per cup of boiling water and steep for 10 to 20 minutes, then strain if you wish.

Safety

It's safe to use small amounts used of clove oil on teeth and gums. However, do not ingest the oil. As little as 1 teaspoon can cause serious toxicity. Externally, clove oil may cause skin irritation.

Some smokers switch to clove cigarettes, thinking that they're safer than tobacco. No. Most clove cigarettes are 50 to 60 percent tobacco, and when clove burns, it releases many carcinogens. The *Journal of the American Medical Association* has reported many toxic reactions to clove cigarettes.

Use clove oil only temporarily for dental pain. See a dentist promptly.

Clove oil may cause allergic reactions or other unexpected side effects. If any develop, reduce your dose or stop taking it. For more on herb safety, see Chapter 2.

Gardening

Native to the Philippines, clove has leathery leaves and reaches 60 feet. The aromatic evergreen does not grow in the United States. Today, Tanzania produces about 80 percent of the world supply. The tree also grows in Indonesia, Sri Lanka, Brazil, and the West Indies.

COCOA (CHOCOLATE)

Great News! Dark Chocolate Is Very
Good for You!

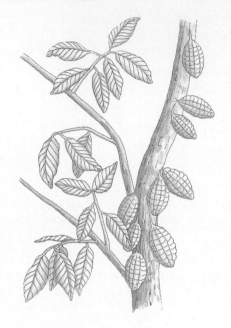

Family: *Sterculiaceae*; other members
include kola

Genus and species: *Theobroma cacao*

Also known as: Chocolate and cacao

Parts used: Seeds (beans)

Chocoholics of the world, rejoice! Your favorite
vice may be just what the doctor ordered for a
long, sweet life with reduced risk of heart attack
and stroke. The only catch is that you must eat
dark chocolate. Milk and white chocolate offer
no health benefits.

Healing History

Imagine the desolation of a world without chocolate. That's how it was in Europe until 1519,
when Spanish conquistador Hernando Cortez
saw Mexico's Aztec ruler, Montezuma, sip a bitter drink called *xocoatl* from a golden goblet.
Cortez was more interested in the goblet's gold
than its contents—until the Aztecs informed
him that the drink was made from beans so
valuable that 100 could buy a healthy slave. The
Aztecs also claimed that *xocoatl* was an aphrodisiac. Montezuma never visited his harem
without it. After conquering Mexico, Cortez
shipped some *xocoatl*, which he called *chocolatl*,
back to Spain as a gift for the king.

The Aztecs and Mayans drank enormous
amounts of *xocoatl* (bitter water). The common
folk could afford it only for special occasions, for
example, at weddings. Priests used it in prayer
offerings. But royalty couldn't get enough. Surviving records suggest that a century before
Cortez, the Aztec royal court consumed an
astonishing 32,000 cocoa beans a day.

Cortez's gift to his king was an instant sensation with the Spanish court. Chocolate proved
so popular that Spanish royalty consumed 200
tons of beans annually. They vowed to keep it
secret from the rest of Europe—and succeeded
for 100 years. But, some ships carrying the
beans were captured by pirates and other European powers, and eventually, the secret got out.

By the mid-17th century, chocolate had
spread throughout Western Europe. It became
especially popular in Switzerland, England, Belgium, and Holland. In 1875, Daniel Peter, a
Swiss candy maker, figured out how to add milk
to cocoa powder. Voila, milk chocolate. Peter and
his neighbor, Henri Nestlé, started a company
that quickly became the world's leading maker
of chocolate candies.

Oddly, until the 19th century, chocolate was
consumed only as a beverage—dark and bitter,

or sweetened with sugar, or made creamier with milk, but always a liquid. It was only about 150 years ago that chocolate was first fashioned into the bars and candies that we love today.

For centuries, Central Americans have used cocoa to treat fever, coughs, and problems associated with pregnancy and childbirth. They also applied cocoa butter to soothe burns, chapped lips, balding heads, and nursing mothers' sore nipples.

America's 19th-century Eclectic physicians, forerunners of today's naturopaths, recommended cocoa butter externally as a wound dressing and salve. They prescribed hot cocoa internally as a treatment for asthma, as a substitute for coffee, and as "a very useful nutritive for invalids and persons convalescing from acute illness."

Therapeutic Uses

Cocoa's generic name, *Theobroma*, means "food of the gods." But its derivative, chocolate, is much more than a sweet treat. It possesses remarkable healing powers, thanks largely to its antioxidants, caffeine, and theobromine.

APHRODISIAC? Cocoa and chocolate contain caffeine, 10 to 20 percent of the amount in coffee, about 13 milligrams per cup of cocoa compared with instant coffee's 65 milligrams and drip coffee's 100 to 150 milligrams. But consume enough and it's a stimulant. In traditional herbal medicine worldwide, stimulant herbs have always been considered sex stimulants.

In addition, chocolate contains a compound (phenylethylamine or PEA) that plays a key role in the biochemistry of feeling in love. PEA is an antidepressant chemically similar to amphetamine. It's what makes lovers feel as if they're walking on clouds. When a love affair ends, PEA levels drop precipitously.

Some scientists argue that chocolate contains too little PEA to produce amorous emotions. But the skeptics can't explain why chocolate is among the world's favorite Valentine's Day gifts. Perhaps it's a coincidence, or maybe this custom developed because chocolate boosts lovers' PEA levels, increasing emotional attachment and erotic interest. It may also explain why those with broken hearts sometimes binge on chocolate—to replace their lost PEA and recoup some of its mood-elevating effects.

ANTIOXIDANT. Although chocolate is high in fat (more on this shortly), oddly, it doesn't spoil when left unrefrigerated. This unexpected observation led researchers to speculate that cocoa might contain antioxidants that prevent fat spoilage. They discovered that cocoa and dark chocolate contain large amounts of flavonoids and phenols, both important categories of antioxidant nutrients. Antioxidants—among them vitamins A, C, and E and the mineral selenium—help prevent the cell damage at the root of heart disease, stroke, and many cancers.

Korean researchers compared the antioxidant content of cocoa with red wine and tea, both high in antioxidants. Cocoa was the clear winner.

- Cocoa powder (2 tablespoons dissolved in 200 milliliters of water): Phenolics, 611 milligrams. Flavonoids, 564 milligrams.

- Red wine (Merlot, 140 milliliters): Phenolics, 340 milligrams. Flavonoids, 163 milligrams.

- Green tea (2 grams steeped in 200 milliliters of water for 2 minutes): Phenolics, 165 milligrams, Flavonoids, 47 milligrams.

🍀 Black tea (2 grams bag steeped in 200 milliliters of water for 2 minutes): Phenolics, 124 milligrams. Flavonoids, 34 milligrams.

Dark chocolate's antioxidant content is similar to cocoa's. But milk chocolate contains considerably less because it is diluted with milk and sugar.

Strong antioxidants like cocoa and dark chocolate aid health so much that they add to longevity. Harvard researchers tracked the diets and lifestyles of 7,800 Harvard graduates for several decades. Compared with those who ate no dark chocolate, those who did lived almost 1 year longer.

HEART DISEASE, BLOOD PRESSURE, CHOLESTEROL. Many studies have shown that tea and red wine (up to two glasses a day) reduce risk of heart attack. When researchers learned that cocoa is richer in antioxidants, they began investigating dark chocolate for prevention of heart disease—often with funding from Nestlé (maker of Kit Kat) or Mars (M&M's).

Swiss researchers used sophisticated tests to measure blood flow through 25 men's arteries, then gave them 1.5 ounces of dark chocolate (74 percent cocoa) or white chocolate. White chocolate had no effect on blood flow, but dark chocolate significantly improved blood flow. The dark chocolate also made blood platelets less likely to form clots. Increased arterial blood flow and reduced clotting both help prevent both heart attack and stroke.

A German study shows that in people with high blood pressure, daily consumption of 3.5 ounces of dark chocolate lowers blood pressure as much as the blood pressure medications atenolol (Tenormin) and propranolol (Inderal). An analysis of five studies by other German researchers agrees: Dark chocolate lowers blood pressure significantly.

Harvard researchers analyzed 136 studies of cocoa's and dark chocolate's effects on cardiovascular health. They found consistent evidence that they reduce blood pressure, raise HDL (good cholesterol), reduce LDL (bad cholesterol), reduce inflammation, and prevent internal blood clots, meaning reduced risk of heart disease and stroke.

CANCER. Cocoa also reduces cancer risk. Panamanian researchers compared cancer deaths among mainland Panamanians and members of the Kuna tribe who live in relative isolation and drink a great deal of cocoa. The Kuna's risk of death from cancer, heart disease, and diabetes was much lower.

Cancer risk reduction may also be inferred from a Harvard study that tracked the diets and health of 7,814 male Harvard graduates for many years. Compared with those who ate no dark chocolate bars, men who ate one to three bars a month had a 36 percent lower death rate from all causes, including cancer.

OVERALL HEALTH. Finnish scientists tracked the physical and emotional health of 1,367 men from their 30s into their 70s. Those who ate the most dark chocolate were the healthiest.

FATIGUE AND LETHARGY. The caffeine in cocoa and chocolate help relieve drowsiness. But their stimulant action does not cause as much jitteriness, insomnia, and irritability as coffee—thanks to the theobromine in the herb. Try some when you feel lethargic (purely as herbal medicine, of course).

DIGESTIVE UPSETS. The theobromine in cocoa relaxes the smooth muscle lining the digestive tract, which may explain why many people have chocolate after heavy meals. Try some to soothe your stomach after eating.

BRONCHIAL CONGESTION. Theobromine and caffeine are close chemical relatives of theophylline, which, until recently, was a standard asthma medication. Theophylline opens the bronchial passages; theobromine and caffeine have similar effects.

If you're really congested or if you have asthma, the large dose of decongestant caffeine in coffee may be more beneficial. But even the low dose in cocoa or chocolate may provide some relief from the chest congestion of colds and flu.

MENTAL ACUITY. A team of English and Australian researchers gave 30 healthy college students cognitive function tests and then one of three cocoa beverages (46 milligrams flavonoids, 520 milligrams, or 994 milligrams). Each participant consumed all three separated by 3-day wash-out periods. The lowest dose had no impact on mental acuity, but the two higher doses, equivalent to a few ounces of dark chocolate, improved mental processing speed.

PRE-ECLAMPSIA. This potentially fatal complication of pregnancy shares many risk factors with heart disease. Since dark chocolate reduces heart disease risk, Yale researchers wondered if it might do the same for pre-eclampsia. Two or three weekly servings of cocoa/dark chocolate reduced pre-eclampsia risk by about 40 percent.

Intriguing Possibilities

Back in the 1960s, teens were told to that chocolate caused acne. Many subsequent studies debunked this, but recently University of Miami, Florida, researchers gave dark chocolate (100 percent cocoa) to 10 young men with histories of acne. The more chocolate they ate, the more pimples they developed. One small study can't be considered definitive, especially in light of all the research showing no chocolate-acne link. But it's a possibility.

A pilot study in Ghana hints that dark chocolate might help prevent malaria.

Rx Recommendations

Kiss guilt goodbye. Brew yourself a heavenly cup of cocoa. Try it as a gentle pick-me-up or digestive aid. And if you have respiratory congestion from a cold, flu, or asthma, there's no harm in sipping steamy hot cocoa, as long as you combine it with appropriate professional medical care.

To make cocoa, use 1 to 2 heaping teaspoons of herb per cup of hot water or low-fat or fat-free milk.

Milk chocolate shows some health benefits, but nowhere near as many as dark chocolate. For those who grew up eating just milk chocolate, the dark variety may not taste as good. Many chocolate makers now label their products based on how much cocoa they contain. Start with dark chocolate that's around 50 percent cocoa and slowly work up to around 70 percent.

Safety

Chocolate cake is sometimes called "devil's food." Chocolate has long been vilified as a cause of obesity, tooth decay, acne, kidney stones, infant colic, headaches, and heartburn. Much of this reputation is undeserved. Chocolate's fat content may contribute to obesity. But a good deal of its fat is in the form of stearic acid, which does not raise cholesterol. Cocoa and dark chocolate contain no cholesterol, but milk chocolate does. So, the chocolate in confections is rarely as much of a problem as the high-fat, high-cholesterol butter and cream added to it.

Chocolate's contribution to tooth decay has been blown way out of proportion. Some research even suggests that the antioxidants in cocoa *inhibit* the bacteria that cause tooth decay. Again, the problem with chocolate candy is not its cocoa content but rather its sugar.

There is no evidence that chocolate causes kidney stones or infant colic. However, it contains compounds (tyramines) that may trigger headaches in some people, particularly those prone to migraines.

Some folks are super-sensitive to the stimulants in cocoa and chocolate. If insomnia, irritability, or hyperactivity becomes a problem, eat less.

Some people sip hot chocolate after meals as a stomach soother. The glitch is that cocoa and chocolate may cause heartburn. The herb relaxes the valve at the end of the esophagus, the tube that carries food into the stomach. When this valve (lower esophageal sphincter) does not shut tightly, stomach acids splash up into the esophagus, causing heartburn pain. If cocoa or chocolate give you heartburn, consume less or give it up.

The real safety issue with cocoa and chocolate has to do with the caffeine content. Caffeine is a powerfully stimulating, classically addictive drug. It has been linked to insomnia, irritability, and anxiety attacks; elevated blood pressure, cholesterol, and blood sugar (glucose) levels; and increased risk of birth defects. (For more on caffeine's many effects, see Coffee, page 165.)

Although cocoa and chocolate contain only 10 to 20 percent as much caffeine as coffee, large amounts may trigger caffeine's effects. People with insomnia, anxiety problems, high cholesterol, high blood pressure, diabetes, or heart disease should limit their caffeine intake.

Cocoa and chocolate may cause allergic reactions or other unexpected side effects. If any develop, reduce your dose or stop taking it. For more on herb safety, see Chapter 2.

If symptoms get worse or persist longer than 2 weeks, consult a health professional promptly.

Gardening

Cocoa (or cacao) should not be confused with coconut or with coca, the source of cocaine. Cocoa trees are small, oval-leafed evergreens that grow in tropical lowlands. They do not grow in the United States.

Wild cocoa trees grow to 30 feet, but growers prune cultivated trees to about 15 feet for ease of harvesting the seeds (beans). Central and South America grow and export cocoa beans, but an estimated 80 percent of the world crop now comes from Africa.

Once harvested, cocoa beans are roasted and ground into a liquid (cocoa liquor). The next step is dutching, the addition of a minute amount of caustic lye as a flavor enhancer. The amount is so small that it poses no hazard. The dutched liquor is further processed to remove the fat (cocoa butter). The final product, chocolate, is a combination of the defatted cocoa powder with some of the butter added back in.

The powder that we know as cocoa is simply dried cocoa liquor, perhaps with a little sugar added. Baker's chocolate is processed cocoa liquor with no sugar added. Bittersweet chocolate has some sugar added, semisweet contains more sugar, and milk chocolate has the most, plus milk to make it creamy.

COFFEE

Beyond the Boost, Many Benefits

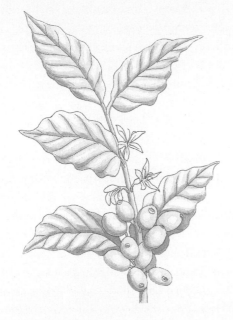

Family: Rubiaceae; other members include gardenia, cat's claw, and cinchona

Genus and species: *Coffea arabica*, *C. liberica*, and *C. robusta*

Also known as: Arabica, mocha, java, espresso, cappuccino, and latté

Parts used: Seeds (beans)

The next time anyone gives you a hard time about using medicinal herbs, here's the perfect comeback: "Do you drink coffee?"

Coffee is America's most widely used herbal medicine. The average American drinks 28 gallons a year, requiring 10 pounds of coffee beans—and for clearly medicinal reasons, to gain the stimulant effects of this herb's caffeine.

But coffee does more than wake us up in the morning. It also helps treat colds, flu, allergies, and asthma. It improves athletic performance and helps prevent kidney stones and jet lag. It relieves pain and combats depression, possibly even reducing the risk of suicide. It may also promote weight loss in those who are obese.

On the other hand, coffee impairs women's fertility and can produce significant side effects. Its active constituent, caffeine, is addictive. Over time, regular users develop a tolerance. If they suddenly give up caffeine, they experience withdrawal.

Caffeine has also been accused, often mistakenly, of causing or contributing to many other health problems. Ironically, its main downside—its effect on women's fertility—has not been well publicized.

Caffeine is definitely not risk-free. No drug is. Authorities generally agree, however, that for most people most of the time, it's safe to drink 1 or 2 cups a day.

Healing History

Our word coffee comes from Caffa, the region in Ethiopia where the fabled beans were first discovered. Archeological evidence suggests that prehistoric East Africans loved coffee's remarkable stimulant properties. They ate the red, unroasted beans (cherries) before tribal wars, extended hunts, and other activities that required alertness, strength, and stamina.

The beverage we love emerged around AD 1000, when Arabs began roasting and grinding coffee beans and sipping the hot drink as we do today. Around the same time, the noted Arab physician Avicenna penned the first medical description of coffee's stimulant effects.

Today coffee is enormously popular, but it took centuries to get there. From 1000 to 1500, only those in the Middle East consumed it. Then, in 1517, Sultan Selim I introduced the beverage into Constantinople (now Istanbul). At around the same time, spice traders introduced it into Italy. Over the next 100 years, it spread throughout Europe.

The first coffeehouse opened at Oxford University in England in 1650. It was remarkably similar to coffeehouses today—places to enjoy coffee, conversation, reading, and writing. Coffeehouses quickly spread to London, where they became hotbeds of political discussion and dissent. In 1675, King Charles II ordered all of London's coffeehouses closed, claiming they fostered sedition.

Coffee arrived in New York City in 1696, 30 years before it reached Brazil, which is now one of the world's major coffee-exporting nations.

Until the 17th century, Arabia supplied all of the world's coffee through the port of Mocha, which became another term for coffee. Then the Dutch introduced the plant into Java. The island and coffee quickly became synonymous.

In 1732, Bach composed the "Coffee Cantata" in celebration of his favorite beverage, despite some feeling that it threatened Germany's traditional brew, beer. As coffee became more popular in Germany, the backlash in favor of beer intensified. In 1777, Frederick the Great of Prussia issued a manifesto denouncing coffee in favor of beer.

In 1904, Fernando Illy of Italy invented the espresso machine. In 1910, Merck, the pharmaceutical manufacturer, introduced decaffeinated coffee. And in 1938, Nestlé introduced Nescafé instant coffee. It is still the leading brand.

Coffee has always been more popular as a beverage than as a healing herb, but European herbalists believed its stimulant effect could help treat opium and alcohol sedation.

In their medical text *King's American Dispensatory* (1898), America's 19th-century Eclectic physicians, forerunners of today's naturopaths, prescribed coffee as "an agreeable stimulant . . . that frequently overcomes the soporific [sedative] effects of opium, morphine, and alcohol." They also recommended it to treat asthma, constipation, menstrual cramps, and dropsy (congestive heart failure).

The Eclectics also recognized coffee's downside. From *King's*: "If taken too freely, [coffee causes] irritability, trembling, confusion, bowel disorders, and ringing in the ears. On the other hand, if one is accustomed to moderate amounts, headache will result if coffee be withdrawn."

Folk healers have used coffee for centuries to treat asthma, fever, headache, colds, and flu. But few modern herbalists consider it a healing herb. How odd, considering that coffee is America's most popular medicinal herb.

Therapeutic Uses

Caffeine, the stimulant in coffee (and in tea, cocoa, chocolate, cola, maté, and guarana), is also an ingredient in many cold, flu, antidrowsiness, and menstrual remedies. These uses reflect coffee's role in traditional herbal healing.

Coffee's caffeine content depends on its preparation. A cup of instant contains about 65 milligrams, a cup of drip or percolated has 100 to 150 milligrams, and a cup of espresso delivers about 350 milligrams.

Caffeine is classically addictive. Regular users develop a tolerance and require increasing amounts to obtain expected stimulation. Deprived of caffeine, java junkies usually develop withdrawal symptoms, primarily headache and constipation that can last for up to 2 weeks.

The media regularly report health problems linked to caffeine and coffee, many of which have been debunked, but they rarely discuss coffee's many potential therapeutic benefits. Herbal medicine users deserve a more balanced perspective.

FATIGUE AND LETHARGY. No doubt about it: Coffee is a powerful central nervous system stimulant. On long drives, it helps prevent dozing at the wheel. It also counteracts the sedative effects of antihistamines, one reason it's included in many cold remedies. However, it does not help drunks sober up.

BEVERAGE OF CHAMPIONS. Attention, athletes: Coffee improves physical stamina and athletic performance. Over 9 days, British researchers gave 18 runners 1 to 2 cups of either regular or decaffeinated coffee, and then timed them running a mile. With caffeine's help, they ran 4.2 seconds faster.

In a similar study, researchers had runners run and cyclists ride until they were clinically exhausted. A few days later, the athletes were retested an hour after drinking 5 cups of coffee. Fortified by caffeine, their stamina improved 44 percent while running, and 51 percent while cycling.

The International Olympic Committee regulates caffeine use by Olympic athletes, allowing no more than 12 micrograms of caffeine per milligram of urine. To reach that level, an athlete would have to drink at least 5 cups of coffee up to 3 hours before events.

To experience performance improvement, you must consume more caffeine than you already tolerate. A person who uses no caffeine might gain athletic benefits by drinking a cup or two, but a 1-cup-a-day athlete might have to drink 2 or 3 before noticing benefit.

COLDS, FLU, AND ALLERGIES. Caffeine is a decongestant, useful in treating chest congestion caused by colds, flu, and allergies. That's another reason it's included in cold formulas.

ASTHMA. Some years ago, North Carolina pharmacists Joe and Terry Graedon, authors of *The People's Pharmacy* books and syndicated column, received a letter from a woman who had just returned from her honeymoon. While in Hawaii, the woman, who had asthma, began wheezing. She reached for her inhaler but couldn't find it. Wheezing more and feeling panicky, she ransacked her luggage. Nothing. In all the wedding and honeymoon commotion, she'd forgotten to pack it.

Then she recalled reading in *The People's Pharmacy* that caffeine is chemically similar to some asthma medications, that it's a bronchodilator, meaning it opens constricted bronchial tubes and eases breathing. In a pinch, the Graedons advised, caffeine can help stop asthma attacks.

The wheezing newlywed rushed to the hotel snack bar and quickly downed 3 cups of coffee. Within minutes, she was breathing easier. She wrote the Graedons: "You saved my honeymoon."

This woman's experience is not unique. A survey of 70,000 Italian households shows that as coffee consumption increases, risk of asthma attacks decreases.

PAIN RELIEF. Compared with plain aspirin or ibuprofen (Motrin, Advil), a combination of pain reliever and a caffeine (60 milligrams, about the amount in 1 cup of instant coffee, or a half cup of brewed coffee, or a strong cup of black tea, or a 12-ounce cola) relieves pain faster and more effectively. Caffeine does not relieve pain. But it's a mild antidepressant. Pain and mood are connected. Pain hurts more when you feel depressed and less when you feel better. Coffee's mood-elevating effect is the reason it boosts the action of pain-relieving drugs. Next time you reach for aspirin or ibuprofen, wash it down with a caffeinated beverage. Or take Excedrin, a combination of aspirin and caffeine.

ANTIOXIDANTS. Like other plants, coffee beans contain antioxidant nutrients. Compared with tea, cocoa (chocolate), fruits, and vegetables, coffee is a lesser source of antioxidants. But coffee is so popular that University of Scranton, Pennsylvania, researchers calculate that it's the top source of antixodants for many Americans. Antioxidants help prevent and reverse the cell damage at the root of heart disease, cancer, and many other conditions.

STROKE. Harvard researchers tracked the diet and lifestyle of 83,076 women nurses. After 24 years, they suffered 2,280 strokes. But the more coffee they drank, the less likely they were to suffer stroke. Compared with nurses who drank less than 1 cup a month, those who consumed 4 or more daily cups had 20 percent less stroke risk.

LONGEVITY. In 1995, researchers with the National Institutes of Health asked 229,119 members of AARP, age 50 to 71, to complete a comprehensive diet and lifestyle survey. During 14 years of follow-up, 52,515 participants died (33,731 men, 18,784 women). After controlling for other variables (smoking, exercise, etc.), the regular coffee drinkers enjoyed a small but significant increase in longevity, which the researchers attributed to the antioxidants in coffee.

DIABETES. Several studies show that coffee reduces risk of Type 2 diabetes. A Harvard study in *Diabetes Care* shows that 1 cup a day reduces diabetes risk 13 percent and 2 or 3 cups reduces risk 42 percent. Other studies show somewhat different findings, but they all agree that moderate coffee consumption reduces risk of Type 2 diabetes. Why would coffee lower risk? That remains unclear, but coffee's antioxidant content may play a role. In addition, coffee helps dieters lose weight (see the opposite page), and Type 2 diabetes is strongly associated with obesity.

SUICIDE. Caffeine's mood-elevating effect also appears to explain why regular coffee drinkers have less-than-expected risk of suicide. For more than 20 years, Harvard researchers have followed the diet, lifestyle, and health of some 85,000 female nurses in the ongoing Nurses Health Study. Compared with nurses who drink 2 or 3 daily cups of coffee, those who drink none are more likely to attempt suicide.

KIDNEY STONES. Kidney stones cause excruciating low-back and groin pain. Doctors urge those with a history of kidney stones to prevent new ones by drinking plenty of water, which keeps urine dilute, and minimizes risk of stone formation. But the Nurses Health Study, just mentioned, shows that compared with no preventive efforts, a daily glass of water cuts kidney stone risk 2 percent, while a daily cup of coffee reduces risk 10 percent. (Tea cuts risk 8 percent.)

GALLSTONES. Gallstones afflict 20 million Americans and send 800,000 to hospitals each year. Harvard researchers followed 46,008 male health professionals who'd never had gallstones. Eight years later, 1,081 had developed them. Compared with those who drank no coffee, participants who consumed 1 cup a day had significantly less gallstone risk. Consuming 2 or 3 daily cups of coffee cut risk 40 percent.

MENSTRUAL FLOW. Coffee appears to

protect against heavy menstrual flow, which is inconvenient and contributes to iron-deficiency anemia. California researchers surveyed 403 healthy premenopausal women about their diet, lifestyle, and health. Compared with those who drank no coffee, women who drank more than 2 cups a day (300 milligrams of caffeine) were significantly less likely to have menstrual periods last at least 8 days. Caffeine is a vasoconstrictor. It narrows blood vessels, including those in the uterus, which apparently explains reduced menstrual flow.

JET LAG. Ever feel disoriented, groggy, and fatigued after flying across time zones? Coffee tricks the body into acting like it's an hour earlier in the day, maintaining bodily functions that naturally power down in the evening. Some jet-lag authorities recommend drinking coffee when traveling west and having longer days. But drinking coffee while traveling east may aggravate jet lag.

WEIGHT LOSS. The caffeine in coffee raises basal metabolic rate (BMR), the rate the resting body burns calories. As BMR increases, fat decreases, and the body sheds unwanted pounds. In medically supervised weight-loss programs, those who supplement a low-calorie diet and regular exercise with caffeine lose a little more weight. Not much, but enough to include caffeine in some weight-loss programs. However, caffeine only helps those who are severely obese, weighing well over 20 percent more than their recommended weight. It does not help those with more modest weight-loss goals—5 to 10 pounds.

GOUT. Harvard researchers correlated gout attacks and coffee drinking in 45,000 men over 12 years. Drinking up to 3 cups a day had no effect on gout risk. But 4 cups a day reduced risk

40 percent, and 6 cups reduced it 59 percent. Decaf produced similar results.

MENTAL ACUITY. Italian researchers found 22 rigorous trials of coffee and tea consumption and cognitive function. Of the 10 short-term studies, most showed that as caffeine consumption increased, so did cognitive function. Of the 12 long-term studies, several showed that regular caffeine intake preserves mental acuity and slows age-related cognitive decline.

In addition, a Finnish study suggests that coffee may reduce risk of dementia. The researchers followed 1,409 Finns age 65 to 79. After 21 years of follow-up, 61 developed dementia. Compared with those who drank no coffee, participants who drank 3 to 5 daily cups during midlife showed 65 percent less dementia risk.

PARKINSON'S DISEASE. Hawaiian researchers have followed the diet and lifestyle of 8,000 Japanese-American Hawaiians since the 1960s. During decades of follow-up, 107 developed Parkinson's. Among those who drank no coffee, the rate was 10.4 per 10,000 person-years. With increasing coffee consumption, the rate steadily declined. Those who drank 3 or 4 cups a day had a Parkinson's rate of only 1.9, a risk reduction of about 80 percent.

BRAIN TUMORS. English scientists compared coffee and tea consumption in healthy controls and among 588 people with brain tumors. Those who drank 1 or 2 daily cups of coffee or tea had 67 percent less risk of stroke—in the men, 59 percent less, in the women, 74 percent less.

Rx for Coffee

Coffee has a wonderful, rich, pleasantly bitter taste. Strong sales of decaf demonstrate that taste alone is sufficient for millions to drink it regularly. Of course, most enjoy regular coffee as a stimulating pick-me-up, and for all the other reasons just mentioned.

For an infusion (otherwise known as a cup of java or joe), use 1 heaping tablespoon of ground beans per cup of water. Brew it using your favorite method, or buy instant and follow directions on the label. Drink as much as you comfortably tolerate.

Coffee-flavored food items (yogurt, ice cream, etc.) also contain some caffeine. If you use them, be aware that they add to your caffeine consumption and may increase your tolerance and side effects.

Safety

Coffee is classically addictive and causes so many side effects that one report noted: "If caffeine were a newly synthesized drug, its manufacturer would almost certainly have great difficulty getting it licensed under current FDA regulations. If it were licensed, it would almost certainly be available only by prescription."

More Than Just Jitters

If you drink coffee, you know that consuming more than you're used to makes you a jittery, irritable, impatient insomniac. If you're concerned about a short temper, consider reducing your consumption or switching to decaf. If you have sleep problems, drink less, switch to decaf, or drink regular only in the morning, so the stimulant effect wears off by bedtime.

Individual reactions to caffeine vary, but over time, large amounts—8 daily or more cups—may cause "caffeinism:" nervousness, irritability, chronic muscle tension, insomnia, heart palpitations, diarrhea, heartburn, and stomach upset. The *American Journal of Psychiatry* reports many people diagnosed with "anxiety disorders" actually suffer caffeinism.

Java Junkies—for Real

The caffeine in coffee is classically addictive. Regular use produces tolerance. Over time, you need increasing amounts to produce the desired stimulation. Once addicted to caffeine, suddenly stopping coffee produces a withdrawal syndrome: headache that may last a week, and often sluggishness and constipation. If you want to cut down on coffee, or stop drinking it, or switch to decaf, do it gradually. This minimizes withdrawal discomforts. To switch to decaf, over several weeks, mix increasing amounts of decaf with decreasing amounts of regular until you're drinking 100 percent decaf.

In addition, coffee increases secretion of stomach acid. Those with ulcers or other chronic digestive disorders should use it sparingly, if at all.

Links to Serious Illnesses?

Coffee has been accused of increasing risk of several serious conditions: cancer, high cholesterol, heart attack, high blood pressure, birth defects, hyperactivity, growth, and stunting in children. The news here is largely reassuring.

CANCER? Roasting coffee introduces carcinogens into the beans. Over the years, coffee has been linked to cancers of the breast, bladder, ovaries, pancreas, and prostate. Subsequent studies have largely debunked these associations. The researchers who accused caffeine of increasing risk of bladder cancer later repudiated their own findings. At this point, there is no evidence that a daily cup or two significantly increases cancer risk. A few studies show that coffee *reduces* risk of liver and breast cancers. Apparently, the antioxidants in coffee neutralize the carcinogens.

HIGH BLOOD PRESSURE? Caffeine narrows the blood vessels (vasoconstrictor), which increases blood pressure. Those using it for the first time show a sharp spike in blood pressure. But several studies agree that in people with normal blood pressure, this increase is temporary and blood pressure soon returns to normal. Harvard researchers tracked the blood pressure and coffee consumption of 155,600 women nurses for 12 years (1991–2003). More than 100,000 were diagnosed with high blood pressure. But there was no association between those diagnoses and the nurses' coffee consumption. If your blood pressure is normal, modest caffeine consumption—1 or 2 daily cups—does not cause chronically high blood pressure (hypertension). But if you take blood pressure medication, discuss your caffeine intake with your doctor.

HIGH CHOLESTEROL? Some years ago, a Scandinavian study that followed 38,500 men and women for 3 years showed that as coffee consumption increased, so did cholesterol and risk of heart attack. Rising coffee consumption was associated with higher cholesterol, and compared with abstainers, those who consumed 9 cups a day had triple the risk of heart attack. Very few drink 9 cups a day. Nonetheless, risk increased with every cup so the association was troubling.

It's considerably less troubling today. The same researchers continued their study for 12 years, and the association between coffee drinking and elevated cholesterol and heart attack plummeted. After 12 years, the 9-cup-a-day coffee drinkers had only 1.3 times the risk of

their no-coffee counterparts, which is barely significant, and those who drink a cup or two showed hardly any elevated risk.

What changed? Scandinavians' brewing method. They used to boil their coffee, which extracts compounds from the beans that raise cholesterol and increase risk of heart attack. But as this study was taking place, Scandinavians switched to drip coffee, which filters out these harmful compounds. So does instant coffee. The vast majority of Americans drink instant or drip coffee. An analysis of long-term data from the ongoing Nurses Health Study shows no association between coffee consumption and risk of heart disease.

Most recently, Swedish researchers discovered that coffee raises blood levels of another risk factor for heart disease, homocysteine. But the increase was small, and the researchers concluded that a daily cup or two poses no heart-disease risk. Public health authorities are no longer concerned that typical coffee consumption increases heart-attack risk.

HEART DISEASE? Despite accusations that coffee increases heart-disease risk, the beans contain antioxidants that help prevent heart disease. As a result, we would not expect it to increase risk of heart disease. That's what Harvard researchers found in two huge studies. In one, they followed 85,747 women nurses for 10 years and found no association between coffee drinking and heart disease risk. In the other, they followed 44,005 men and 84,488 women for 14 years and again found no evidence that drinking up to 6 cups a day increases risk.

OSTEOPOROSIS? Caffeine pulls calcium from bone. As a result, coffee drinking has been accused of increasing risk of osteoporosis. Dozens of studies have investigated caffeine as a risk factor for osteoporotic fractures. About half show that caffeine increases fracture risk. Around 40 percent show no effect on fracture risk. The rest are inconclusive. The evidence tilts slightly toward caffeine as a risk factor for fractures. But it's far from compelling.

There may be a simple explanation for the studies' disagreement. There may be a caffeine threshold for fracture risk. Up to 2 cups of coffee a day (4 cups a day of tea or cola) do not increase risk. But any more does. Most coffee drinkers consume only 1 or 2 daily cups, below the threshold for caffeine-related bone damage. If you limit coffee to two cups a day (four cups of tea), you're probably okay. But if you drink more, you might consider cutting down to protect your bones.

MISCARRIAGE? University of Utah researchers analyzed stored blood samples of 3,000 pregnant women, 600 of whom had miscarriages. They checked for a compound produced by caffeine metabolism and used that information to estimate the women's daily caffeine intake. Women consuming the equivalent of 1 cup of brewed coffee a day showed no increased miscarriage risk. But as caffeine consumption increased, so did risk of pregnancy loss.

BIRTH DEFECTS? Studies from the early 1980s showed that animals fed extraordinarily high doses of caffeine bear young with an increased risk of birth defects. But no human study has ever shown that a daily cup or two of coffee increases this risk. Still, the Food and Drug Administration warns pregnant women to limit their caffeine intake. Nature seems to have the same opinion. Many women lose their taste for coffee while pregnant.

CHILDHOOD HYPERACTIVITY? Caffeine is a powerful stimulant, but there is no evidence that it contributes to hyperactivity. In fact, stimulants are often used to treat this condition (Ritalin). It's not clear why stimulants calm hyperactive children, but they often do. Researchers at the University of Chicago analyzed 12 studies of caffeine and behavior in children. None showed any increase in hyperactivity. A few showed calming benefits.

STUNTING CHILDREN'S GROWTH? Many parents tell their kids: "Don't drink coffee. It will stunt your growth." Actually, the research shows that coffee has no effect on children's growth.

Problems for Women

For all the publicity of coffee side effects, the media have generally underreported the problems caffeine can cause women.

FEMALE FERTILITY IMPAIRMENT. In a 10-year study, Johns Hopkins researchers followed the diets and lifestyles of 1,430 mothers, including their coffee consumption. During the study, the women experienced 2,501 pregnancies. The more coffee they drank, the longer it took them to get pregnant. A 3-cup-a-day coffee habit reduced fertility 26 percent. Why would coffee reduce fertility? In animal studies conducted at the University of Nevada, Reno, researchers discovered that caffeine reduces muscle activity in the fallopian tubes, impairing eggs' ability to reach the uterus.

If you're trying to get pregnant, drink decaf. However, even in large amounts, coffee should not be considered a contraceptive because its fertility-reducing effect is highly unreliable.

FIBROCYSTIC BREASTS? A few studies have linked caffeine to painful, noncancerous breast lumps (fibrocysts), a normal but annoying condition. Women bothered by fibrocystic breasts might try eliminating all caffeine—in coffee, tea, cocoa, chocolate, soft drinks, and over-the-counter drugs. It might help.

PREMENSTRUAL SYNDROME? In one study, compared with abstainers, women who drank 2 to 4 cups of brewed coffee a day suffered five times the rate of premenstrual syndrome (PMS) symptoms. If PMS is a problem for you, consider cutting back or switching to decaf.

STRESS INCONTINENCE. Coffee contributes to stress incontinence, urine leakage with coughing, laughing, or sneezing. For reasons that remain unclear, coffee consumption is associated with weakening of the muscles that hold the urine tube (urethra) closed (detrusor instability). Brown University researchers surveyed 259 women with various types of urinary incontinence. Compared with those who drank little or no coffee, the women who consumed 5 cups a day were 2.4 times more likely to suffer stress incontinence.

A Cup or Two a Day

As America's most popular herbal medicine, the debate over coffee's safety is sure to continue with headlines trumpeting any findings of harm. But public health experts generally agree that for people with no medical reason to abstain, it's safe to drink 1 or 2 cups a day. Beyond that, risk of side effects increases.

Inform health professionals of the amount of coffee you drink. Problematic herb-drug interactions are possible.

Coffee may cause allergic reactions or other unexpected side effects. If any develop, reduce your dose or stop taking it. For more on herb safety, see Chapter 2.

Gardening

Coffee grows in tropical areas around the world. The Arabian *arabica* species comprises most of the world's supply, but *liberica*, from Liberia, and *robusta*, from the Congo, are also cultivated worldwide.

It's an evergreen shrub or small tree with bright crimson fruits containing two green seeds. The seeds (beans) are extracted and roasted to produce the dark brown, oily beans recognized the world over.

Coffee may also be grown as an ornamental in sunny, humid locales where the temperature does not dip below 60°F. The plant requires full sun, moist air, moist soil, good drainage, and regular feeding.

Coffee plants can also be grown as houseplants. They require full sun and high humidity. They grow well in greenhouses, but not in homes with forced-air heating—too dry. Consult your local nursery or plant store.

COMFREY

Controversial Wound Treatment

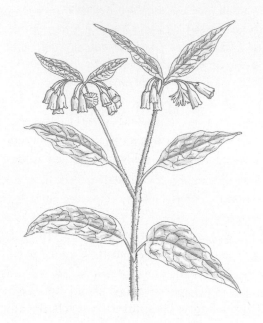

Family: Boraginaceae; other members include borage and forget-me-not

Genus and species: *Symphytum officinale*

Also known as: Bruisewort, knitbone, boneset, and healing herb

Parts used: Roots

Well into the 1980s, many herbalists touted comfrey as "an absolute must" that's "perfectly safe and harmless." Then the herb was found to contain compounds that damage the liver. Today, responsible herbalists recommend comfrey for external use only.

Healing History

The early Greeks used juicy comfrey root externally to treat wounds, believing that it encour-aged torn flesh to knit. The Roman naturalist Pliny encouraged this, observing that boiling comfrey in water produces a sticky paste capable of binding chunks of meat together. Comfrey paste hardens like plaster, and on ancient battlefields, cloths soaked in it were wrapped around broken bones. When the paste dried, the result was a primitive but effective cast. This treatment earned comfrey the popular names knitbone and boneset (not be confused with the herb boneset).

During the 1st century AD, the Greek physician Dioscorides prescribed comfrey tea internally for respiratory and gastrointestinal problems.

By the 1500s, herbalists recommended comfrey tea, not paste, to mend broken bones. One early English herbal suggested that it "helpeth [people who have] broken the bone of the legge."

The 17th-century English herbalist Nicholas Culpeper recommended comfrey roots, "full of glutinous and clammy juice," for "all inward hurts, and for outward wounds and sores in [all] fleshy or sinewy parts of the body. . . . [It] is especially good for ruptures and broken bones." Culpeper also prescribed the herb for fever, gout, hemorrhoids, gangrene, and respiratory and menstrual problems.

As plaster replaced comfrey paste for casting broken bones, names like knitbone were discarded. Comfrey came to be used internally to soothe inflamed mucous membranes. America's 19th-century Eclectic physicians, forerunners of today's naturopaths, prescribed it for diarrhea, dysentery, cough, bronchitis, and "female debility" (menstrual discomfort).

Mexican midwives still apply comfrey to torn vaginal tissue. In the Philippines, the herb is used to treat arthritis, diabetes, anemia, lung infections, and even leukemia.

By the mid-1990s, responsible herbalists had stopped recommending comfrey internally because of its potential for liver damage. Today, it's primarily used to heal wounds and provide pain relief for musculoskeletal injuries.

Therapeutic Uses

The ancient Greeks and Romans were right about comfrey aiding wound healing. But the herb's stickiness has nothing to do with it.

WOUNDS. Russian researchers gave 108 children suffering burns or other wounds standard medical care. In addition, half received an ointment with 10 percent comfrey (Traumaplant), while the other half applied the same ointment diluted to contain 1 percent comfrey. The wounds treated with the 10 percent comfrey ointment healed significantly faster. Traumaplant, a German product, is available at health food stores in the United States. Or mix powdered comfrey with skin cream or with honey, which also aids wound healing.

Comfrey contains allantoin, a compound that promotes the growth of new skin cells. This validates the herb's 2,500 years of external use on everything from minor cuts and burns to major battle wounds. Comfrey also helps relieve inflammation, adding to its wound-treating action. Wash wounds thoroughly with soap and water before applying the herb.

The FDA considers allantoin safe in concentrations of up to 2 percent. It is an ingredient in many over-the-counter products for dry skin, diaper rash, and herpes.

Such widespread commercial use of allantoin suggests that whole comfrey root preparations may provide similar benefits. Commission E, the expert panel that evaluates herbal medicines for the German counterpart of the FDA, approves comfrey root powder for treatment of minor wounds.

Comfrey is absorbed through the skin but if not digested, poses no risk of liver damage.

ARTHRITIS. German researchers gave 220 people with arthritis of the knee either a placebo ointment or a comfrey cream (2 grams three times a day). After 3 weeks, the comfrey cream provided significantly greater pain relief. Another German team gave a placebo or comfrey ointment to 142 men with sprained ankles. Again, the herb group reported significantly greater pain relief.

BACK PAIN. In a Czech study, researchers had 215 chronic back pain sufferers, age 18 to 70, apply either 10 percent comfrey Traumaplant or the same ointment diluted to contain 1 percent comfrey. Five days later, the 10 percent group reported significantly less back pain.

Rx Recommendations

Wash minor wounds with soap and water, then sprinkle some dried, powdered root or make a paste from powdered root and a little water. Apply the paste to the wound and cover with a clean bandage. Change the bandage and reapply the comfrey daily.

For pain relief, buy a comfrey lotion or add powdered root to any skin cream.

Safety

Comfrey contains pyrrolizidine alkaloids (PAs), which, in large amounts, cause serious liver damage. Animals fed plants containing PAs showed symptoms of poisoning, and some died. In humans, several cases of poisoning have also been reported after long-term ingestion of comfrey.

FDA research shows that comfrey's PA content varies greatly, with roots—the part most widely used in herbal medicine—containing the most. Some herbalists have claimed that PAs are not water-soluble and that, as a result, comfrey tea should be free of PAs. But FDA scientists have found PAs in comfrey tea.

The American Herbal Products Association, the herb industry trade organization, recommends that all comfrey products be labeled for external use only. Do not ingest comfrey. Use it topically only.

Gardening

Comfrey is a hardy 5-foot perennial with large, hairy, lance-shaped leaves; thick, spreading roots; a hollow, bristly stem; and bell-like white, blue, or purple flowers.

Comfrey can be started from seed, but it grows best from root cuttings taken in spring or fall. An inch-long piece of root planted in 3 inches of soil almost always produces a plant. Set cuttings 3 feet apart. The herb grows in any well-drained soil and tolerates full sun or partial shade. It spreads vigorously, so contain it in a pot or border it with sheet metal to a depth of 12 inches.

Harvest roots in autumn, after the first frost, or in spring before leaves appear. Wash harvested roots thoroughly and cut them into slices to dry. Grind them to a powder in a blender or coffee grinder and store in a sealed container.

CORDYCEPS
The Parasitic "Worm" That Heals

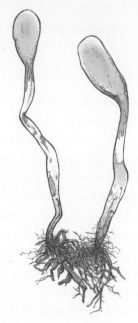

Family: Clavicipitaceae; other members include mushrooms

Genus and species: *Cordyceps sinensis*

Also known as: Caterpillar fungus and *dong chong xia cao*, which means summer plant/winter worm

Parts used: Whole fungus

Cordyceps is native to Asia at elevations above 10,000 feet. It's a parasite that infests and kills insect larvae and caterpillars, hence the name caterpillar fungus. The fungus emerges from its dying host looking like a worm. Oddly, ancient Chinese physicians considered cordyceps fungus a plant during the summer and an animal in winter, hence the name summer plant/winter worm.

Healing History

Cordyceps has long been popular in traditional Himalayan healing. An ethnomedical survey published in 2006 shows that its popularity endures in parts of Nepal.

Not much cordyceps found its way from the Himalayas to lowland China. The fungus was so rare in China that only the Emperor's family used it. Its first mention in a Chinese medical text dates from 1757. In 1843, an American physician called cordyceps similar to ginseng, boosting energy and stamina, improving sexual vitality, and enhancing longevity.

Therapeutic Uses

IMMUNE STIMULATION. Canadian scientists have discovered that cordyceps activates infection-fighting white blood cells. In a Chinese study of cancer sufferers, it improved immune function and quality of life.

ANTIOXIDANT. A Japanese study shows that cordyceps possesses "potent antioxidant activity." Antioxidants help prevent the cell damage at the root of heart disease, cancer, and many other conditions. Hong Kong researchers agree, calling the fungus a "strong antioxidant."

HEART ATTACK AND STROKE. A Chinese report shows that cordyceps reduces both cholesterol and blood fats (triglycerides), meaning less risk of heart attack and stroke. A Japanese study shows that it slows the growth of cholesterol-rich deposits that narrow the arteries and increase risk of heart attack and stroke. Other Chinese studies show that cordyceps (3 grams/day) normalizes heart rhythm and improves congestive heart failure by reducing shortness of breath.

KIDNEY DISEASE. Chinese scientists have found that cordyceps reduces risk of kidney failure and rejection of transplanted kidneys. They called the fungus "ideal" for people receiving kidney transplants.

Other Chinese researchers have discovered that cordyceps prevents lupus-related kidney inflammation (lupus nephritis). They studied 61 lupus sufferers with this condition. Half received a Chinese herb formula and half cordyceps (3 grams/day before meals) plus another Chinese herb, artemisinin (0.6 grams/day after meals). After 3 years, the herb-formula group reduced lupus nephritis recurrences in 77 percent of users, while the figure for the cordyceps/artemisinin group was 97 percent.

LIVER DISEASE. Chinese studies show that cordyceps improves liver function in people with chronic hepatitis and cirrhosis.

ASTHMA, BRONCHITIS. Several Chinese studies show that cordyceps improves lung function in asthma and bronchitis sufferers. In a review of five studies, 4 weeks of cordyceps treatment (3 to 4.5 grams/day) improved lung function in 78 to 92 percent of participants.

FATIGUE, STAMINA. In the elderly, cordyceps appears to live up to its traditional use as a fatigue fighter and stamina builder. Chinese researchers tested the endurance of 30 elderly Chinese and then gave them either a placebo or the fungus (3 grams/day). Six weeks later, the placebo-users showed no improvement in stamina, but those taking cordyceps showed significantly improvement. In another Chinese study, compared with those who took a placebo, elderly people who used corcyceps (3 grams/day) reported significantly less fatigue, dizziness, ringing in the ears (tinnitus), and intolerance to cold.

However, four studies show that cordyceps (3 grams/day for 2 to 5 weeks) does not improve athletic performance in younger people. Two trials involved competitive cyclists tested before and after taking the fungus. It's possible that cordyceps helps the elderly, but not young adults.

Intriguing Possibilities

Korean scientists have shown that cordyceps treatment kills liver cancer cells, presumably because it's an antioxidant and stimulates the immune system. It's too early to call cordyceps a cancer treatment, but one day it might be.

In a Chinese study of 155 people with unspecified sex problems, almost two-thirds reported improvement after taking cordyceps.

Rx Recommendations

Most studies have used 3 grams/day (approximately 1 tablespoon). For weakness, debility, and recovery from illness, Chinese medical practitioners recommend 3 to 9 grams/day (1 to 3 tablespoons) of powdered fungus. It can also be mixed into soup and eaten.

Safety

Animal studies show low toxicity, if any.

Pregnant and nursing women should not use cordyceps.

Do not give cordyceps to children under 2. In older children, adjust the recommended dose based on the child's weight. Give a 50-pound child one-third of the dose a 150-pound adult would take.

If you're over 65, start with a low dose, and increase only if necessary.

Inform health professionals of the herbs you use. Problematic herb-drug interactions are possible.

Cordyceps may cause allergic reactions or other unexpected side effects. If any develop, reduce your dose or stop taking it. For more on herb safety, see Chapter 2.

If symptoms get worse or persist longer than 2 weeks, consult a health professional promptly.

Gardening

Medicinal *Cordyceps sinensis* is not found outside of the Himalayas. A related species, *C. militaris*, parasitizes some caterpillars in North America.

Aloha Medicinals of Carson City, Nevada (alohamedicinals.com) grows *Cordyceps sinensis* in the United States under simulated high-altitude conditions—low temperature and low oxygen equivalent to an elevation of 18,000 feet. The company claims to be the world's largest producer of the fungus.

CRANBERRY

Not Just for UTIs

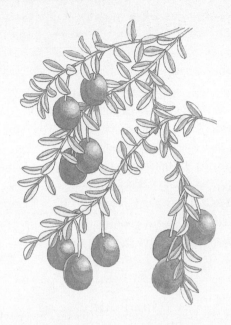

Family: Ericaceae; other members include azalea, blueberry, and uva-ursi

Genus and species: *Vaccinium macrocarpon* or *Oxycoccus quadripetalus*

Also known as: No other common names

Parts used: Berries

Cranberry—actually cranberry juice—is the herbal choice for preventing urinary tract infections (UTIs). The berries are also rich in antioxidant nutrients, which help prevent degenerative diseases, particularly those that affect the eyes.

Healing History

In 1621, the Pilgrims reportedly dined on cranberry dishes at the first Thanksgiving. But cranberry sauce did not become a national tradition until after the Civil War. General Ulysses S. Grant considered cranberry sauce an essential part of Thanksgiving and ordered it served to Union troops in 1864 during the siege of Petersburg. Soldiers unfamiliar with the tart berries loved them, and the custom stuck.

The Pilgrims had no idea that cranberries are high in vitamin C, but New England sailors who ate the bright red berries did not develop scurvy.

America's 19th-century Eclectic physicians, forerunners of today's naturopaths, did not consider cranberry particularly medicinal. However, their text, *King's American Dispensatory* (1898), contained this curious prescription: "A split cranberry, held in position by a daub of starch paste, will quickly relieve the pain and inflammation attending boils on the tip of the nose."

Today, Americans eat cranberries not only at Thanksgiving but year-round—2 pounds annually per capita. Annual American consumption is 9 million barrels, worth almost $400 million.

Therapeutic Uses

Cranberry's claim to fame as a UTI preventive comes not from herbal tradition but rather from 19th-century German chemists.

URINARY TRACT INFECTIONS. During the 1840s, German researchers discovered that the urine of cranberry eaters contains bacteria-fighting hippuric acid. Sixty years later, American researchers speculated that urine acidified by a steady diet of cranberries might prevent UTIs, a common, recurrent, and often chronic health problem among women.

Women plagued by UTIs began drinking cranberry juice with gusto, and several studies endorsed the practice. But by the late 1960s, nay-sayers claimed that the tart berries did not significantly acidify urine and therefore could not prevent UTIs.

More recent research shows that cranberry juice does, indeed, reduce risk of UTI. A 1984 study, in the *Journal of Urology*, showed that after drinking a pint of commercial cranberry juice cocktail daily for 3 weeks, 73 percent of recurrent UTI sufferers experienced significant protection. The researchers theorized that urinary acidity has nothing to do with the herb's effectiveness. Instead, they explained, the juice prevents the germs that cause UTIs from adhering to the lining of the urinary tract, reducing likelihood of infection.

Since then, dozens of studies have reached the same conclusion. British researchers analyzed 10 studies involving 1,049 women. Their conclusion: "Compared with placebo treatment, cranberry products reduce incidence of UTI by 35 percent." The reason: Cranberries contain antioxidant compounds called proanthocyanidins that inhibit bacterial adherence in the bladder.

ANTIOXIDANT. Proanthocyanidins are members of the family of antioxidants known as anthocyanosides. Antioxidants help prevent and reverse the cell damage at the root of heart disease, most strokes, many cancers, and other degenerative diseases. Tufts University researchers analyzed and ranked dozens of common plant foods according to their total antioxidant content. The best sources turned out to be brightly colored fruits and berries, such as cranberries with their generous amount of anthocyanosides.

CATARACTS. Cataracts are a major cause of vision impairment and blindness among older adults in the United States. The condition results from oxidative damage when the normally clear lens of the eye develops cloudy spots.

For reasons that remain unclear, anthocyanosides have unusually powerful effects on the eyes. In one Italian study, 50 people with early-stage cataracts were given an extract of bilberry (another berry rich in anthocyanosides) three times a day, along with antioxidant vitamin E. The treatment stopped cataract progression in 97 percent of the study participants. Like bilberries, cranberries also contain similar generous amounts of anthocyanosides, so they, too, appear helpful in cataract prevention.

MACULAR DEGENERATION. Macular degeneration involves deterioration of the macula, the part of the nerve-rich retina in the back of the eye responsible for discerning fine detail and seeing what's directly in front of you (central vision).

In a European study, 31 people with retinal problems including macular degeneration were given an extract of bilberry. Those with macular degeneration experienced significant vision improvement. Cranberries contain many of the same eye-friendly nutrients as bilberries, so odds are they may also help this condition.

DIABETIC RETINOPATHY. Diabetes damages the blood vessels, including the tiny capillaries that nourish the retina. When injured, these capillaries can leak blood into the eye, causing the blurred vision of diabetic retinopathy.

Anthocyanosides strengthen retinal blood vessels, reducing leakage. In the study of retinal eye problems mentioned above, people with diabetic retinopathy showed significant improvement when taking the bilberry extract. Cranberries should also help.

INCONTINENCE. Cranberry juice helps deodorize urine. A report in the *Journal of Psy-*

chiatric Nursing suggests that people with urinary incontinence incorporate cranberry juice into their diets to reduce embarrassing odor.

Intriguing Possibilities

A Czech study suggests that cranberry may help treat prostate enlargement.

A study by University of Florida researchers hints that a daily glass of cranberry juice may reduce the severity of cold symptoms.

And a report from Taiwan suggests that cranberry reduces cholesterol.

Rx Recommendations

Most studies showing UTI prevention have used cranberry juice cocktail, available in supermarkets. Pure cranberry juice is highly acidic and too sour to drink. Ocean Spray and other marketers add water and sugar, turning pure juice into a "cocktail." If you're prone to UTIs, try drinking a daily glass or two. It may help prevent recurrences.

In the study of UTIs reported in the *Journal of Family Practice*, participants did not drink juice. Instead, they took one capsule of cranberry extract (400 milligrams of cranberry solids) twice a day for at least a month. The solids were as effective as the juice. If you'd like to try an extract, they are available in many health food stores. Or munch on dried cranberries. Many health food stores and supermarkets sell them as Craisins, a snack food similar to raisins.

Safety

Cranberries are unlikely to cause allergic reactions or other unexpected side effects. But if any develop, reduce your dose or stop taking them.

Inform health professionals of the herbs you use. Problematic herb-drug interactions are possible. For more on herb safety, see Chapter 2.

If symptoms get worse or persist longer than 2 weeks, consult a health professional promptly.

Gardening

Cranberry is a small evergreen shrub that grows in mountain forests and damp bogs from Alaska to Tennessee. Its pink or purple flowers bloom from late spring to late summer and produce bright red fruits in fall.

Few gardeners have the conditions necessary to grow this herb. It requires wet, boggy, acidic soil amended with peat moss or leaf mold. Check with your local nursery to see if cranberry is viable in your area.

DANDELION

Much More Than a Weed

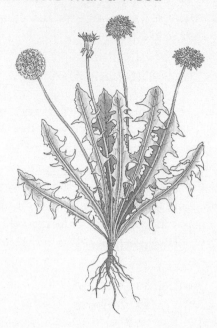

Family: Compositae; other members include daisy and marigold

Genus and species: *Taraxacum officinale*

Also known as: Lion's tooth, wild endive, and piss-abed

Parts used: Primarily roots, also leaves

Dandelion is so widely despised as a weed that many people have a hard time seeing that it's a nutritious healer with a medicinal reputation dating back more than 1,000 years.

Dandelion is a diuretic that may help relieve premenstrual syndrome, high blood pressure, and congestive heart failure, among other benefits.

Healing History

Chinese physicians have prescribed dandelion since ancient times to treat colds, bronchitis, pneumonia, hepatitis, boils, ulcers, obesity, dental problems, itching, and internal injuries. They also used poultices of chopped dandelion to treat breast cancer. India's traditional Ayurvedic physicians used the herb similarly.

Tenth-century Arab physicians were the first to recognize that dandelion increases urine production.

During the Middle Ages, Europeans believed in the Doctrine of Signatures, the idea that plants' physical characteristics reveal their healing virtues. Under the Doctrine, yellow plants were linked to the liver's yellow bile and considered liver remedies, which is why dandelion gained a reputation as a treatment for jaundice and gallstones.

The Doctrine of Signatures also supported the observation that dandelion is diuretic. The plant has a juicy root, stem, and leaves. Anything juicy was linked to urination.

By the 17th century, dandelion was so renowned as a diuretic that the English referred to it as piss-abed, from the French pissenlit. Meanwhile, the French thought the herb's toothed leaves resembled lion's teeth and dubbed it *dent de lion*, Anglicized as dandelion.

Thanks to herbal exaggerators like 17th-century English herbalist Nicholas Culpeper, dandelion's medicinal reputation spread as widely as the plant itself across an untended lawn. Culpeper recommended the herb for every "evil disposition of the body."

In fact, dandelion was used for so many ailments that it became known as "the official remedy for disorders." This designation lives on today in dandelion's genus name, Taraxacum, from the Greek *taraxos*, meaning "disorder," and *akos*, for "remedy."

American colonists introduced dandelion to North America, and Native Americans quickly adopted it as a tonic. Dandelion root was an ingredient in Lydia E. Pinkham's Vegetable Compound, a popular 19th-century patent medicine for menstrual discomforts. Because it's a diuretic, dandelion no doubt helped relieve the bloating that many women experience before menstrual periods.

Although dandelion was listed in the *U.S. Pharmacopoeia*, a standard drug reference, from 1831 to 1926, many 19th-century herbalists despised it for the weed it had become. According to *King's American Dispensatory* (1898), the text used by Eclectic physicians, forerunners of today's naturopaths, dandelion was "overrated. . . . Dandelion root possesses little medicinal virtue [except] slightly diuretic action."

Contemporary herbalists recommend dandelion almost exclusively as a diuretic for premenstrual syndrome, menstrual discomforts, swollen feet and ankles, high blood pressure, congestive heart failure, and weight loss.

Therapeutic Uses

Before reviling dandelion, read Ralph Waldo Emerson. "What is a weed?" the distinguished author wrote. "A plant whose virtues have not yet been discovered." As far as dandelion is concerned, truer words were never penned, although this plant's virtues have been well documented.

GALLSTONES. The Doctrine of Signatures was right on at least one count. Two German studies suggest that dandelion stimulates the flow of bile, which helps digest fats.

In Germany, where herbal medicine is more mainstream than in the United States, physicians routinely recommend dandelion to help improve the flow of bile and prevent gallstones. A German preparation, Chol-Grandelat, a combination of dandelion, milk thistle, and rhubarb,

is prescribed for gallbladder disease. (It's not available in the United States.)

Commission E, the expert panel that evaluates herbal medicines for the German counterpart of the FDA, endorses dandelion root and leaves as bile flow stimulants.

PREMENSTRUAL SYNDROME (PMS). Animal studies suggest that dandelion does, indeed, possess diuretic action. Findings in animals don't always apply to people, but this one seems to.

Commission E recognizes dandelion as an effective diuretic. Since diuretics may help relieve the bloated feeling of PMS, women may want to try some before menstrual periods.

HIGH BLOOD PRESSURE. As the fluid volume of blood decreases, so does blood pressure. That's why physicians often prescribe diuretics. Dandelion may help. Of course, high blood pressure is a serious condition that requires professional treatment. Use dandelion in consultation with your physician.

CONGESTIVE HEART FAILURE. Congestive heart failure involves chronic fatigue of the muscular heart. The condition is often treated with diuretics because they reduce blood volume, so the weakened heart has less fluid to pump. As a natural diuretic, dandelion may be appropriate when taken in conjunction with other prescribed therapies. Like high blood pressure, congestive heart failure is a serious condition that cannot be self-treated. If you'd like to try dandelion, discuss it with your physician.

CANCER. Dandelion leaves contain large amounts of beta-carotene and vitamin C. Both nutrients are antioxidants that help prevent the cell damage that sets the stage for cancer, not to mention other degenerative diseases.

OVERWEIGHT. In one study, animals fed dandelion lost significant weight. As a diuretic, the herb may help eliminate water weight, but experts discourage diuretics for permanent weight control. Most advocate a low-calorie, low-fat diet, moderate portion size, and regular exercise. Lost water weight eventually returns as the body, which is mostly water, adjusts to ongoing treatment with diuretics and decreases its urine output.

Intriguing Possibilities

Dandelion may help reduce the amount of sugar in the blood, meaning possible value in managing diabetes. If you have diabetes, use dandelion only in consultation with your physician.

In some studies, dandelion root has shown anti-inflammatory properties, suggesting its possible value in treating arthritis.

And a Japanese study hints at antitumor activity, though it's much too early to consider the herb a cancer treatment.

One study found that dandelion inhibits the growth of *Candida albicans*, the fungus responsible for vaginal yeast infections.

Rx Recommendations

Eat fresh leaves in salads or steam them as a vegetable.

If using dandelion as a diuretic (for premenstrual syndrome, high blood pressure, or congestive heart failure) or as a digestive aid, take it as a leaf infusion, root decoction, or tincture. The taste is reasonably pleasant, with a slightly bitter sharpness.

To make a leaf infusion, use ½ ounce of dried leaves per cup of boiling water. Steep for 10 minutes, then strain. Drink up to 3 cups a day.

For a root decoction, gently boil 2 to 3 tea-

spoons of powdered root per cup of water for 15 minutes, let cool, and strain if you wish. Drink up to 3 cups a day.

With a homemade tincture, take 1 to 2 teaspoons up to three times a day.

When using commercial preparations, follow package directions.

Safety

Long-term use of diuretics such as dandelion can be hazardous. Diuretics deplete the body of potassium, an essential nutrient. People using them should be sure to eat foods rich in potassium, such as bananas and fresh vegetables. Fortunately, dandelion causes less potassium loss than other diuretics because the herb itself is high in potassium. Nevertheless, if you use dandelion for long periods, be sure to eat potassium-rich foods.

Women who are pregnant or nursing should not take diuretics in any form without a doctor's approval.

Do not give medicinal preparations of dandelion to children under 2. In older children, adjust the recommended dose based on the child's weight. Give a 50-pound child one-third of the dose a 150-pound adult would take.

If you're over 65, start with a low dose, and increase only if necessary.

Inform health professionals of the herbs you use. Problematic herb-drug interactions are possible.

Dandelion may cause skin rash, allergic reactions, or other unexpected side effects. If any develop, reduce your dose or stop taking it. For more on herb safety, see Chapter 2.

If symptoms get worse or persist longer than 2 weeks, consult a health professional promptly.

Gardening

If you cultivate dandelions, be careful whom you tell. You may end up with unhappy neighbors.

As every gardener knows, dandelions grow like weeds. This low-growing perennial has a deep taproot, a rosette of jaggedly toothed leaves that radiate from its base, and a smooth, hollow, 6- to 12-inch stem capped by a single yellow flower that gives rise to hundreds of tufted single-seed fruits. The root, leaves, and stem contain a milky fluid.

Harvest young leaves as they develop. As they mature, they become unpleasantly bitter. Herbalists generally recommend harvesting the root at the end of the second growing season. To prevent spreading, clip the flowers before seed tufts form.

Dandelion seeds may not be readily available, but check seed catalogs. Better yet, check nearby lawns or vacant lots. It's unlikely that anyone will mind if you take a few. Plant the seeds in early spring. They grow in almost any soil but prefer moist, well-drained loam.

DEVIL'S CLAW

An Angel of a Pain Reliever

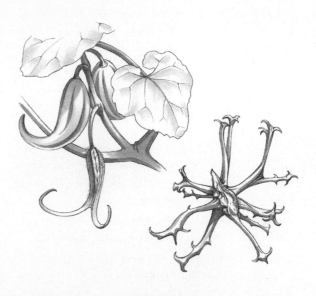

Family: Pedaliaceae; other members include sesame

Genus and species: *Harpagophytum procumbens*

Also known as: Grapple plant, harpago

Parts used: Tubers

Are you bothered by stiff, achy, arthritic joints or low-back pain? Then devil's claw can be an angel of a healer.

Devil's claw is a perennial ground cover that grows only in the dry highlands of Angola, Zimbabwe, Namibia, Botswana, and South Africa. Its fierce-looking, hook-shaped fruits are the source of its satanic name and its other name, grapple plant. The herb's Latin generic, *Harpago*, means hook. The plant's taproot produces secondary tubers, the part used medicinally.

Healing History

Indigenous Southern Africans have used devil's claw for centuries to treat upset stomach, fever, inflammation, and pain. German researchers first became interested in the plant 50 years ago. Since then, European researchers have amassed considerable evidence that the herb is a safe, effective treatment for low-back pain and osteoarthritis, the form of joint pain most people call "arthritis."

Therapeutic Uses

The active constituent in devil's claw tubers is the compound harpagoside.

LOW-BACK PAIN. In a 6-week study at the University of Freiburg, Germany, researchers gave 44 back-pain sufferers either the standard dose of an arthritis drug (Vioxx) or devil's claw (60 milligrams harpagoside/day). Compared with the drug takers, those who used devil's claw were more likely to report a 50 percent decrease in pain and more likely to become pain-free. Several other studies show similar results—with devil's claw generally causing few side effects. Several other German studies have reached the same conclusion. One team concluded that the herb "appears to be an effective alternative for the treatment of chronic back pain." Commission E, the German counterpart of the FDA, approves devil's claw for treating pain and inflammation.

OSTEOARTHRITIS. Several studies show that devil's claw relieves the aches, pain, and stiffness of osteoarthritis, the most common cause of joint pain. French researchers gave 122 people with osteoarthritis of the knee or hip either a pharmaceutical pain reliever—a nonsteroidal anti-inflammatory drug—or the

herb (6 capsules a day, 435 milligrams/capsule, 2,610 milligrams total, containing approximately 54 milligrams hapragoside/day). Four months later, both treatments produced the same relief, but the herb group reported fewer side effects.

Intriguing Possibilities

A South African animal study suggests that devil's claw reduces blood sugar. It's too early to call the herb a treatment for diabetes, but one day it might be.

Rx Recommendations

Studies showing relief of osteoarthritis and low-back pain have used doses in the range of 50 to 60 milligrams/day of harpagoside, which corresponds to 2,400 to 2,900 milligrams of devil's claw extract. Follow label directions, or take 2,400 to 2,900 milligrams of extract per day divided into two or three doses.

Safety

Devil's claw causes no serious side effects, though mild stomach distress is possible.

Unlike the nonsteroidal anti-inflammatory drugs (NSAIDs) often prescribed for osteoarthritis and low back pain, devil's claw causes no significant abdominal distress. In addition, it does not interfere with blood clotting, so it can be used safely by those taking blood-thinning drugs, or those with clotting disorders.

Devil's claw may stimulate secretion of stomach acid. People with stomach or duodenal ulcers should not use it.

Pregnant and nursing women should not use devil's claw.

Do not give this herb to children under 2. In older children, adjust the recommended dose based on the child's weight. Give a 50-pound child one-third of the dose a 150-pound adult would take.

If you're over 65, start with a low dose, and increase only if necessary.

Inform health professionals of the herbs you use. Problematic herb-drug interactions are possible.

Devil's claw may cause allergic reactions or other unexpected side effects. If any develop, reduce your dose or stop taking it. For more on herb safety, see Chapter 2.

If symptoms get worse or persist longer than 2 weeks, consult a health professional promptly.

Gardening

Not grown in the United States.

DILL

Beyond Pickles, a Potent Stomach Soother

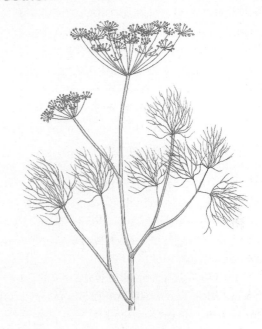

Family: Umbelliferae; other members include carrot, parsley, celery, fennel, and angelica

Genus and species: *Anethum graveolens*

Also known as: No other common names

Parts used: Fruits (seeds); leaves are used in cooking

Dill does more for pickles than provide flavor. It's also a natural preservative. In fact, food preservation was pickling's original purpose.

Dill has been used in herbal healing since the dawn of Egyptian civilization, and for good reason. In addition to its preservative action, the herb is an infection fighter and a soothing digestive aid.

Healing History

Records discovered in 3,000-year-old Egyptian tombs show that ancient physicians used fragrant dill as a digestive aid and remedy for intestinal gas. The 1st-century Greek physician Dioscorides prescribed dill so frequently that it was known for centuries as "the herb of Dioscorides." The Romans chewed dill seeds to promote digestion, and they hung dill garlands in their dining halls, believing that the herb prevented stomach upset.

Traditional Chinese physicians have used dill as a digestive aid for more than 1,000 years. They recommend it especially for children because its action is milder than that of other digestive herbs such as caraway, anise, and fennel.

The Vikings were well aware of dill's digestive benefits. The word "dill" comes from the Old Norse *dilla*, meaning to soothe.

The 17th-century English herbalist Nicholas Culpeper claimed dill "stayeth the belly . . . and is a gallant expeller of wind." Culpeper also recommended the herb for hiccups and swelling and to "strengthen the brain."

Colonists brought dill to North America. Its seed infusion, known as dillwater, became a favorite among American folk healers for childhood ailments such as colic, cough, indigestion, gas, stomachache, and insomnia. In adults, the herb was used to treat hemorrhoids, jaundice, scurvy, and dropsy (congestive heart failure).

Contemporary herbalists still tout dill as the herb of choice for infant colic. They recommend chewing the seeds for bad breath and drinking dill tea both as a digestive aid and to stimulate nursing mothers' milk production.

Therapeutic Uses

If you use dill only in pickling spices or on salmon, you're missing out on a marvelous healer. While it won't cure hemorrhoids or increase milk production, some of its other traditional applications are supported by science.

DIGESTIVE PROBLEMS. Research has validated dill's 3,000 years of use as a digestive aid. The herb relaxes the smooth muscles of the digestive tract. One study found dill to be an antifoaming agent, meaning that it helps prevent the formation of intestinal gas bubbles. Dill seed oil also inhibits the growth of several types of bacteria that attack the intestinal tract, suggesting that it may help prevent infectious diarrhea.

Commission E, the expert panel that evaluates herbal medicines for Germany's counterpart of the FDA, endorses dill for indigestion.

URINARY TRACT INFECTIONS. Dill inhibits *Escherichia coli*, the bacteria usually responsible for urinary tract infections.

Intriguing Possibilities

When injected into laboratory animals, dill extract stimulates respiration, slows heart rate, and opens blood vessels, all of which reduce blood pressure. Of course, people don't inject dill preparations, but these effects suggest that there's more to learn about dill's healing potential.

Rx Recommendations

To benefit from dill's breath-freshening effects, chew ½ to 1 teaspoon of seeds.

When using the herb as a digestive aid, take it as an infusion or tincture. To make a pleasant-tasting infusion, use 2 teaspoons of crushed seeds per cup of boiling water, steep for 10 minutes, and strain. Drink up to 3 cups a day.

As a homemade tincture, take $\frac{1}{2}$ to 1 teaspoon up to three times a day.

When using commercial preparations, follow package directions.

Safety

Never ingest dill seed oil. As little as a teaspoon may be toxic.

Dill leaves and seeds are generally considered nontoxic, but sensitivity is possible and may cause skin rash.

Inform health professionals of the herbs you use. Problematic herb-drug interactions are possible.

Dill may cause allergic reactions or other unexpected side effects. If any develop, reduce your dose or stop taking it. For more on herb safety, see Chapter 2.

If symptoms get worse or persist longer than 2 weeks, consult a health professional promptly.

Gardening

Dill is an annual with a long taproot like its close relative, carrot. It has a delicate, fast-growing, spindly stem with lacy leaves. Yellow flowers appear in summer and produce great quantities of tiny, ridged fruits (seeds).

Dill grows vigorously from seeds sown $\frac{1}{4}$ inch deep in early spring. Germination takes about 2 weeks. Thin seedlings to 12-inch spacing. The plants grow to 3 feet in rich, moist, slightly acidic soil under full sun, or in partial shade in the South. Shelter plants from the wind.

Harvest the leaves once plants have become established. Fresh dill leaves are much more aromatic than dried. To guarantee a supply of fresh leaves from late spring to late fall, plant seeds throughout your growing season.

The seeds mature in about 2 months. Harvest them when they begin to turn brown.

Dill self-sows, so if you leave a few plants unharvested, you'll have this tasty healing herb every year.

ECHINACEA

The Immune-Boosting Cold Remedy

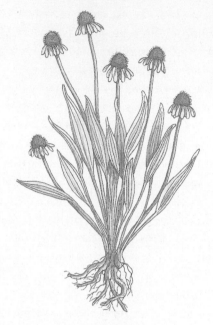

Family: Compositae; other members include daisy, dandelion, and marigold

Genus and species: *Echinacea angustifolia* and *E. purpurea*

Also known as: Purple coneflower

Parts used: Primarily roots; also leaves and flowers

Echinacea (eh-kin-AY-sha) has had its ups and downs on the way to becoming one of the nation's bestselling herbal medicines. Since the 1870s, it has been reviled, then lionized, then forgotten, and finally resurrected.

Today, echinacea is widely accepted as an effective remedy for colds and flu. Many—but not all—studies published in mainstream medical journals agree that it's a safe, effective immune stimulant that helps the body combat all manner of infections, particularly upper respiratory viruses.

Healing History

Echinacea is a tall, daisy-like flower native to the American Great Plains. It was the primary medicine of the region's Native Americans. They applied root poultices to wounds, snakebites, and insect bites and stings. They used echinacea mouthwash for toothache and drank echinacea tea to treat colds, smallpox, measles, mumps, and arthritis.

Plains settlers adopted the herb, but it remained a folk remedy until 1870, when a cantankerous patent-medicine purveyor, Dr. H. C. F. Meyer of Pawnee City, Nebraska, used it in his Meyer's Blood Purifier. He promoted the remedy as "an absolute cure" for rattlesnake bite, blood poisoning, and a host of other ills. Claims like Dr. Meyer's are what earned patent medicines the derisive name, snake oil.

But Dr. Meyer truly believed that echinacea could cure rattlesnake bite and wanted to prove it. In 1885, he sent a sample to John Uri Lloyd, professor at the Eclectic Medical Institute in Cincinnati. Lloyd was an early pharmacologist, one of the first presidents of the American Pharmaceutical Association, and a cofounder (with his brothers) of Lloyd Brothers Pharmacists, a prominent 19th-century drug company. Lloyd identified the plant as echinacea, but after one look at Dr. Meyer's label with its claim of "absolute cure" for rattlesnake bite, he dismissed Meyer as a crackpot.

Dr. Meyer wrote back, insisting that echinacea *was* a cure for rattlesnake bite. He was so confident that he offered to bring a live rattlesnake to Cincinnati and let it bite him in Lloyd's presence to demonstrate his Blood Purifier's effectiveness. Lloyd declined the offer.

Undaunted, Dr. Meyer shipped some echinacea to Lloyd's Eclectic colleague, John King, who, in the 1850s, had mentioned the plant's Native American uses in the first edition of his pharmacological text, *King's American Dispensatory*. King tested the herb, and after successfully using it to treat bee stings, chronic nasal congestion, leg ulcers, and a variety of infections, he extolled the plant in subsequent editions of his book.

Eventually, Lloyd also accepted echinacea, declaring it useful for treating wounds, venomous bites and stings, blood poisoning (septicemia), diphtheria, meningitis, measles, chickenpox, malaria, scarlet fever, influenza, syphilis, and gangrene.

Lloyd's enthusiasm transcended academics. His family business, Lloyd Brothers Pharmacists, developed several echinacea products, which enjoyed tremendous popularity throughout the United States as infection treatments from the 1890s to the 1920s. During the early 20th century, it was a rare medicine cabinet that didn't contain tincture of echinacea. (The Lloyd brothers also owned the New York Giants baseball team and founded the Lloyd Library in Cincinnati, currently one of the world's largest collections of botanical literature.)

Unfortunately, echinacea became a casualty of the war between mainstream physicians (known prior to World War I as "regulars"), who favored the emerging laboratory-synthesized drugs, and the Eclectics, who were more herbally inclined. Each side was hostile to the other's medicines. In 1909, the following statement appeared in the *Journal of the American Medical Association*: "Echinacea . . . has failed to sustain the reputation given it by its enthusiasts . . . [who] make use of early unverified reports to endow their nostrums with remarkable therapeutic properties."

By World War II, as modern antibiotics became available, echinacea's popularity waned. The *National Formulary*, a standard pharmacy reference, listed it from 1916 until 1950. But from the 1940s on, it was largely forgotten—until the herbal revival of the 1970s.

Contemporary herbalists are as enthusiastic about echinacea as the Eclectics were. They tout it as a botanical antibiotic and immune-system stimulant for boils, colds and flu, bladder infections, tonsillitis, and other infections. Some recommend taking the herb daily as a tonic and immune-system enhancer.

Therapeutic Uses

Old Dr. Meyer would be tickled to learn how potent his favorite herb actually is. Echinacea has never been shown to cure rattlesnake bite, but from the 1950s through the 1980s, many studies (almost all of them German) concluded that the plant is a remarkable immune stimulator and infection fighter. By the 1990s, American researchers were studying the herb and coming to the same conclusion.

ENHANCED IMMUNITY. Echinacea helps treat infection by revving up the immune system. When disease-causing microorganisms attack, infected cells secrete compounds that attract infection-fighting white blood cells (macrophages). The macrophages (literally, "big eaters") engulf and digest the invaders. Echinacea boosts their ability to destroy germs.

The herb also energizes other important white blood cells, natural killer cells and T lymphocytes. And it increases secretion of interleukin-1, another component of the immune system.

Ultra-strenuous athletics, for example, triathlons, suppress the immune system. German researchers gave 42 triathletes one of three daily treatments: a placebo, mineral supplements, or echinacea. A month later, shortly after a triathlon, those who had taken the echinacea showed the least immune suppression.

INFECTIONS. In addition to immune stimulation, echinacea helps combat a broad range of disease-causing viruses, bacteria, fungi, and protozoa. Echinacea fights infection in several ways. It contains echinacoside, a natural antibiotic with broad-spectrum antimicrobial activity. It strengthens the body against assault by invading microorganisms. Our cells contain hyaluronic acid (HA), a chemical that, in part, shields against germ attack. Many germs produce the enzyme hyaluronidase to dissolve the HA shield so they can penetrate tissues and cause infection. Echinacea contains another compound, echinacein, that counteracts the germs' tissue-dissolving enzyme and prevents their entry into the body's cells. In addition, echinacea mimics interferon, the body's own virus-fighting compound. Before a virus-infected cell dies, it releases a tiny amount of interferon, which boosts the ability of surrounding cells to resist the infection. Echinacea appears to do the same thing. Researchers bathed cells in echinacea extract, then exposed them to two potent viruses (influenza and herpes). Compared with untreated cells, only a small number of the treated cells became infected.

German researchers report success in using echinacea to treat tonsillitis, bronchitis, tuberculosis, meningitis, wounds, abscesses, whooping cough (pertussis), ear infections, and especially colds and flu.

COLD TREATMENT. By the late 1990s, more than a dozen studies had investigated echinacea as a cold treatment. While most showed significant benefit—shorter, milder colds—enough showed no benefit to keep critics carping that echinacea offered more hype than substance.

Then, in a 1999 report in the *Journal of Family Practice*, two mainstream M.D.s from the University of Wisconsin and one from Bastyr University, the naturopathic medical school near Seattle, analyzed eight studies of echinacea for treatment of upper-respiratory infections that involved more than 1,000 participants All eight were double-blind—neither the participants nor the researchers knew who took the placebo or the echinacea. Those taking the herb used tablets, capsules, juices, or tinctures of the herb's immune-boosting roots, leaves, and flowers.

Among the eight studies, this one was typical. In a large Swedish furniture factory, researchers identified 60 workers with sore throat, the first symptom of most colds. Half took placebos, the rest took tincture of echinacea (20 drops in water every 2 hours on day one, then the same amount three times a day for up to 10 days). In the placebo group, recovery time averaged 8 days. But those taking echinacea recovered in half the time, 4 days.

All eight studies showed similar results. Six were statistically significant. Two were not, but showed a clear trend in the direction of benefit. The reviewers' verdict: Echinacea is a solid winner as a treatment for colds and flu. In all eight studies, compared with placebos, the herb cut colds' severity and duration in half.

The researchers concluded that treatment with echinacea should begin as soon as you feel the first twinges of a cold or flu coming on. Take it several times a day, then taper off as you begin to feel better.

Commission E, the expert panel that evaluates herbal medicines for the German counterpart of the FDA, also endorses echinacea as a treatment for colds and flu.

Unfortunately, echinacea remains controversial. In 2005, a study by Austrian researchers published in the prestigious *New England Journal of Medicine* showed the herb useless against colds. The researchers squirted live cold virus up the noses of 399 college students and then treated them with a placebo or the herb. It neither prevented colds nor reduced the severity of those that developed. This study was widely publicized. The *New York Times* story was headlined: "Study Says Echinacea Has No Effect on Colds." But the study had a fatal flaw. The researchers used a dose that many herbal medicine experts considered too low to have any benefit.

In 2007, researchers at the University of Connecticut School of Pharmacy analyzed 14 studies of echinacea for prevention and treatment of colds. They found that the herb significantly reduced cold severity and cut duration 1.4 days.

Finally, German and American researchers analyzed 24 double-blind American, Canadian, and European trials involving 4,631 subjects. Compared with placebo treatment, those who took echinacea experienced substantially milder, briefer colds ($p < 0.001$).

COLD PREVENTION. Traditional herbalists never claimed that echinacea prevents colds. They considered it only a treatment. But now it appears that the herb has cold-preventive value—though that remains controversial.

The *Journal of Family Practice* study discussed above also analyzed four prevention studies involving 1,152 participants. Again, the studies were double-blind and used various preparations of all parts of the herb. How many showed statistically significant preventive value? None.

On the other hand, the German-American team whose analysis of 24 treatment trials showed substantial preventive value also found that echinacea *prevents* colds, reducing risk by 58 percent.

A more recent Australian study supports echinacea for cold prevention. The researchers studied 175 adults flying from Australia to the United States, Europe, or Africa. Participants took either a placebo or echinacea (112.5 milligrams of *E. purpurea* plus 150 milligrams of *E. angustifolia*) twice a day starting 2 weeks before flying and ending 2 weeks after landing. Those taking the herb developed significantly fewer colds.

Researchers with the Common Cold Center at the University of Cardiff, Wales, gave 755 healthy adults a placebo or tincture of echinacea (0.9 milliliters in water three times a day, five times a day if they had colds). After 4 months, the placebo takers reported 188 colds lasting 850 total days, but the echinacea group experienced only 149 colds lasting a total of 672 days—significant preventive efficacy.

Finally, Austrian and German investigators reviewed three prevention trials and found that compared with placebo treatment, echinacea reduced the risk of catching colds by 55 percent.

No doubt, echinacea will continue to be a controversial cold remedy. But the evidence shows that it's effective for both treatment and prevention.

WOUNDS. Science has confirmed echinacea's traditional use in wound healing. Echinacein—the same compound that prevents germs from penetrating tissues—also helps broken skin knit faster by spurring the cells that form new tissue (fibroblasts) to work more efficiently.

Echinacea preparations can be applied to cuts, burns, psoriasis, eczema, genital herpes sores, and cold sores. Commission E supports the use of echinacea for wound treatment.

YEAST INFECTION. In a German study, 203 women with recurrent vaginal yeast infections were treated with either a standard pharmaceutical antiyeast cream or the cream plus oral echinacea. Within 6 months, 60 percent of the women who used just the cream experienced recurrences. Among those who also took echinacea, the figure was only 16 percent, a highly significant difference.

GASTROINTESTINAL INFECTION. University of Arkansas researchers analyzed 12 volunteers' stool samples for evidence of bacteria that cause food poisoning and other gastrointestinal infections. Then the participants took echinacea (1,000 milligrams/day for 10 days). Subsequent stool analysis showed significantly fewer bacteria, enough of a decrease to reduce risk of GI infections.

CANCER CHEMOTHERAPY AND RADIATION THERAPY. Cancer chemotherapy typically reduces white blood cell counts, increasing risk of infection. German researchers gave chemotherapy to 15 people with advanced esophageal or colorectal cancer. They also took echinacea and an extract of the thymus gland, a component of the immune system. Instead of falling, as would be expected, their white blood cell counts increased.

Radiation treatments also depress white blood cell counts, suggesting that echinacea may help. If you're receiving cancer chemotherapy or radiation therapy, ask your medical and radiation oncologists about incorporating echinacea into your treatment plan.

Intriguing Possibility

In animals, echinacea has demonstrated promising anticancer activity against leukemia and a few tumors. It would be premature to describe the herb as a cancer treatment, but that day may come.

Rx Recommendations

Use either a decoction or tincture. To make a decoction, use 2 teaspoons of root material per cup of water. Bring it to a boil, then simmer for 15 minutes. Drink up to 3 cups a day. You'll find the taste initially sweet, then bitter.

As a homemade tincture, take 1 teaspoon up to three times a day.

When using commercial preparations, follow package directions.

Safety

Echinacea tincture often causes transient tongue numbing or tingling. This is harmless and goes away in about 30 minutes. Headache, dizziness, fatigue and stomach upset have also been reported.

AUTOIMMUNE DISEASES. Through the mid-1990s, herbal medicine authorities agreed that echinacea should not be used by people who are HIV-positive or those who have autoimmune conditions such as lupus, multiple sclerosis, or rheumatoid arthritis. The thinking was that stimulating the immune system might aggravate these conditions. But echinacea has become so popular that many people with HIV or autoimmune diseases have used it, and a 1999 report in the *European Journal of Herbal Medicine* claims there have been no published reports that the herb aggravated AIDS or autoimmune conditions.

If you are HIV-positive or have an autoimmune disease, ask your physician about the advisability of using echinacea to treat your colds.

PREGNANCY. Medical authorities advise pregnant and nursing women not to take drugs or medicinal herbs without consulting their physicians. This is sound advice. Drugs and medicinal herbs might harm the fetus, particularly during the first trimester. However, two studies of echinacea use by pregnant women—a 2000 report in *Archives of Internal Medicine* and a 2006 study in the *Canadian Journal of Clinical Pharmacology*—showed no increased risk of birth defects. Pregnant and nursing women should still consult their physicians before using echinacea. But these reports should reassure pregnant women who use this herb.

LONG-TERM USE. Traditional herbalists recommended echinacea only for short-term treatment of wounds or acute illnesses (colds, flu, etc.), not for regular use over long periods. However, some people take it daily, like a vitamin. No published trials of daily, long-term echinacea use have been published. But herb-medical authorities discourage regular long-term use and recommend echinacea only for short-term treatment of wounds or acute illnesses.

Do not give echinacea to children under 2. In older children, adjust the recommended dose based on the child's weight. Give a 50-pound child one-third of the dose a 150-pound adult would take.

If you're over 65, start with a low dose, and increase only if necessary.

Inform health professionals of the herbs you use. Problematic herb-drug interactions are possible.

Echinacea may cause allergic reactions or other unexpected side effects. If any develop, reduce your dose or stop taking it. For more on herb safety, see Chapter 2.

If symptoms get worse or persist longer than 2 weeks, consult a health professional promptly.

Gardening

Echinacea is a 2- to 5-foot perennial whose flowers resemble black-eyed Susans, with purple rays radiating from a cone-shaped center (hence its common name, purple coneflower). The herb has black roots, a single stem covered with bristly hairs, and narrow leaves.

Echinacea grows from seeds or root cuttings taken in spring or fall. Don't cover the seeds. When the temperature is in the 70s, simply tamp them into moist, sandy soil.

Echinacea grows in poor, rocky, slightly acidic soil under full sun. It also thrives in richer soils.

It takes 3 to 4 years for the roots to grow large enough to harvest. Pull them in autumn after the plant has gone to seed. Roots larger than $\frac{1}{2}$ inch in diameter should be split before drying.

ELDERBERRY

Herbal Flu-Fighter—and More

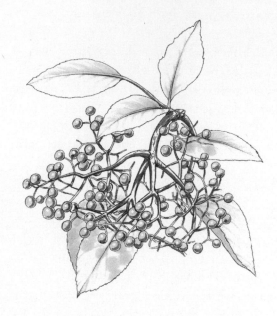

Family: Caprifoliaceae; other members include honeysuckle

Genus and species: *Sambucus nigra* (European) and *S. canadensis* (American)

Also known as: Sweet elder, common elder, sambucus

Parts used: berry, flower extract

An old Austrian saying goes: "Tip your hat to the elder." It refers not to older adults but to the elder tree, in honor of its many traditional medical uses.

Elder is two related plants, an American shrub that grows to 12 feet and a European tree that reaches 30. Both plants produce dark purple berries.

Elderberry was used medicinally in the ancient world, but fell into obscurity. In the 1990s, researchers resurrected it by discovering its remarkable flu-fighting action. Now the elderberry product, Sambucol, is widely available as an herbal flu treatment.

Healing History

As early as 400 BC, Hippocrates called the elder his "medicine chest." Other ancient physician/herbalists, among them, the Greek physician/botanists Theophrastus and Dioscorides and the Roman Galen also considered elder a great healer. They recommended the flowers and leaves—but not the berries—to treat many maladies: arthritis, asthma, colds, constipation, and even cancer.

From the Middle Ages into the 19th century, European and American herbalists used the berry as a laxative and diuretic, to treat diabetes, and to treat infections, such as flu.

Beyond medicine, elderberry has also been used for centuries to make preserves and wine.

Therapeutic Uses

FLU. Fascinated by folk use of elderberry to treat flu, in the 1990s, Israeli researchers discovered that the purple berry substantially reduces replication of flu viruses. The researchers turned the berries into a syrup and in 1993, used it to treat a flu outbreak on an Israeli kibbutz. Among those who did not receive elderberry, it took 6 days to recover. But 90 percent of the group that received the herbal syrup recovered in just 3 days. The elderberry syrup, Sambucol, is now available at health food stores and some pharmacies.

During the 1999–2000 flu season, the researchers who developed Sambucol journeyed to Scandinavia and gave 60 Norwegian flu sufferers either a placebo or Sambucol (2 teaspoons four times a day for 5 days). The Sambucol group recovered an average of 4 days faster.

Subsequent studies have shown that elderberry does not attack the flu virus directly. Instead, it boosts the immune system against the virus. Elderberry increases production of important immune compounds (cytokines).

ANTIOXIDANT. Dark-colored fruits, among them elderberry, have been shown to contain potent antioxidants called anthocyanins. Antioxidants help prevent and reverse the cell damage at the root of heart disease, cancer, and many other conditions associated with aging.

HEART ATTACK AND STROKE. At Tufts University, U.S. Department of Agriculture researchers tested elderberry on the cells that line human arteries. Damage to these cells initiates a cascade of reactions that eventually leads to the arterial blockages that trigger heart attack and most strokes. The herb protected the arterial cells from damage. The researchers concluded that elderberry reduces risk of cardiovascular disease.

GUM DISEASE. Elderberry also boosts the immune system's ability to combat the bacteria responsible for gum disease. Louisiana State University researchers incubated infection-fighting white blood cells and gum-disease bacteria with or without elderberry extract. The herb-exposed white blood cells "potently inhibited" the bacteria. Elderberry toothpaste and mouthwash can't be too far away.

Intriguing Possibilities

To date no studies have shown that elderberry reduces cancer risk. But given the berries' antioxidant content, that's a good bet.

In addition to inhibiting flu virus, elderberry also fights the herpes and AIDS viruses. It's too early to call the herb a treatment for these conditions, but in the future, that's possibile.

Rx Recommendations

The most popular elderberry product is Sambucol (produced in Israel, distributed in North America by Nature's Way). For general health and cardiovascular disease prevention, the recommended adult dose is 2 teaspoons a day, 1 for children. For flu symptoms—fever, aches, malaise—adults should take 2 teaspoons four times a day, children 1 teaspoon four times a day.

Safety

No significant side effects have been reported among people using Sambucol.

If an elderberry bush or tree grows near you, the ripe berries are safe to eat. However, eating unripe, uncooked berries may produce nausea.

Elderberry leaves and stems contain cyanide. Ingestion has caused poisonings.

Gardening

The European tree has been naturalized to the United States, so both varieties are found here. Elder thrives in shady, moist, temperate locations. It tolerates marginal soils. Fragrant white flowers appear in early summer, and by autumn, produce purple-black berries that must be cooked before eating. Ingestion of uncooked berries may cause diarrhea and vomiting.

ELECAMPANE

Goodbye, Intestinal Parasites

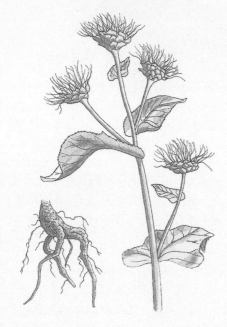

Family: Compositae; other members include daisy, dandelion, and marigold

Genus and species: *Inula helenium*

Also known as: Wild sunflower, velvet dock, scabwort, and horseheal

Parts used: Roots

Legend has it that Helen of Troy carried a handful of elecampane on the fateful day that the Trojan prince, Paris, abducted her from Sparta, igniting the Trojan War. Perhaps the woman whose face launched 1,000 ships had amoebic dysentery, pinworms, hookworms, or giardiasis.

We'll never know. But elecampane, whose Latin name, *Inula helenium*, memorializes the Greek beauty, may help expel intestinal parasites.

Healing History

Hippocrates, father of Western medicine, believed that elecampane stimulates the brain, kidneys, stomach, and uterus. The ancient Romans used it to treat indigestion. The Roman naturalist Pliny wrote, "Let no day pass without eating some roots of elecampane to help digestion, expel melancholy, and cause mirth." And the Roman physician Galen recommended the herb as "good for passion of the hucklebone [sciatica]."

Traditional Chinese and Indian Ayurvedic physicians recommended elecampane to treat respiratory problems, particularly bronchitis and asthma.

During the Middle Ages, European herbalists prescribed elecampane to treat coughs, bronchitis, and asthma. But it was more popular as a veterinary medicine, reputed to cure scab disease in sheep, hence one of its popular names, scabwort. Herbalists also considered it a panacea for horses, hence the name horseheal.

In medieval Europe, elecampane was the main ingredient in a digestive drink, *potio Paulina*.

The 17th-century London herbalist Nicholas Culpeper touted elecampane "to relieve cough, shortness of breath, and wheezing." Echoing Galen, he also endorsed it for sciatica and claimed that it restored vision and cured gout, sores, and "worms in the stomach."

In Culpeper's day, elecampane root was candied and enjoyed as a confection. Lozenges combining elecampane and honey were a popular treatment for whooping cough (pertussis).

Early American colonists introduced elecampane and used it as an expectorant, digestive aid, menstruation promoter, and diuretic for treating the fluid retention of dropsy (congestive heart failure). Native American tribes in the Northeast adopted the plant for respiratory problems.

America's 19th-century Eclectic physicians, forerunners of today's naturopaths, also used elecampane as a diuretic and menstruation promoter. Primarily, however, they prescribed the herb for "asthma, bronchial and chronic pulmonary [lung] affections, weakness of the digestive organs, itching, dyspepsia [indigestion], night sweats, and severe colds."

Today, herbalists generally recommend elecampane only for respiratory ailments: cough, asthma, bronchitis, and emphysema. Some recommend it as a digestive aid, as a treatment for menstrual and skin problems, and to banish intestinal parasites.

Therapeutic Uses

Elecampane has not been well researched, but studies to date show that for once, Nicholas Culpeper wasn't completely off the deep end.

INTESTINAL PARASITES. European scientists have discovered that elecampane contains a compound (alantolactone) that helps expel intestinal parasites, as Culpeper claimed. The herb also kills some bacteria and fungi, adding to its potential therapeutic action in the intestine.

The United States faces growing problems from intestinal parasites, especially pinworms and *Giardia lamblia*, the protozoan that causes giardiasis. Families with children in day care are particularly susceptible. Intestinal parasites are common in the tropics. If you venture there, act like Helen of Troy. Take elecampane with you.

Intriguing Possibilities

In European animal trials, elecampane reduced blood pressure. People with high blood pressure might try it, in consultation with their physicians.

Elecampane has also been shown to sedate laboratory animals. People with insomnia might try it before bed.

Rx Recommendations

To prepare a decoction, gently boil 1 to 2 teaspoons of dried, powdered root in 3 cups of water for 30 minutes, then strain if you wish. The taste is bitter. Take 1 to 2 tablespoons at a time with honey, up to 2 cups a day.

As a homemade tincture, use $1/4$ to $1/2$ teaspoon up to three times a day.

When using commercial preparations, follow package directions.

Safety

People who are sensitive to elecampane may develop a rash from skin contact with the herb or its oil. Otherwise, no harmful effects have been reported.

Pregnant and nursing women should not use elecampane.

Do not give elecampane to children under 2. In older children, adjust the recommended dose based on the child's weight. Give a 50-pound child one-third of the dose a 150-pound adult would take.

If you're over 65, start with a low dose, and increase only if necessary.

Inform health professionals of the herbs you

use. Problematic herb-drug interactions are possible.

Elecampane may cause allergic reactions or other unexpected side effects. If any develop, reduce your dose or stop taking it. For more on herb safety, see Chapter 2.

If symptoms get worse or persist longer than 2 weeks, consult a health professional promptly.

Gardening

Elecampane is a striking, wooly-haired perennial that reaches 5 feet and produces a large flower, hence its common name, wild sunflower. The medicinal roots are large, branching, and fleshy.

Elecampane may be started from seeds sown indoors in late winter, then transplanted. Once established, however, the herb is best propagated from 2-inch root cuttings taken in fall from the buds (eyes) of 2-year-old roots. Cover cuttings with moist, sandy soil and store them for the winter in a cool indoor room. Plant them 3 feet apart after frost danger has passed. Deeply cultivated soil produces the largest roots.

Elecampane likes rich, moist, well-drained, slightly acid loam and full sun or partial shade. Harvest the roots during the fall of their second year. Older roots become too woody. To speed drying, slice roots into pieces.

ELEUTHEROCOCCUS

Ginseng's Siberian Cousin Offers Similar Benefits

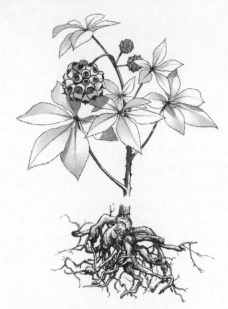

Family: Araliaceae; other members include ginseng and English ivy

Genus and species: *Eleutherococcus senticosus*

Also known as: Siberian ginseng, eleuthero

Parts used: Primarily root, sometimes leaves and berries

Eleutherococcus, often called eleuthero, looks nothing like ginseng. It's a deciduous shrub that grows to 6 feet, while ginseng is an ivy-like ground cover. Eleuthero stems have thorns. Ginseng does not. And eleuthero has a woody root. Ginseng's is fleshy. But these plants offer similar benefits. They are both adaptogens, medicinal herbs with a remarkable number of healing actions. Their benefits are so similar that some call eleuthero "Siberian ginseng."

Healing History

Eleuthero is native to China, Japan, and Russia. But Asians, particularly the Chinese and Koreans, who have revered ginseng for thousands of years, largely ignored shrubby eleuthero.

That began to change in 1947, when Russian scientist N. V. Lazarev became interested in drugs that helped the body adapt to physical and emotional stress and coined the term *adaptogen* to describe them. Ginseng was the prime adaptogen, but Lazarev's student Israel I. Brekhman wondered if there might be a less expensive substitute and investigated folk claims for eleuthero. He discovered similar actions. His research popularized eleutherococcus.

Adaptogens increase energy, relieve stress, boost resistance to many diseases, and have a normalizing effect on the body, improving many parameters of health while causing few, if any, side effects.

"Adaptogens give body a tune-up," says Salt Lake City herb researcher Daniel Mowrey, Ph.D. "They help the cells produce energy and use it more efficiently. Over time, adaptogenic herbs are very beneficial to health. But unlike many drugs, their effects are subtle, which makes these herbs controversial."

Therapeutic Uses

ENERGY AND STAMINA. Polish researchers evaluated the health and physical fitness of 50 men and women and then gave them either the well-known immune booster, echinacea, or eleuthero (25 drops of tincture three times a day). After 1 month, the echinacea group showed no changes in fitness. But the eleuthero group showed enhanced muscle use of oxygen, which improves fitness and stamina. Some eleuthero studies show no increase in stamina or reduced fatigue, but University of Iowa researchers gave 96 people suffering chronic fatigue either a placebo or eleuthero. After 2 months, the herb group reported significantly more energy. Commission E, the German counterpart of the FDA, approves eleuthero for invigoration during convalescence and for fatigue and debility.

IMMUNE FUNCTION. German researchers measured the immune function of 36 people and then gave them eleuthero (10 milliliters of tincture three times a day). After 4 weeks, the herb increased their number of T-cells, a key component of the immune system. Eleuthero also increases production of interleukin-1 and -6, important immune proteins. A Russian report concludes that eleuthero "stimulates immunological vigor."

COMMON COLD. In a cell-culture study published in *Antiviral Research*, German scientists have documented eleuthero's "strong antiviral" action. Russian researchers gave 40 children with colds either conventional treatment or an herbal preparation that included eleuthero (and andrographis, page 60). The herb group recovered faster.

DIABETES. Eleuthero lowers blood sugar, which may help prevent and treat diabetes.

ANTIOXIDANT. Russian researchers have identified six antioxidants in eleuthero. Antioxidants help prevent and repair the cell damage at the root of heart disease, cancer, and many other conditions associated with aging.

HEART DISEASE. A Polish study shows that eleuthero reduces LDL ("bad") cholesterol and triglycerides (blood fats), both risk factors for heart disease. It also helps prevent the internal blood clots that trigger heart attacks and most strokes. Eleuthero's effects on blood sugar also help reduce the likelihood of heart disease because diabetes is a major risk factor for heart attack. Finally, a Russian animal study shows that the herb helps normalize heart rhythm.

MEMORY AND VISUAL ACUITY. Eleuthero improves short-term memory and visual acuity, according to Russian research. It increases the sensitivity of the retina, which improves color perception and the ability to see clearly in low light.

QUALITY OF LIFE. Add up all these effects, and like ginseng, eleuthero improves quality of life. In a study by Italian researchers at the University of Bologna published in *Archives of Gerontology and Geriatrics*, 20 elderly people completed a health status survey and then took either a placebo or eleuthero. Four weeks later, the herb group scored higher on mental health and social functioning.

Intriguing Possibilities

BONE STRENGTH. Pilot studies by Russian researchers at Vladivostok State Medical University have shown that eleuthero treats osteoporosis as well as soy protein.

RADIATION EXPOSURE. Bulgarian research hints that eleuthero speeds recovery from radiation exposure.

LIVER. Korean animal studies suggest that the herb improves liver function.

CANCER. A Russian study shows eleuthero contains four compounds with anticancer action. Another Russian report finds that in animals with drug-induced tumors, the herb extends survival. A third Russian study shows that eleuthero boosts the immune systems of people with cancer. These results suggest that eleuthero may help treat human cancers.

Rx Recommendations

Follow package directions. If using dry powdered root, the recommended dose is 2 to 3 grams/day. To make a tea, steep 2 to 3 grams (approximately 2 teaspoons) per cup of boiling water for 10 minutes.

Safety

Eleuthero causes few side effects, but drowsiness, anxiety, irritability, headache, insomnia, and depressed mood are possible. Large doses have caused irritability, insomnia, and anxiety. Commission E says it should not be used by people running a fever or suffering high blood pressure.

Pregnant and nursing women should not use this herb.

Do not give eleuthero to children under 2. In older children, adjust the recommended dose based on the child's weight. Give a 50-pound child one-third of the dose a 150-pound adult would take.

If you're over 65, start with a low dose, and increase only if necessary.

Inform health professionals of the herbs you use. Problematic herb-drug interactions are possible.

Eleuthero may cause allergic reactions or other unexpected side effects. If any develop, reduce your dose or stop taking it. For more on herb safety, see Chapter 2.

If symptoms get worse or persist longer than 2 weeks, consult a health professional promptly.

Gardening

Eleuthero can be grown in the United States, though most medicinal roots are imported.

This herb grows in coniferous and mixed mountain forests, forming shrubby undergrowth or thickets at forest edges. It prefers rich, well-drained soil, but can grow in sandy, loamy, rocky, and heavy clay soils, with acid, neutral, or alkaline pH. It tolerates sun or dappled shade, but likes protection from wind. Eleuthero tolerates cold to -15 degrees C. Seeds may be slow to germinate. Start seeds in pots in fall. Seedlings should be kept in a greenhouse or cold frame for at least the first winter. Plant out in late spring or summer.

EPHEDRA
An Ancient, Controversial Healer

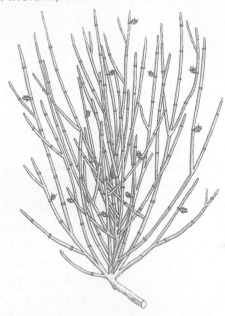

Family: Ephedraceae; other members include broom and horsetail

Genus and species: *Ephedra sinica, E. vulgaris, E. nevadensis, E. antisyphilitica,* and other species

Also known as: *Ma huang,* Mormon tea, and whorehouse tea

Parts used: Stems and branches

Ephedra—in Chinese, *ma huang*—is a powerful bronchial decongestant and stimulant. Many herbalists call ephedra the world's oldest medicine. It's certainly one of the oldest.

Sadly, few people who take over-the-counter cold remedies containing the herb's laboratory equivalent (pseudoephedrine) have any idea that they are part of an herbal healing tradition that dates back some 5,000 years. More sadly, a small but widely publicized group who've used irresponsibly large amounts of ephedra have experienced serious consequences, including death.

Healing History

The origins of Chinese medicine are lost in legend. However, authorities generally agree that Chinese physicians began prescribing a tea made from Chinese ephedra for colds, asthma, and hay fever around 3000 BC. The Indian and Pakistani species of the herb have been used medicinally for almost as long.

When the Mormons reached Utah in 1847, local Native Americans introduced them to American ephedra, a piney-tasting tonic beverage. The Mormons adopted it as a substitute for coffee and tea, and around the West it became known as Mormon tea, a name that survives today.

American ephedra is a mild diuretic. In the Old West, it developed a reputation as a cure for syphilis and gonorrhea. It was served in many Western brothels, hence another of its common names, whorehouse tea, and the Latin name for one species, *E. antisyphilitica*.

Contemporary herbalists recommend ephedra, just as the ancient Chinese did, to treat asthma, hay fever, and the nasal and chest congestion of colds and flu.

Therapeutic Uses

When people say "ephedra," they usually mean the Chinese variety *ma huang* (*E. sinica*). However, some herb marketers mistakenly refer to American ephedra as *ma huang* and the Chinese herb as Mormon tea. Check labels for species. Medicinal ephedra is *Ephedra sinica* or *E. sinica*.

American ephedra is just a refreshing beverage. It contains none of the pharmacologically active compounds (ephedrine, pseudoephedrine, and norpseudoephedrine) found in Chinese ephedra.

The active compounds in Chinese ephedra are powerful stimulants, more powerful than caffeine but less potent than amphetamine. All three open the bronchial passages (meaning that they're bronchodilators). They also stimulate the heart and uterine contractions; increase blood pressure, metabolic rate, and perspiration and urine production; and reduce secretion of both saliva and stomach acids.

RESPIRATORY PROBLEMS. From the 1920s through the 1940s, Chinese ephedra's active constituent, ephedrine, was added to cold, asthma, and hay fever products as a decongestant and bronchodilator. Ephedrine was generally effective and reasonably safe, but it caused potentially hazardous side effects: increased blood pressure and rapid heartbeat (palpitations). It was eventually replaced by a close chemical relative, pseudoephedrine, also found in *ma huang*.

Scientists consider pseudoephedrine as effective as ephedrine but with fewer side effects. Pseudoephedrine is the active ingredient in many over-the-counter cold and allergy products, notably Sudafed, whose name comes from its active ingredient.

Ephedra continues to be used in herbal cold, flu, allergy, and decongestant products. Chinese physicians prescribe it to treat asthma. Commission E, the expert panel that evaluates herbal medicines for the German counterpart of the FDA, endorses *ma huang* for the treatment of bronchial congestion.

OVERWEIGHT. *Ma huang* increases metabolic rate, the speed the body burns calories. It also depresses appetite a bit. This combination of effects led to studies of the herb (actually chemically isolated ephedrine) for weight control, usually in combination with another stimulant, caffeine.

In physician-supervised weight-loss programs that include a low-fat diet and regular exercise, treatment with a combination of ephedrine and caffeine has increased weight loss by about 5 percent. In other words, a person who loses 100 pounds without *ma huang* might lose 105 with it.

In a 3-month trial, Danish researchers showed that compared with overweight women taking medically inactive placebos, those taking oral ephedrine (20 milligrams three times a day) lost somewhat more weight. And in a 2-month study, Italian researchers found that overweight women lost more weight if they supplemented a low-calorie diet with oral ephedrine (50 milligrams three times a day).

To experience ephedra's weight-reduction benefits, you must be clinically obese, that is, at least 20 percent heavier than your recommended weight. Ephedrine has shown no benefit in people who want to lose 5 to 10 pounds.

When used for weight control, ephedra typically causes side effects that may be unpleasant (see Safety).

Experts generally agree that the keys to permanent weight loss are a low-fat, low-calorie diet and daily exercise. Nonetheless, ephedra is an ingredient in many herbal weight-loss formulas sold in health food stores and drugstores.

Intriguing Possibility

Ephedrine causes uterine contractions in laboratory animals. Women may want to try ephedra to initiate menstruation. But do not take large doses to trigger abortion.

Medicinal Myths

SEXUAL INFECTIONS. Although American ephedra was popular in the Old West as a remedy for syphilis and gonorrhea, in reality, the herb has no effect on either disease. Anyone who develops a genital sore or discharge should consult a physician.

ATHLETIC PERFORMANCE. Some stimulants—for example, coffee—increase stamina. Some athletes believe that ephedra enhances performance. Little evidence supports this.

Rx Recommendations

In decoctions or tinctures, ephedra tastes pleasantly piney.

For a decoction, use 1 teaspoon of dried herb per cup of water. Bring it to a boil, then simmer for 10 to 15 minutes. Drink up to 2 cups a day.

As a homemade tincture, take $\frac{1}{4}$ to 1 teaspoon up to three times a day.

When using commercial preparations, follow package directions.

Safety

During the 1990s, products that promised a legal methamphetamine-like high included huge doses of Chinese ephedra. Brand names included Herbal Ecstasy, Cloud 9, and Ultimate X-phoria. Large doses of ephedra do, indeed, produce effects similar to methamphetamine. They also cause serious—possibly fatal—heart problems and stroke.

Researchers at the New England Medical

Center in Boston used data supplied by the FDA to document 14 cardiac arrests, 13 strokes, 9 heart attacks, and more than 900 other adverse reactions associated with high-dose ephedra. Most victims were dieters using the herb to lose weight or young people seeking speed-like intoxication.

Subsequently, however, an audit of the FDA's ephedra database by the Government Accountability Office (GAO), the investigative arm of Congress, accused the FDA of "questionable" science and unsubstantiated statistical information. The GAO concluded that the FDA's database of adverse reactions was "open to question."

Despite the GAO's criticism, in 2003 the FDA announced tough new labeling rules. Critics charged that the agency in effect banned ephedra. In 2005, a federal judge struck down the FDA's rules. Since then, the U.S. government has taken no action to reduce the use of this herb.

Even recommended doses have powerful stimulant action and may also cause nervousness, jitters, irritability, anxiety, insomnia, dizziness, heart palpitations, and skin flushing.

Some compounds in *ma huang* have been shown to raise blood pressure and blood sugar. Other compounds have been shown to lower them. People with diabetes or high blood pressure should err on the side of caution and not use the herb. Nor is ephedra appropriate for people with heart disease, glaucoma, or kidney conditions, because of the risk of elevated blood pressure.

People with overactive thyroid (hyperthyroidism or Graves' disease) should avoid all stimulants, including ephedra.

Ephedra constricts the urethra and can lead to difficulty urinating. Men with benign prostate enlargement, which also causes urinary problems, should not use it.

Ephedra often causes insomnia. People who have difficulty sleeping should use the herb early in the day, if at all.

Ephedra may cause dry mouth. Increase your intake of nonalcoholic liquids.

Ephedra appears on the United States Olympic Committee's list of banned substances. Even if you're not an Olympian, think twice before using ephedra in hot weather. It may increase risk of potentially fatal heatstroke.

Pregnant and nursing women should not use ephedra.

Do not give ephedra to children.

If you're over 65, start with a low dose, and increase only if necessary.

Inform health professionals of the herbs you use. Problematic herb-drug interactions are possible.

Ephedra may cause allergic reactions or other unexpected side effects. If any develop, reduce your dose or stop taking it. For more on herb safety, see Chapter 2.

If symptoms get worse or persist longer than 2 weeks, consult a health professional promptly.

Gardening

Ephedra is not a garden herb. It is an odd-looking, botanically primitive, almost leafless shrub that resembles horsetail. It has tough, jointed, barkless stems and branches, with small scale-like leaves and tiny yellow-green flowers that appear in summer. Male and female flowers appear on different plants. The seeds develop in cones.

EUCALYPTUS

The Australian Cold and Flu Remedy

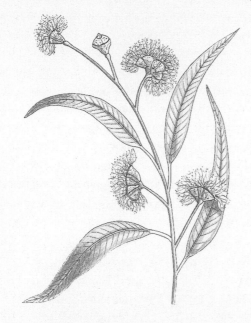

Family: Myrtaceae; other members include myrtle, tea tree, and clove

Genus and species: *Eucalyptus globulus*

Also known as: Gum tree, blue gum, and Australian fever tree

Parts used: Leaves

Eucalyptus is Australia's contribution to herbal healing. It's even won FDA approval for treatment for colds and flu.

If you've ever used Listerine mouthwash or a decongestant such as Vicks VapoRub, you're familiar with the unique, refreshing scent of eucalyptus. And if you've ever seen a koala in a zoo, you've probably seen eucalyptus, because the plant's long, scythe-shaped leaves are the sole food source for the cute, furry marsupial.

Healing History

Eucalyptus roots hold an astonishing amount of water. Australia's aborigines chewed them for water in the dry outback. They also drank eucalyptus leaf tea to treat fevers.

In the 1780s, when England declared Australia a penal colony and started shipping convicts to what is now Sydney, it took a while for the new arrivals to appreciate eucalyptus' water-laden roots. Some early outback explorers died of thirst within sight of eucalyptus groves.

Around 1840, crew members of a French freighter anchored off Sydney developed high fevers. Eucalyptus tea cured them. Reports of similar incidents prompted Europeans to dub the plant "Australian fever tree."

By the 1860s, eucalyptus leaves and oil were being used around the Mediterranean area to treat "intermittent fever" (malaria), which had plagued the area for millennia. Some physicians reported curing the disease with eucalyptus, but others dismissed it as worthless.

Eucalyptus has no direct effect on the protozoan that causes malaria. Ironically, however, the eucalyptus tree was responsible for virtually eradicating the devastating disease throughout Italy, Sicily, and Algeria, where it had raged unchecked since ancient times. Mosquitoes that live in swampy areas transmitted malaria. Europeans planted eucalyptus trees in the marshlands bordering the Mediterranean, and as the trees grew, their roots soaked up water and drained the swamps, eliminating malarial mosquitoes' habitat—and the disease they carried.

In 19th-century British hospitals, eucalyptus oil was a popular antiseptic on urinary catheters. It became known as catheter oil.

In America, 19th-century Eclectic physicians, forerunners of today's naturopaths, used eucalyptus oil as an antiseptic on wounds and medical instruments. They also recommended inhaling the vapors in steam to treat bronchitis, asthma, whooping cough (pertussis), and emphysema.

Contemporary herbalists recommend eucalyptus as a topical antiseptic, a gargle for sore throat, and a treatment for the nasal and chest congestion of colds, flu, bronchitis, croup, and asthma.

Therapeutic Uses

Eucalyptus leaf oil contains eucalyptol, a compound that provides the herb's pleasant aroma and healing value.

COLDS AND FLU. Eucalyptol loosens chest phlegm so it's easier to cough up. That's why eucalyptus is an ingredient in so many cough lozenges. The FDA approves it for cough and colds. Commission E, the expert panel that evaluates herbal medicines for the German counterpart of the FDA, also endorses the herb as a cold and flu treatment.

Russian animal studies show that eucalyptol kills some bacteria and influenza A, the virus that causes the most serious form of flu. Inhaling the vapors of a strong eucalyptus infusion may help prevent bacterial bronchitis, a possible complication of colds and flu.

WOUNDS. The antibacterial action of eucalyptol makes it an effective treatment for minor cuts and scrapes.

PERIODONTAL HEALTH. Japanese researchers gave 97 people with gum disease either a placebo chewing gum or a gum containing eucalyptus extract. After 12 weeks, those who chewed the eucalyptus gum showed significantly fewer symptoms of gum disease.

HEADACHES. In two similar studies, German researchers treated people who were prone to tension headaches with either medically inactive placebos or different combinations of eucalyptus and peppermint oils. Participants rubbed the preparations on their foreheads and temples. The herb treatments produced better relief. The formula that was mostly eucalyptus oil produced the greatest muscle relaxation, while the formula that was mostly peppermint oil yielded the greatest pain relief. The researchers suggested trying an herbal treatment instead of or in addition to an over-the-counter pain reliever.

Intriguing Possibilities

Science News reports that eucalyptol repels cockroaches. And a Korean study suggests that inhaled vapors reduce post-surgical pain.

Rx Recommendations

To make a eucalyptus inhalant, boil a handful of leaves or a few drops of the oil in water.

For minor cuts and scrapes, thoroughly wash the wound with soap and water, then apply a drop or two of eucalyptus oil.

To relieve headaches, rub the oil on your forehead and temples.

To prepare a eucalyptus bath, wrap a handful of leaves in a cloth and run bath water over it.

For a cool, spicy, refreshing infusion to treat colds and flu, use 1 to 2 teaspoons of dried, crushed leaves per cup of boiling water. Steep for 10 minutes. Drink up to 2 cups a day. You can also make an infusion by using 1 to 2 drops of eucalyptus oil.

When using commercial preparations, follow package directions.

If your home is infested with cockroaches and you don't want to use insecticides, try soaking small cloths in eucalyptus oil and placing them around your cabinets.

Safety

Used externally, eucalyptus oil is considered nonirritating, but rash is possible in those with unusual sensitivity. If you use it on infants and children, they may rebel against the pungent aroma.

If you use eucalyptus oil, be very careful not to ingest more than a drop or two. Like other herb oils, it's poisonous. Fatalities have been reported from ingestion of as little as a teaspoon.

Pregnant and nursing women should not use eucalyptus.

Do not give eucalyptus to children under 2. In older children, adjust the recommended dose based on the child's weight. Give a 50-pound child one-third of the dose a 150-pound adult would take.

If you're over 65, start with a low dose, and increase only if necessary.

Inform health professionals of the herbs you use. Problematic herb-drug interactions are possible.

Eucalyptus may cause allergic reactions or other unexpected side effects. If any develop, reduce your dose or stop taking it. For more on herb safety, see Chapter 2.

If symptoms get worse or persist longer than 2 weeks, consult a health professional promptly.

Gardening

The 500 species of eucalyptus account for three-quarters of Australia's native vegetation. Eucalyptus varies from 5-foot shrubs to the tallest trees on earth—up to 475 feet, the height of a 40-story building.

As long as temperatures don't dip below freezing, eucalyptus grows anywhere with loamy soil and adequate water. Obtained saplings at nurseries. If leaves begin to blister, reduce watering.

Eucalyptus often kills surrounding vegetation (except other Australian plants), which is why the trees are usually found in stands with little between them. They grow extremely rapidly, up to several feet per year, and their trunks eventually attain enormous girth.

Horticulturists discourage planting eucalyptus. The plant's roots destroy water and sewer lines. Its trunks buckle sidewalks. And its limbs may break off in gusting winds, damaging property and endangering lives.

EVENING PRIMROSE

A Therapeutic Powerhouse

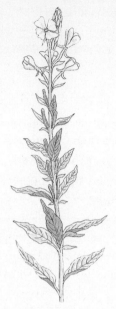

Family: Onagraceae; other members include fuchsia

Genus and species: *Oenothera biennis*

Also known as: Evening star

Part used: Seeds

Have you ever seen an evening primrose bloom? It's beautiful. Each flower opens for only one night. Just before dusk, all that's visible is the ripe, unopened bud. As the light of day begins to fade, the bud starts quivering. All of a sudden, the four green sepals flick out perpendicular to the flower stem, revealing a tight bundle of dainty yellow petals. The petals tremble as they emerge from their tight cocoon. With jerky, dancing contortions that take about a minute, the golden 2-inch petals spread, radi-ant in the sunset. By morning, the flower with-ers and dies.

Fortunately, the healing power of evening primrose seed oil lasts much longer than the plant's flowers. Evening primrose oil (EPO) is a relative newcomer to herbal medicine. It began attracting research attention only in the 1970s. Since then, many studies have shown that it helps treat cardiovascular disease, premen-strual syndrome, rheumatoid arthritis, eczema, and possibly even breast cancer and multiple sclerosis.

Healing History

Evening primrose is native to North America. Native Americans used the plant as both food and medicine. Many tribes ate the boiled roots. Others ate the young leaves and seeds.

Medicinally, Native Americans applied the whole evening primrose plant externally to con-trol wound inflammation. They also drank root tea to treat coughs.

Early colonists adopted evening primrose enthusiastically. They ate the boiled roots and used the seeds to garnish breads. They also adopted the Native American practice of apply-ing the plant to wounds.

The Shakers, whose enormous gardens sup-plied many early Americans with medicinal herbs, used a tea made from evening primrose seeds to treat digestive upsets.

America's 19th-century Eclectic physicians, forerunners of today's naturopaths, picked up on the Native American and Shaker recommenda-tions. They advised mixing a strong tea with lard and applying it to wounds and other skin conditions. They also prescribed the tea for digestive problems and suggested evening primrose for "sallow skin when the patient's mentality is of a gloomy and despondent character."

Until the 1980s, evening primrose was a minor medicinal herb. Herbalists recommended it mostly for indigestion. But since researchers discovered a key essential fatty acid in its seed oil, evening primrose has become much more widely studied and recommended.

Therapeutic Uses

Evening primrose seed oil (and borage oil, page 107) contains a compound rarely found in plants, gamma-linolenic acid (GLA), an essential fatty acid or EFA. Essential fatty acids are involved in the synthesis of prostaglandins, compounds that regulate dozens of body functions. They are also anti-inflammatory and help regulate metabolism.

EFA cannot be synthesized by the body and must be obtained from diet. Fish—especially cold-water fish (salmon, halibut, etc.)—contain these fatty acids, most notably the omega-3's. People who eat meat daily tend to have low EFA levels.

Laboratory animals placed on EFA-deficient diets develop infertility, immune suppression, cardiovascular disease, liver abnormalities, lingering wounds, and eczema-like skin conditions. These findings spurred researchers to try EFA supplementation for conditions linked to its deficiency. The results have been remarkably positive.

The *Review of Natural Products*, a scientific publication that monitors herbal medicine research, has concluded that for conditions related to EFA deficiencies, the value of evening primrose oil "cannot be overstated . . . [and produces] excellent results."

HEART DISEASE AND STROKE. The GLA in evening primrose oil reduces cholesterol substantially. In one Scottish study, 79 people with high cholesterol took evening primrose oil (4,000 milligrams/day for 3 months). Their cholesterol fell 31.5 percent. Cardiologists have found that for every 1 percent decrease in total cholesterol, the risk of heart attack drops 2 percent. So these subjects' risk of heart attack plummeted more than 60 percent.

Other research has shown that evening primrose oil reduces blood pressure and helps prevent the internal blood clots that lead to heart attacks and most strokes.

PREMENSTRUAL SYNDROME (PMS). The research goes both ways on evening primrose oil as a treatment for the mood swings, fluid retention, and breast tenderness of PMS. Some studies show benefit. Others do not. Those showing benefits generally last five cycles or longer. In one, 19 women took evening primrose oil during the 2 weeks before their menstrual periods for 5 months. Their symptoms declined significantly, with the greatest benefit occurring during the final month.

BREAST PAIN. PMS may trigger breast pain or tenderness, but other conditions unrelated to the menstrual cycle may also cause it. In a 17-year study that involved more than 400 women, University of Wales researchers prescribed either one of two standard drugs (Danazol or bromocriptine) or evening primrose oil. All three treatments produced similar results: significant relief for about 90 percent of the women whose pain came and went with their menstrual cycles as well as for 60 percent of the women with constant breast pain.

RHEUMATOID ARTHRITIS (RA). Several studies have shown that evening primrose helps relieve the joint pain, swelling, and tenderness of RA. At the University of Pennsylvania, researchers gave 37 people with rheumatoid arthritis either GLA or medically inactive placebos. After 6 months, the placebo group's symptoms remained unchanged, while those taking the herbal oil reported 36 percent fewer tender joints and 45 percent less joint pain—without side effects.

Two British studies produced similar findings. In one, 40 RA sufferers added either a placebo or evening primrose oil to their drug regimens. After 6 months, those taking the placebo reported symptoms unchanged, but the evening primrose group recorded significant improvement.

ECZEMA AND OTHER SKIN CONDITIONS. Finnish researchers gave 25 eczema sufferers either a placebo or evening primrose oil. Three months later, the herb group showed significantly less severe skin inflammation. Several other studies have confirmed this finding.

BREAST CANCER. Animal studies show that, when injected under the skin, evening primrose oil reduces the size of breast tumors. British researchers gave 38 women with breast cancer either a standard dose of the drug, tamoxifen, or tamoxifen plus GLA (8 capsules/day totaling 2.8 grams). Biopsies before and after assessed changes in estrogen receptors. Those receiving the herb oil showed a significant decrease in estrogen receptors, the desired clinical response.

Intriguing Possibilities

Pilot trials hint that the oil may improve symptoms of multiple sclerosis. If you have MS, discuss this with your physician. Evening primrose oil causes no significant side effects, so why not try it?

It has also been used successfully to treat diabetic nerve damage (neuropathy) and alcohol-related liver damage.

Rx Recommendations

Evening primrose oil comes in 500-milligram capsules containing 320 to 480 milligrams of GLA. Studies showing benefit from supplementation have used 3 to 12 capsules a day. Follow package directions.

Safety

Evening primrose oil causes no significant side effects. Still, allergic reactions and digestive upsets are possible. If problematic side effects develop, reduce your dose or stop taking it.

Pregnant women wishing to use evening primrose oil should discuss it with their physicians.

Breast milk is rich in GLA, so nursing women may use it in consultation with their physicians.

Do not give evening primrose oil to children under 2. In older children, adjust the recommended dose based on the child's weight. Give a 50-pound child one-third of the dose a 150-pound adult would take.

If you're over 65, start with a low dose, and increase only if necessary.

Inform health professionals of the herbs you use. Problematic herb-drug interactions are possible. For more on herb safety, see Chapter 2.

If, despite evening primrose oil treatment, symptoms get worse or persist longer than 2 weeks, or, for PMS, 6 months, consult a health professional.

Gardening

Botanically, evening primrose is not a true primrose. It's an annual or biennial very popular with gardeners and grows throughout the United States.

Depending on conditions, the plants reach from 3 to 9 feet. Flowers bloom from June through September for one night each.

Commercial farming in California, Oregon, Texas, and the Carolinas produces about 400 tons of seed annually.

FENNEL

Great for Digestion

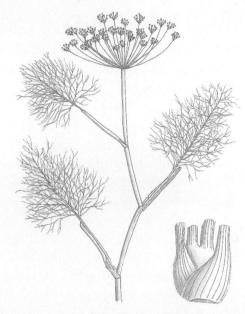

Family: Umbelliferae; other members include carrot, parsley, celery, dill, and angelica

Genus and species: *Foeniculum vulgare* and *F. vulgare dulce*

Also known as: Finocchio, carosella, and Florence fennel

Parts used: Fruits (seeds); stalks and bulbs are used in cooking

Colonial New England Puritans called fennel "meeting seeds." The meetings were their endless church services, and some experts believe that they used fennel as an appetite suppressant. Others theorize that many Puritans steeled themselves for church with whiskey and then chewed fennel seeds to mask the odor.

The Puritans also used fennel as a digestive aid. This has been the herb's primary purpose in herbal healing from the time of the Pharaohs to the present day.

Healing History

In Greek mythology, humanity received knowledge from Mount Olympus as a fiery coal encased in a fennel bulb.

The ancient Greeks had different ideas about fennel's medicinal value. During the third century BC, Hippocrates prescribed it as a stomach soother to treat infant colic. Four hundred years later, Dioscorides deemed it an appetite suppressant and gave the seeds to nursing mothers to boost milk production. The Greeks also called fennel *maraino*, meaning "to grow thin." They thought the herb helped control weight.

The Roman naturalist Pliny loved fennel and included the plant in 22 medicinal recipes. He noted that some snakes rubbed against the plant after shedding their skins and that soon after, their glazed eyes cleared. Pliny took this as a sign that fennel could cure human eye problems, including blindness.

Ancient India's Ayurvedic physicians revered fennel as a digestive aid.

Under the medieval Doctrine of Signatures— the medieval notion that plants' physical characteristics revealed their medicinal value— fennel's yellow flowers were linked to the liver's yellow bile. Thus, the herb was recommended for jaundice.

The emperor Charlemagne ordered fennel grown in all of his imperial "physic" (medicinal) gardens. The household of King Edward I of England consumed 8 pounds of the herb a month. The Church permitted the seeds to be nibbled on fast days as an appetite suppressant.

Fennel was one of Hildegard of Bingen's favorite herbs. The 12th-century German abbess/herbalist recommended it for colds, flu, the heart, and to "make us happy, [with] good digestion . . . and good body odor."

The Anglo-Saxons who settled England around the 5th century used fennel as both a spice and a digestive aid. They also hung fennel over their doors to protect against witchcraft.

By the 17th century, fennel was a mainstay of herbal healing and a standard seasoning for fish. Seventeenth-century English herbalist Nicholas Culpeper, apparently not a fish lover, wrote that fennel "consumes the phlegmatic humour which fish . . . annoys the body with." Culpeper also echoed the ancient recommendations, prescribing fennel to "break wind, increase milk, cleanse the eyes from mists that hinder sight, take away the loathings which oftentimes happen to stomachs of sick persons . . . [and] in drink or broth to make people lean that are too fat." He also claimed that it "brought women's courses" (menstruation).

Folk herbalists often mixed fennel with laxative herbs (buckthorn, senna, rhubarb, and aloe) to reduce the intestinal cramps the laxatives often caused.

Colonists brought fennel to North America. Henry Wadsworth Longfellow alluded to Pliny when he wrote:

> *Above the lower plants it towers*
> *The Fennel with its yellow flowers;*
> *And in an earlier age than ours*
> *Was gifted with wondrous powers*
> *Lost vision to restore.*

America's 19th-century Eclectic physicians, forerunners of today's naturopaths, prescribed fennel as a digestive aid, milk and menstruation promoter, and flavoring agent to "conceal the unpleasantness of other medicines."

Latin Americans still boil the seeds in milk as a milk promoter for nursing mothers. Jamaicans use fennel to treat colds. And Africans take the herb for diarrhea and indigestion.

Contemporary herbalists recommend fennel as a digestive aid, milk promoter, expectorant, eyewash, and buffer for herbal laxatives.

Therapeutic Uses

Fennel won't cure blindness, but science supports some of its other traditional uses.

DIGESTIVE PROBLEMS. Like other aromatic herbs, fennel relaxes the smooth muscle lining the digestive tract (antispasmodic). It also expels gas and promotes the secretion of bile, which speeds the digestion of fats. And European research shows that fennel kills some bacteria, lending some support to its traditional role in treating diarrhea.

In Germany, where herbal medicine is more mainstream than it is in the United States, fennel is used like caraway to treat indigestion, gas pains, irritable bowel syndrome, and infant colic. Many Indian restaurants keep a bowl of candied fennel seeds by the door as a digestive aid for departing diners.

German researchers gave either a standard pharmaceutical stomach settler (metoclopramide) or a combination of herbs (fennel, peppermint, caraway, and wormwood) to 60 people ages 18 to 85, who had complained of indigestion, heartburn, nausea, or unusual belching or fullness. The participants were instructed to take their medicine 20 minutes before meals. After 2 weeks of treatment, those taking the herbal combination reported significantly greater relief and fewer side effects. Commission E, the expert panel that evaluates herbal medicines for the German counterpart of the FDA, endorses fennel for the treatment of digestive upsets.

INFANT COLIC. Russian researchers gave either a placebo or a fennel seed preparation to colicky infants, with notably persistent crying. In the placebo group, 24 percent showed significantly less crying; but in the fennel group, 65 percent.

WOMEN'S HEALTH. Antispasmodics soothe not only the digestive tract but also other smooth muscles, including the uterus. Fennel, however, was traditionally used not to relax the uterus but to stimulate it into menstruation. This contradiction remains scientifically unresolved.

OVERWEIGHT. Animal studies show that fennel has diuretic action. This probably accounts for the herb's traditional role in weight control. Diuretics eliminate only water weight. Weight-loss experts discourage routine use of diuretics for weight management. They recommend a low-calorie, low-fat diet and daily exercise.

Intriguing Possibility

One study suggests that fennel has a mild estrogenic effect, meaning that it acts like the female sex hormone estrogen. This action may have something to do with its traditional use as a milk and menstruation promoter.

Rx Recommendations

To use fennel as a digestive aid, either chew a handful of seeds or try an infusion or tincture.

To make a pleasant, licorice-flavored infusion, steep 1 to 2 teaspoons of bruised seeds in 1 cup of boiling water for 10 minutes. Drink up to 3 cups a day.

As a homemade tincture, take ½ to 1 teaspoon up to three times a day.

When using commercial preparations, follow package directions.

Safety

Fennel has only a mild estrogenic effect. But estrogen, a key ingredient in birth control pills, has many effects on the body. Women advised by their doctors not to take the Pill should not use medicinal amounts of fennel. The same is true for anyone with a history of abnormal blood clotting or estrogen-dependent breast tumors.

Pregnant women should not use medicinal amounts of fennel.

Nursing women may give dilute fennel preparations to colicky infants in consultation with the child's physician.

Fennel seeds are safe, but fennel oil may cause skin rash in those who are sensitive.

When taken internally, even small amounts of the oil—a teaspoon or so—may cause nausea, vomiting, and possibly seizures. Don't ingest it.

Inform health professionals of the herbs you use. Problematic herb-drug interactions are possible. For more on herb safety, see Chapter 2.

If symptoms get worse or persist longer than 2 weeks, consult a health professional promptly.

Gardening

Native to southern Europe and Asia Minor, fennel is a striking 6-foot perennial with feathery leaves and tall stalks capped by large umbrella-like clusters of tiny yellow flowers. The tiny oval-shaped fruits (seeds) are ribbed and greenish gray. All parts of the plant have the herb's characteristic anise/licorice fragrance.

Fennel grows easily from seeds sown in rich, moist soil in fall or after the danger of frost has passed. Germination takes about 2 weeks. Thin seedlings to 12-inch spacing. Do not overwater the seedlings, but as plants develop, extra water increases stem succulence. Leaves may be harvested once plants are established.

When the stems are about 1 inch thick, hill the soil over them to cause blanching, which results in milder flavor. Harvest about 10 days after hilling.

Harvest the seeds in late summer as they turn greenish gray.

Fennel may damage some neighboring plants: bush beans, tomatoes, caraway, and kohlrabi. If you plant coriander nearby, fennel will not fruit.

Warning: In the wild, fennel can be easily confused with poison hemlock (wild parsley), which can be fatal. Don't eat wild fennel unless you're sure you've identified it correctly.

FENUGREEK

The Cholesterol Controller

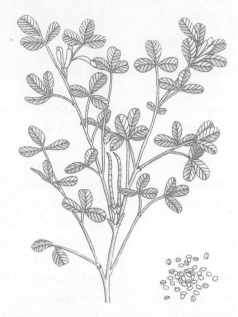

Family: Leguminosae; other members include beans and peas

Genus and species: *Trigonella foenum-graecum*

Also known as: Greek hay, foenu greek, and fenigreek

Parts used: Seeds

In 1922, when archeologists opened the 3,000-year-old tomb of Egypt's King Tutankhamen (Tut), they found fenugreek seeds inside. From ancient times through the late 19th century, fenugreek played a major role in herbal healing. Then it fell by the wayside.

Lately, however, the herb that tastes like an odd combination of bitter celery and maple syrup has been resurrected. Fenugreek helps reduce cholesterol and blood sugar.

Healing History

The early Greeks used fenugreek to heal sick livestock long before the seeds became popular for human ills. They mixed the plant into moldy or insect-damaged animal forage to make it more palatable. In the process, they discovered that sick horses and cattle would eat fenugreek when they wouldn't eat anything else. The Egyptians and Romans subsequently adopted "Greek hay." The plant's Latin name, *foenum graecum*, evolved into "fenugreek."

Today fenugreek is widely used to flavor horse and cattle feed. Some veterinarians still use it to encourage sick livestock to eat.

As fenugreek spread around the Mediterranean, ancient physicians learned that its seeds contain a special type of fiber, mucilage. When immersed in water, mucilage becomes gelatinous and soothes inflamed or irritated tissue. Egyptian physicians put fenugreek into ointments to treat wounds and abscesses. They also recommended the herb internally to treat fevers and respiratory and intestinal complaints. Hippocrates and other ancient Greek and Roman physicians used it similarly.

Ancient Chinese healers recommended fenugreek to treat fevers, hernias, gallbladder problems, muscle aches, and even impotence.

In India, where the herb is an ingredient in curry spice blends, Ayurvedic physicians prescribed it to treat arthritis, bronchitis, and digestive upsets.

Indian mothers ate fenugreek seeds to increase milk production. Arab women from Libya to Syria ate the roasted seeds to help them gain weight, enlarge their breasts, and attain the Rubenesque proportions that were synonymous with beauty from ancient times through the 19th century.

Fenugreek is the only healing herb ever used as a weapon of war. During the Roman siege of Jerusalem (AD 66–70), general and future emperor Vespasian ordered his troops to scale the city's imposing walls. The standard defense was to pour boiling water or oil on the attackers as they ascended their ladders. According to *The History of the Jewish War* by Flavius Josephus, Jerusalem's defenders added fenugreek to their oil, making anything it touched more slippery and hindering Romans ladder climbers.

Around the 9th century, Benedictine monks, who were avid herb gardeners and creators of fine liqueurs, popularized fenugreek throughout Europe. Like ancient cultures, folk herbalists used it to treat wounds, fevers, and digestive and respiratory ailments.

Early settlers brought fenugreek to North America and used it as forage and in folk medicine, where it gained a reputation as a treatment for menstrual complaints and menopausal discomforts. Lydia E. Pinkham incorporated it into her Vegetable Compound, one of 19th-century America's most popular patent medicines for "female weakness" (menstrual cramps and menopausal discomforts). Pinkham's advertising proclaimed her remedy "the greatest medical discovery since the dawn of history." Health authorities were outraged, and their outcries played a part in creating the FDA, which regulates drug claims.

Modern herbalists recommend fenugreek poultices and plasters to treat wounds, boils, and rashes. They prescribe warm fenugreek gargles to sooth sore throat. They also suggest using the herb internally to treat coughs, bronchitis, and menstrual and menopausal complaints. Some even claim that eating fenugreek—especially sprouts—enlarges women's breasts.

Today, fenugreek is most widely used in the United States as a source of imitation maple flavor.

Therapeutic Uses

Some of fenugreek's traditional uses have been supported by science, but the herb's most important potential benefit has only recently come to light.

HIGH CHOLESTEROL. Indian researchers measured the cholesterol levels of 60 people not taking any cholesterol-lowering medications. Then the participants were instructed to eat a bowl of soup containing about 1 ounce of powdered fenugreek seed with lunch and dinner daily. After 4 weeks, participants' cholesterol levels began to decline. After 6 months, their average total cholesterol dropped 14 percent. For every 1 percent decrease in total cholesterol, the risk of heart attack risk drops around 2 percent, so in this study, fenugreek cut participants' risk of heart attack by about 28 percent.

In another Indian trial, 2 teaspoons (5 grams) of powdered fenugreek seed a day for 3 months had no effect on the cholesterol levels of 30 people with normal readings—but in 30 others with elevated cholesterol, it reduced cholesterol significantly.

DIABETES. Animal studies show that fenugreek reduces blood sugar. In the first Indian study above, all participants had Type 2 diabetes. Besides lowering their cholesterol, daily consumption of about an ounce of powdered fenugreek seed also lowered their blood sugar levels. Other Indian reports have confirmed these results.

SORE THROAT. Fenugreek's soothing mucilage helps relieve sore throat pain and cough, as well as some indigestion.

WOUNDS. Fenugreek's mucilage also soothes minor wounds. Commission E, the expert panel that evaluates herbal medicines for Germany's counterpart of the FDA, approves fenugreek as a topical wound treatment.

WOMEN'S HEALTH. Fenugreek seeds contain diosgenin, a compound similar to the female sex hormone estrogen. Estrogen causes fluid retention and weight gain, validating Arab women's age-old practice of eating the seeds to gain weight. The diosgenin in fenugreek also stimulates breast tissue growth, which is why many women who take estrogen-based birth control pills report weight gain and breast swelling.

ARTHRITIS. Belgian researchers have discovered that fenugreek has mild anti-inflammatory action. This lends some credence to the herb's traditional role in treating arthritis, wounds, and other inflammatory conditions.

Intriguing Possibilities

BREAST AUGMENTATION. The discovery of a plant estrogen in fenugreek suggests that the herb might one day be used as natural hormone replacement therapy to treat menopausal hot flashes.

Fenugreek's phytoestrogen content also supports the American folk practice of eating the seeds for breast augmentation. James A. Duke, Ph.D., retired USDA herbal medicine authority, has observed that fenugreek sprouts contain much more diosgenin than the unsprouted seeds. He has recommended the sprouts to women interested in nonsurgical breast augmentation and says he's received several thank-you notes from satisfied users. Only one study has been published on fenugreek's effects, if any, on breast size. It was an animal study, and the animals' breast weight increased, indicating increased size.

Rx Recommendations

To soothe a sore throat, relieve menstrual or menopausal discomforts, or possibly relieve arthritis pain, try a fenugreek decoction. In consultation with your physician, you might also use the herb to lower your cholesterol or blood sugar.

For a bitter, maple-flavored decoction, gently boil 2 teaspoons of crushed seeds in 1 cup of water, then simmer for 10 minutes and strain. Drink up to 3 cups a day. To improve the flavor, add sugar, honey, lemon, anise, or peppermint.

As a homemade tincture, use $\frac{1}{4}$ to $\frac{1}{2}$ teaspoon up to three times a day.

When using commercial preparations, follow package directions.

Safety

Because fenugreek may be a uterine stimulant, pregnant women should not ingest it. Nursing women should also avoid it.

Do not give fenugreek to children under 2. In older children, adjust the recommended dose based on the child's weight. Give a 50-pound child one-third of the dose a 150-pound adult would take.

If you're over 65, start with a low dose, and increase only if necessary.

Inform health professionals of the herbs you use. Problematic herb-drug interactions are possible.

Fenugreek may cause allergic reactions or other unexpected side effects. If any develop, reduce your dose or stop taking it. For more on herb safety, see Chapter 2.

If symptoms get worse or persist longer than 2 weeks, consult a health professional promptly.

Gardening

Fenugreek is an annual that reaches 18 inches and resembles large clover. It has three-lobed leaves and white, triangular, pea-like flowers that produce the long seed pods characteristic of the bean family. Fenugreek's sickle-shaped seed pods are 2 inches long and contain 10 to 20 hard, smooth, oblong, somewhat flattened seeds.

After the danger of frost has passed and soil temperature has reached 55°F, sow seeds in almost any soil in full sun. Germination typically takes a few days. To prevent root rot, do not overwater.

The plants flower in about 3 weeks and produce seeds 3 weeks later. Harvest pods when they're fully formed but before they begin to crack. Remove the seeds and sun-dry them.

FEVERFEW
Prevent Migraines

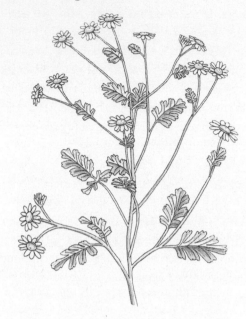

Family: Compositae; other members include daisy, dandelion, and marigold

Genus and species: *Chrysanthemum parthenium*; *Matricaria parthenium*; *Tanacetum parthenium*

Also known as: Febrifuge plant, wild quinine, and bachelor's button

Parts used: Leaves

From the 19th century to the late 1970s, feverfew was washed up as a healing herb. In 1974, in *The Herb Book,* herbalist John Lust noted, "Feverfew has fallen into disuse. It is hard to find, even at herb outlets."

Shortly after Lust penned this obituary, however, feverfew experienced a renaissance. It became clear that the herb is remarkably effective at preventing migraines.

Healing History

Many sources claim that this herb's name comes from the Latin *febrifugia*, meaning "driver-out of fevers." They add that feverfrew has been used since ancient times to treat fever.

Actually, the plant was never called febrifugia. Ancient physicians, including Dioscorides and Galen, referred to it by its Greek name, *parthenion*, and prescribed it for menstrual and recovery from childbirth, not fever.

During the Middle Ages, the plant was renamed featherfoil because of its feathery leaf borders. "Featherfoil" evolved into "featherfew" and eventually "feverfew."

But once the name feverfew became popular, herbalists decided that the herb was, in fact, a fever treatment. They sowed the strong-smelling plant around their homes hoping to purify the air and prevent malaria, which they mistakenly believed was caused by foul air ("malaria comes from the Italian *mala*, "bad," and *aria*, "air").

Malaria had plagued Europe since prehistoric times. It was untreatable until Spanish explorers returned from Peru with cinchona bark and early chemists isolated the bark's anti-malarial constituent, quinine. Quinine proved so successful at curing malaria that for a brief period, other herbs prescribed for fever basked in reflected glow. That's how feverfew became known as wild quinine. But the name didn't stick. Quinine proved so superior as a malaria treatment that herbalists stopped recommending feverfew.

Meanwhile, some herbalists recommended feverfew for headache. Seventeenth century English herbalist John Parkinson called it "very effectual for paines in the head." More than a century later, John Hill wrote, "In the worst headache, this herb exceeds whatever else is known."

Most herbalists stuck with feverfew's traditional gynecological uses, however. Seventeenth-century English herbalist Nicholas Culpeper called it a "general strengthener of wombs" and prescribed it in tea form for colds and chest congestion. Culpeper also recognized the herb's decline, declaring it "not much used in present practice."

Early colonists introduced feverfew into North America, where malaria was also a major problem. But as the herb fell from fashion in England, it stopped being used here as well.

America's 19th-century Eclectic physicians, forerunners of today's naturopaths, prescribed feverfew mainly as a menstruation promoter and as a treatment for "female hysteria" (menstrual discomforts).

Therapeutic Uses

In the 1970s, a chance meeting of two migraine sufferers made earlier observations about feverfew's benefit for "paines in the head" appear prophetic.

MIGRAINES. The wife of the chief medical officer of Britain's National Coal Board suffered migraines. A miner heard about her problem. When she accompanied her husband on a visit to his mine, the miner told her that he'd also been plagued by migraines-—until he started chewing a few feverfew leaves every day. The woman tried the herb and noticed immediate improvement. Fourteen months later, she was headache-free.

The medical officer brought his wife's experience to the attention of Dr. E. Stewart Johnson of the City of London Migraine Clinic. In a pilot study, Dr. Johnson gave feverfew leaves to 10 of his patients. Three pronounced themselves cured, and the other seven reported significant improvement.

Next, Dr. Johnson gave feverfew to 270 migraine sufferers. Seventy percent reported significant relief—and for many, standard treatment had done nothing at all.

Finally, Dr. Johnson arranged a scientifically rigorous double-blind, placebo-controlled trial in which some of the participants took feverfew, while others took medically inactive placebos. Neither the participants nor the researchers knew who got what until after the trial ended—a "double-blind" trial. Feverfew significantly outperformed the placebos.

Soon after Dr. Johnson completed his research, the British medical journal *Lancet* reported the results of an even more rigorous double-blind experiment. Seventy-two people with chronic migraines were randomly assigned to take either a daily placebo or capsules of powdered, freeze-dried feverfew (85 milligrams, equivalent to two medium-size leaves). After 2 months, the groups switched treatments. Those who had been taking placebos were given feverfew and vice versa—a "cross-over trial." The results were striking: Feverfew cut migraines 24 percent, and those that occurred were comparatively mild, with significantly less nausea and vomiting.

Since then, many other studies have shown feverfew to be effective for migraine prevention. In 1996, however, one highly publicized Dutch study found the herb ineffective. As it turned out, this trial used a tincture (alcohol extract) of feverfew, not the leaf material that had been used in the other studies.

In 1998, British researchers reviewed five studies of feverfew for migraine prevention, using sophisticated statistical techniques, a "meta-analysis." Their conclusion: Feverfew works.

In the 21st century, many more studies have confirmed feverfew's value in migraine prevention.

DIGESTIVE PROBLEMS. Like its close botanical relative, chamomile, feverfew contains chemicals that calm the smooth muscles of the digestive tract (antispasmodic). Try feverfew after meals to protect against digestive upset.

MENSTRUAL CRAMPS. Antispasmodic herbs soothe not only the digestive tract but also other smooth muscles, such as the uterus. In addition, feverfew has the ability to neutralize certain prostaglandins, substances that have been linked to pain and inflammation. (This may be another reason that feverfew helps prevent migraines.) Prostaglandins also play a role in menstrual cramps. Feverfew's possible antispasmodic and antiprostaglandin actions support its traditional use in treating menstrual discomforts.

Intriguing Possibilities

One animal study suggests that feverfew has a mild tranquilizing effect. Another report hints that feverfew has tumor-fighting action. It's too early to deem the herb a cancer treatment, but that day may come.

Rx Recommendations

For migraine prevention, chew two fresh (or freeze-dried) leaves a day or take a pill or capsule containing 85 milligrams of whole-leaf material. Since feverfew is very bitter, most people prefer the pills or capsules to chewing the leaves.

To improve digestion or promote menstruation, take feverfew as an infusion. Use ½ to 1 teaspoon of herb per cup of boiling water, steep for 5 to 10 minutes, then strain. Drink up to 2 cups a day.

Do not give feverfew to children under age 2. For older children and adults over age 65, start with low-strength preparations and increase the strength if necessary.

Safety

Feverfew prevents migraines, but does not cure them. If you stop taking it, migraines typically return, so migraine sufferers might take it for decades. At this writing, the herb has been used in migraine prevention for some 40 years with no reports of significant problems.

Feverfew has not been shown to cause uterine contractions, but it has a long folk history as a menstruation promoter. Pregnant women should err on the side of caution and not take it. Nursing women should also avoid it.

Chewing fresh feverfew leaves may cause mouth sores. Some people also report abdominal pain from using the herb.

Feverfew may inhibit blood clotting. People with clotting disorders and those who are taking anticoagulant (blood-thinning) medications or supplements (vitamin E) should consult a physician before using it.

Do not give feverfew to children under 2. In older children, adjust the recommended dose based on the child's weight. Give a 50-pound child one-third of the dose a 150-pound adult would take.

If you're over 65, start with a low dose, and increase only if necessary.

Inform health professionals of the herbs you use. Problematic herb-drug interactions are possible.

Feverfew may cause allergic reactions or other unexpected side effects. If any develop, reduce your dose or stop taking it. For more on herb safety, see Chapter 2.

If symptoms get worse or persist longer than 2 weeks, consult a health professional promptly.

Gardening

Feverfew is a perennial that reaches 3 feet and has lovely daisy-like flowers with yellow centers and up to 20 white rays. For personal migraine prevention, a few plants should suffice.

Feverfew grows from seeds, but most authorities recommend planting root cuttings when the temperature reaches 70°F. Space plants 18 inches.

Feverfew does best in partial shade. Compost stimulates growth. Pinch buds to encourage bushiness. Harvest leaves when they mature.

Bees generally avoid feverfew, so don't grow it around other plants that require bee pollination. Feverfew can also be grown indoors year-round as a houseplant.

FLAX

From Linen to Healing

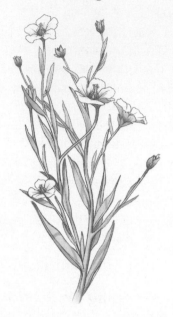

Family: Linaceae; other members include the more than 200 species of flax

Genus and species: *Linum usitatissimum*

Also known as: flaxseed, linseed, linum

Parts used: Seed oil

Ten thousand years ago, flax was one of the first plants farmed for purposes other than food. Flax has a fibrous stem, and the fibers were woven into cloth, called linen. But flax seeds also produce an oil (flaxseed or linseed oil) that has been used medicinally for almost as long.

Flax was among the most important crops to colonial American farmers. It was grown in almost every state east of the Mississippi River, and some beyond. Before the invention of the cotton gin in the early 1800s, most Americans wore clothing made from either wool or linen. Even after cotton became affordable, linen remained a commercially important fiber.

Healing History

More than 1,000 years ago, French king Charlemagne decreed that all his subjects should eat flaxseed to stay healthy. In the 1600s, British herbalist Nicholas Culpeper hailed flaxseed as having "great use against inflammations and tumors."

Flaxseed is rich in mucilage, a soluble fiber that becomes spongy when immersed in water. In ancient Europe, flax mucilage and flaxseed oil were used topically to soothe irritated skin. Flaxseed oil was used internally as a laxative and treatment for cough, colds, and urinary tract infections.

America's 19th-century Eclectics, forerunners of today's naturopaths, prescribed it for colds, cough, and digestive and urinary problems.

Therapeutic Uses

BREAST CANCER. Flaxseed is extraordinarily rich in plant estrogens (lignans), containing up to 800 times as much other vegetable sources. But lignans are chemically weaker than the body's own hormone. Estrogen stimulates the growth of breast cancer. Lignans bind to cellular estrogen receptors, locking out the body's own estrogen, thus reducing risk of breast cancer.

In animal studies, flaxseed oil inhibits growth of mammary tumors. Finnish researchers compared lignan consumption (from flax and other foods) in 194 women with breast cancer and 208 controls. As lignan intake increased, breast cancer risk decreased. Compared with women who consumed little or no lignan, those who ate the most had 62 percent less risk. Canadian researchers asked women newly diagnosed with breast cancer to eat one muffin a day containing about an ounce of flaxseed, while other recently diagnosed women ate muffins without flaxseed. A month later, the flaxseed group showed biomarkers reflecting slower tumor growth. Swedish researchers conducted a similar study and came up with the same findings. "Our results suggest that flaxseed and its lignans may prove beneficial in breast cancer prevention."

PROSTATE CANCER. Lignans have also shown benefit against prostate cancer. Duke researchers drew blood from 25 men with prostate cancer who were awaiting prostate removal, then gave them gave flaxseed daily (30 grams/day, about an ounce) for a month. After prostatectomy, their prostates were compared with those of similar men who had not eaten flaxseed. The tumors of men who had taken the herb showed less aggressive cancer.

CHOLESTEROL. Flaxseed is rich in soluble fiber. Many studies show that a diet high in soluble fiber, for example, oatmeal, lowers cholesterol. Oklahoma State researchers gave 55 women with high cholesterol either a placebo or flaxseed (30 grams/day). Three months later, the flaxseed group had significantly lower cholesterol. Several other studies have shown similar results.

HEART ATTACK. Flaxseed oil is one of the richest plant sources of alpha-linolenic acid (ALA, also known as omega-3 fatty acids). Harvard scientists assessed ALA intake (from flaxseed and foods) among 76,283 women nurses and then followed them for 10 years. As ALA intake increased, deaths from heart attack decreased. Compared with nurses who consumed the least ALA, those who ate the most were 45 percent less likely to suffer fatal heart attack.

DIABETES. Soluble fiber also reduces blood sugar. Studies by Chinese and Canadian researchers have shown that flaxseed lowers blood sugar, suggesting utility in diabetes prevention and treatment.

HOT FLASHES. Lignans have an estrogenic effect, and estrogen minimizes hot flashes. Mayo Clinic researchers gave flaxseed (40 grams/day) to women complaining of hot flashes. After 6 weeks, the frequency and severity of hot flashes decreased 50 percent. In a similar study, Canadian researchers came up with similar findings: "Compared with placebo, hot flashes were significantly less severe with flaxseed."

Intriguing Possibilities

A pilot study at Oklahoma State University suggests that in postmenopausal women, flaxseed may prevent bone loss. If confirmed, flaxseed might help prevent osteoporosis.

Some research suggests that ALA may help treat attention deficit hyperactivity disorder (ADHD). Indian scientists gave flaxseed to children diagnoses with ADHD: "There was significant improvement in ADHD symptoms."

Rx Recommendations

Flaxseeds can be found in bulk at most health food stores. They have a mild wheat-like flavor and can be generously sprinkled on cereals, baked into bread, or ground up and added to soups, casseroles, and many other dishes. Once ground, flaxseeds spoil quickly. Use them immediately.

Flaxseed oil supplements typically contain 1,000 milligrams of oil (500 to 600 milligrams of alpha-linolenic acid). Follow package directions.

Safety

Flaxseed contains a tiny amount of cyanide, not enough to harm an adult, but possibly enough to harm a fetus or infant. Pregnant and nursing women should not use it.

Do not give flaxseed to children under 2. In older children, adjust the recommended dose based on the child's weight. Give a 50-pound child one-third of the dose a 150-pound adult would take.

If you're over 65, start with a low dose, and increase only if necessary.

Inform health professionals of the herbs you use. Problematic herb-drug interactions are possible.

Flaxseed may cause allergic reactions or other unexpected side effects. If any develop, reduce your dose or stop taking it. For more on herb safety, see Chapter 2.

If symptoms get worse or persist longer than 2 weeks, consult a health professional promptly.

Gardening

Flax is a slender annual that reaches 3 feet. Its branches produce one or two delicate blue flowers that bloom from February to September. It likes well-drained soil. Plant in spring. Late frosts rarely damage seedlings, but yields suffer when it's planted in the same field year after year.

GARLIC
The Wonder Herb

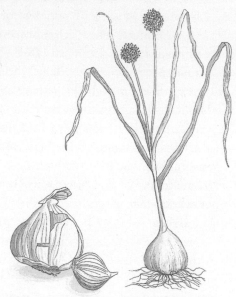

Family: Liliaceae; other members include lily, tulip, onion, and chive

Genus and species: *Allium sativum*

Also known as: Stinking rose, heal-all, and rustic's or poor man's treacle

Parts used: Bulbs

If the term wonder drug can be applied to any healing herb, garlic deserves the honor. It's one of the world's oldest medicines—and still among the best.

Within the genus *Allium*, garlic is the most powerful (and most thoroughly researched) healer. But traditional herbalists also valued garlic's close botanical relatives—onion, scallion, leek, chive, and shallot—though they were considered less medicinal. Modern research agrees. Onions are almost as therapeutic as garlic, but the other plants are less medicinal.

Healing History

Remains of garlic have been discovered in caves inhabited 10,000 years ago, but the first prescription for the herb, chiseled in cuneiform on a Sumerian clay tablet, dates from 3000 BC.

Garlic appears prominently in the world's oldest surviving medical text, the Ebers Papyrus (1500 BC). The herb was an ingredient in 22 ancient Egyptian remedies for headache, insect and scorpion bites, menstrual discomforts, intestinal worms, tumors, and heart problems.

From Spain to China, the ancient world loved garlic. However, no one enjoyed it more than the Egyptians. Greek writers called them "the stinking ones" because of their garlic breath. Egyptians taking solemn oaths swore on garlic like we swear on the Bible. King Tut's tomb contained garlic. Egyptians could trade 15 pounds of the herb for a healthy male slave.

The Egyptians believed the herb prevented illness and increased strength and endurance. They gave their slaves a daily ration, and over time, the slaves who built the pyramids also came to revere the herb. Legend has it that during the construction of one pyramid, a garlic shortage forced the Egyptians to cut the slaves' ration. The result was a labor revolt, the world's first recorded strike.

Around 1200 BC, after Moses led the Hebrew slaves out of Egypt, they complained of missing the finer things of life in bondage. "We remember the fish we ate in Egypt, and the cucumbers, melons, leeks, onions, and garlic" (Numbers 11:5).

For Combat and Competition

Greek athletes ate garlic before races, and Greek soldiers munched it before battle. In his play *Knights*, Aristophanes wrote: "Now bolt down garlic. You will have greater mettle for the fight."

In Homer's *Odyssey*, the sorceress Circe turns Ulysses' men into swine. Fortunately, Hermes, god of science (whose symbol, the serpent-wrapped staff, came to symbolize medicine), gave Ulysses garlic, which thwarted Circe's spells.

Greek midwives hung garlic cloves around birthing rooms to protect newborns from disease and witchcraft. As the centuries passed, Europeans fastened braided garlic plants to their doorposts to deter evil spirits, a custom that survives in the garlic braids hung in many kitchens.

Greek and Roman physicians loved garlic. Hippocrates recommended it for infections, wounds, cancer, leprosy, and digestive problems. Dioscorides prescribed it for heart problems. And Pliny listed it in 61 remedies for ailments ranging from the common cold to epilepsy and from leprosy to tapeworm. Science supports many of these uses.

Eventually, upper-class Greeks and Romans came to hate the stinking rose, viewing garlic breath as a sign of low social status. Antipathy to garlic breath is still with us today.

Despite the scourge of garlic breath, many Roman emperors couldn't eat enough. The ancients considered the herb an antidote to poisons, which were widely employed in ancient Rome to dispatch political rivals. Many Roman herbalists specialized in poisons—and in antidotes that usually included garlic.

Like the Greeks, ancient India's Ayurvedic healers prescribed garlic for leprosy, a practice that continued for thousands of years. When India became a British colony and adopted English, leprosy became known as "peelgarlic" because lepers spent so much time peeling and eating the cloves. Indians also used garlic to treat cancer. Modern research supports garlic's ability to treat leprosy and prevent certain cancers.

Tenth-century Arab physicians inherited the Greco-Roman ambivalence toward garlic. One Persian herbal said that the herb should be "despised because of its unpleasant odor," then affirmed that it "acts as an antidote to deadly poisons. It drives away toothache if you bruise it and lay it upon the tooth. No kitchen should be without it."

The same ambivalence persisted in medieval Europe. The well-to-do shunned garlic, but the peasantry consumed tons, viewing the herb as a cure-all—hence one of its names, heal-all.

By the Elizabethan era, the Latin term for antidote, *theriaca*, had evolved into the English word treacle, meaning "panacea." Garlic was commonly called the poor man's treacle.

From Social Scourge to Saving Grace

As the centuries passed, the upper class returned to using garlic, but only medicinally and sparingly. The 17th-century English herbalist Nicholas Culpeper endorsed it as "a remedy for all diseases and hurts. . . . It helpeth the biting of mad dogs and other venomous creatures, killeth worms in children, cutteth tough phlegm, purgeth the head . . . and is a good remedy for any plague."

However, Culpeper also embraced upper-class disdain for garlic and criticized folk healers for "quoting many diseases this [herb] is good for, but concealing its vices." Culpeper warned against garlic's "offensiveness on the breath" and wrote, "Its heat is very vehement, [and it] sends up ill-favoured vapours to the brain. Let it be used inwardly with moderation."

Culpeper's call for moderation fell on deaf ears. As a Welsh rhyme advised, "Eat leeks in March, and garlic in May/And all the year after, physicians may play."

During Culpeper's time, the typical breakfast for French peasants consisted of dark bread and garlic. French folk healers considered the herb a strengthener and cure-all.

In 1721, French reverence for garlic soared when a plague struck Marseilles, killing most of its population. Legend has it that convicted thieves were assigned to bury the dead, a task certain to infect them, thus saving the government the bother of executing them. But four enterprising thieves mixed garlic into wine and survived. They not only escaped the guillotine, they grew rich robbing all the bodies. This tale is mythological, but to this day, southern Europeans drink a garlic medicine called Four Thieves Vinegar (*Vinaigre des Quatre Voleurs*).

America's 19th-century Eclectic physicians, forerunners of today's naturopaths, shared the Victorian prejudice against garlic's "strong, offensive smell . . . and acrimonious, almost caustic taste." But they conceded its effectiveness in treating colds, coughs, whooping cough, and other respiratory ailments. They also believed that garlic juice applied to the ear cured deafness.

During World War I, British, French, and Russian army physicians used garlic juice to treat infected battle wounds. They also prescribed the herb to prevent and treat amoebic dysentery.

Alexander Fleming's 1928 discovery of penicillin launched the age of antibiotics. By World War II, penicillin and sulfa drugs had largely replaced garlic for treatment of infected wounds. In Russia, however, the needs of more than 20 million World War II casualties overwhelmed its antibiotic supply. Red Army physicians relied heavily on garlic, which was dubbed Russian penicillin.

Modern herbalists recommend garlic (as well as other *Allium* vegetables) for colds, coughs, flu, fever, bronchitis, ringworm, intestinal worms, and cardiovascular disease.

Therapeutic Uses

Garlic does not cure epilepsy or deafness, but an enormous amount of scientific evidence proves that the "poor man's treacle" is an herbal wonder.

INFECTIONS. During World War I, garlic's success in treating infected wounds and dysentery showed that the herb has potent antimicrobial action, validating millennia of healing tradition. But garlic's antibiotic constituent remained a mystery until the 1920s, when researchers at Sandoz Pharmaceuticals in Switzerland isolated alliin (pronounced AL-lee-in).

By itself, alliin has no medicinal value, but when garlic is chewed, chopped, bruised, or crushed, its alliin reacts with an enzyme, allinase, which transforms alliin into allicin, a powerful antibiotic.

Since the 1920s, garlic's broad-spectrum antibiotic properties have been confirmed in dozens of animal and human studies. Garlic kills the bacteria that cause tuberculosis (*Mycobacterium tuberculosis*), food poisoning (*Salmonella*), and women's bladder infections (*Escherichia coli*). The herb may also deter the influenza virus.

Chinese researchers report success in using garlic to treat 21 cases of cryptococcal meningitis, an often fatal fungal infection. Several studies have shown garlic effective against the fungi that cause athlete's foot (*Trichophyton mentagrophytes*) and vaginal yeast infections (*Candida albicans*). Commission E, the expert panel that evaluates herbal medicines for the German counterpart of the FDA, recognizes garlic's antibiotic value.

COLDS. Garlic also has antiviral action. British scientists gave 146 healthy volunteers either a daily placebo or a commercial garlic supplement. After 12 weeks, the garlic group reported significantly fewer and milder colds.

ULCERS. In one study, garlic inhibited the germ that causes most ulcers (*Helicobacter pylori*). The researchers estimate that two daily cloves may provide significant protection against *H. pylori* infection.

HIGH CHOLESTEROL. Dozens of studies document garlic's ability to reduce cholesterol. In one published in the British journal *Lancet*, researchers fed volunteers a meal rich in butter, which raises cholesterol. Half the subjects also ate garlic (nine cloves). Three hours later, controls' average cholesterol increased 7 percent. But in the garlic group, it decreased 7 percent. The researchers concluded, "Garlic has very significant protective action [against elevated cholesterol]."

Two groups of researchers—one Australian, the other American—have published analyses of garlic-cholesterol studies. The Australians reviewed 16 trials involving 952 people. They concluded that 10 fresh cloves or 1 gram of a dried high-allicin preparation reduces total cholesterol about 12 percent. The Americans reviewed five rigorous trials involving 365 people, concluding that one fresh clove a day or 1 gram of a dried high-allicin preparation can lower total cholesterol by 9 percent.

Chinese researchers analyzed 26 studies and concluded that garlic significantly reduces both cholesterol and triglycderides (blood fats).

Experts estimate that for every 1 percent decrease in total cholesterol, the risk of heart attack drops 2 percent. These studies suggest that daily garlic consumption may reduce heart attack risk by up to 24 percent. Compared with drugs, garlic is safer and substantially less expensive.

Over the years, a few highly publicized studies have shown that garlic has no effect on cholesterol. These reports have been criticized for poor methodology. The scientific consensus is that garlic lowers cholesterol. Commission E endorses it for that purpose.

If you take cholesterol medication, ask your doctor about including garlic in your treatment program.

HIGH BLOOD PRESSURE. Many animal and human studies confirm garlic's ability to reduce blood pressure. British researchers analyzed 10 studies and Australian scientists analyzed 11. Their conclusion: Garlic reduces blood pressure significantly. More recently (2015), Swiss, Australian, and Russian researchers analyzed 9 garlic trials involving 482 people who took 240 to 2,400 milligrams/day for 8 to 256 weeks. The herb significantly reduced blood pressure.

INTERNAL BLOOD CLOTS. These trigger heart attacks and most strokes. Garlic has anticoagulant action that helps prevent them. One researcher compared call the herb as effective as aspirin, a standard anticlotting heart attack preventive.

HEART ATTACK AND STROKE. Garlic continues to be controversial for cardiovascular health. Every time a study shows that it reduces cholesterol only slightly or not at all, critics call it useless. But no pharmaceutical simultaneously reduces cholesterol and blood pressure, while helping to prevent internal blood clots. Garlic does all three. If you want to reduce your risk of heart attack and stroke, eat more garlic.

Garlic also helps treat heart disease. German researchers gave 152 people with severe heart disease either medically inactive placebos or 900 milligrams of a standardized powdered garlic preparation (Kwai). Four years later, the placebos group showed 16 percent more arterial narrowing. But in the garlic group, arterial blockages receded 3 percent.

CANCER. Garlic's antibiotic allicin is also a potent antioxidant that helps prevent the cell damage underlying cancer. Many cell culture, animal, and human studies have shown that garlic inhibits various cancers, notably stomach and colon cancers.

Researchers coordinating the Iowa Women's Health Study have tracked the diet, lifestyle, and health status of 41,387 middle-aged Iowa women since 1985. Those who eat the most garlic are the least likely to develop colon cancer. Eating just a few cloves a week cut risk 35 percent. Fruits and vegetables help prevent cancer, but in this study, of all plant foods analyzed, garlic was the best preventive.

In the Netherlands Cohort Study, Dutch researchers have followed more than 120,000 middle-aged adults for decades. Their findings: As participants' consumption of garlic's close relative, onion, increases, their risk of stomach cancer significantly decreases.

Meanwhile, a study of 1,800 Chinese found that those most likely to develop stomach cancer eat the least garlic. The researchers' conclusion: A diet high in garlic "can significantly reduce risk of stomach cancer."

DIABETES. In both animals and human, garlic reduces blood sugar. Diabetes is a serious condition that requires professional treatment, but if you're diabetic, why not use garlic combined with prescribed medication.

LEAD POISONING. European studies show that garlic speeds elimination of lead and other toxic heavy metals. Children are particularly susceptible to lead toxicity. Add garlic to spaghetti sauces and other foods kids enjoy.

BENIGN PROSTATE ENLARGEMENT. Italian researchers surveyed 1,369 men with enlarged prostates and 1,451 controls. Compared with those who ate little or no garlic, the men who at the most were 28 percent less likely to develop prostate enlargement. (A diet high in onions reduced risk 59 percent.)

Intriguing Possibilities

ALOPECIA AREATA. This condition causes substantial hair loss. Iranian researchers gave 40 alopecia areata sufferers either a topical placebo gel or a garlic gel (applied twice daily). After 3 months, the garlic group experienced significantly greater hair regrowth.

LEPROSY. Ancient Ayurvedic healers were onto something when they used garlic to treat leprosy, now called Hansen's disease. Indian researchers gave people with Hansen's a garlic ointment made and foods containing the herb. Compared with those who did not receive garlic treatment, those who did showed significant improvement.

AIDS. In addition to anti-HIV medications, garlic helps treat AIDS. In one study, people with AIDS who ate a clove a day for 3 months showed significantly improved immune function, less diarrhea, and fewer herpes sores.

Rx Recommendations

For minor skin infections, garlic juice applied externally may prove sufficient. But unless you're working with an experienced herbalist, don't rely exclusively on garlic to treat infections.

Researchers have found that 1 medium garlic clove packs the antibacterial punch of about 100,000 units of penicillin. Depending on the type of infection, oral penicillin doses typically range from 600,000 to 1.2 million units. The garlic equivalent would be 6 to 12 cloves. Chew 3 cloves at a time two to four times a day.

To help reduce blood pressure, cholesterol, and the likelihood of blood clots, experts recommend eating 3 to 10 fresh cloves of garlic a day. The herb must be chewed, chopped, bruised, or crushed to transform its medicinally inert alliin into antibiotic allicin. For greatest benefit, use fresh garlic. But the herb retains healing benefits when lightly cooked.

Raw garlic has a sharp, biting flavor, which cooking eliminates. Use it in foods to taste.

To prepare an infusion, put six chopped cloves in 1 cup of cool water and steep for 6 hours.

For a tincture, soak 1 cup of crushed cloves in 1 quart of brandy. Shake the mixture daily for 2 weeks, then take up to 3 tablespoons a day.

When using commercial preparations, follow package directions.

What About the Smell?

Since 3000 BC, the main drawback to garlic has been its odor. The stinking rose continues to bother many people. However, garlic-rich Italian and Asian cuisines are very popular. Some of the nation's finest restaurants now proudly serve dishes heavily flavored with garlic.

Gilroy, California, near Monterey, is the garlic capital of America. Every year, garlic lovers gather for the annual Garlic Festival, which features such delights as garlic soup, garlic cake, and garlic ice cream. A popular festival bumper sticker proclaims "Fight Mouthwash. Eat Garlic."

Still, most of us are a long way from promoting garlic breath. To eliminate it, try chewing traditional herbal breath fresheners: parsley, fennel, or fenugreek.

Today, deodorized medicinal garlic preparations are available in health food stores and some pharmacies. Many scientists believe that the herb's medicinal value comes from its odor-causing sulfur compounds, which has raised doubts about the medicinal effectiveness of deodorized garlic. Still, some studies have shown that even without the stink, garlic retains its healing benefits.

Safety

Garlic's anticlotting action may help prevent heart attacks and some types of stroke—but cause problems for those with clotting disorders. If you're among them, or if you take anticoagulant (blood-thinning) medication or vitamin E, consult your physician before using garlic in medicinal amounts.

Garlic's genus name, *Allium*, comes from the Celtic word *all,* meaning "burning." Fresh garlic can cause a burning sensation in the mouth that some people find unpleasant.

Allergic reactions are possible. Rashes have been reported after touching or eating the herb. If garlic gives you a rash, don't eat it. Garlic-induced stomach upset has also been reported.

Garlic has been used as a food and medicine for thousands of years by people of all ages,

including pregnant women. It has never been implicated in miscarriage or birth defects.

However, garlic enters the milk of nursing mothers and may contribute to infant colic.

Inform health professionals of the herbs you use. Problematic herb-drug interactions are possible, particularly given garlic's anti-clotting action.

Garlic may cause allergic reactions or other unexpected side effects. If any develop, reduce your dose or stop taking it. For more on herb safety, see Chapter 2.

If symptoms get worse or persist longer than 2 weeks, consult a health professional promptly.

Gardening

Garlic grows easily from seeds or cloves. It's easier to start with cloves. Plant them 2 inches deep and 6 inches apart in early spring.

Garlic is cold tolerant and can be planted up to 6 weeks before the final frost date. It thrives best in rich, deeply cultivated, well-drained soil. Do not overwater. Full sun produces the largest bulbs, but garlic tolerates some shade. During summer, cut back the flower stalks so the plant devotes all its energy to producing fat, aromatic bulbs.

Harvest bulbs in late summer and store them in a cool, dark place.

Take care to protect bulbs from bruising, which invites mold and insects. Braid the leaves into a wreath or rope and display it in your kitchen, removing bulbs as needed.

GENTIAN

Feel Better with Bitter Moxie

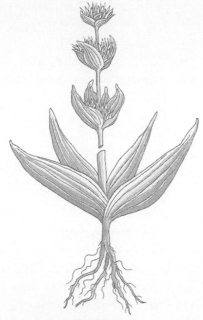

Family: Gentianaceae; other members include other gentians and marsh felwort

Genus and species: *Gentiana lutea*

Also known as: Yellow gentian, bitter root, and bitterwort

Parts used: Roots

In Depression-era slang, "moxie" meant reckless courage. Teddy Roosevelt, Charles Lindbergh, Al Capone—they all had moxie. The term comes from Moxie, a bitter soft drink available only in New England since the 1890s.

Moxie owes its bite to gentian root, a healing herb with a 3,000-year history as a digestive "bitter." Modern research shows that gentian stimulates digestion.

Healing History

The ancient Egyptians, Greeks, and Romans used gentian primarily as an appetite stimulant, but also as an antiseptic and treatment for intestinal worms, digestive disorders, liver ailments, and "female hysteria" (menstrual discomforts).

Sixth-century Arab physicians adopted the herb and introduced its medicinal uses to Asia. Since then, Chinese physicians have prescribed the herb to treat digestive disorders, sore throat, headache, and arthritis. India's Ayurvedic physicians recommended it for fevers, venereal diseases, and liver problems.

During the Middle Ages, European herbalists prized gentian because it caused less intestinal irritation than other digestive bitters.

Seventeenth-century English herbalist Nicholas Culpeper wrote that gentian "strengthens the stomach exceedingly, helps digestion, comforts the heart, helps agues [fevers] of all sorts, kills worms, and preserves against fainting and swooning. It provokes urine and terms [menstruation] exceedingly; therefore, let it not be given to women with child."

When colonists arrived in Virginia and the Carolinas, they found Native Americans applying a root decoction of American gentian (*Gentiana puberula*) to relieve back pain.

America's 19th-century Eclectic physicians, forerunners of today's naturopaths, considered gentian a powerful tonic and prescribed it to "improve appetite and stimulate digestion." But their text *King's American Dispensatory* (1898) warned, "When taken in large doses, it is apt to oppress the stomach, irritate the bowels, and produce nausea, vomiting, and headache."

Gentian was listed as a digestive stimulant

in the *U.S. Pharmacopoeia*, a standard drug reference, from 1820 to 1955.

Before the introduction of hop (page 268), gentian root was an ingredient in beer. The herb is still used in liqueurs, vermouths, and many digestive bitters popular in Europe.

In 1885, Augustin Thompson of Union, Maine, introduced his gentian-laced beverage, Moxie Nerve Food. The original label proclaimed the bitter brew cured "brain and nervous exhaustion, loss of manhood, helplessness, imbecility, and insanity"—claims that took a lot of moxie even in the pre-FDA heyday of patent medicines.

Thompson peddled Moxie from town to town in New England. Eventually it caught on—not as medicine but as a beverage. That was fine with Thompson, who retracted his medicinal claims and repositioned Moxie as a soft drink. For years, Moxie outsold Coca-Cola in New England. It's still available there, and gentian is still an ingredient.

In the 1930s, Maude Grieve, author of *A Modern Herbal*, called gentian "one of our most useful bitter tonics, especially in general debility, weakness of the digestive organs, or want of appetite. It is one of the best strengtheners of the human system."

Contemporary herbalists echo Grieve. One suggests chewing gentian root as a substitute for smoking cigarettes.

Therapeutic Uses

Forget gentian for "loss of manhood, helplessness, imbecility, and insanity." But the bitter root lives up to its ancient reputation as a digestive aid.

DIGESTIVE PROBLEMS. Gentian contains gentianine, a bitter-tasting compound that stimulates salivation and the secretion of stomach acid

and bile, lending credence to the herb's 3,000-year history as a digestive aid. Try some before meals.

Commission E, the expert panel that evaluates herbal medicines for the German counterpart of the FDA, endorses gentian for loss of appetite and digestive complaints.

ARTHRITIS. Several studies have shown that gentian has anti-inflammatory action, suggesting that traditional Chinese physicians may have been correct prescribing the herb for arthritis.

Rx Recommendations

Use gentian decoction or tincture to stimulate digestion or treat arthritis.

To make a decoction, boil 1 teaspoon of powdered root in 3 cups of water for 30 minutes, then strain if you wish and let cool. Take 1 tablespoon before meals. Gentian tastes very bitter, so you may want to add sugar or honey.

As a homemade tincture, take $\frac{1}{4}$ to 1 teaspoon before meals.

When using commercial preparations, follow package directions.

Safety

Gentian digestive bitters are popular in Germany, where herbal medicine is considerably more mainstream than in the United States. German physicians discourage the herb's use by people with high blood pressure. They also echo the Eclectics' warning that large amounts may cause stomach irritation, with possible nausea and vomiting.

Gentian has never been shown to stimulate the uterus. In fact, it relaxes smooth muscle tissue, the type of tissue that forms the uterus. Nonetheless, for centuries, herbalists have considered it a powerful menstruation promoter. Pregnant and nursing women should err on the side of caution and not use it.

Do not give gentian to children under 2. It may taste too bitter for older children. But if they can tolerate it, adjust the recommended dose based on the child's weight. Give a 50-pound child one-third of the dose a 150-pound adult would take.

If you're over 65, start with a low dose, and increase only if necessary.

Inform health professionals of the herbs you use. Problematic herb-drug interactions are possible.

Gentian may cause allergic reactions or other unexpected side effects. If any develop, reduce your dose or stop taking it. For more on herb safety, see Chapter 2.

If symptoms get worse or persist longer than 2 weeks, consult a health professional promptly.

Gardening

Gentian is a striking 6-foot perennial with branching medicinal roots, deeply veined, pointed oval leaves, and large, beautiful yellow flowers.

Once established, it requires little care other than abundant water and shelter from wind and full sun. But establishing gentian can be a problem. The seeds need frost to germinate, and even with frost, germination may take a year, if it occurs at all. Most authorities recommend using root cuttings instead.

Gentian prefers rich, loamy, slightly acidic soil. An annual dressing of peat moss helps. Harvest the roots in late summer. Desirable roots are dark reddish brown, tough, and flexible, with a strong, unpleasant odor. They taste sweet initially, then very bitter. Dry the roots, then powder them.

GINGER

Stop Motion Sickness and Morning Sickness

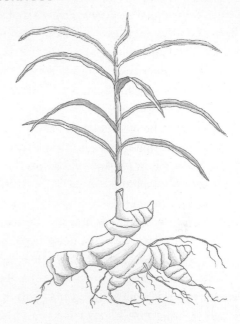

Family: Zingiberaceae; other members include turmeric and cardamom

Genus and species: *Zingiber officinale*

Also known as: Jamaican, African, and Cochin (Asian) ginger

Parts used: Rhizomes (commonly called roots)

An Indian proverb says, "Every good quality is contained in ginger." That's not much of an exaggeration.

Fleshy and aromatic, ginger has played a role in cooking and healing since the dawn of history. Modern research has supported its traditional use against nausea and has added several benefits ancient herbalists never dreamed of.

Healing History

Ancient Indians used their native ginger in cooking, to preserve food, and to treat digestive problems. They also considered the herb a physical and spiritual cleanser. Indians shunned strong-smelling garlic and onions before religious celebrations for fear of offending their deities, but they ate lots of ginger, which left them smelling sweet and presentable to the gods.

Ginger figured prominently in China's first great herbal, the *Pen Tsao Ching* (*Classic of Herbs*), supposedly compiled by the mythical emperor-sage Shen Nung around 3000 BC. As the story goes, the wise herbalist tested hundreds of medicinal herbs on himself—until he took a little too much of a poisonous herb and died. Shen Nung recommended ginger for colds, fever, chills, tetanus, and leprosy. The *Pen Tsao Ching* also echoed Indian practice, saying that fresh ginger "eliminates body odor and puts a person in touch with the spiritual [realm]."

Over time, Chinese women began taking ginger for menstrual discomforts. Then they noticed that the herb relieved the nausea of morning sickness. Chinese sailors adopted ginger, chewing the root at sea to prevent seasickness. Chinese physicians prescribed it to treat arthritis, ulcers, and kidney problems.

The Chinese also consider ginger an antidote to shellfish poisoning. This is why Chinese fish and seafood dishes are often seasoned with the herb.

Ancient Greek traders liked the Asian practice of using ginger as a nausea-preventing digestive aid. They brought it to Greece, where, after big meals, it was wrapped in sweetened bread and eaten as a stomach-settling dessert. Eventually, the Greeks began baking the herb into the sweet bread, and the herbal seasickness remedy evolved into the world's first cookie, gingerbread.

The Romans also used ginger as a digestive aid. After the fall of Rome, however, the herb became scarce in Europe and quite costly.

Once renewed Asian trade made ginger more available, European demand proved almost insatiable. The ancient Greeks' modest gingerbread cookies evolved into sugary gingerbread men and elaborate confections like the witch's gingerbread house in Hansel and Gretel.

In England and her American colonies, ginger was incorporated into a stomach-soothing drink called ginger beer, the forerunner of today's ginger ale. Ginger ale is still a popular home remedy for upset stomach, diarrhea, nausea, and vomiting.

America's 19th-century Eclectic physicians, forerunners of today's naturopaths, prescribed ginger powder, tea, wine, and beer for infant diarrhea, indigestion, nausea, dysentery, flatulence, fever, headache, toothache, and "female hysteria" (menstrual complaints).

Contemporary herbalists recommend ginger for colds, flu, and motion sickness and as a digestive aid.

Therapeutic Uses

Break out the gingerbread and ginger ale. Scientific research has lent support to several of ginger's traditional uses—and has revealed even more benefits.

NAUSEA, MOTION SICKNESS, MORNING SICKNESS. The ancient Chinese were right. Ginger does indeed prevent nausea associated with seasickness, other types of motion sickness, and the morning sickness of pregnancy.

Ginger's antinausea action first received scientific validation in 1982 in a study conducted by researchers at Brigham Young University published in the British medical journal *Lancet*. The researchers gave 36 volunteers with a history of motion sickness either 100 milligrams of the popular anti–motion sickness drug dimenhydrinate (Dramamine) or ginger powder (940 milligrams). A short time later, the participants were seated in a motorized rocking chair programmed to move so occupants would develop motion sickness. The chair was equipped with a switch that allowed its riders to stop the movement when they began to feel queasy.

Compared with those who took Dramamine, participants in the ginger group stayed in the chair 57 percent longer.

Since that study, many others have confirmed ginger's value for the prevention of motion and morning sickness. Here's a small sampling.

❧ Swedish Navy researchers gave ginger to 80 naval cadets who were sailing turbulent seas. Compared with a group that took a medically inactive placebo, those who took ginger experienced 72 percent less seasickness.

❧ British surgeons gave 60 women about to have gynecological surgery either ginger or the prescription antinausea drug metoclopramide (Reglan). Those who received ginger experienced significantly less postsurgical nausea and vomiting.

❧ Danish researchers gave 30 pregnant women, all battling morning sickness, either a placebo or ginger for 4 days. Then the women switched treatments for another 4 days. While taking ginger, 70 percent of participants reported significant relief from nausea. Doctors discourage moms-to-be from taking any drugs, including antinausea medications, but ginger is safe to use during pregnancy.

❧ Italian researchers asked passengers boarding a cruise ship if they were prone to seasickness. Sixty said they were. The ship's doctor gave them either a standard dose of Dramamine or ginger (500 milligrams before embarking and 500 milligrams every 4 hours during 2 days of rough seas). Among those taking Dramamine, 50 percent reported "very good" or "excellent" results. But in the ginger group, the figure was 70 percent.

❧ Other Italian scientists studied 28 children who took a 2-day class trip that involved travel by car, boat, and airplane. All were given either a standard children's dose of Dramamine or ginger (for those younger than 6, 250 milligrams before departure and every 4 hours thereafter; for those 6 or older, 500 milligrams). A physician rated their motion sickness symptoms. Among those taking Dramamine, 31 percent showed "good" benefits, while 69 percent demonstrated "modest" benefits. Among those who took ginger, 100 percent had "good" results.

❧ Cancer chemotherapy is notorious for causing nausea and vomiting. Indian researchers gave 60 children being treated for bone cancer standard antinausa medication plus a placebo or ginger (1,000 or 2,000 milligrams/day depending on their weight). After 3 days, 93 percent of the placebo group reported nausea and 77 percent vomited, but in the ginger group, just 56 percent developed nausea and only 33 percent vomited, highly significant differences. An American trial confirms ginger's ability to prevent chemotherapy-induced nausea.

Commission E, the expert panel that evaluates herbal medicines for the German counterpart of the Food and Drug Administration, endorses ginger for the prevention and treatment of motion sickness. In addition, many cancer specialists recommend it for the nausea associated with chemotherapy.

DIGESTIVE PROBLEMS. Ginger is a gastrointestinal antispasmodic. It prevents indigestion and abdominal cramping by soothing the muscles that line the intestines. It also contains some compounds similar to digestive enzymes that break down proteins. Commission E approves ginger to prevent and treat indigestion.

HEART DISEASE AND STROKE. Few people in the ancient world were sedentary or ate a diet high in animal fat or lived long enough to develop heart disease or stroke. Today, these conditions account for half of all deaths in the United States.

Ginger helps prevent heart disease and stroke by controlling three key risk factors. The herb helps reduce cholesterol, according to a study published in the *New England Journal of Medicine*. It also helps lower blood pressure, and it prevents the internal blood clots that trigger heart attacks and most strokes.

ULCERS. Research confirms the ancient Chinese practice of using ginger to treat ulcers. In experiments involving animals that were given drugs known to produce ulcers, pretreatment with a ginger preparation prevented ulcers.

Ginger does not cure ulcers, nor has it been well researched in humans. But a small pilot study involving 10 ulcer sufferers who took ginger (6 grams/day) showed that the herb helps relieve symptoms.

DIABETES. Iranian researchers gave 64 Type-2 diabetics either a placebo or ginger (2 grams/day). After 8 weeks, the ginger group showed improved insulin sensitivity, that is, more sugar moved into the cells and less stayed in the bloodstream. Another Iranian team gave 88 Type-2 diabetics either a placebo or ginger (3,000 milligrams/day). Eight weeks later, the ginger group's blood sugar dropped 21 percent.

ARTHRITIS. Ginger congtains anti-inflammatory compounds, lending support to the herb's traditional use in treating arthritis.

MENSTRUAL CRAMPS. Antispasmodics soothe not only the digestive tract but also other smooth muscles, including the uterus. As an antispasmodic, ginger helps ease menstrual cramps. Iranian scientists gave 122 university students plagued by cramps either ibuprofen or ginger (250 milligrams every 6 hours). After two cycles, both treatments produced the same relief—but ginger was less likely to cause stomach upset.

COLDS AND FLU. Chinese studies show that ginger helps kill influenza virus, and Indian researchers report that the herb increases the immune system's ability to fight infection. These findings lend some support to ginger's traditional role in treating colds, flu, and other infectious illnesses.

OSTEOARTHRITIS. Ginger contains pain-relieving compounds known as COX-2 inhibitors. Russian scientists gave 43 osteoarthritis sufferers daily glucosamine (500 milligrams) plus either ibuprofen or ginger (2,000 milligrams). After 1 month, both groups reported similar pain relief, but those taking ginger experienced significantly less stomach distress.

Intriguing Possibilities

In animal studies, ginger reduces blood sugar levels, suggesting that the herb may help control diabetes.

Other animal studies have shown that ginger shrinks certain tumors. While these findings don't necessarily apply to humans, ginger may someday be used in cancer treatment. And if you have cancer, there's no harm in eating more ginger in consultation with your doctor.

A Russian pilot study suggests that ginger may help relieve post-exercise muscle soreness.

Rx Recommendations

Use ginger to taste in cooking to create warm, spicy, aromatic dishes.

For motion sickness, the recommended dose is 1,000 milligrams 30 minutes before travel. Commercial capsules are usually most convenient, but a 12-ounce container of ginger ale also provides the recommended amount, provided that it's made with real ginger and not artificial flavor. Check the label to be sure.

Or try a ginger infusion. To make it, use 2 teaspoons of powdered or fresh grated root per cup of boiling water, steep for 10 minutes, and strain if you wish.

To ease other digestive upsets or to treat colds or flu, make an infusion. To help relieve arthritis or prevent heart disease and stroke, use the herb in cooking or drink ginger ale or ginger tea.

You may give weak ginger preparations to children under 2 for colic.

Inform health professionals of the herbs you use. Problematic herb-drug interactions are possible.

Ginger may cause allergic reactions or other unexpected side effects. If any develop, reduce your dose or stop taking it. For more on herb safety, see Chapter 2.

If symptoms get worse or persist longer than 2 weeks, consult a health professional promptly.

Safety

Ginger's antinausea effects may prevent morning sickness, but the herb has a long history as a menstruation promoter. Might it cause miscarriage? One study suggests that its uterine effects depend on the amount used.

In the *Lancet* study mentioned earlier, less than 1 gram of ginger was needed to prevent nausea. To trigger menstruation, Chinese physicians recommend 20 to 28 grams. A strong cup of ginger tea contains about 500 milligrams, and an 8-ounce glass of ginger ale contains approximately 1,000 milligrams. None of these come close to the amount that promotes menstruation.

There have been no reports in the scientific literature of ginger triggering abortion or causing birth defects. Pregnant women with no history of miscarriage should feel free to try modest amounts of ginger tea or ginger ale to treat morning sickness.

Although ginger generally relieves indigestion, some people who take it to prevent motion sickness report heartburn.

Gardening

Ginger is a tropical perennial that grows from a tuberous underground stem, or rhizome. Each year, the plant produces a round, 3-foot stem with thin, pointed, lance-shaped, 6-inch leaves and a single, large, yellow and purple flower.

Ginger grows outdoors in Hawaii, Florida, southern California, New Mexico, Arizona, and Texas. It does best when well watered in partial shade in raised beds deeply cultivated with composted manure and kelp.

Propagate ginger from young fresh roots, which contain eyes similar to those in potatoes. The ginger root sold in most supermarkets, with tough, tan skin, is neither young nor fresh, so its propagation potential is low. The best place to obtain growable ginger root is at an Asian specialty market, though some nurseries also carry it. Look for roots with light green skin.

Plant roots about 3 inches deep and 12 inches apart. After 12 months, uproot the plant, harvest some roots, and replant the rest.

You can also grow ginger indoors in deep pots with a soil mixture of loam, sand, compost, and peat moss. Indoors, it needs warmth, plenty of water, and high humidity. A greenhouse environment is best.

GINKGO

For Alzheimer's Disease and Many Other Conditions

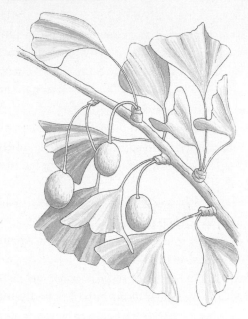

Family: Ginkgoaceae; no other members

Genus and species: *Ginkgo biloba*

Also known as: Maidenhair tree

Parts used: Leaf extract

Ginkgo, a 200-million-year-old relic of the dinosaur age, is the oldest surviving tree on earth. Appropriately enough, as a healing herb, ginkgo aids the oldest surviving people. It helps prevent and treat many conditions associated with aging, including Alzheimer's disease, stroke, heart disease, deafness, blindness, memory loss, and erectile dysfunction.

Healing History

Ginkgo was deemed "good for the heart and lungs" in China's first great herbal, the *Pen*

Tsao Ching (*The Classic of Herbs*), attributed to the mythical emperor-sage Shen Nung around 3000 BC.

Traditional Chinese physicians used ginkgo to treat asthma and chilblains, swelling of the hands and feet due to damp cold. The ancient Chinese and Japanese ate roasted ginkgo seeds as a digestive aid and to prevent drunkenness. Even today, some bars in Japan serve the roasted seeds to prevent intoxication.

India's traditional Ayurvedic healers associated ginkgo with long life. They reportedly used the herb as an ingredient in soma, a longevity elixir.

Asian Buddhists considered the ginkgo tree sacred and often planted it around their temples.

Ginkgo was introduced into Europe in 1730. Today, the trees thrive throughout the temperate world. But as 18th-century horticulturists tended saplings, herbalists ignored the tree. As a result, ginkgo's fan-shaped leaves have no history in Western herbal medicine.

But since the 1970s, researchers have discovered an enormous number of medical uses. Today, ginkgo is a top-selling medicinal herb in the United States and Europe, with sales approaching $1 billion annually. It is particularly popular in Europe, where it ranks among the most widely prescribed medications. Many older Americans use it daily.

Therapeutic Uses

Ginkgo is medically exciting for two reasons. First, it's rich in potent antioxidants (ginkgo flavone glycosides and terpene lactones). Antioxidants help prevent and reverse the cell damage at the root of many degenerative conditions associated with aging, including heart disease, stroke, many cancers, and Alzheimer's disease.

In addition, ginkgo inhibits a compound produced by the body, platelet activation factor (PAF). Discovered in 1972, PAF is involved in an enormous number of biological processes, including arterial blood flow, asthma attacks, organ graft rejection, and the blood clots involved in heart attacks and most strokes.

ALZHEIMER'S DISEASE AND MULTI-INFARCT DEMENTIA (MID). In the United States, ginkgo made its biggest splash in 1997, when the *Journal of the American Medical Association* published a study by researchers at Albert Einstein College of Medicine in the Bronx, New York showing that it not only slows mental deterioration in people with Alzheimer's disease but also, in some cases, actually improves their cognitive abilities.

The researchers gave 202 people in various stages of Alzheimer's either a medically inactive placebo or ginkgo (120 milligrams/day of a standardized extract). One year later, compared with those who received the placebo, participants who took ginkgo retained significantly more mental function.

Many other studies have corroborated ginkgo's effectiveness for slowing the progression of Alzheimer's. Some examples:

- Belgian researchers gave 65 Alzheimers' sufferers a pharmaceutical (Aricept), ginkgo (240 milligrams/day), or both. After 22 weeks, all three treatments showed about the same benefit. In other words, the herb was as effective as the drug.

- European researchers gave 60 Alzheimer's sufferers either a placebo or ginkgo (120 or 240 milligrams/day). After 3 months, compared with the placebo takers, both ginkgo groups performed significantly better on cognitive function tests.

❧ Another European team gave 156 people with either Alzheimer's or multi-infarct dementia (MID, an Alzheimer's-like condition caused by mini strokes) either a placebo or ginkgo (240 milligrams/day). Six months later, the ginkgo group retained greater cognitive function.

❧ German researchers gave 404 people with mild to moderate Alzheimer's or MID either a placebo or ginkgo (240 milligrams/day). After 6 months the ginkgo group showed better cognitive function, fewer behavior problems (wandering, anxiety, angry outbursts, etc.), and greater ability to perform activities of daily living.

In all these studies, the response to ginkgo was similar to what physicians would expect from the pharmaceuticals currently approved to slow the progression of Alzheimer's or MID. It's still not entirely clear how ginkgo works, but it's a powerfully antioxidant that improves blood flow through the brain.

Several studies show ginkgo ineffective in slowing dementia, but the weight of the evidence supports the herb. Commission E, the expert panel that evaluates herbal medicines for the German counterpart of the FDA, approves ginkgo for the treatment of Alzheimer's disease and MID.

Currently, no treatment, either pharmaceutical or herbal, permanently halts or reverses the progression of Alzheimer's disease or MID. But ginkgo slows the progression of conditions as well as pharmaceuticals and causes few, if any, side effects.

CEREBRAL INSUFFICIENCY. As people get older, blood flow through the brain declines (cerebral insufficiency), which slows reaction time and impairs memory, concentration, and problem-solving ability—effects called "senior moments." Many studies show that ginkgo improves blood flow through the brain and, as a result, reduces cerebral insufficiency.

MEMORY LOSS. Animal studies show that ginkgo improves memory. Human trials have produced similar findings.

❧ A European research team gave 241 otherwise healthy elderly people who had memory problems either a placebo or ginkgo. After 6 months, those taking the herb showed memory improvement.

❧ British researchers gave 31 middle-aged people who reported memory problems either a placebo or ginkgo (120 milligrams/day). After 6 months, the ginkgo group showed significant improvement in memory and reaction time.

❧ In another English study, researchers tested the short-term memory skills and reaction times of eight women in their 20s and 30s before and after they were given either a placebo or ginkgo (600 milligrams). After taking the herb, their memory and reaction time improved "very significantly."

MENTAL FUNCTION IN HEALTHY ADULTS. In addition to the study just mentioned, a few other reports also show that ginkgo provides cognitive benefits in healthy adults. A German study showed that after taking gingko (500 milligrams), keystroke errors by middle-aged computer users dropped 30 percent. And English scientists gave a placebo or ginkgo (50 or 100 milligrams three times a day or singles doses of 120 or 240 milligrams). After a month, the herb significantly improved scores in half of memory tests. Meanwhile, other British researchers analyzed 15 studies of ginkgo in nondemented adults and found little evidence of benefit. This issue remains unresolved, but the evidence tilts in the herb's favor. Ginkgo causes few side effects. If you'd like to try it for memory enhancement, feel free.

Commission E approves ginkgo as a treatment for memory problems.

STROKE. As blood flow through the brain decreases with age, brain cells receive less food and oxygen. If blood flow becomes blocked, the result is a stroke, the third leading cause of death in the United States. Europe physicians often prescribe ginkgo to support recovery from stroke. Commission E approves the herb for stroke treatment and rehabilitation.

HEART DISEASE. In addition to improving blood flow through the brain, ginkgo boosts blood flow through the heart. It also contains antioxidants that help prevent heart disease. It reduces blood pressure. And it helps prevent the internal blood clots that trigger heart attack. Add 'em up and the herb reduces risk of heart disease. A French study shows that taking ginkgo after coronary artery bypass surgery speeds recovery.

INTERMITTENT CLAUDICATION (IC). When cholesterol deposits narrow the arteries in the legs, the result is intermittent claudication, which causes pain, cramping, and weakness, particularly in the calves. Ginkgo improves blood flow through the legs, relieving IC symptoms.

German researchers gave a standard medication or ginkgo to 36 people with IC. After a year, the herb produced significantly greater pain relief. Another German team measured how far people with IC could walk before developing leg pain. Then the participants began taking either a placebo or ginkgo. After 6 months, the placebo group showed scant improvement, while those taking ginkgo were able to walk 50 percent farther. Commission E approves ginkgo as a treatment for intermittent claudication.

ERECTILE DYSFUNCTION (ED). A study in the *Journal of Urology* shows that ginkgo helps relieve ED caused by narrowed arteries in the penis. In the study, 60 men with ED caused by impaired penile blood flow were instructed to take ginkgo (60 milligrams/day). After 12 months, half reported erection improvement.

ANTIDEPRESSANT-RELATED SEXUAL PROBLEMS. Pharmaceutical antidepressants work. Unfortunately, many cause sex problems: ED in men, loss of vaginal lubrication in women, and in both sexes, loss of libido and difficulty with orgasm. At the University of California, San Francisco, an elderly man taking antidepressants who also used ginkgo for his memory told his doctor that the herb seemed to give him a sexual boost. This comment led to a study of ginkgo's effects in 63 people who were experiencing antidepressant-related sex problems. In addition to prescribed medications, the patients took ginkgo (207 mg/day). Ninety-one percent of the women and 76 percent of the men reported significant improvement: enhanced sexual desire, greater ability to have erections or produce lubrication, and generally more pleasurable sex.

In this study, the researchers didn't test ginkgo against a placebo, so the study was not scientifically rigorous. Placebos usually benefit about one-third of users. But the response rate in this study was much greater than a typical placebo response, evidence that ginkgo has real ability to relieve antidepressant-related sex problems.

MENOPAUSAL LIBIDO LOSS. During menopause, many women experience mild to severe libido loss. Iranian scientists surveyed desire among 63 sexually active menopausal women. Then participants took either a placebo or ginkgo (120 milligrams/day for a week, then 240 milligrams/day for 3 weeks). Thirty-four percent of the placebo group reported increased sexual desire, but among those taking ginkgo, the figure was 65 percent.

ANXIETY. Ginkgo reduces anxiety in people with Alzheimer's, so German researchers wondered if it might do the same for other older adults. They gave 107 anxious elders either a placebo or ginkgo (240 or 480 milligrams/day). After 4 weeks, both ginkgo groups showed significantly less anxiety.

MACULAR DEGENERATION. Macular degeneration, a leading cause of adult blindness, involves deterioration of the macula, the part of the eye's nerve-rich retina responsible for central vision (what you see right in front of you). In a French study, people with macular degeneration who took ginkgo experienced "significant vision improvement."

DIABETIC RETINOPATHY. Another leading cause of adult blindness, this complication of diabetes involves substantially reduced blood flow through the retina. Researchers in Taiwan gave 25 Type-2 diabetics with retinopathy either a placebeo or ginkgo (240 milligrams/day). After 3 months, the ginkgo group showed signifidantly improved retinal blood flow.

COCHLEAR DEAFNESS. Researchers believe that cochlear deafness results from decreased blood flow to the nerves involved in hearing. A French study that compared ginkgo with standard therapy showed significant improvement in both groups, but greater benefit in the ginkgo group.

Intriguing Possibilities

INSOMNIA. In a Swiss pilot study, researchers gave 14 people with depression-related insomnia either a pharmaceutical antidepressant or ginkgo (320 milligrams/day). After a week, they slept better.

CHRONIC DIZZINESS (VERTIGO). French researchers gave 70 vertigo sufferers either a placebo or ginkgo. After 3 months, 18 percent of the placebo group reported improvement, but in the ginkgo group, 47 percent, a highly significant difference. Commission E approves ginkgo as a treatment for vertigo.

CHRONIC RINGING IN THE EARS (TINNITUS). A 13-month French study involving 103 people deemed ginkgo "conclusively effective" for chronic tinnitus. According to the researchers, the herb improved all the patients who took it. Commission E approves ginkgo as a treatment for tinnitus. However, other studies have shown no benefit. Ginkgo's effect on tinnitus remains to be determined. But if you have this condition, it can't hurt to try the herb.

INTOXICATION. There may be some truth to the age-old Asian belief that ginkgo minimizes drunkenness. Japanese researchers have discovered an enzyme in ginkgo seed that accelerates metabolism of alcohol. Faster metabolism means less alcohol in the bloodstream and less likelihood of intoxication. Of course, munching roasted ginkgo seeds is no substitute for responsible drinking.

MULTIPLE SCLEROSIS. In a pilot study, researchers at the University of North Carolina, at Charlotte, gave either a placebo or ginkgo (240 milligrams/day) to 22 people with MS. After 4 weeks, the ginkgo group showed "significant" decreases in fatigue and symptom severity, and improved ability to perform activities of daily living.

Preliminary reports also suggest that ginkgo may improve immune function and reduce rejection risk in transplanted organs. It may also be effective against allergies, high blood pressure, migraines, kidney problems, and dyslexia in children.

Rx Recommendations

The medicinal compounds in ginkgo leaf occur in concentrations too small for infusions or tinctures to provide any benefit. Commercial preparations use a concentrated 50:1 extract— 50 pounds of leaves processed into 1 pound of standardized extract containing 24 percent ginkgo flavone glycosides and 6 percent terpene lactones.

Buy a standardized ginkgo product and take according to package directions. Most studies have used 120 or 240 milligrams a day, typically divided into three doses—40 or 80 milligrams 3 times a day.

Safety

BLEEDING HAZARD? Platelet activation factor plays a role in blood clotting. Ginkgo's PAF-inhibiting action may cause problems for people with clotting disorders and those taking anticoagulant (blood-thinning) medications. Several cases of hemorrhage have been reported in people taking ginkgo. As a result, surgeons have placed it on the list of herbs that should not be taken for at least 2 weeks before scheduled surgery.

But how much of a bleeding hazard is ginkgo? Not much, it turns out. Turkish researchers measured clotting times in 40 elderly folks with mild cognitive impairment, a condition treated with ginkgo. Then subjects took ginkgo (80 milligrams three times a day). A week later, the researchers retested clotting times. Ginkgo delayed clotting time, but only slightly—17.1 seconds before ginkgo, 17.5 seconds after.

More evidence that ginkgo is not a major bleeding hazard comes from a German analysis of 75 million German prescription users from 1999 to 2002, including 320,644 who took ginkgo. When taking no medication at all, 1.63 bleeding episodes occurred per 100 person-years; when taking any medication, 3.51; when taking other Alzheimer's drugs, 1.44; and when taking ginkgo, less than 1.0. In other words, ginkgo posed *less* of a bleeding hazard than drugs in general, notably other Alzheimer's medications. The authors suggest that ginkgo has been falsely accused of causing bleeding problems. Unfortunately, once erroneous information gets into the medical literature, it's very difficult to erase. Undoubtedly, ginkgo will continue to be called a bleeding hazard and surgeons will continue to urge people to stop taking it before surgery. But the best evidence shows that ginkgo is not a significant bleeding hazard.

No serious side effects have been associated with ginkgo, but stomach upset, headache, and rash are possible. Some people who take large doses have reported irritability, restlessness, diarrhea, nausea, and vomiting. Allergic reactions or other unexpected side effects are also possible. If any develop, reduce your dose or stop taking this herb.

Pregnant and nursing women should not use ginkgo.

There is no reason to give ginkgo to children, except as a treatment for dyslexia. Discuss this with the child's doctor.

Inform health professionals of the herbs you use. Problematic herb-drug interactions are possible. For more on herb safety, see Chapter 2.

Gardening

Ginkgo is a stately, deciduous tree that reaches 100 feet with a 20-foot girth. Trees can live for up to 1,000 years. Its flat, fan-shaped leaves have two lobes, hence its Latin species name, *biloba*. Ginkgoes are dioecious—male and female flowers appear on different trees. The females produce apricot-size, orange-yellow fruits that contain edible seeds.

Ginkgoes are attractive street or yard trees that can be grown throughout much of the United States. Obtain saplings through nurseries. However, plant only males. Fruits produced by female trees are messy and foul-smelling.

Plant saplings in well-drained soil and stake them to ensure straight growth. Young trees are oddly proportioned and often look gawky, but over time become stately. Water regularly until trees are 20 feet tall. After that, they are self-sufficient.

Ginkgoes grow up to 2 feet per year. They resist insects and disease. In autumn, the leaves turn a beautiful gold color before falling.

GINSENG

Asia's Most Revered Adaptogen

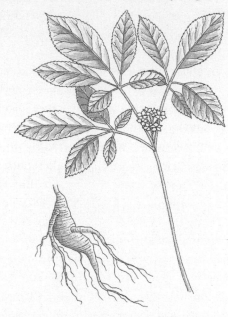

Family: Araliaceae; other members include ivy

Genus and species: *Panax ginseng* (Chinese/Korean/Japanese); *Panax quinquefolius* (American)

Also known as: Man root, life root, root of immortality, Tartar root, heal-all, 'seng, and 'sang

Parts used: Roots

Ginseng is fascinating—and controversial. The root of an unassuming, ivy-like groundcover, this herb has been the subject of more than 1,500 books and scientific papers, yet its effects continue to be debated.

Herbalists call ginseng the ultimate tonic, in Chinese medicine, a strengthener of the entire body. Western scientific supporters call it an "adaptogen," an herb that helps the body resist physical and emotional challenges, combat illness, and stay healthy.

Critics counter that no drug could possibly provide the enormous variety of benefits claimed for ginseng, therefore, advocates exaggerate the herb's value.

But as an increasing number of rigorous scientific studies have confirmed ginseng's many benefits, blanket dismissals of its therapeutic value—and other adaptogens, notably, eleuthero (page 200) and rhodiola (pages 393)—have diminished. Critics continue to take shots at ginseng. Not every study supports it. But the weight of the evidence shows that this herb ranks among the most potent healing herbs.

Healing History

Ginseng is not one herb but two: Chinese, Korean, or Japanese (*Panax ginseng*) and American (*P. quinquefolius*). Chinese physicians draw distinctions between the two plants' effects, but Western scientists generally consider them equivalent.

Ginseng has a fleshy, multibranched root. If you stretch your imagination, some roots resemble the human form, with limb-like branches suggesting arms and legs. The ancient Chinese called the plant "man root," or *jen shen*, which eventually entered English as "ginseng."

Ginseng figured prominently in the first great Chinese herbal, the *Pen Tsao Ching* (*The Classic of Herbs*), purportedly compiled by the mythical emperor-sage Shen Nung around 3000 BC. Shen Nung recommended the herb for "enlightening the mind and increasing wisdom." He noted that "continuous use brings longevity."

Like medieval European physicians, the ancient Chinese embraced the Doctrine of Signatures, the belief that a plant's physical characteristics revealed its healing powers or "signature." Ginseng's fancied resemblance to the human form led to the ancient Chinese belief that it was a whole-body tonic.

For centuries, Chinese physicians have revered ginseng, particularly for the elderly. It was widely used to treat infirmities of old age: lethargy, arthritis, senility, menopausal complaints, and loss of sexual interest and function. The Chinese, Koreans, and Japanese still consider ginseng among the best health promoters, though "root of immortality" is a stretch.

As the popularity of ginseng spread throughout ancient Asia, demand soared and rapacious collection decimated the wild supply. Chinese ginseng became increasingly rare and more valuable than gold. Unscrupulous merchants sold other roots as ginseng. Adulteration remains a problem today.

Unlike other Asian herbs that became favorites in the West (ginger, cinnamon, ephedra), ginseng remained relatively unknown in Europe until the 18th century, when missionaries in China informed early European botanists of its reputation as a longevity promoter. Europeans scoffed at this claim, but those familiar with Asia, particularly the Jesuits who had missions in China, appreciated the herb's great value there.

In 1704, a French explorer returned to Paris from Canada with what turned out to be American ginseng. Jesuits in France alerted their brethren in Canada to its enormous value in China. Jesuits in Montreal shipped a boatload to Canton, where other Jesuits sold it to the Chinese for what was then a king's ransom, $5 a pound.

Immediately, Jesuits in Canada asked their

Native American acolytes to find as much as they could. The Jesuits shipped tons of the herb to China and made a fortune. They also kept the lucrative trade a secret. But eventually, word leaked out that the celibate fathers seemed to take an unusual interest in a certain low-growing herb that was reputed to be an aphrodisiac in far-off Cathay.

Once ginseng's reputation spread, the herb was discovered growing as far south as Georgia. It enjoyed a brief burst of popularity among American colonists interested in sexual stimulation. Most were disappointed. Virginia plantation owner William Byrd sniffed that ginseng "frisks the spirits" but causes none "of those naughty effects that might make men too troublesome and impertinent to their wives."

America's "Ginseng Rush"

By the 1740s, news of the herb's incredible value in China hit the 13 colonies like news of the California gold strike a century later. Shippers offered to buy the herb for the then-fabulous sum of $1 a pound. Foragers scoured the countryside, and frontier scouts, surveyors, and fur trappers collected ginseng as a sideline to their other work. Ginseng quickly became the colonies' most valuable export—more precious pound for pound than even the finest furs.

By the 1770s, ginseng fever had wiped out the plant along the Eastern seaboard, forcing collectors into the trackless wilderness across the Appalachians. The search for ginseng played a significant role in the exploration of western Pennsylvania, West Virginia, Kentucky, and Tennessee. One intrepid pioneer who combined trapping and scouting with ginseng hunting was none other than Daniel Boone. According to Scott Persons' *American Ginseng: Green Gold*,

in 1788, a boat owned by Boone capsized in the Ohio River—and lost 12 tons of ginseng.

Native Americans learned of ginseng from the Jesuits and used it to combat fatigue, stimulate appetite, and aid digestion. Some tribes mixed it into love potions.

America's 19th-century Eclectic physicians, forerunners of today's naturopaths, called ginseng a stimulant for "mental exhaustion from overwork" and prescribed it for loss of appetite, indigestion, asthma, laryngitis, bronchitis, and tuberculosis. The Eclectic textbook *King's American Dispensatory* (1898) added that the herb "invigorates the virile powers."

Contemporary herbalists echo the Chinese, recommending ginseng as a tonic stimulant that promotes vitality, longevity, virility, and resistance to stress and illness. The world ginseng market is estimated at $2 billion a year. Americans growers export ginseng worth $77 million a year. Various experts estimate that Americans, mainly Asian-Americans, currently spend $500 million a year on ginseng products.

Wild American ginseng is officially an endangered species, but in Appalachia, collectors still forage for it. According to a *New York Times* report (2005), wild American ginseng roots sell for $100 apiece or around $300 per pound. Most collectors never use the herb themselves. In the words of Georgia ginseng trader Jake Plott, "I never found it worth a damn for anything but to get money out of." Well, Jake, if you read the research, you'd feel differently.

"Tonic" in the East, "Adaptogen" in the West

Ginseng owes its healing power to several compounds (ginsenosides). Scientists do not fully understand their actions, which can be downright confusing. Some ginsenosides stimulate the central nervous system, others depress it. Some raise blood pressure, others lower it. These observations need to be clarified, but there's no doubt that this herb offers many health benefits.

Among the first Western scientists to seriously investigate ginseng were two Russian pharmacologists, N. V. Lazarev, Ph.D., and his student, Israel I. Brekhman, Ph.D., of the former Soviet Union's Academy of Sciences. In 1947, they coined the term "adaptogen" to describe ginseng and other herbs that help the body resist physical and emotional stresses. They discovered that ginseng increases resistance to disease and offers subtle but significant body-strengthening benefits, while causing few, if any, side effects.

Brekhman and researchers in China, Korea, and Japan conducted hundreds of studies showing that ginseng combats fatigue, improves stamina, repairs damage caused by physical and emotional stress, and prevents the depletion of stress-fighting adrenal hormones. Brekhman came to concur with what traditional Asian herbalists had said for more than 1,000 years—that ginseng is a tonic. Eventually, Western scientists became interested in the herb. Today scientists around the world study ginseng.

(Brekhman eventually focused on another plant, eleuthero (*Eleutherococcus senticosus*), a less expensive adaptogen sometimes called "Siberian ginseng." Eleuthero is *not* a ginseng, but it offers similar benefits. See page 200.)

"Adaptogens give the body a tune-up," says Salt Lake City herb researcher Daniel Mowrey, Ph.D. "They help the cells produce energy and use it more efficiently. But adaptogens don't overpower the cells as drugs often do. Their effects are subtle, which accounts for the contro-versy these herbs arouse. Over time, adaptogenic herbs are very beneficial to health."

Adpatogenic Value

INCREASED ENERGY. Ginseng is a noncaffeine stimulant that helps counteract fatigue. European researchers studied 232 people, age 25 to 60, who complained of fatigue. Half took a daily placebo. The rest tried a vitamin formula containing ginseng (80 milligrams/day). After 7 weeks, the group taking the ginseng formula showed significantly less lethargy. The researchers concluded that ginseng combats fatigue by supporting the adrenal glands.

ENHANCED ATHLETIC PERFORMANCE. For decades, Russian, Chinese, and Korean Olympic athletes have included ginseng in their training. They take the herb before events just as American Olympians load up on coffee (page 165). Some American athletes have also adopted ginseng. Research shows that the herb enhances athletic performance.

Italian researchers gave 50 male physical education teachers, age 21 to 47, either placebos or a vitamin formula containing ginseng, then tested them running on treadmills. Subsequently, the two groups switched treatments. Those who'd taken the placebo switched to the ginseng formula, and vice versa. While using ginseng, the men's hearts and lungs worked more efficiently and their stamina increased.

COGNITIVE FUNCTION. Danish researchers tested 112 healthy middle-aged adults' memory, reaction times, and ability to learn, concentrate, and reason. Then the participants took either a placebo or ginseng (400 milligrams/day). After 9 weeks, the ginseng group showed significant improvement in reaction time and reasoning. In a similar Italian study ginseng significantly improved attention, reaction time, and ability to perform mental arithmetic.

ENHANCED IMMUNITY. In animal studies, Chinese researchers have found that ginseng revs up the white blood cells (macrophages and natural killer cells) that devour disease-causing microorganisms. Researchers at the University of Southern California have shown that ginseng spurs synthesis of immune-boosting antibodies and interferon, the body's own virus fighter.

German researchers demonstrated ginseng's immune-enhancing action in a study involving 36 healthy volunteers who took either a placebo or ginseng (2 teaspoons of tincture three times a day). After 4 weeks, the ginseng group showed significantly more activated T-lymphocytes (T-cells), a type of infection-fighting white blood cell.

Italian researchers gave people with chronic bronchitis either a placebo or ginseng (100 milligrams every 12 hours). After 8 weeks, the researchers took respiratory mucus samples and analyzed them for macrophages, the white blood cells that engulf and devour invading germs. Those taking ginseng developed significantly more active white blood cells that killed more germs.

The same Italian team gave flu (influenza) shots to 227 adults. Then some took a placebo while others received ginseng (100 milligrams/day). Flu shots do not act directly on flu virus. They stimulate an immune response that kills the virus. The researchers reasoned that if ginseng enhances immune function, the herb should boost flu vaccine's effectiveness. That's exactly what they found. After 3 months, the ginseng group was significantly less likely to develop flu. Researchers at Eastern Virginia Medical School in Norfolk confirmed these results by giving flu shots plus either a placebo or ginseng (200 milligrams/day) to 198 nursing home residents, average age 82. After 12 weeks, the ginseng group was 89 percent less likely to develop flu.

Enhanced immune function means greater resistance to illness, speedier recovery, and improved well-being, all of which support the Chinese belief that ginseng is a whole-body tonic. Commission E, the expert panel that evaluates herbal medicines for the German counterpart of the FDA, approves ginseng for invigoration, convalescence, and support of work capacity and concentration.

IMPROVED WELL-BEING. At the Medical School of the National Autonomous University of Mexico, researchers surveyed 500 people about their health, well-being, pain, mood, energy, sex life, sleep quality, and personal satisfaction. Then some were given a daily vitamin supplement, while the rest consumed the same supplement plus ginseng (standardized extract, 80 milligrams/day). Four months later, both groups reported enhanced quality of life, but those taking ginseng showed significantly greater improvement.

Several other similar studies agree that ginseng improves quality of life. Researchers at Hartford Hospital in Connecticut analyzed nine studies of ginseng's effects on quality of life. Their conclusion: "Nearly every study (eight of the nine) demonstrated some degree of quality of life improvement."

Therapeutic Uses

In addition to its tonic-adaptogen benefits, ginseng's immune-enhancing action helps prevent and treat many conditions.

CANCER. Korean researchers surveyed the diets and lifestyles of 4,634 Korean adults over 40, including their use of ginseng. Five years later, some of the group had developed cancer. Compared with those who did not use ginseng, those who took it regularly had 60 percent less risk of all cancers. Another Korean study involving 1,467 participants showed similar results—in the ginseng users, 44 percent less cancer risk. A third Korean study showed the regular ginseng use reduced cancer risk by half.

Meanwhile, a study at the Mayo Clinic in Rochester, Minnesota, shows that ginseng helps treat the fatigue cancer patients typically develop while taking chemotherapy. The researchers gave either a placebo or ginseng (2,000 milligrams/day) to 364 people with breast, lung, or colon cancer. After 8 weeks, those taking ginseng reported significantly less fatigue.

Finally, a study at Vanderbilt University in Nashville shows that in women with breast cancer, ginseng improves survival and quality of life. The researchers tracked 1,455 participants in the Shanghai Breast Cancer Study for 2 years. Compare with those who shunned ginseng, those who used it regularly had 29 percent less risk of death and reported significantly greater quality of life.

COLDS. In the Italian flu-shot study mentioned previously, the ginseng group also gained some protection against colds. Other studies have confirmed this.

- University of Connecticut researchers gave 43 people over 65 either a placebo or ginseng (400 milligrams/day). For the first 2 months (September and October), both groups caught the same number of colds. But during November and December, the ginseng group developed only half as many colds. In addition, colds in the ginseng users cleared up significantly faster.

- Canadian scientists gave 323 adults, age 18 to 65, either a placebo or ginseng (400 milligrams/day). After 4 months, 23 percent of the placebo group developed two or more colds, but in the ginseng group, just 10 percent—and colds in the ginseng group were milder and briefer.

- Korean researchers gave 100 healthy adults, age 30 to 70, either a placebo or Korean red ginseng (boiled root, 1 gram/day). After 12 weeks, 44 percent of the placebo group reported colds, but among those taking ginseng, just 25 percent.

HIGH BLOOD PRESSURE. According to studies at Yale, ginseng increases the body's synthesis of nitric oxide, which opens (dilates) blood vessels. As arteries dilate, blood pressure drops. At Seoul National University College of Medicine, Korean researchers gave 34 middle-aged high-blood-pressure sufferers either a placebo or ginseng (1,500 milligrams three times a day). Eight weeks later, those taking the placebo showed no change in blood pressure, but the ginseng group registered a significant decrease.

Some of this study's participants took ginseng combined with a pharmaceutical blood pressure medication (beta-blocker or calcium channel-blocker). Compared with ginseng alone, the addition of the pharmaceutical produced no greater drop in pressure.

Meanwhile, a few reports show that ginseng *raises* blood pressure. If you have high blood pressure and want to include ginseng in your treatment regimen, work closely with your physician and monitor your pressure regularly. If it rises, stop taking ginseng.

HOT FLASHES. Korean researchers gave 72 menopausal women either a daily placebo or Korean red ginseng. After 12 weeks, the ginseng group reported significantly fewer hot flashes—and lower cholesterol.

Japanese scientists surveyed 20 women about their menopausal discomforts then gave them ginseng (6,000 milligrams/day). A month later, their symptoms had declined significantly.

DIABETES. In a Finnish study, 36 people newly diagnosed with type 2 diabetes took either a placebo or ginseng (100 or 200 milligrams/day). Compared with the placebo group, both ginseng groups showed reduced blood sugar—and improved mood and enhanced performance on physical and cognitive tests. The high-dose group showed the greatest benefit.

EMPHYSEMA. Israeli researchers tested the lung function of 15 emphysema sufferers, average age, 67) and then asked them to walk as far as they could in 6 minutes. Then all participants were instructed to take ginseng (200 milligrams/day). Three months later, the participants' lung function improved significantly, meaning that more oxygen entered their bloodstreams. The distance they could walk in 6 minutes increased 42 percent, from 600 meters to 854 meters.

ERECTILE DYSFUNCTION (ED) AND LOW SEXUAL DESIRE. Ginseng dilates the arteries, including the ones that carry blood into the penis. More blood in the penis means greater likelihood of erection. Korean researchers gave 90 ED sufferers one of three treatments: a placebo, an antidepressant (trazodone), or ginseng. The placebo and antidepressant groups showed 30 percent improvement in erection rigidity and

libido, but the ginseng group experienced 60 percent improvement. This study supports the traditional Chinese belief that ginseng is a mild aphrodisiac.

Other Korean scientists repeated this study, giving a placebo or ginseng (2,700 milligrams/day) to 45 men with ED. After 8 weeks, the men taking ginseng reported significantly firmer erections. "Ginseng," the researchers concluded, "is an effective alternative for treating male erectile dysfunction."

MALE INFERTILITY. University of Rome researchers gave ginseng (4,000 milligrams/day) to 30 men, age 26 to 41, who had very low sperm counts, and to 20 men with normal counts. After 3 months, counts in the infertile men rose 93 percent, from 15 million to 29 million per milliliter. The men with initially normal sperm counts showed a 9 percent increase, from 85 million to 93 million per milliliter.

LONGEVITY. Add up all of ginseng's benefits and a reasonable conclusion would be that it extends life. That's what Korean researchers discovered in a study of 9,378 people over 55 tracked for 19 years. As ginseng use increased, death from all causes decreased—but oddly, only in men. Compared with abstainers, men who took it regularly were 10 percent less likely to die. While ginseng did not reduce all-cause mortality in women, regular use reduced their cancer mortality by 39 percent.

Intriguing Possibilities

APPETITE LOSS. Asians have long considered ginseng particularly helpful for the elderly. As people age, senses of taste and smell deteriorate, reducing appetite. In addition, the intestine's ability to absorb nutrients declines. As a result, some elders suffer malnutrition. Ginseng enjoys a thousand-year-old reputation as an appetite stimulant. One study showed that it increases the ability of the intestine to absorb nutrients, thus helping to prevent malnutrition.

LIVER DAMAGE. Ginseng protects the liver from the harmful effects of drugs, alcohol, and other toxic substances. In one experiment, researchers gave what should have been fatal doses of various narcotics to experimental animals pretreated with ginseng extract. Most of the animals survived. And in a pilot human study, ginseng improved liver function in 24 elderly people with alcohol-induced cirrhosis.

RADIATION THERAPY. Ginseng can minimize cell damage from radiation. In two studies, researchers injected animals with various protective agents, then subjected them to radiation in doses used to treat cancer. Ginseng did the best job of protecting healthy cells, suggesting that the herb may be beneficial during radiation therapy.

Adulteration and Maturity

While many studies attest to ginseng's therapeutic value, critics cite other studies showing no benefit at all. Why such disparate results? Adulteration appears to be a big part of the answer. Because of ginseng's rarity and enormous value, adulteration has been a problem for centuries—and still is. It's quite possible that some researchers have used "ginseng" that in fact contained little or none of the herb.

One study from the 1980s evaluated 54 ginseng products sold in health food stores in the United States. Sixty percent contained too little herb to have any biological effect. Twenty-five percent contained no ginseng at all.

The health food industry denounced the study, and the health food trade journal *Whole Foods* commissioned an independent test. It produced very similar results.

The most notorious of the nonginseng "ginsengs" was wild red American ginseng or wild desert ginseng, which appeared in health food stores from the 1970s through the 1980s. Ginseng is a shade-loving, moisture-demanding plant, which means that desert ginseng is a botanical impossibility. Nonetheless, many consumers fell for the fraud. The phony ginseng was actually red dock, a laxative.

An outcry from responsible herbalists forced wild desert ginseng off the shelves, but problems with adulteration and fraud have persisted. That's why the American Herbal Products Association, a trade group, and the American Botanical Council, the nation' leading nonprofit herb education organization, both periodically analyze ginseng products to help ensure quality, a program rarely undertaken with other herbs.

Meanwhile, even if you start with real ginseng, it may not provide medicinal benefits if it's not mature. Ginseng roots should not be harvested until they are 6 years old, but sometimes, younger roots are mixed in to stretch the amount—a form of adulteration that may render the product useless.

Unfortunately, the only way to be absolutely certain of ginseng's purity and age is to grow it yourself, which is much easier said than done. If you buy ginseng, read labels carefully. Look for products that are identified by species and specify 6-year-old roots.

Rx Recommendations

Ginseng tastes sweetish and is slightly aromatic. To take advantage of its many therapeutic powers, use root powder, teas, tinctures, capsules, or tablets available in health food stores, herb shops, supplement centers, and some drugstores. You can even buy ginseng soft drinks that promise a lift similar to that of caffeinated sodas.

To prepare a tea, use ½ to 1 teaspoon of powdered root per cup of boiling water, simmer for about 15 minutes, and strain if you wish. Drink up to 2 cups a day.

When using a tincture or any other commercial preparation, follow package directions.

Safety

Ginseng is a stimulant. People taking large doses have reported nervousness and restlessness, symptoms similar to those experienced by people who drink too much coffee. Ginseng may also enhance the effects of other stimulants, such as ephedra and caffeine, causing overstimulation.

Other problems with ginseng are rare, but the medical literature contains a few dozen reports of adverse reactions: insomnia, breast soreness, allergy symptoms, asthma attacks, increased blood pressure, and heart rhythm disturbances (cardiac arrhythmias). People with insomnia, fibrocystic breasts, or hay fever should use ginseng with caution. Those with asthma, high blood pressure, cardiac arrhythmia, or fever should use ginseng in consultation with their doctors, if at all.

Some studies show that ginseng has anticoagulant (blood-thinning) action. Many physicians discourage it in people with clotting problems or who take anticoagulant medications, and surgeons ask patients to stop using it 2 weeks before scheduled surgery. However, Korean researchers gave stroke survivors either warfarin, a pharmaceutical anticoagulant or warfarin plus ginseng. They expected the combination to have greater anticoagulant action—but it didn't. The ginseng did not potentiate the warfarin, suggesting no blood-thinning action for the herb. Ginseng may have anticoagulant action, but it remains to be clarified.

Studies at Harvard, and in Korea and Hong Kong show that like soy (page 439), ginseng is weakly estrogenic. This helps prevent breast cancer. But it may cause problems for those advised to avoid exposure to this hormone. Talk to your doctor.

In Asia, ginseng has long been considered an herb for the elderly. Don't give it to children.

While Asian studies have concluded that ginseng does not cause birth defects in the offspring of rats, rabbits, or lambs, pregnant and nursing women should err on the side of caution and not use it.

Ginseng may cause allergic reactions or other unexpected side effects. If any develop, reduce your dose or stop taking it.

A 1979 article in the *Journal of the American Medical Association* documented a condition its authors dubbed "ginseng abuse syndrome," with symptoms including diarrhea. This study was seriously flawed. Real ginseng does not cause diarrhea—but red dock, the laxative plant called wild desert ginseng, does. In other words, the study documenting purported ginseng abuse syndrome *did not use ginseng*. Herb authorities immediately pointed this out, but herb critics cited ginseng abuse syndrome as a reason to shun ginseng well into the 1990s.

If you ever see a reference to ginseng abuse syndrome, ignore it.

Inform health professionals of the herbs you use. Problematic herb-drug interactions are possible. For more on herb safety, see Chapter 2.

If symptoms get worse or persist longer than 2 weeks, consult a health professional promptly.

Gardening

Ginseng is extremely difficult and expensive to grow. Prospective ginseng gardeners should heed the words of one frustrated horticulturist: "God and the growers know what they're doing, but neither one is talking."

During the 20th century, almost all cultivated American ginseng was grown in Wisconsin. It was by far the state's most lucrative crop per acre, valued at almost $100 million a year. Today, competing British Columbian growers have snatched some of the market.

Ginseng requires shade, so growers plant it under frames fitted with nylon mesh. It's a struggle to keep young plants alive. They're prone to several fungal infections. And growers must be patient. Roots shouldn't be harvested until they're 6 years old.

The harvesting process is painstaking. Roots' value in Asia depends in part on the arrangement of the root limbs. The more human-like the root, the higher the price. Breaking off an "arm" or "leg" during harvesting or drying cuts the price.

Root cuttings are often diseased, so most growers start with seeds, which are costly. Before planting, seeds must be disinfected in a solution of one part chlorine bleach and nine parts water.

If you want to try your hand at growing ginseng, plant the seeds in early autumn in well-prepared, humus-rich beds at a depth of $\frac{1}{2}$ inch and 6-inch spacing. Ginseng grows poorly in sandy or clay soils. Maintain soil pH in the range of 5.0 to 6.0.

Seed germination can take up a year. The plants must be shaded, ideally under trees, although the covered frames work, too.

Harvest roots after 6 years, digging carefully to avoid breaking the root limbs. Dry them for 1 month.

GOLDENSEAL

A Potent Antibiotic

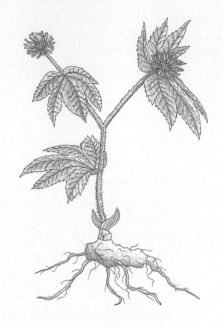

Family: Ranunculaceae; other members include buttercup, larkspur, and peony

Genus and species: *Hydrastis canadensis*

Also known as: Yellow root, yellow puccoon, Indian turmeric, Indian dye, Indian paint, jaundice root, eye balm, eye root, golden root, and poor man's ginseng

Parts used: Rhizomes and roots

Goldenseal is popular and powerful, a combination that virtually guarantees controversy. It should come as no surprise that many contemporary herbalists view goldenseal as one of our most useful herbs, while several scientific authorities continue to quote one pharmacologist's opinion—from 1948—that it has "few, if any, rational indications" and may cause "death from respiratory paralysis or cardiac arrest" (see Safety).

On balance, there's no cause for alarm. Goldenseal is definitely beneficial, but potentially harmful side effects are also possible. Informed home herbalists who use it carefully can take advantage of its many benefits.

Healing History

The Native Americans of the northeastern United States pounded goldenseal's yellow roots (the source of most of its names) and used the yellow juice as a dye. They also used the herb medicinally as an eyewash (hence the names eye balm and eye root), as a treatment for skin wounds, sore throat, and digestive complaints, and for recovery from childbirth. The Cherokees mixed the herb with bear grease to make an insect repellent.

European colonists did not do much with this herb until the early 19th century, when Samuel Thomson, founder of Thomsonian herbal medicine, popularized it as an antiseptic. Thomson disliked the herb's Indian name, yellow root. So he changed it to goldenseal, combining "golden" from its color and "seal" from the circular scars left on the plant's root by each year's stems. Thomson thought the scars resembled the circular wax seals that were used to keep correspondence private in the days before glued envelopes.

By the Civil War, Thomsonian medicine had fallen from fashion, but America's 19th-century Eclectic physicians, forerunners of today's naturopaths, embraced goldenseal. They called it hydrastis, after its Latin name, and greatly expanded its uses. They prescribed it externally to relieve wounds, hemorrhoids, rectal fissures, pinkeye (conjunctivitis), eczema, and boils. They also recommended it internally to treat colds, tonsillitis, diphtheria, uterine problems, postpartum hemorrhage, and digestive ailments and as a tonic during convalescence from any major illness.

After the Civil War, the golden herb enjoyed a golden age. Goldenseal was an ingredient in many patent medicines, notably Dr. Pierce's Golden Medical Discovery, a popular tonic. Demand for the herb soared. Its price jumped to $1 a pound, making it almost as costly as America's most valuable healing herb, ginseng. But while most American ginseng was exported to China, goldenseal remained in the United States. And like ginseng, goldenseal was collected almost to the point of extinction.

Over time, goldenseal acquired some of ginseng's medicinal reputation as a panacea and longevity tonic (hence another of its popular names, poor man's ginseng). The herb was listed as an astringent and antiseptic in the *U.S. Pharmacopoeia*, a standard drug reference, from 1831 to 1936, and in the *National Formulary*, the pharmacists' reference, from 1936 to 1960, when modern antibiotics pushed it aside.

Still, goldenseal has remained a favorite among herbalists. In the late 1940s, Jethro Kloss, author of *Back to Eden*, described the herb as "one of the most wonderful remedies in the entire herb kingdom . . . A real cure-all."

Modern herbalists recommend goldenseal externally to disinfect wounds and treat eczema, ringworm, athlete's foot, itching, and conjunctivitis. They prescribe it internally for digestive upset and colds, as a douche, and to stop excessive menstrual flow and postpartum uterine bleeding—though most also caution that the herb may cause restlessness and trigger uterine contractions.

Goldenseal is a favorite of homeopaths, who prescribe microdoses for alcoholism, asthma, indigestion, cancer, hemorrhoids, and liver ailments.

The herb remains a popular folk medicine as well. In "Hoosier Home Remedies," a 1985 survey of Indiana folk medicine, the late herb expert Varro E. Tyler, Ph.D., reported that goldenseal was used extensively as an astringent and antiseptic to treat canker sores, chapped lips, and many other external problems.

Therapeutic Uses

In the late 1970s, heroin addicts came to believe that goldenseal tea could prevent the detection of opiates in urine specimens. Much to their chagrin, they were mistaken. Goldenseal absolutely does not prevent the detection of opiates or any other drugs. Nor is it a cure-all.

Scientists have determined that goldenseal contains two active constituents: berberine and hydrastine. Berberine, the more important, is also the active compound in barberry. As a result, barberry and goldenseal have similar uses (and similar hazards), though goldenseal is more popular—and more expensive. Those interested in a "poor person's goldenseal" might try barberry.

INFECTIONS. Berberine kills many of the bacteria that cause diarrhea (*Escherichia coli, Salmonella, Shigella, Klebsiella,* and even *Vibrio cholerae,* which causes cholera). In one study, 165 adults with diarrhea resulting from either *E. coli* or cholera were given either a placebo or berberine (400 milligrams). After 24 hours, among those with *E. coli* diarrhea, 20 percent of the placebo group was cured, but in the berberine group, 43 percent. Among those with cholera, berberine also produced significant benefit. These results support goldenseal's long history as a treatment for infectious diarrhea.

Goldenseal has also shown benefit against the bacteria that cause ulcers (*Helicobacter pylori*) and the protozoa that cause amoebic dysentery (*Entamoeba histolytica*) and giardiasis (*Giardia lamblia*). In addition, it kills the protozoan that causes trichomoniasis (*Trichomonas vaginalis*) and the fungus that causes yeast infections *(Candida albicans)*. This lends credence to goldenseal's traditional use as a treatment for fungal infections.

ENHANCED IMMUNITY. In addition to killing germs, some research shows that berberine boosts the immune system by revving up macrophages, the white blood cells that devour disease-causing microorganisms.

HEAVY MENSTRUAL FLOW. In some animal studies, berberine calms the uterus, supporting its traditional use in stopping excessive menstrual flow and postpartum hemorrhage. Other studies, however, show that it stimulates uterine contractions. Women troubled by heavy menstrual flow might try the herb, but women who are pregnant or trying to conceive should avoid it.

Postpartum hemorrhage is a potentially serious condition that requires prompt professional attention. If you'd like to try goldenseal in addition to standard therapy, discuss it with your obstetrician or midwife.

DIGESTIVE PROBLEMS. Goldenseal stimulates bile secretion in humans, which means that it helps digest fats.

Intriguing Possibilities

Some naturopaths claim that goldenseal helps restore digestive and liver function in people with alcoholism.

Cell culture studies have shown that the herb kills tumor cells, lending support to its traditional role as a cancer treatment. Some day, it may complement other cancer treatments.

A Chinese report suggests that berberine lowers cholesterol.

Medical Myth

Because goldenseal treats so many infectious diseases, some herbalists have recommended it for colds and flu. Herbal cold formulas often pair it with echinacea (page 190). However, there is no evidence that goldenseal is effective against cold or flu viruses. In traditional herbal folklore, goldenseal was used almost exclusively as an oral treatment for digestive tract infections or topically for bacterial and fungal infections. Modern research validates these benefits, but goldenseal should not be expected to shorten the duration of colds or flu.

Rx Recommendations

For an infusion, use ½ to 1 teaspoon of powdered root per cup of boiling water, steep for 10 minutes, and strain if you wish. Drink up to 2 cups a day. Goldenseal tastes bitter; you may add honey, sugar, or lemon or mix it with a beverage tea to improve its flavor.

As a homemade tincture, take ½ to 1 teaspoon up to twice a day.

When using a commercial preparation, follow package directions.

Safety

The active compounds in goldenseal have opposite effects on blood pressure: Berberine lowers it, but hydrastine raises it. People with high blood pressure, heart disease, diabetes, glaucoma, kidney disease, or history of stroke should err on the side of caution and not take goldenseal. If you have a home blood pressure monitor, though, you might try it and see how it affects you. If it doesn't raise your blood pressure, feel free to use it in recommended amounts in consultation with your physician.

Because of goldenseal's high cost and scarcity, adulteration has long been a problem. One traditional adulterant is bloodroot (*Sanguinaria canadensis*). When fresh, bloodroot is red, but when dried, it turns yellow like goldenseal and tastes equally bitter. Bloodroot is a powerful laxative. In high doses, it also causes dizziness, gastrointestinal burning, intense thirst, and vomiting. If your "goldenseal" causes purging or any of these symptoms, stop using it. It's probably bloodroot.

Large doses of goldenseal may irritate the skin, mouth, and throat and cause nausea and vomiting. Goldenseal douches may cause vaginal irritation.

The medical literature contains no reports of serious harm from goldenseal, but hydrastine stimulates the central nervous system, and in animals, unusually large doses have caused death from respiratory paralysis and cardiac arrest. Do not use more than recommended amounts.

Pregnant and nursing women should not use goldenseal.

Do not give goldenseal to children under 2. In older children, adjust the recommended dose based on the child's weight. Give a 50-pound child one-third of the dose a 150-pound adult would take.

If you're over 65, start with a low dose, and increase only if necessary.

Inform health professionals of the herbs you use. Problematic herb-drug interactions are possible.

Goldenseal may cause allergic reactions or other unexpected side effects. If any develop, reduce your dose or stop taking it. For more on herb safety, see Chapter 2.

If symptoms get worse or persist longer than 2 weeks, consult a health professional promptly.

Gardening

Wild goldenseal is an endangered species. It grows wild from Vermont to Arkansas, if you can find it. Today, the herb is farmed but still costly, and adulteration continues to be a problem.

Goldenseal is a small, erect perennial with a hairy, purplish, annual stem that rises from a short, knotty rhizome with yellow-brown bark and bright yellow pulp. The herb's lobed leaves resemble raspberry. Its small, greenish white flowers bloom in spring and produce orange-red berries.

Plants may be started from seed, but it takes 5 years for roots to become medicinally mature. Most authorities recommend buying 2-year-old rhizomes from specialty nurseries so you can harvest the roots 3 years later.

Viable rhizomes should have a sweet, licorice aroma. Plant them in early fall at a depth of 1 inch with 8-inch spacing. The soil should be amended with compost, leaf mold, sand, and bone meal. Frequently, top growth will not appear until the second summer.

Goldenseal requires moisture with good drainage and about 70 percent shade. It grows best under tree cover or shade frames.

Harvest rhizomes in late fall, after frost has killed the top growth. Wash the roots and dry them until they become brittle, then powder them and store the powder in airtight containers.

GOTU KOLA

Soothes Skin Problems and More

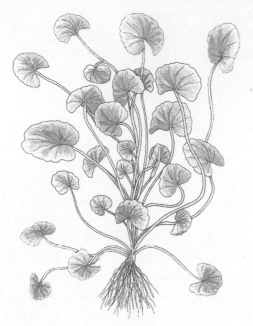

Family: Umbelliferae; other members include carrot, parsley, celery, fennel, dill, and angelica

Genus and species: *Centella asiatica* or *Hydrocotyle asiatica*

Also known as: Sheep rot, Indian pennywort, marsh penny, water pennywort, and hydrocotyle

Part used: Leaves

Long ago, the native Sinhalese of Ceylon (Sri Lanka) noticed that elephants, renowned for their longevity, loved the rounded leaves of the diminutive gotu kola. The herb gained a reputation as a longevity promoter, and a Sinhalese proverb advised, "Two leaves a day keeps old age away."

Don't expect gotu kola to extend your life, but it accelerates wound healing, relieves psoriasis, prevents varicose veins, and may even boost memory.

Healing History

India's Ayurvedic herbalists first used gotu kola the way the Chinese used ginseng—to promote longevity, aid mental acuity, and treat problems associated with aging. But over time, the herb became a popular treatment for skin diseases, including leprosy.

Philippine healers prescribed gotu kola to treat wounds and gonorrhea. Chinese physicians recommended it for fever and colds.

Gotu kola got a bum rap in Europe, where several species grow. Europeans believed that it caused foot rot in sheep (hence the name, sheep rot). No evidence supports this.

Close relatives of gotu kola grow in the United States. America's 19th-century Eclectic physicians, forerunners of today's naturopaths, recognized the herb's Asian use as a treatment for leprosy. Their text, *King's American Dispensatory,* notes, "In 1852, Dr. Boileau of India, having been for many years afflicted with leprosy . . . experimented with [it] and recovered."

The Eclectics considered gotu kola safe and effective when used externally to treat skin problems. But they deemed it a poison when taken internally, asserting that large doses produce "headache, dizziness, stupor, itching, and bloody passages from bowels."

During the early 20th century, gotu kola faded. But after World War II, it surfaced in an herbal tea blend called Fo-Ti-Tieng, touted to boost longevity. The story was that ancient Chinese herbalist Li Ching Yun had sipped the blend regularly and lived for 256 years, surviving 23 wives. The tea caught on, and gotu kola re-emerged from obscurity as an herbal tonic.

Contemporary herbalists recommend gotu kola externally as a poultice for wounds. Internally, they prescribe small doses as a tonic stimulant and large doses as a sedative.

Therapeutic Uses

Longevity claims for gotu kola are as farfetched as the tale of Li Ching Yun. But modern science has found support for other traditional therapeutic powers of this ancient herb.

WOUNDS. One compound in gotu kola, asiaticoside, speeds wound healing. Another, madecassoside, is an anti-inflammatory. A study in *Annals of Plastic Surgery* asserts that gotu kola accelerates the healing of burns and minimizes scarring. Other studies have shown that the herb accelerates the healing of skin grafts and surgical enlargement of the vagina during childbirth (episiotomy).

STRETCH MARKS. Pregnancy-related stretch marks are not wounds, but they bother many women. British researchers gave 100 pregnant women either a placebo cream or one containing gotu kola extract. Those using the gotu kola cream were less than half as likely to develop stretch marks.

PSORIASIS. Validating gotu kola's traditional role as a treatment for skin diseases, one Asian study showed that a cream made with the herb can help relieve the scaly red welts of psoriasis. Seven people with psoriasis were instructed to apply the cream. In five, welts healed within 2 months. Only one of the five experienced any recurrence within 4 months after stopping treatment. The gotu kola cream used in this study is not available commercially. But those with pso-riasis might try compresses of a strong gotu kola infusion.

HIGH BLOOD PRESSURE. In one study, researchers gave either placebos or gotu kola extract to 89 people with high blood pressure. Those taking the herb experienced a significant drop in pressure.

ANXIETY. Canadian researchers gave anxiety sufferers either a placebo or gotu kola (12 grams/day) then subjected them to sudden loud noises. The gotu kola group reacted with significantly less physiological stress.

MEMORY, MOOD. Thai researchers administered cognitive function tests to 28 healthy elderly and then gave them gotu kola daily (250, 500, or 750 milligrams). Two months later, retesting showed significant improvement in memory and mood.

DIABETES. Diabetes impairs circulation through the smallest blood vessels, which over time causes most of the disease's complications. Several British studies have shown that gotu kola improves circulation through these blood vessels. In one, 40 people with diabetes were treated with either a placebo or gotu kola extract (60 milligrams twice a day). After 8 weeks, the herb group had significant better circulation.

VARICOSE VEINS. Gotu kola improves blood flow through the lower limbs, which helps prevent varicose veins. In one study, 94 people with swelling, heaviness, and pain from poor circulation in the legs (venous insufficiency) took either a daily medically inactive placebo or gotu kola (60 milligrams). After 2 months, the herb group showed significantly improved circulation and less swelling. The researchers concluded that the herb strengthened veins.

LEPROSY. Gotu kola's traditional use in treating leprosy (now called Hansen's disease) was supported by a study in the British journal *Nature*. The bacteria that cause leprosy have a waxy coating that protects them from the immune system. The asiaticoside in gotu kola dissolves the waxy coating, allowing the immune system to destroy the bacteria.

Intriguing Possibilities

There may be something to the Ayurvedic belief that gotu kola improves memory. Animal studies show improvement in learning and memory. And an Indian pilot study found that treatment with the herb improves the intellectual performance of mentally challenged children.

An Indian cell-culture study shows that gotu kola extract destroys cancer cells without harming other cells. In the future, gotu kola may be included in cancer treatment regimens.

Rx Recommendations

To prepare an infusion, steep ½ teaspoon of the herb in a cup of boiling water for 10 to 20 minutes, then strain. Drink up to 2 cups a day. Gotu kola tastes bitter and astringent. Add sugar, honey, and/or lemon or mix it into an herbal beverage blend.

To help treat wounds or psoriasis topically, apply compresses made from a gotu kola infusion. If the results are disappointing, try a stronger infusion.

When using commercial preparations, follow package directions.

Safety

The only confirmed side effect of gotu kola is skin rash in people who are sensitive.

In laboratory animals, gotu kola acts as a sedative. Large doses are narcotic, causing stupor and possibly coma. Sedation has never been reported in humans, but some scientists claim that it's possible.

Ironically, reports have appeared claiming that gotu kola causes restlessness and insomnia, odd for a purported sedative. Apparently, these cases involved mislabeling of another herb, kola, which contains caffeine.

Pregnant women may use gotu kola topically to prevent stretch marks. But pregnant and nursing women should not ingest it.

Do not give gotu kola to children under 2. In older children, adjust the recommended dose based on the child's weight. Give a 50-pound child one-third of the dose a 150-pound adult would take.

If you're over 65, start with a low dose, and increase only if necessary.

Inform health professionals of the herbs you use. Problematic herb-drug interactions are possible.

Gotu kola may cause allergic reactions or other unexpected side effects. If any develop, reduce your dose or stop taking it. For more on herb safety, see Chapter 2.

If symptoms get worse or persist longer than 2 weeks, consult a health professional promptly.

Gardening

Gotu kola is not related to true kola (*Cola nitida*), the caffeine-containing nut used in cola drinks. Nor is it cultivated in North America, although several related species grow wild.

As a member of the Umbelliferae family, gotu kola is related to carrot, dill, and fennel, but it has neither the characteristic feathery leaves nor the umbrella arrangement (umbel) of tiny flowers. Instead, gotu kola's creeping stem grows in marshy areas and produces fan-shaped leaves about the size of an old British penny (hence its names Indian pennywort, marsh penny, and water pennywort). A cuplike clutch of inconspicuous flowers develops near the ground. Leaves may be harvested year-round.

HAWTHORN
Mayflower for Heart Disease

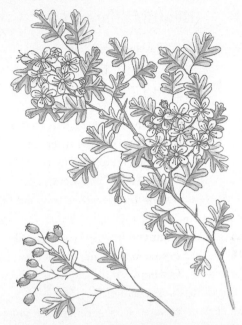

Family: Rosaceae; other members include rose, peach, almond, apple, and strawberry

Genus and species: *Crataegus oxycantha*

Also known as: Hawthorne, haw, may, mayblossom, and mayflower

Parts used: Flowers, leaves, and fruits

American schoolchildren learn that the Pilgrims' ship was the Mayflower. But few Americans know that the name refers to hawthorn, which, in England, flowers in May. Even fewer know that the herb is remarkably beneficial to the heart.

Today, European physicians often prescribe hawthorn to treat congestive heart failure, serious heart-muscle fatigue that causes shortness of breath after mild exertion, and fluid buildup around the body, notably in the ankles and lungs. Now hawthorn is starting to catch on in this country as well.

Healing History

Archeologists have discovered hawthorn seeds at Neolithic sites, suggesting that our ancestors ate the fruits.

To the ancient Greeks and Romans, hawthorn was rich in symbolism, linked to hope, marriage, and fertility. Greek brides carried hawthorn boughs and bridesmaids wore fragrant hawthorn blossoms. The Romans placed hawthorn leaves in babies' cradles to ward off evil spirits.

Christianity changed hawthorn's image dramatically. Christ's crown of thorns was reputedly hawthorn, and as a result, the herb became a symbol of bad luck and death.

The flowers of some European species smell foul, which bolstered the plant's association with death. These trees are pollinated by carrion-eating insects, and to attract them, their flowers emit the odor of rotting meat. During periods of bubonic plague, so many died so quickly that many bodies rotted—and smelled a bit like hawthorn. As a result, the herb was associated with plague and shunned.

As time passed, hawthorn shed its bad reputation and was embraced as a medicinal herb. Seventeenth-century English herbalist Nicholas Culpeper praised it as "a singular remedy for the stone [kidney stones], and no less effectual for dropsy [congestive heart failure]."

Despite Culpeper's influential endorsement, hawthorn was not widely recommended to treat heart problems until the close of the 19th century. An Irish doctor popularized it to treat congestive heart failure. In 1896, an article touting the Irish physician's work appeared in a medical journal for Eclectic physicians, forerunners of today's naturopaths. The Eclectics began prescribing the herb for congestive heart failure and the chest pain of angina.

Modern herbals echo these recommendations. Most would agree with David Hoffmann's *Holistic Herbal*: "Hawthorn [is] one of the best tonics for the heart . . . .It may be used safely in long-term treatment for heart weakness or failure . . . palpitations . . . angina pectoris . . . and high blood pressure."

Therapeutic Uses

Many studies support the traditional use of hawthorn as a heart stimulant.

CONGESTIVE HEART FAILURE. Hawthorn supports the heart in several ways. It opens (dilates) the coronary arteries, improving the heart's blood supply and allowing it to pump blood more efficiently, which is what people with congestive heart failure need. Here's a sampling of the research:

❧ German researchers gave heart function tests to 3,664 people with congestive heart failure. Then everyone took hawthorn (300 milligrams standardized to contain 2.2 percent flavonoids, three times a day). After 2 months, their heart function improved significantly, about as much as would be expected from standard pharmaceuticals. In addition, the proportion of participants experiencing heart palpitations dropped from 40 percent to 18 percent. Leg swelling declined 37 percent. And work capacity, measured as the ability to expend effort by riding a stationary cycle, increased 15 percent.

✤ Another German team gave 136 congestive heart failure sufferers either medically inactive placebos or hawthorn (80 milligrams twice a day). After 8 weeks, the placebo group's heart function had deteriorated somewhat, but those taking hawthorn showed significant improvement.

✤ A third German trial involved 78 people with congestive heart failure. The researchers documented their work capacity using a stationary cycle, then gave them either a placebo or hawthorn (600 milligrams/day). After 2 months, the placebo group's work capacity improved slightly. But among those in the hawthorn group, it increased almost *six times* as much.

Hawthorn caused no significant side effects in any of these studies.

British researchers analyzed 14 trials of hawthorn for congestive heart failure. In addition to standard medications, the 1,110 participants took 160 to 1,800 milligrams/day for 3 to 16 weeks. The researchers concluded that hawthorn offers "significant benefit" in heart failure.

Commission E, the expert panel that evaluates herbal medicines for the German counterpart of the FDA, approves hawthorn as a treatment for congestive heart failure. German doctors prescribe several hawthorn-based heart medicines. Noted German medical herbalist Rudolph Fritz Weiss, M.D., says the herb "has become one of [our] most widely used heart remedies." German physicians rely on hawthorn to normalize heart rhythm, reduce the likelihood and severity of angina attacks, and prevent cardiac complications in elderly patients with influenza and pneumonia.

However, Dr. Weiss cautions that hawthorn is not a quick fix. "One cannot expect rapid improvement in cardiac function," he writes. "[Hawthorn] has a long-term, sustained effect."

Although hawthorn is considered safe and may be effective in the treatment of congestive heart failure, angina, and cardiac arrhythmias, these are serious, potentially life-threatening conditions that require professional care. Consult your physician if you'd like to use hawthorn as part of your treatment regimen.

BLOOD PRESSURE. Part of the reason hawthorn treats congestive heart failure is that it lowers blood pressure, which relieves strain on the heart. Iranian researchers gave either a placebo or hawthorn to 92 men and women with high blood pressure. After 4 months, the herb group's blood pressure was significantly lower. A British study confirms this finding.

CHOLESTEROL AND HEART RHYTHM. Some evidence also shows that hawthorn helps reduce cholesterol and corrects some types of heart rhythm disturbances (arrhythmias).

Intriguing Possibility

A French pilot study suggests that hawthorn may help treat anxiety.

Rx Recommendations

If you use a homemade tincture, German physicians recommend taking 1 teaspoon upon waking and one at bedtime for up to several weeks. To mask the bitter taste, add sugar, honey, and/or lemon or mix with an herbal beverage blend.

To prepare an infusion, herbalists recommend using 2 teaspoons of crushed leaves or fruits per cup of boiling water. Steep for 20 minutes. Drink up to 2 cups a day.

When using commercial preparations, follow package directions.

Safety

In the 14-study analysis discussed above, one-third of trials reported no side effects. Two-thirds reported some dizziness, vertigo, and upset stomach.

Large amounts of hawthorn may cause sedation and/or a significant drop in blood pressure, possibly causing faintness.

Pregnant and nursing women should not use hawthorn.

Do not give hawthorn to children.

If you're over 65, start with a low dose, and increase only if necessary.

Inform health professionals of the herbs you use. Problematic herb-drug interactions are possible.

Hawthorn may cause allergic reactions or other unexpected side effects. If any develop, reduce your dose or stop taking it. For more on herb safety, see Chapter 2.

If symptoms get worse or persist longer than 2 weeks, consult a health professional promptly.

Gardening

Hawthorn is a small deciduous tree with white bark, extremely hard wood, sharp thorns, clusters of white, aromatic flowers, and brilliant red fruits that look like small apples. It blooms from April to June, depending on latitude. In England, blossoms appear in May (hence the names, may, mayblossom, and mayflower).

With some 900 North American species, hawthorn is well adapted to many environments, from urban areas to windswept wilderness hillsides. The tree tolerates a variety of soils but prefers somewhat alkaline, rich, moist loam. Some species prefer full sun, others grow well in partial shade. Consult a nursery for the species best suited to your area.

HIBISCUS

This Beautiful Tropical Flower Lowers Blood Pressure

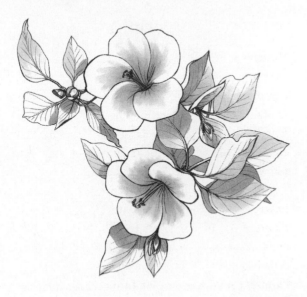

Family: Malvaceae; other members include cotton and mallow

Genus and species: *Hibiscus sabdariffa*

Also known as: Red tea, sour tea, red sorrel, Jamaica sorrel, roselle

Part used: flower

Have you ever enjoyed a cup of Red Zinger tea? Its red color comes from hibiscus flowers (hence the "red" in some of its common names). But don't confuse hibiscus with African red bush tea, often called rooibos, which is a different plant. Native to Africa, hibiscus now grows around the world.

Hibiscus is remarkably useful. For centuries, its leaves have been eaten like spinach. Its fibrous stems can be used to make rope. And its fragrant flowers have been used in perfumes and teas. But hibiscus was a minor medicinal herb until the 21st century, when studies showed that it reduces blood pressure.

Healing History

In tropical Africa, hibiscus leaves were used topically as a skin soother for bites, stings, and wounds, and internally as a laxative. In Egypt, hibiscus is a popular folk treatment for heart disease. In Iran, traditional herbalists prescribed it to treat high blood pressure. Iranian researchers wondered about this. In 1999, they published the first study showing that hibiscus lowers blood pressure.

Therapeutic Uses

BLOOD PRESSURE. In the original Iranian study, the researchers measured the blood pressure of 54 adults with high blood pressure, and then had them drink either black tea or hibiscus tea daily. After 15 days, the hibiscus group showed significantly lower blood pressure. Since then, several other studies around the world have confirmed this effect. In the most recent report, Mexican scientists gave 193 people with high blood pressure either a standard medication (Zestril) or hibiscus. After 4 weeks, the drug was more effective, but the herb reduced blood pressure significantly.

Intriguing Possibilities

An Indian animal study suggests that hibiscus has immune-stimulating action.

Rx Recommendations

Use 1 to 3 teaspoons of chopped or powdered flowers per cup of boiling water. Steep for 2 to 5 minutes.

Safety

No significant side effects. Safe for children and pregnant and nursing women.

Hibiscus may cause allergic reactions or other unexpected side effects. If any develop, reduce your dose or stop taking it.

Gardening

Hibiscus grows outdoors in the southern United States and Hawaii. It's an annual that grows to 5 feet in full sun. It tolerates many soils, but thrives in sandy, slight acidic loam. Add compost. Water frequently until the plant is established. Mulching helps. Propagate using seed or cuttings. In colder areas, this herb can be grown indoors in containers. Drainage is crucial for potted plants. For best results, soil should be 80 percent potting mix and 20 percent sand, then add some compost. Water frequently.

HOP

Not Just for Beer

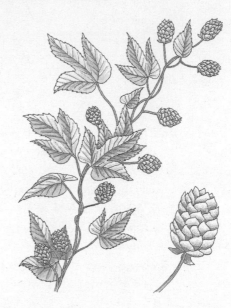

Family: Cannabaceae; other members include hemp and marijuana

Genus and species: *Humulus lupulus*

Also known as: Humulus

Parts used: Strobiles (glandular hairs of female fruits)

"Hop" comes from the Anglo-Saxon term *hoppan*, meaning "to climb," a reference to the vine's growth. Hop, also known as hops, is the bitter, aromatic ingredient in beer. Today, 98 percent of the world's hop harvest is used in beer brewing. But hop also has a long history in herbal healing, and some of its traditional uses have been supported by modern science.

Healing History

Chinese physicians have prescribed hop for centuries to aid digestion and to treat dysentery, tuberculosis, and leprosy, now called Hansen's disease.

Ancient Greek and Roman physicians also recommended the herb as a digestive aid and treatment for intestinal ailments. The Roman naturalist Pliny touted it as a vegetable. He recommended eating young shoots in spring before they matured and grew tough and bitter. (Prepare young shoots like asparagus.)

Hop was a minor herb until about 1,000 years ago, when brewers began using it to preserve the fermented barley beverage we know as beer.

Beer was an accidental offshoot of bread baking. As agriculture developed, late-prehistoric homemakers noticed that bread made from raw grain did not keep as well as bread made from sprouted grain. So before pounding their grain into flour, they soaked it in water to sprout it. If the water happened to become contaminated with yeast from fruit skins, it fermented into a crude, sweet beer, very different from today's brews.

Ancient beers were amazingly popular. Around 2500 BC, an estimated 40 percent of the Sumerian grain crop was used in brewing. And the world's first written legal code, Babylonia's Code of Hammurabi (1750 BC), described punishments for ale houses that sold overpriced or diluted beer.

As the centuries passed, brewers used several herbs—marjoram, yarrow, wormwood—for flavoring. Around the 9th century, the Germans began adding hop, both for its pleasantly bitter flavor and because it preserved the brew, extending shelf life in an age before refrigeration. By the 14th century, most European beers contained hop.

England's Brew Battle

The hop vine grew wild in England, where folk herbalists recommended it as a appetite-stimulating digestive bitter.

England's fermented beverage of choice was ale, a sweet beer that contained other herbs, but not hop. Around 1500, British brewers began making European-style, hop-flavored bitter beer. Brewers and innkeepers loved it. Hop's preservative action extended beer's shelf life. But among British beer drinkers, the addition of hop provoked outrage.

Legions of hop haters petitioned Parliament to ban the herb from beer. Henry VIII, an ale traditionalist, agreed, calling hop "a wicked weed that endangers the people." Hop remained illegal in English beer until Henry's son, Edward VI, rescinded the ban (1552).

But the furor refused to die. A century later, English writer John Evelyn declared, "Hop transmuted our wholesome ale into beer. This one ingredient preserves the drink indeed, but repays the pleasure in tormenting diseases and a shorter life."

Beer brewing transformed hop from a spring vegetable into a cash crop, but hop farmers noticed that it had two odd effects on harvesters. They fatigued easily, and the women got their menstrual periods early. Over time, the herb gained a reputation as a sedative and menstruation promoter.

Hop has been used ever since as a sedative, not only in tea but also sewn into pillows. The herb's warm fragrance was said to induce sleep.

Seventeenth-century English herbalist Nicholas Culpeper recommended hop "in opening obstructions of the liver and spleen . . . cleansing the blood . . . helping cure the French disease [syphilis], and bringing down women's courses [menstruation]." Culpeper also added his two pence to the lingering beer-ale controversy, writing that hop's medicinal uses made beer "better than ale."

More Than a Sedative

Meanwhile, in North America, Native Americans were using American hop as a sedative and digestive aid. America's 19th-century Eclectics, forerunners of today's naturopaths, deemed hop a digestive aid and a treatment for the "morbid excitement of delerium tremens." But they were unimpressed with its reputation as a sedative, warning that it "often failed."

Still, hop was listed as a sedative in the *U.S. Pharmacopoeia*, a standard drug reference, from 1831 to 1916. Throughout the 19th century, it was a popular ingredient in many patent medicines, including Hop Bitters, a popular digestive tonic (containing 30 percent alcohol). Its advertising slogan typified patent-medicine claims in the era before the FDA: "Hop Bitters three times a day, and no doctor bills to pay."

Hop is botanically related to marijuana. During the 1950s, pot-smoking jazz musicians were called "hopheads," and cannabis was said to make users "hopped up." But smoking hop does not produce intoxication.

Contemporary herbalists recommend hop primarily as a sedative, tranquilizer, and digestive aid.

Therapeutic Uses

Those old brewers were right about hop preserving beer. It contains two compound, humulone and lupulone, that kill food- and beer-spoiling bacteria.

INFECTIONS. The bacteria fighters in hop may help prevent infection in humans. Hop is not a major herbal antibiotic, but if you cut yourself near a hop vine, grab some leaves, crush them, and press them into the wound until you can wash it with soap and water. One laboratory study has shown hop to be effective against the bacteria that cause tuberculosis, lending some credence to one of the herb's traditional Chinese uses.

INSOMNIA AND ANXIETY. Scientists were skeptical of hop's age-old reputation as a sedative—until 1983, when they discovered a sedative compound in the plant (2-methyl-3-butene-2-ol). Fresh leaves contain only trace amounts, but as the herb dries and ages, concentration increases. If you want to try hop as a sedative, stick with the dried, aged herb. Herbal sleep aids often combine hop with valerian (page 473). German researchers gave 42 middle-aged insomniacs either a placebo or tincture of hop (460 milligrams valerian and 460 milligrams of hop in alcohol). The valerian/hop formula produced significantly deeper, longer sleep.

Commission E, the expert panel that evaluates herbal medicines for the German counterpart of the FDA, approves hop for treatment of anxiety and sleep disturbances.

MENOPAUSAL DISCOMFORTS. German researchers have identified a compound in hop similar to the female sex hormone estrogen (8-prenylnaringenin), which may explain women hop harvesters' menstrual changes. Estrogen relieves hot flashes and so does hop. Finnish researchers gave 36 menopausal women either a placebo or hop (standardized to 100 micrograms of its estrogenic constituent) daily. After 8 weeks, the groups switched treatments. While taking hop, the women reported significantly fewer hot flashes and other menopausal complaints.

DIGESTIVE PROBLEMS. French researchers have shown that hop relaxes the smooth muscle lining the digestive tract, supporting the herb's traditional use as an antispasmodic digestive herb.

Rx Recommendations

For infection prevention and digestive support, use the freshest hop you can find. For insomnia, use hop that has been dried and aged.

For an infusion, use 2 teaspoons of herb per cup of boiling water and steep for 5 minutes. Drink up to 3 cups a day. Hop tastes warm and pleasantly bitter.

When using commercial preparations, follow package directions.

Safety

Some hop pickers develop a rash, hop dermatitis. Otherwise, there are no reports of the herb causing harm.

Women who are pregnant or who have estrogen-dependent breast cancer should not use it. There is no evidence that these women should abstain from beer, but prudence dictates caution.

Do not give hop to children under 2. In older children, adjust the recommended dose based on the child's weight. Give a 50-pound child one-third of the dose a 150-pound adult would take.

If you're over 65, start with a low dose, and increase only if necessary.

Inform health professionals of the herbs you use. Problematic herb-drug interactions are possible.

Hop may cause allergic reactions or other unexpected side effects. If any develop, reduce your dose or stop taking it. For more on herb safety, see Chapter 2.

If symptoms get worse or persist longer than 2 weeks, consult a health professional promptly.

Gardening

Hop is a resinous, hairy, climbing perennial vine that resembles grape. Grown commercially in Bavaria, Germany, and in the Pacific Northwest in pole-studded fields, hop yards, mature vines reach 25 feet.

Hop can be raised from seed, but most growers use root cuttings taken in spring or fall. Plant the cuttings in hills, three roots per hill, with hills 18 inches apart.

Hop needs deeply cultivated, rich, moist soil, full sun, and frequent watering.

Harvest female flowers in fall when they feel firm, turn amber-colored, and are covered with yellow dust. Dry them immediately in an oven no hotter than 150°F.

HOREHOUND
For Coughs, Colds, and Flu

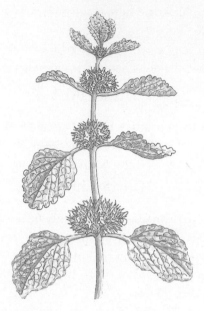

Family: Labiatae; other members include mints

Genus and species: *Marrubium vulgare*

Also known as: Hoarhound, white horehound, and marrubium

Parts used: Leaves and flowers

For 2,000 years, horehound was a popular herbal expectorant and cough remedy. Even skeptics of herbal medicine acknowledged its safety and effectiveness. Then, in 1989, out of the blue, the FDA banned it from over-the-counter cough remedies, claiming that it was ineffective. Worse, over the objections of many scientists, the FDA decreed another expectorant, guaifenesin, effective. Herbalists rolled their eyes.

Healing History

Horehound was first used medicinally in ancient Rome as an ingredient in the multi-ingredient (and ineffective) poison antidotes known as theriaca. Medieval Europeans extended this to believing that the herb protected against witchcraft.

The Roman physician Galen was the first to prescribe horehound for coughs and respiratory problems. It's been used as an expectorant ever since. The ancients also relied on it to soothe upset stomachs.

The medieval German abbess/herbalist Hildegard of Bingen considered horehound among the best herbs for colds. And England's John Gerard wrote, "Syrup made of the greene fresh leaves and sugar is a most singular remedie against cough and wheezings of the lungs."

Seventeenth-century English herbalist Nicholas Culpeper wrote that in addition to curing "those that have taken poison . . . a decoction of the dried herb taken with honey is a remedy for those that are short-winded, have a cough, or are fallen into consumption . . . .It helpeth to expectorate tough phlegm from the chest."

Colonists introduced horehound into North America, where it was a popular cough, cold, and tuberculosis remedy. Folk herbalists also considered it to be a digestive aid, laxative, and treatment for hepatitis, malaria, intestinal worms, and menstrual problems.

America's 19th-century Eclectic physicians, forerunners of today's naturopaths, prescribed horehound for coughs, colds, asthma, intestinal worms, and menstrual complaints.

Most contemporary American herbalists recommend horehound only for cough, colds, and bronchitis. European herbalists also consider it a digestive aid.

Therapeutic Uses

The FDA order to remove horehound from cough and cold remedies says more about the watchdog agency's shortcomings than it does about the herb's.

COUGHS. Horehound contains a compound (marrubiin) that Russian and German researchers have found to loosen phlegm (expectorant). In Europe, the herb has been used for decades in a large number of cough syrups and lozenges. It has been widely used in the United States as well. Even the late herb conservative Varro Tyler, Ph.D., author of *Tyler's Honest Herbal*, describes horehound as an effective expectorant.

The FDA's horehound ban followed the recommendation of an agency advisory panel, which decreed that only one expectorant, guaifenesin, is safe and effective. Ironically, many pulmonologists question guaifenesin's effectiveness.

The FDA order applies only to horehound preparations marketed as cough remedies. The herb is still available in bulk and in some sore throat products and herbal cough and cold supplements.

DIGESTIVE PROBLEMS. Commission E, the expert panel that evaluates herbal medicines for the German counterpart of the FDA, approves horehound for the treatment of indigestion, bloating, and flatulence.

Intriguing Possibilities

European animal studies show that horehound opens (dilates) blood vessels, which lowers blood pressure. It might help treat high blood pressure.

Other animal studies show that in small amounts, horehound helps normalize irregular heart rhythm (arrhythmia), but in large amounts, the herb may cause them.

Rx Recommendations

For an infusion, use ½ to 1 teaspoon of dried leaves per cup of boiling water. Steep for 10 minutes, then strain. Drink up to 3 cups a day. To offset horehound's bitter taste, add sugar or honey.

As a homemade tincture, take ¼ to ½ teaspoon up to three times a day.

When using commercial preparations, follow package directions.

Safety

No significant adverse reactions. But in light of animal studies suggesting that large doses may cause cardiac arrhythmias, people with this condition should avoid it.

Horehound's traditional use as a menstruation promoter has not been confirmed scientifically. Still, pregnant women should exercise caution and not take it. Nursing women should also avoid horehound.

Do not give horehound to children under 2. In older children, adjust the recommended dose based on the child's weight. Give a 50-pound child one-third of the dose a 150-pound adult would take.

If you're over 65, start with a low dose, and increase only if necessary.

Inform health professionals of the herbs you

use. Problematic herb-drug interactions are possible.

Horehound may cause allergic reactions or other unexpected side effects. If any develop, reduce your dose or stop taking it. For more on herb safety, see Chapter 2.

If symptoms get worse or persist longer than 2 weeks, consult a health professional promptly.

Gardening

Horehound is a spreading, pleasantly aromatic perennial with square annual stems that reach 18 inches. The leaves are rounded, wrinkled, and deeply veined. Tiny white flowers develop at the stem-leaf stalk junctions. The entire plant is covered with soft hairs, giving it a woolly appearance and a grayish white cast.

A self-seeder that tolerates poor soil, horehound grows so easily that it may become a pest. It thrives in full sun but tolerates partial shade.

Plant seeds just under the surface in either spring or fall. Thin seedlings to 9-inch spacing. Horehound does not bloom until its second year, but you can harvest the leaves and top growth after one growing season.

In the soil, the herb exudes a musky odor that some people dislike. As the plant dries, the odor disappears.

HORSE CHESTNUT
Victory Over Varicose Veins

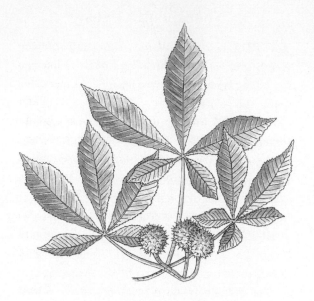

Family: Hippocastanaceae; other members include Ohio buckeye

Genus and species: *Aesculus hippocastanum*

Also known as: Chestnut and buckeye

Parts used: Seeds

The ancients thought this tree's large seeds (nuts) resembled horse eyes, hence the name. Horse chestnut seeds also resemble the eyes of stags, hence the common name buckeye.

Healing History

Since ancient times, horse chestnut wood has been used in construction and furniture-making. Bark extracts produce a yellow dye long used in weaving. Ancient herbalists also applied seed preparations topically to treat arthritis.

In 1615, a French traveler returned from Constantinople (now Istanbul) with horse chestnut seeds he planted in Paris. Within 100 years, the tree had spread throughout Europe.

When ingested, all parts are poisonous—especially the seeds. Fortunately, seeds can be detoxified. Native Americans buried them for months. The soil absorbed the poisons. Then tribes unearthed the detoxified seeds, boiled them, and ate them as food. Some tribes combined crushed seeds with bear fat and applied the mixture to treat hemorrhoids, a type of varicose veins.

California Native Americans crushed the fresh seeds and scattered them in lakes and streams to stupefy fish, making them easier to catch.

In 1896, a French researcher reported that horse chestnut seed extract helped relieve hemorrhoids. America's 19th-century Eclectic physicians, forerunners of today's naturopaths, embraced this. The Eclectic textbook *King's American Dispensatory* (1898) noted that horse chestnut helps treat "vascular fullness and capillary engorgement," in other words, varicose veins.

The Eclectics also used horse chestnut topically to relieve joint pain, and they detoxified the seed extract for internal use to treat fevers, including malaria.

Contemporary herbalists recommend horse chestnut seed almost exclusively for varicose veins and hemorrhoids.

Therapeutic Uses

Horse chestnut seed contains aescin, a compound that strengthens the walls of veins and promotes elasticity. This helps prevent the pooling of blood in weakened veins that causes varicosities and hemorrhoids.

VARICOSE VEINS. Leaky veins (venous insufficiency) are an early sign of varicose veins. German researchers gave 22 people with venous insufficiency, either a medically inactive placebo or horse chestnut (600 milligrams of extract containing 50 milligrams of aescin). Three hours later, the placebo showed just as much fluid leakage but in those who had taken horse chestnut, leakage decreased 22 percent, demonstrating that the herb had strengthened their veins.

Another German research team gave 240 people with venous insufficiency one of three treatments: a placebo, compression therapy (support stockings, a standard treatment), or horse chestnut seed extract (50 milligrams of aescin twice a day). After 3 months, leg swelling increased among those taking the placebo, but it decreased 25 percent in both the people wearing support stockings and those taking horse chestnut. The researchers concluded that compression therapy and herbal therapy produced equivalent benefits.

British researchers analyzed 13 studies of horse chestnut for venous insufficiency. Their conclusion: It works. For varicose veins, they called horse chestnut seed extract is "an option worth considering."

Commission E, the expert panel that evaluates herbal medicines for the German counterpart of the FDA, endorses horse chestnut extract as a treatment for varicose veins.

HEMORRHOIDS. Horse chestnut research has focused on varicose veins in the legs, but initially, herbalists used the herb to strengthen weak veins around the anus, hemorrhoids. Horse chestnut seed extract should help heal varicosities in the anal area.

HEARING PROBLEMS. Poor blood circulation in the inner ear is associated with hearing loss and ringing (tinnitus). German researchers gave either a standard medication (pentoxyfyllin) or a treatment that included horse chestnut (125 milligrams aescin/day) to 68 people with hearing difficulties. After 44 days, those taking the horse chestnut preparation experienced significantly greater hearing restoration.

ARTHRITIS. Horse chestnut seed has anti-inflammatory action, lending credence to its traditional use as a treatment for joint pain.

Rx Recommendations

In the varicose vein studies, the typical dose has been 50 milligrams of aescin two or three times a day.

Safety

Warning: All parts of horse chestnut trees are poisonous unless detoxified. Poisoning from the fresh, unprocessed plant causes muscle weakness and spasms, loss of coordination, pupil dilation, vomiting, diarrhea, and paralysis. Adults have become quite ill from drinking tea made from fresh leaves and twigs. Children have died. Never ingest any part of this tree. Use only commercial medicinal preparations. They're detoxified. Follow label directions.

Pregnant women should not ingest aescin. If you develop varicose veins during pregnancy, try compression stockings and a topical cream made with horse chestnut seed extract. Nursing women should also avoid horse chestnut.

Do not give horse chestnut to children under 2. In older children, adjust the recommended dose based on the child's weight. Give a 50-pound child one-third of the dose a 150-pound adult would take.

If you're over 65, start with a low dose, and increase only if necessary.

Inform health professionals of the herbs you use. Problematic herb-drug interactions are possible.

Horse chestnut may cause allergic reactions or other unexpected side effects. If any develop, reduce your dose or stop taking it. For more on herb safety, see Chapter 2.

If symptoms get worse or persist longer than 2 weeks, consult a health professional promptly.

Gardening

Native to the Balkans and the Middle East, majestic horse chestnut trees now grow worldwide. Trees grow to 75 feet, producing large leaves and attractive pink and white flowers in spring or summer, depending on latitude. The fruit has a thick, leathery husk that contains up to six nuts.

HORSETAIL

An Herbal Gold Mine

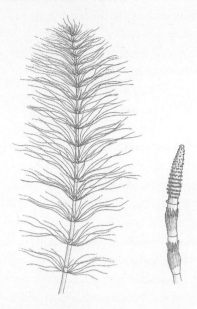

Family: Equisetaceae; the family is extinct except for horsetail

Genus and species: *Equisetum arvense*

Also known as: Equisetum, scouring rush, pewterwort, shave grass, corncob plant, and bottlebrush

Parts used: Stems

All that's gold does not necessarily glitter. Take horsetail. The bamboo-like marsh dweller absorbs gold dissolved in water. Doctors once prescribed preparations containing gold for rheumatoid arthritis—and horsetail has a long history as a remedy for joint pain.

Healing History

Centuries before anyone realized that horsetail contains gold, the ancients discovered its value as an abrasive cleanser. Over time, the herb was used to scour pots, polish pewter, and sand or "shave" wood—hence its popular names scouring rush, shave grass, and pewterwort (wort is Old English for "plant").

During ancient famines, Romans ate horsetail shoots, which look like asparagus but are neither as tasty nor as nutritious. (Backpacking guides still commend the tough, stringy shoots to wilderness foragers.) The Roman physician Galen claimed that horsetail healed severed tendons and ligaments and stopped nosebleeds.

Ancient Chinese physicians recommended horsetail as a treatment for wounds, hemorrhoids, arthritis, and dysentery.

Seventeenth-century English herbalist Nicholas Culpeper called horsetail "very powerful to stop bleeding . . . and heal ulcers . . . the juice or decoction being drunk . . . or applied outwardly . . . It solders together wounds and cures all ruptures."

Later, horsetail gained a reputation as a diuretic. America's 19th-century Eclectic physicians, forerunners of today's naturopaths, prescribed the herb for incontinence, gonorrhea, kidney stones, kidney infections, urinary complaints, and congestive heart failure, which causes fluid retention and swelling.

Contemporary herbalists recommend horsetail externally for wounds and internally for urinary and prostate problems. Homeopaths prescribe microdoses for urinary complaints: bladder infections, bed-wetting, incontinence, and urethritis.

Therapeutic Uses

Horsetail is a minor medicinal herb and has not been well researched. But available evidence suggests that it lives up to its traditional reputation.

WOUNDS. Commission E, the expert panel that evaluates herbal medicines for the German counterpart of the FDA, approves horsetail compresses for treating wounds.

URINARY PROBLEMS. Horsetail contains a weak diuretic compound (equisetonin), which lends support to the herb's traditional use in stimulating urination. Commission E approves horsetail as a treatment for urinary tract infections and kidney stones.

ARTHRITIS. Horsetail absorbs gold dissolved in water better than most plants, as much as 4 ounces per ton of fresh stalks. Of course, the amount of gold in a cup of horsetail tea is tiny, but small amounts may help treat rheumatoid arthritis (RA). Chinese herbalists recommend horsetail for RA. If you have RA, ask your physician about adding it to your treatment regumen. *Note:* Mainstream physicians no longer use gold to treat rheumatoid arthritis. Drugs that work better have been developed.

Medicinal Myth

Horsetail contains nicotine, so some herbalists recommend it to smokers attempting to quit. But compared with cigarettes, horsetail's nicotine content is minute. It's unlikely to satisfy a smoker's craving. Prescription nicotine gum (Nicorette) is a better alternative.

Rx Recommendations

To treat a urinary condition, use either an infusion or a tincture. For wounds, try a topical application of either preparation.

To make an infusion, use 1 to 2 teaspoons of dried herb per cup of boiling water, steep for 10 minutes, and strain. Drink up to 2 cups a day. Horsetail has little taste.

As a homemade tincture, use ½ to 1 teaspoon up to twice a day.

When using commercial preparations, follow package directions.

Safety

Horsetail may cause rashes in those who are sensitive.

In addition to absorbing an unusually large amount of gold, horsetail also absorbs relatively large amounts of selenium. Selenium is an important nutrient, a potent antioxidant that has been shown to help prevent several cancers. But excessive selenium may cause birth defects. In marshes downstream from heavily fertilized agricultural areas, horsetail may have hazardously high selenium levels. Pregnant women should not use the herb. Nursing women should also avoid it.

Horsetail contains equisetine. In large amounts, it's a nerve poison. Animals fed the herb have lost weight and developed fever, muscle weakness, and abnormal heart rhythm. Some have died. Children have reportedly suffered nonfatal reactions after ingesting the juice while using the hollow stems as toy blowguns. Don't let children play with this herb.

If you're over 65, start with a low dose, and increase only if necessary.

Inform health professionals of the herbs you use. Problematic herb-drug interactions are possible.

Horsetail may cause allergic reactions or other unexpected side effects. If any develop, reduce your dose or stop taking it. For more on herb safety, see Chapter 2.

If symptoms get worse or persist longer than 2 weeks, consult a health professional promptly.

Gardening

Horsetail is the sole surviving descendant of the giant fernlike plants that covered the earth some 200 million years ago. Its creeping rhizome sends up hollow, jointed, virtually leafless, bamboo-like stalks that reach 6 feet. At their ends, spore-bearing structures (catkins) develop that resemble horse tails, corncobs, or bottle-brushes, hence some of the herb's names.

Horsetail may be purchased from specialty nurseries, or root cuttings may be taken from wild plants in spring when the spear-like stems have reached a few inches. Set plants or cuttings just under the surface of marshy soil. Keep it wet. If you don't want the plant to spread, surround it with embedding sheet metal to a depth of 18 inches. Harvest stalks in fall. Make that sure children do not suck on the hollow stems.

HYSSOP

The Biblical Antiseptic

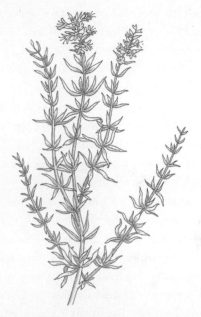

Family: Labiatae; other members include mints

Genus and species: *Hyssopus officinalis*

Also known as: No other names, but many other plants are called hyssop

Parts used: Leaves and flowers

The Biblical book of *Psalms* (51:9) says, "Purge me with hyssop and I shall be clean." But this herb does more than clean. It may work as an antiseptic for infections such as cold sores and genital herpes.

Healing History

Some 2,500 years ago, Jewish priests used strong-smelling hyssop to clean the temple in Jerusalem. But back then, so many plants were called hyssop that we have no way to know if the cleanser and the medicinal herb (*Hyssopus officinalis*) were the same.

Despite the confusion, the Greeks adopted hyssop. The noted Greek physician Dioscorides prescribed the herb in a tea for cough, wheezing, and shortness of breath and in plasters and chest rubs for congestion.

The medieval German abbess/herbalist Hildegard of Bingen wrote that hyssop "cleanses the lungs." She also recommended a meal of chicken cooked in hyssop and wine as a treatment for sadness (depression).

In 17th-century Europe, hyssop was a popular air freshener or "strewing herb." At the time, people rarely bathed and farm animals often shared human living quarters. To mask odors, crushed hyssop leaves and flowers were scattered (strewn) around homes. When bathing became popular and strewing ceased, hyssop was placed in scent baskets in sickrooms.

Seventeenth-century English herbalist Nicholas Culpeper echoed Dioscorides' endorsement of hyssop for chest ailments: "It expelleth tough phlegm and is effectual for all griefs of the chest and lungs." He also claimed, "It killeth worms in the belly . . . .Boiled with figs, it makes an excellent gargle for quinsey [tonsillitis] . . . Boiled in wine, it is good to wash inflammations . . . the head being anointed with the oil, it killeth lice."

Colonists introduced hyssop into North America and continued using it to treat chest congestion. It developed a reputation for promoting menstruation and inducing abortion—but doesn't do either.

As time passed, hyssop's popularity waned. America's 19th-century Eclectic physicians, forerunners of today's naturopaths, prescribed the herb externally to relieve the pain of bruises and

as a gargle for cough, sore throat, tonsillitis, and asthma.

Contemporary herbalists recommend hyssop compresses and poultices for bruises, burns, and wounds and suggest infusions for colds, coughs, bronchitis, flatulence, indigestion, menstruation promotion, and even seizures. As proof of the herb's effectiveness for wounds and respiratory infections, some herbalists point to the fact that the microorganism that produces penicillin (*Penicillium*) grows on hyssop leaves.

Therapeutic Uses

Hyssop can't compete with modern cleansers, but its main traditional medical uses have some scientific support.

COUGHS. Hyssop is a member of the aromatic mint family, and its volatile oil contains several soothing camphor-like constituents, plus one expectorant (marrubiin) that loosens phlegm so it's easier to cough up. Scientific sources agree that hyssop is a "reasonably effective" treatment for the cough and respiratory irritation of colds and flu.

HERPES. Hyssop inhibits the growth of herpes simplex virus, which causes genital herpes and cold sores. Try the infusion in a compress if you have this chronic, recurring infection.

VARICOSE VEINS. Hyssop contains diosmin, a compound that helps strengthen veins. The herb can be up to 6 percent diosmin (dry weight). It takes only about 5 grams of hyssop (approximately 2 teaspoons) to provide the 300 milligrams of disomin considered necessary for vein-strengthening.

HEMORRHOIDS. Hemorrhoids are a type of varicose vein. Hyssop may help treat them.

Intriguing Possibility

A few laboratory studies have shown that hyssop extract disables HIV, the virus that causes AIDS. It's too early to call hyssop an AIDS treatment, but in the future, that's possible.

Medicinal Myth

Penicillium does indeed grow on hyssop. But the assertion that hyssop heals because it carries this microorganism is mistaken.

Rx Recommendations

To make a compress for treating herpes, use 1 ounce of dried herb per pint of boiling water. Steep for 15 minutes and let cool. Soak a clean cloth in the infusion and apply it to cold sores and genital herpes sores as needed.

For an infusion to treat cough, varicose veins, or hemorrhoids, use 2 teaspoons of herb per cup of boiling water, steep for 10 minutes, and strain. Drink up to 3 cups a day. Hyssop has a strong, camphor-like smell and tastes bitter. Add sugar, honey, or lemon or mix it with an herbal beverage blend to improve the flavor.

As a homemade tincture, take 1 teaspoon up to three times a day.

When using commercial preparations, follow package directions.

Safety

Make sure you use *Hyssopus officinalis*. Several other North American plants go by the same name, including hedge hyssop (*Gratiola officinalis*), the giant hyssops (several species of *Agastache*), and the water hyssops (several species of *Bacopa*). Except for one species of bacopa (*Bacopa monnieri*, page 80), these plants should not be ingested. Buy hyssop only from sources that identify it by Latin binomial.

Hyssop has not been shown to stimulate the uterus, but its traditional use to induce abortion should discourage pregnant women from taking it. Nursing women should also avoid it.

No reports of harm from hyssop appear in the world medical literature. However, laboratory animals injected with the herb's essential oil have developed convulsions that caused some deaths. Do not ingest the oil.

Do not give hyssop to children under 2. In older children, adjust the recommended dose based on the child's weight. Give a 50-pound child one-third of the dose a 150-pound adult would take.

If you're over 65, start with a low dose, and increase only if necessary.

Inform health professionals of the herbs you use. Problematic herb-drug interactions are possible.

Hyssop may cause allergic reactions or other unexpected side effects. If any develop, reduce your dose or stop taking it. For more on herb safety, see Chapter 2.

If symptoms get worse or persist longer than 2 weeks, consult a health professional promptly.

Gardening

If you want bees, plant this pretty, hardy, shrubby perennial. Hyssop also has a reputation for enhancing the flavor of grapes and increasing the yield of cabbages planted nearby.

Hyssop has small, lance-shaped leaves and the square stems characteristic of mints. The plant reaches 2 feet and has a medicinal odor that becomes more mint-like when the leaves are crushed. Dense clusters of blue or violet flowers form on 6-inch spikes atop the stems in summer and early fall.

Hyssop enjoys dry, sunny locations and tolerates most soils. In partial shade, it tends to become leggy. It may be propagated from seeds, cuttings, or root divisions. Seeds should be sown ¼ inch deep after the danger of frost has passed. Cuttings and divisions may be rooted either indoors or outdoors in a cool, shady place.

Thin established plants to 12-inch spacing. Add compost each spring. Water seedlings every few days. Mature plants prefer a drier environment and require little care.

Once hyssop reaches 18 inches and exudes its characteristic aroma, prune tops to stimulate leaf growth. The leaves may be harvested at any time. If you don't plan to use the flowers, cut back the entire plant to 4 inches above ground just before it blooms. Dry the herb and store it in airtight containers.

JUNIPER

The Gin-Flavored Healer

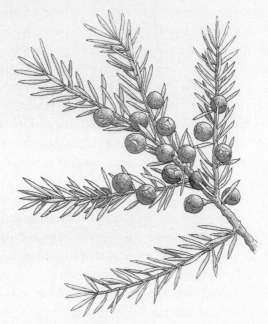

Family: Cupressaceae; other members include cypress

Genus and species: *Juniperus communis*

Also known as: Genvrier and geneva

Parts used: Berries (actually miniature female cones)

If you've ever sipped a martini, you've had juniper. Aromatic juniper berries supply the flavor in gin. Juniper also increases urine production, making the herb a potential treatment for premenstrual syndrome, high blood pressure, and congestive heart failure.

Healing History

During the Middle Ages, Europeans believed that planting a juniper beside the front door kept witches out. Unfortunately, it did not provide complete protection. A witch could still enter if she correctly guessed the number of needles on the tree.

As time passed, juniper's protective reputation evolved into the belief that its smoke prevented leprosy and bubonic plague. As recently as World War II, French nurses burned juniper in hospital rooms to fumigate them.

By the 17th century, juniper was a popular diuretic. English herbalist Nicholas Culpeper wrote that the herb "provokes urine exceedingly . . . .[juniper] is so powerful a remedy against dropsy [congestive heart failure], it cures the disease." In addition, Culpeper prescribed juniper for "cough, shortness of breath, consumption [tuberculosis] . . . to provoke terms [menstruation] . . . and give safe and speedy delivery to women with child."

Native Americans independently discovered juniper's childbirth-assisting properties. In 1540, when the Spanish explorer Coronado entered what is now New Mexico looking for the mythical Seven Cities of Cibola, he found Zuni women using juniper berries to promote uterine recovery after childbirth. They also used the herb to treat wound infections and arthritis.

America's 19th-century Eclectic physicians, forerunners of today's naturopaths, dismissed juniper as a childbirth aid but endorsed it for congestive heart failure. The Eclectics also prescribed juniper externally for eczema and psoriasis and internally for gonorrhea, bladder and kidney infections, and other genito-urinary conditions.

Contemporary herbalists recommend juniper externally as an antiseptic, internally for arthritis, gout, bladder infections, intestinal cramps, and as a urinary deodorant in cases of chronic incontinence because it adds the fragrance of violets to urine.

But all medicinal claims for juniper take a back seat to its use in gin, invented in the 17th century by a Dutch professor of medicine, Franciscus Sylvius, who was interested in creating a diuretic tincture. Our word gin comes from the Dutch term for juniper, *geniver*. The English took to gin so enthusiastically that references to its native land still pepper the English language. Drink a little gin, and you obtain "Dutch courage." Drink too much, and you get in trouble, "in Dutch."

Therapeutic Uses

Juniper's aromatic oil contains terpinen-4-ol, a diuretic compound that increases fluid-filtering in the kidneys. This supports the herb's traditional role as a diuretic.

HIGH BLOOD PRESSURE. Physicians often prescribe diuretics to treat high blood pressure (hypertension). This is a serious condition requiring professional care. If you'd like to use juniper as part of your treatment plan, consult your physician.

CONGESTIVE HEART FAILURE. Culpeper exaggerated when he said that juniper "cures" congestive heart failure. As a diuretic, however, the herb can be part of an overall treatment plan. Congestive heart failure is a serious condition requiring professional care. If you'd like to try juniper, discuss it with your doctor.

PREMENSTRUAL SYNDROME. Diuretics can help relieve the bloated feeling caused by premenstrual fluid retention. Women bothered by premenstrual syndrome might try juniper before their periods.

MENSTRUATION. In animal studies, juniper stimulates uterine contractions. For this reason, pregnant women should not take it (except at term under the supervision of a physician, when it may help stimulate labor). Other women might try it to help start their menstrual periods.

ARTHRITIS. Juniper has anti-inflammatory properties, suggesting possible value in treating arthritis. Native Americans used the herb for this purpose. Likewise, in Germany, where herbal medicine is considerably more mainstream than in the United States, physicians prescribe juniper preparations for arthritis and gout.

Intriguing Possibility

Animal studies show that juniper reduces blood sugar levels. It's too early to call it a treatment for diabetes, but in the future, that's possible.

Medicinal Myth

Juniper has never been shown to be effective against gonorrhea or bladder or kidney infections.

Rx Recommendations

Use 1 teaspoon of crushed berries per cup of boiling water. Steep for 10 to 20 minutes, then strain. Drink up to 2 cups a day for no more than 6 weeks. Juniper has a strong, pleasantly aromatic taste.

When using commercial preparations, follow package directions.

Safety

Diuretics deplete the body of potassium, an essential mineral. If you use juniper, be sure to eat foods rich in potassium, such as bananas and fresh vegetables.

In large doses, the diuretic compound in juni-per irritates the kidneys. It may cause kidney damage in people who are particularly sensitive or have kidney disease. Those with kidney infections or a history of kidney impairment should not take it.

Even low doses taken over long periods may cause problems. "The rule," notes distinguished German medical herbalist Rudolph Fritz Weiss, M.D., "is never take juniper for longer than 6 weeks."

Symptoms of overdose include diarrhea, intestinal pain, kidney pain, protein in the urine (albuminuria), blood in the urine (hematuria), purplish urine, rapid heartbeat, and elevated blood pressure. If you notice any of these symptoms while taking juniper, stop taking it.

Many elderly have kidney impairment. Those over age 65 should have their kidney function checked before taking juniper and then start with a low dose, increasing it only if necessary.

Up to one-third of people with hay fever develop allergy symptoms from exposure to juniper, according to a study in *Clinical Allergy*. If you have hay fever, you may want to avoid the herb. It may also trigger rash.

Pregnant and nursing women should not use juniper.

Do not give juniper to children under 2. In older children, adjust the recommended dose based on the child's weight. Give a 50-pound child one-third of the dose a 150-pound adult would take.

Inform health professionals of the herbs you use. Problematic herb-drug interactions are possible.

Juniper may cause allergic reactions or other unexpected side effects. If any develop, reduce your dose or stop taking it. For more on herb safety, see Chapter 2.

If symptoms get worse or persist longer than 2 weeks, consult a health professional promptly.

Gardening

The genus *Juniperus* contains more than 70 species of aromatic evergreens. Most are small trees, but some grow to 40 feet. The species most widely used in herbal healing, common juniper (*J. communis*), reaches 6 to 20 feet, depending on locale. Its close, tangled, spreading branches are covered with reddish brown bark, sticky gum, and pointed ½-inch needles. Males produce yellow flowers, females green blossoms. The females also produce scaly, green, aromatic ¼-inch cones (berries) that turn blue-black during their two-year maturation. If you want berries, be sure to plant both male and female plants.

Junipers usually prefer sandy soil and full sun, but adapt to many soil and climate conditions. Consult a nursery for advice specific to yours.

Females produce immature (green) and mature (blue-black) berries simultaneously. Harvest only the mature berries in fall. Dry them in the sun. When dried, they turn a dull black. Store berries in airtight containers to preserve their volatile oil.

KAVA

The South Pacific Soother

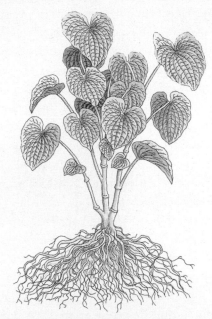

Family: Piperaceae; other members include black pepper

Genus and species: *Piper methysticum*

Also known as: Kava kava, awa, kew, tonga

Parts used: Rhizome and root

For centuries, the peoples of the South Pacific have used kava the way Americans use beer—as a mild social intoxicant. In the mid-1990s, kava became popular in the United States as a treatment for stress and anxiety. But at the turn of the 21st century, this herb became a hazard. Almost 100 users worldwide developed liver damage. Some suffered liver failure and died. Headlines called kava "a killer" and its popularity plummeted. Since then, scientists have deduced what happened. Their conclusion: Kava root does not cause liver toxicity.

Healing History

For centuries, Polynesians from New Guinea to Tahiti have enjoyed this herb in "kava circles" of several people. One places a few tablespoons of white, powdered kava root in half of a coconut shell and adds about a cup of water to form a milky solution. Then the circle claps once in unison as the drinker downs the brew in a big gulp. The shell passes to the next person in the circle, who repeats the ceremony until each participant has taken several gulps. As the festivities continue, the conversation and laughter flow more easily, like after a few beers.

In the South Pacific, kava has also been used as a treatment for headache, colds, and arthritis and as a sedative and aphrodisiac. Hawaiians used it to control asthma.

The 18th-century British explorer Captain James Cook and his crew tried kava during their voyage to the South Pacific (1768–1771). They enjoyed its peppery taste and the mild intoxication it produced. They also noticed that elderly kava drinkers, who had consumed the herb over many decades, had oddly scaly skin. They identified kava dermopathy (more on page 289).

Around 1990, kava began attracting the attention of American herbalists. German studies had shown that at doses lower than those used in the South Pacific, the root produces little or no euphoria but acts as a mild tranquilizer.

Therapeutic Uses

The active compounds in kava, kavalactones, have a mild tranquilizing effect similar to a low dose of Valium (diazepam). But unlike the drug, kava is much less likely to cause sedation, and it's not addictive. (However, the combination of kava and alcohol or other depressants is powerfully sedative.)

ANXIETY AND STRESS. Many studies, mostly German, show that kava is an effective treatment for stress and anxiety.

🍀 German researchers gave 100 people complaining of anxiety, agoraphobia, or social phobia either a placebo or kava (300 milligrams/day). After 8 weeks, the herb group showed significantly less anxiety and depression. The benefits continued for the 6-month duration of the study. Only 5 of the 50 kava users reported side effects, mostly mild digestive upsets.

🍀 In another German study, 58 people with anxiety disorders took either a placebo or kava (100 milligrams three times a day). In the kava group, anxiety symptoms began to decline after just 1 week of treatment and continued to diminish throughout the month-long study. The kava takers reported no side effects.

🍀 At the Medical College of Virginia, researchers gave either a placebo or kava (240 milligrams/day) to 60 adults plagued by stress and anxiety. After 4 weeks, the placebo group showed no significant change in anxiety symptoms, but those taking kava reported fewer anxiety symptoms, less stress, and fewer interpersonal problems—without side effects.

🍀 In a study involving 172 people, German scientists compared kava (100 milligrams three times a day) with standard doses of two drugs similar to Valium. After 6 weeks, all three treatments were equally effective.

☘Italian researchers gave one of three treatments to 68 women complaining of menopause-induced anxiety: a placebo, low-dose kava (100 milligrams/day) or high-dose kava (200 milligrams/day). Both kava treatments were significantly more effective than the placebo.

☘Two research teams, one British, the other German, performed sophisticated statistical analyses (meta-analyses) on studies of kava for anxiety. The English group reviewed seven trials, the Germans six. In both meta-analyses, kava proved effective for anxiety.

Commission E, the expert panel that evaluates herbal medicines for the German counterpart of the FDA, endorses kava as a treatment for stress and anxiety problems. The herb is best used for periods of up to a few months. If you feel that you still need antianxiety medication after that, consult your physician.

MENOPAUSE-RELATED MOOD SWINGS. Italian researchers gave 80 menopausal women one of three treatments: a placebo, a low-dose of kava (100 milligrams/day) or a high-dose (200 milligrams/day). After 3 months, both kava groups reported significantly reduced anxiety and depression.

Intriguing Possibility

Many people suffering major depression also feel quite anxious. In a pilot study, Australian researchers gave 28 people, age 18 to 60, with depression and anxiety a placebo for 2 weeks, then continued with the placebo while the rest took St. John's wort (page 415) and kava (1,800 milligrams of tincture). Then the groups switched treatments. The herb combination produced significant mood elevation and anxiety relief.

Rx Recommendations

You may be able to purchase powdered kava root in bulk, but most Americans take commercial capsules.

Look for a standardized extract that contains 60 to 75 milligrams of kavalactones per capsule. The dose used in most studies is 300 milligrams of standardized extract (the equivalent of about 200 milligrams of kavalactones), taken in divided doses. Follow package directions.

The Liver Toxicity Scare of 2000 and 2001 And Its Resolution

In 2000, a 14-year-old American girl developed persistent nausea, vomiting, fatigue, weight loss, and loss of appetite, symptoms that suggested hepatitis. She consulted a doctor, who prescribed rest and liver-function tests. The tests showed considerably more liver damage than hepatitis typically causes. The girl was hospitalized with liver failure and received an emergency liver transplant.

Liver failure is extremely rare in otherwise healthy teenagers. This girl did not use alcohol, which, in large amounts, is toxic to the liver, and she took no medication implicated in liver damage, just ibuprofen (Motrin, Advil) occasionally. However, to treat anxiety, she'd taken kava daily for 6 weeks.

This was just one of more than 100 reports from around the world of kava users developing liver disease ranging from mild liver impairment (elevated liver enzymes) to jaundice, to hepatitis, to acute liver failure requiring an estimated dozen transplants. Nine of these people died.

By early 2001, kava generated headlines. *USA Today*: "Herb Kava Linked to Liver Problems." The *New York Times*: "Questions about Kava's Safety." They also prompted several countries to ban the herb: Germany, Austria, Canada, France, Ireland, Singapore, Switzerland, and the UK. Kava was not banned in the United States, but the Food and Drug Administration (FDA) warned consumers about the possibility of life-threatening liver damage.

Kava sales plummeted. As sales fell, so did reports of kava-induced liver damage. The controversy became yesterday's news—but not to herb researchers. Studies continued as scientists searched for the reason behind the herb's liver toxicity.

Kava has been used throughout Polynesia for at least 1,500 years with few reports of significant side effects and no reports of liver damage (jaundice) in the ethnopharmacological literature.

Various reports showed that in laboratory animals and isolated human liver cells, powdered kava root mixed with water is not liver-toxic.

Furthermore, many of the case reports of kava-related liver damage turned out to be less than compelling. Researchers at the University of Munster, Germany, analyzed 78 European cases of alleged kava toxicity. Only a few could be persuasively linked to kava alone, compared with an estimated 450 million doses taken in Europe during the decade before the German ban. In most cases, the herb was just one of several liver-threatening drugs the victims had used: alcohol, aspirin, Prozac, Paxil, and birth control pills.

Even if every case were totally attributable to kava, risk worked out to 0.3 cases per 1 million doses, a low rate of serious side effects comparable to many FDA-approved drugs.

An analysis by University of Sydney, Australia, researchers reached the same conclusion: "Only a negligible fraction of the case reports are attributable to kava."

However, many drugs considered safe in recommended amounts can cause liver damage when taken in large amounts, for example, acetaminophen (Tylenol). Two studies have looked at kava use among Australia's aboriginal population. Heavy users occasionally developed elevated liver enzymes, the first sign of liver damage. But none developed liver failure—and the native Australians had used *several ounces of kava a week for decades*, thousands of times more than the amounts that caused liver toxicity in the United States and Europe.

But if recommended doses of kava are reasonably safe, why did several dozen people around the world develop serious liver disease while taking it? The reason turned out to be adulteration.

Kava is slow-growing. It takes 4 to 5 years for roots to mature. During the 1990s, when kava became suddenly popularity as an herbal tranquilizer, demand substantially exceeded supply, and reports surfaced that some growers had stretched their supply by including not just the root but also the plant's aerial parts, which have never been used in South Pacific kava circles. The aerial parts contain a liver-toxic alkaloid, pipermethystin. Contamination of root material with these other parts of the plant caused the liver toxicity.

The toxicity story generated headlines in 2001, after which kava sales plummeted and reports of toxicity evaporated. As demand fell, growers felt less pressure to stretch the supply and stopped adulterating the root with liver-toxic parts of the plant. As evidence mounted that adulteration had caused the toxicity, the countries that had banned it rescinded their prohibitions.

Compared with Valium and other pharmaceutical tranquilizers, kava is *safer*. German researchers estimate that kava produces 0.008 adverse event reports per million doses. Valium produces 2.12. But Valium does not cause liver failure.

The American Botanical Council (ABC) in Austin, Texas, the nation's leading herb education organization, developed guidelines for safe use of kava.

- Don't use kava if you have been diagnosed with liver disease or have a history of liver disease.

- Don't use it if you take drugs with potential liver toxicity, including alcohol. Take a list of your medications to your physician or pharmacist and ask if any might cause liver toxicity. If so, do not use kava.

- Kava-related liver damage is associated with long-term use of the herb. Don't take it daily for more than 4 weeks without consulting a medical professional for a liver-function test. "Periodic liver-function tests are required for those who take statin drugs to lower cholesterol," ABC Executive Director Mark Blumenthal says. "I'd recommend them for long-term kava users."

- Stop taking kava if you experience nausea, vomiting, unusual fatigue, loss of appetite, darkening of urine, or yellowing of the eyes. These are all symptoms of liver disease. If you develop these symptoms, consult a physician promptly.

- Look for kava products that specify only root/rhizome material. This is no guarantee that you'll get only root/rhizome material. But care in labeling suggests care in harvesting.

- Kava affects the body's cytochrome P450 system. This system, little known by the non-physician public, involves a group of 50 enzymes, six of which facilitate metabolism of many drugs, including several medicinal herbs. Simultaneously taking drugs and herbs that both affect the cytochrome P450 enzyme system may cause unusual side effects including liver damage. Cytochrome P450 problems are most likely in those with a genetic deficiency in a certain enzyme, CYP2D6. A test is available, but it's costly and most health insurers don't cover it. If you or your doctor suspect a CYP2D6 deficiency, use other herbal tranquilizers instead of kava: chamomile, hop, lavender, passionflower, or scullcap.

Safety

In unusually large doses—considerably larger than those necessary to treat anxiety—kava causes inebriation similar to alcohol. Thinking and coordination become impaired. The eyes become bloodshot. Walking becomes difficult, and stumbling and falling become more likely.

Taking unusually large doses for many years leads to the development of scaly skin (kava dermopathy). But this is highly unlikely in the doses recommended to treat anxiety. For kava dermopathy, experts recommend stopping the herb.

Do not use kava at the same time as alcohol or other tranquilizing, sedative, or psychoactive medications, including antidepressants. It potentiates the sedative action of other drugs.

Commission E says people taking kava shouldn't drive.

Kava may cause numbing in the mouth. This is harmless. Allergic reactions are also possible.

People who have conditions that impair coordination, such as Parkinson's disease and those taking sedative or antidepressant medications should not use kava.

Pregnant and nursing women should not use kava.

Do not give kava to children under 2. In older children, adjust the recommended dose based on the child's weight. Give a 50-pound child one-third of the dose a 150-pound adult would take.

If you're over 65, start with a low dose, and increase only if necessary.

Inform health professionals of the herbs you use. Problematic herb-drug interactions are possible.

Kava may cause allergic reactions or other unexpected side effects. If any develop, reduce your dose or stop taking it. For more on herb safety, see Chapter 2.

If symptoms get worse or persist longer than 2 weeks, consult a health professional promptly.

Gardening

Kava is not a garden herb in the United States, though cultivation in Hawaii is possible. A botanical relative of black pepper, kava is a perennial shrub with heart-shaped leaves that grows throughout the South Pacific at altitudes of 500 to 1,000 feet. It does best in stony ground under full sun. Plants can climb to 20 feet, but the roots are usually harvested when the shrub reaches about 8 feet.

KOLA

Breathe Deeply

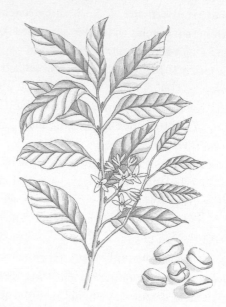

Family: Sterculiaceae; other members include cocoa

Genus and species: *Cola nitida*, *C. vera*, and *C. acurninata*

Also known as: Cola

Parts used: Nuts (actually seed leaves, or cotyledons)

Cola drinks account for most of the enormous U.S. soft drink market. Americans might consume even more if they knew that the tropical nut responsible for colas' flavor can help relieve asthma.

Healing History

Since prehistoric times, West Africans have chewed kola seed for its stimulant effect and to treat fever.

West African slaves introduced the kola tree into Brazil and the Caribbean. In the Caribbean, the herb became a popular diuretic, digestive aid, and remedy for diarrhea, fatigue, and heart problems. Over time, kola's stimulant properties led to the belief that it was an aphrodisiac.

Kola arrived in the United States after the Civil War. Nineteenth-century Eclectic physicians, forerunners of today's naturopaths, noted that the Caribbean people revered kola's "innumerable fabulous virtues."

The Eclectics correctly identified the stimulants in kola—notably caffeine—as the same ones in cocoa, coffee, and tea. They prescribed kola to "overcome mental depression" and prepare for "severe physical and mental exertion." They also recommended it to relieve diarrhea, pneumonia, typhoid fever, migraines, seasickness, and morning sickness and for anyone who "attempts to break the tobacco habit."

Kola's medicinal use meant that 19th-century pharmacists stocked it. Legend has it that on May 8, 1886, Atlanta pharmacist John Styth Pemberton was experimenting with herbs for a new headache remedy. He mixed sugar with extracts of kola and coca (source of cocaine), and then added carbonated water. He liked the taste, and so did his bookkeeper, who dubbed it Coca-Cola.

Two years later, for $2,300, Pemberton sold all rights to his herbal brew to Atlanta businessman Asa Candler. Candler was an imaginative marketer, and by 1895, Coca-Cola had become America's first national soft drink.

Today, Coca-Cola ranks among the world's best-known brand names. People request it some 250 million times a day in 80 languages in 135 countries.

Since its development, Coca-Cola's formula has been a closely guarded secret that has evolved over the years. When the United States outlawed cocaine (1914), the drug was removed from the formula. Today, Coca-Cola is known to contain de-cocainized coca leaf extract and a small amount of kola.

Modern herbalists recommend kola for its "marked stimulating effect on human consciousness," according to medical herbalist David Hoffmann's *Holistic Herbal*. It's also prescribed as a treatment for diarrhea, depression, nervous debility, migraines, and loss of appetite.

Therapeutic Uses

STIMULANT. Some herbals claim that kola contains more caffeine than coffee. Actually, a 6-ounce cup of brewed coffee contains 100 to 150 milligrams of caffeine. A cup of instant coffee has 65 milligrams. By comparison, a 12-ounce can of Coke contains about 50 milligrams of caffeine, most of which comes not from kola but from added caffeine. (For more on the health benefits and risks of caffeine, see coffee, page 165.)

ASTHMA. Coffee can help control asthma, but many children don't like its taste. That's why an article in the *Journal of the American Medical Association* recommended using cola beverages when kids start wheezing without their medicine handy or as tasty adjuncts to standard asthma medication.

Rx Recommendations

Cola beverages are the most convenient way to enjoy this pleasant-tasting herb.

If you prefer a decoction, place 1 to 2 teaspoons of powdered kola nuts in 1 cup of water. Bring to a boil and simmer for 10 minutes, then strain if you wish. Drink up to 3 cups a day.

Safety

Women hoping to become pregnant should avoid herbs containing caffeine, which reduce the likelihood of conception. However, this fertility-impairing effect is not sufficiently reliable to be considered contraceptive.

Pregnant and nursing women should not use kola.

Inform health professionals of the herbs you use. Problematic herb-drug interactions are possible.

People with any of the conditions mentioned in the discussion of the safety of coffee (page 165) should avoid kola.

Don't give kola preparations to children under 2.

Kola may cause allergic reactions or other unexpected side effects. If any develop, reduce your dose or stop taking it. For more on herb safety, see Chapter 2.

If symptoms get worse or persist longer than 2 weeks, consult a health professional promptly.

Gardening

Not grown in the United States.

Kola is a 40-foot tree that grows in West Africa, the Caribbean, Brazil, Sri Lanka, and Indonesia. Kolas have beautiful, purple-spotted yellow flowers that produce chocolate-colored seed pods in spring and fall.

"Nut" usually refers to the whole seed, but the kola nut is only part of the seed, the embryonic leaves (or cotyledons) inside the seed coat. These are dried and powdered.

KUDZU

From Miracle, to Pest, to Medicine

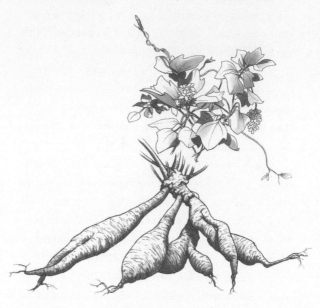

Family: Fabaceae; other members include beans, peas, alfalfa

Genus and species: *Pueraria montana* (formerly *P. lobata*)

Also known as: *kuzu*, *gat gun*, *ge gan*, miracle vine, foot-a-night vine, mile-a-minute vine, and the vine that ate the South

Parts used: primarily root, also flowers

Our word, kudzu, comes from the Japanese name of this fragrant-flowered vine, *kuzu*. It arrived in the United States in 1876. During the 1930s, it became a nightmare in the Southeast, where it still causes major environmental problems. But slowly, the much-reviled vine is becoming appreciated as an herbal medicine. It contains compounds that can help treat menopausal discomforts, high cholesterol, heart disease, and stroke. It might even help alcoholics stop drinking.

Healing History

Kudzu is native to southern Japan and southeast China, where it's known as *gat gun* and *ge gan*. In Asia, it has been used for centuries as a food, animal feed, and treatment for a variety of conditions including vertigo, tinnitus, and hangover.

Kudzu was introduced into the United States in 1876 at the Philadelphia Centennial Exposition, where it was touted as "miracle vine," a fast-growing forage crop, a boon to farmers and ranchers, and a lovely ornamental for gardeners. It never caught on as a livestock feed, but as a garden plant, it was well suited to the Southeast, where it became popular thanks to its large attractive leaves and spikes of fragrant of purple flowers.

Kudzu also has an extensive root system, the kind that can be used to prevent erosion. Starting in 1935, the federal Soil Conservation Service encouraged farmers from Virginia to Arkansas to Texas to plant it near streambeds to prevent loss of topsoil. The Depression-era Civilian Conservation Corps joined in this effort, planting the vine all over the South.

What a mistake. The Southeast has perfect conditions for kudzu: lots of rain, hot summers, no hard freezes, and no natural kudzu predators. As a result, the vine ran amok, growing out of control and earning such names as: foot-a-night vine, mile-a-minute vine, and the vine that ate the South. Kudzu choked streambeds, and strangled crops, often completely covering full-grown trees and multistory buildings. In 1953 the U.S. Department of Agriculture dubbed it a pest. Kudzu now covers 12,000 square miles of the United States and costs an estimated $500 million a year in lost cropland and removal costs.

Therapeutic Uses

Kudzu may be the vine that ate the South, but it's also an herb with a surprisingly large number of medicinal uses.

MENOPAUSAL COMPLAINTS. Kudzu root contains two powerful plant estrogens (phytoestrogens), puerarin and daidzin. Treatment of menopausal discomforts with phytoestrogens does not carry the same potential for serious side effects as hormone replacement therapy, so herbs containing phytoestrogens, chief among them soy (page 439), have emerged as effective but safer alternatives for menopausal complaints. Researchers in Thailand assessed the menopausal symptoms of 48 women and then gave them kudzu root (50 or 100 milligrams/day). After 6 months, both dosage groups reported significantly reduced symptoms. The researchers concluded that kudzu shows "great promise" for treatment of menopausal complaints.

CHOLESTEROL. Chinese researchers gave 120 people with high cholesterol one of three treatments: a standard pharmaceutical (pravastatin), kudzu, or a combination of the two. The drug and herb produced virtually the same benefit—on the drug, 81 percent of participants' cholesterol fell significantly, on the herb, 80 percent. The combination of the two worked best—97 percent showed significantly reduced cholesterol.

ANGINA. This form of heart disease causes chest pain with little or no exertion. Asian doctors often treat angina with injections of puerarin. Chinese researchers analyzed 20 studies of this practice involving 1,240 angina sufferers. The results were published in *Cochrane*

Systematic Database Reviews, a worldwide research collaboration whose conclusions are considered authoritative. Puerarin controlled angina as well as standard pharmaceuticals. And combinations of the herbal extract and drugs controlled it better than any standard drug by itself.

STROKE. Chinese animal studies show that puerarin improves blood flow through the brain and spurs recovery from stroke. In a Chinese study, cerebral hemorrhage survivors were treated with a standard pharmaceutical (nimodipine) or kudzu root (2 milligrams/kilograms/day, or 136 milligrams/day for a person weighing 150 pounds). For restoration of memory and spatial judgment, the herb was more beneficial than the drug. This is just 1 of 14 Asian studies of kudzu for stroke recovery. A review of all of them, totaling 1,141 people, shows that the herb improves memory and reasoning ability.

Intriguing Possibilities

ALCOHOL CRAVINGS. Kudzu's use in Asia as a hangover treatment piqued the curiosity of Western researchers. A major contributor to hangover misery is the compound acetaldehyde. It accumulates in drinkers' bloodstreams and causes "the moaning after." Kudzu contains compounds that make acetaldehyde build up in the blood more quickly, so drinkers develop hangover symptoms not the next morning, but *while drinking*. Now, a hangover is still a hangover no matter when it occurs. But animal studies have suggested that a hangover while drinking reduces alcohol consumption.

Two studies have tested kudzu for deterrence of drinking in alcoholics. One showed no benefit, but the other produced intriguing results.

Researchers at McLean Hospital in Belmont, Massachusetts, monitored 14 alcoholics as they drank at a bar, counting the number of drinks and the time it took them to drink them. Then the researchers gave the participants either a placebo or kudzu root (1,000 milligrams three times a day). After 1 week, the participants returned to the bar. Those in the placebo group consumed just as many drinks just as quickly. But the kudzu group consumed significantly fewer drinks more slowly.

Kudzu is no miracle cure for alcoholism, and one beneficial study doesn't prove that it works. But alcoholism is a major public health problem that's difficult to treat. Kudzu offers real possibilities.

LIVER PROTECTION. Animal studies showing that kudzu reduces alcohol cravings also show that the herb protects the liver from alcohol-induced damage and may even reverse that damage.

OSTEOPOROSIS. In premenopausal women, estrogen helps protect bone. But with menopause, estrogen declines, and osteoporosis becomes a major issue. Several animal studies show that kudzu helps prevent bone loss.

DIABETES. Animal studies suggest that kudzu lowers blood sugar levels.

CLUSTER HEADACHE. These headaches cause such searing pain that some sufferers have attempted suicide. A Yale researcher surveyed alternative therapies used by cluster headache sufferers. Some say that kudzu helps.

Rx Recommendations

At this writing, there is no standard dosage for kudzu. Human trials have used from 50 to 136 milligrams/day.

Safety

Kudzu root is starchy, like potato. For centuries, it has been used in cooking in Asia, with no reports of harm.

However, this herb affects the cytochrome p450 system. This metabolic path way is too complicated to explain here, but kudzu's action on it means that the herb might cause harmful interactions if used in combination with drugs that also affect this system. If you want to try kudzu, first check with your doctor to make sure that you are not taking other drugs that affect the cytochrome p450 system.

Pregnant and nursing women should not use kudzu.

Do not give kudzu to children.

If you're over 65, start with a low dose, and increase only if necessary.

Inform health professionals of the herbs you use. Problematic herb-drug interactions are possible.

Kudzu may cause allergic reactions or other unexpected side effects. If any develop, reduce your dose or stop taking it. For more on herb safety, see Chapter 2.

If symptoms get worse or persist longer than 2 weeks, consult a health professional promptly.

Gardening

Kudzu can be grown in pots indoors almost any-where from seed or cuttings. It likes rich, moist soil, full sun, and heat. Outdoors, kudzu grows outdoors from southern New Jersey to Texas. Because it so readily becomes a pest, gardening authorities recommend against planting it.

LAVENDER

The First Herb of Aromatherapy

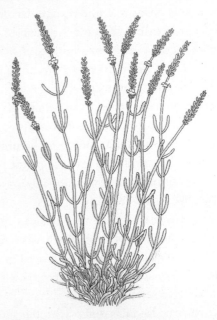

Family: Labiatae; other members include mints

Genus and species: *Lavandula angustifolia*; also known as *L. officinalis* and *L. spica*

Also known as: True lavender, spike lavender, lavandin, and aspic

Parts used: Flower

Lavender grew in abundance around the ancient Syrian city of Nardus. As a result, the ancient Greeks called the plant "nard." The Bible refers to it as spikenard, a reference to its flower spikes.

Our word lavender comes from the Latin *lavare*, meaning "to wash." Lavender was a frequent addition to baths and was also considered a purifier for both body and mind.

Healing History

Since ancient times, lavender has been used as a digestive aid, sleep aid, and tranquilizer for people who are anxious, restless, or troubled.

English farmers wore spikes of lavender flowers under their hats to prevent headache and sunstroke. Insomnia sufferers dried the flowers and sewed them into pillows as a fragrant sleep inducer. The herb was also used to treat acne, migraines, diabetes, lightheadedness, headache, and muscle spasms. Until World War I, lavender infusions and tinctures were used to disinfect wounds.

For centuries, lavender has been an ingredient in sachets and potpourris to freshen the air, especially in sickrooms. Sprigs placed in wardrobes and closets added fragrance to clothing and may have repelled moths.

During the Middle Ages, sprinkling lavender water on a lover's head was said to keep the person faithful, a reputed effect that generated great demand for the herb.

There was also a persistent rumor that the asp, a poisonous snake, nested in lavender bushes, which made people think twice about gathering it. This was pure fiction, apparently promoted by herbalists to drive up lavender's price.

In his *Herball* or *Generall Historie of Plantes*, 16th-century British herbalist John Gerard wrote of lavender's use in treating palsy (tremors or paralysis): "It profiteth them much that have the palsy if they be washed with water of lavender flowers, or are anointed with the oil made from the flowers and olive oil."

Fifty years later, Nicholas Culpeper prescribed lavender for "all the grief and pains of the head . . . it strengthens the stomach . . . two spoonfuls of the distilled water of the flowers help them that have lost their voice . . . ."

America's 19th-century Eclectic physicians, forerunners of today's naturopaths, recommended lavender as a digestive aid. They cautioned, however, that immoderate use of lavender infusions might cause stomach upset.

The Birth of Aromatherapy

During the 1920s, French fragrance chemist Rene-Maurice Gattefosse was in his laboratory trying to develop a new perfume. Lost in thought while blending several herbs' essential oils, he set off a small explosion that burned his arm. Frantic with pain, he plunged his burned limb into the nearest cold liquid, a bowl of lavender oil.

Immediately, Gattefosse felt surprising relief. In addition, instead of the extended healing process he'd known from previous burns—accompanied by inflammation, blisters, and scarring—this burn healed remarkably quickly, with little pain and no scarring. Perhaps, the perfumer thought, he had discovered a powerful healer that had literally been right under his nose.

Gattefosse devoted the rest of his life to studying the role of essential oils in health and healing. In 1928, he published the book *Aromatherapie*, coining the term that's now used to describe the healing discipline that involves inhaling aromatic plant oils or massaging them into the skin for physical or emotional benefits.

Today, aromatherapists use dozens of essential oils, but they still consider lavender one of the best for treating anger, anxiety, burns, depression, indigestion, infection, insomnia, irritability, muscle aches, and wounds.

Therapeutic Uses

Exposure to lavender is no guarantee of a lover's faithfulness. But modern research has validated many of the herb's traditional medicinal uses.

The essential oil extracted from lavender flowers is chemically very complex, containing more than 150 compounds. When rubbed on the skin, it penetrates quickly and can be detected in the blood in as little as 5 minutes.

ANXIETY AND STRESS. After exposure to the scent of lavender, mice become calmer. Studies at the Smell and Taste Research Foundation in Chicago have shown that some scents, including lavender, increase the type of brain waves associated with relaxation. This lends support to the age-old practice of using lavender to treat restlessness, anxiety, and insomnia.

- At a British hospital, researchers divided patients in 90 intensive-care units into three groups. One group received standard care, another got standard care plus up to three massages, while the third had standard care plus massages with lavender oil. All three groups experienced similar reductions in blood levels of stress-related hormones, but those who received lavender massages reported the greatest mood elevation and anxiety relief.

- At the University of Miami, Florida, mothers of fussy, crying infants bathed their babies in water with or without lavender-scented bath oil. In the lavender group, the infants cried less.

- German researchers gave 221 adults with anxiety disorders either a placebo or lavender (80 milligrams/day). Ten weeks later, the placbo group showed just as much anxiety, but the lavender group became significantly calmer.

- Iranian investigators assessed the mood of 141 third-trimester pregnant women, age 18 to 40, and then instructed them to use one of three treatments: a skin lotion with nothing added, a lotion with added lavender, or the lavender lotion plus half-hour foot baths. After 8 weeks, both lavender groups reported significantly better mood. The foot baths made no difference. Lavender without foot baths provided as much relief as the herb plus foot baths.

- Many people with dementia become so agitated that they are difficult to control. At a nursing home housing 15 severely demented and agitated people, British researchers released either water vapor or lavender oil into the day room. When exposed to the herb oil, 60 percent of the residents became calmer.

- Agitated nursing home residents are at high risk of falling, which can be life-threatening. Japanese researchers taped patches to the collars of 175 nursing home residents' clothing. Half the patches emitted no odor, half released a faint but discernible fragrance of lavender. After a year, in the placebo group, 50 percent fell at least once, and 47 percent more than once. But in the lavender group, only 36 fell at all, with just 24 percent experiencing recurrent falls.

Commission E, the expert panel that evaluates herbal medicines for the German counterpart of the FDA, approves lavender as a treatment for anxiety and restlessness.

INSOMNIA. In the baby study previously mentioned, the infants exposed to lavender bath oil slept better afterward.

At the University of Leicester in England, researchers monitored the sleep habits of nursing home residents who had taken sleeping pills for years. For the first 2 weeks, they took their sleep medication as usual. For the next 2 weeks, they stopped using their medications—and slept poorly. For the final 2 weeks, they took no medications, but the researchers infused the fragrance of lavender oil into the air after dark. The participants slept just as long as they had while taking medication—and they slept more soundly. This study involved only four people, but it lends credence to lavender's traditional role as a sleep aid—especially because another small English study in younger people corroborates these results. Commission E endorses lavender for treating insomnia. Several English hospitals offer lavender baths or lavender pillows to help patients sleep.

WOUNDS. Like most aromatic herb oils, lavender oil has antimicrobial action.It can protect wounds from infection and help them heal.

DIGESTIVE PROBLEMS. Like its close botanical relatives, the mints, lavender helps calm the smooth muscle lining the digestive tract. It also promotes the secretion of bile, which helps digest fats. Commission E endorses lavender as a digestive aid and antiflatulent.

PREMENSTRUAL SYNDROME (PMS). Japanese scientists surveyed the symptoms of 17 young adult women who complained of PMS. Then the women sat near a source of steam or lavender vapor. Ten minutes of inhaling water vapor didn't change PMS symptoms, but 10 minutes of lavender provided significant relief.

MENSTRUAL CRAMPS. Herbs that soothe the digestive tract may also calm another smooth muscle, the uterus. Korean researchers asked 67 young women with severe cramps to massage their abdomens with either almond oil or that plus lavender oil (and a little rose and clary sage oil). The herb oil group reported significantly less painful cramps.

RECOVERY FROM CHILDBIRTH. British researchers divided 635 new mothers who had normal, uncomplicated deliveries into three groups. One added true lavender oil to their baths, another used synthetic lavender oil, and used an unscented bath oil placebo. During the 10-day study, all three groups reported reduced pain between the legs, but the true lavender group experienced the speediest recoveries.

EPISIOTOMY RECOVERY. To prevent vaginal tearing during delivery, some obstetricians cut the perineum (episiotomy). Iranian investigators treated 60 episiotomy wounds with either a standard antiseptic (iodine) or lavender oil (five to seven drops of oil in baths twice a day). After 10 days, 22 percent of the iodine group had healed, but in the herb group, 52 percent.

INSECT REPELLENT. Modern research has shown that some of the compounds in lavender oil repel insects. This validates the centuries-old practice of strewing lavender flowers for insect control.

Intriguing Possibility

According to a report in the *Journal of the National Cancer Institute*, a compound in lavender oil (perillyl alcohol) shows remarkable action against a variety of tumors in animals, notably, cancers of the breast, lung, liver, colon, and pancreas. Perillyl alcohol is being tested as a possible cancer treatment.

Rx Recommendations

To prepare an infusion, use 1 to 3 teaspoons of lavender flowers per cup of boiling water, steep for 10 minutes, and strain. Drink up to 3 cups a day.

To treat a minor wound or burn, wash it with soap and water, then apply a compress made with a lavender infusion.

As a homemade tincture, take 1 teaspoon up to three times a day. You may also apply the tincture topically to wounds and burns.

When using commercial preparations, follow package directions.

For a relaxing bath, place a handful of lavender flowers in a cloth bag and run hot water over it, or add lavender infusion, tincture, or oil to your bath.

For an aromatherapy massage, apply a few drops of lavender oil directly to the skin or blend it into a commercial massage lotion (10 drops of oil per ounce of lotion).

To make a lavender pillow, put powdered flowers into a cloth bag and place the bag inside your pillowcase.

Safety

Do not ingest lavender oil. A drop or two is probably harmless, but as little as a teaspoon can be toxic, especially to children and the elderly.

Researchers at the National Institute of Environmental Health Sciences in North Carolina investigated three preteen boys who had inexplicably developed enlarged breasts (gynecomastia). All three had been using a skin lotion that contained lavender and tea tree oil. Shortly after discontinuing the lotion, their breasts reverted to normal. Lavender and tea tree oils have effects that mimic the female sex hormone estrogen. If you use lavender oil regularly, inform your doctor of its estrogenic action and discuss the implications based on your medical situation.

Pregnant and nursing women should not use lavender oil.

Inform health professionals of the herbs you use. Problematic herb-drug interactions are possible.

Lavender may cause allergic reactions or other unexpected side effects. If any develop, reduce your dose or stop taking it. For more on herb safety, see Chapter 2.

If symptoms get worse or persist longer than 2 weeks, consult a health professional promptly.

Gardening

Lavender is a popular ornamental all over the temperate world, but almost the entire commercial crop is used in perfumes, soaps, cosmetics, and hair care products. Some flavors vinegars, vegetable oils, cheeses, and honey. Lavender scones are popular in England, and in France, lavender sorbet is a summer treat.

Native to the Mediterranean, lavender is a pleasantly aromatic, woody, branching perennial shrub that grows to about 3 feet. Its narrow, fuzzy leaves change color from gray to green as they mature. In summer, lavender produces small blue or purple flowers that develop on spikes 6 to 8 inches long, creating beautiful, aromatic bouquets.

The more than 25 species of lavender grow easily in sunny locations. They prefer sandy soil but tolerate a wide range of soil conditions.

If you'd like to grow lavender for medicinal purposes, herbalists consider *Lavandula angustifolia* the best species. But other species have similar benefits. Consult a nursery for the species that grows best in your area.

The fragrance of lavender remains potent long after the flowers have dried.

LEMON BALM

For Herpes, Insomnia, and More

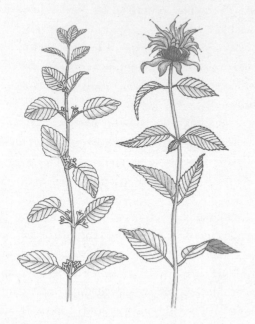

Family: Labiatae; other members include mints

Genus and species: *Melissa officinalis*

Also known as: Balm, bee balm, melissa, sweet balm, and cure-all

Parts used: Leaves

Bees love lemon balm, which has been a favorite among beekeepers for more than 2,000 years. Not surprisingly, its genus, *Melissa*, is Greek for "bee."

Lemon balm is also a honey of a healer. It calms the stomach, soothes the nerves, promotes restful sleep, and helps treat herpes.

Healing History

The ancient Greek physician Dioscorides applied lemon balm leaves to wounds and added the herb to wine to treat many illnesses. The Roman naturalist Pliny recommended lemon balm to stop bleeding.

During the 10th century, Arab doctors recommended lemon balm for nervousness and anxiety. The great 11th-century Arab physician Avicenna wrote, "Balm causeth the mind and heart to become merry."

Medieval Europeans adopted the Arab practice of using lemon balm for nervousness and anxiety. Melissa water, or eau de Melisse, became so popular as a tranquilizer and sedative that the emperor Charlemagne ordered the plant grown in every medicinal ("physic") garden in his realm to guarantee supply.

During the Middle Ages, European herbalists greatly expanded on lemon balm's earlier uses, prescribing it for just about everything: insomnia, arthritis, headache, toothache, sores, digestive problems, and cramps and other menstrual problems. In fact, they recommended the herb for so many ailments that lemon balm was referred to as cure-all.

In his influential herbal, 17th-century English herbalist Nicholas Culpeper echoed Avicenna, commenting, "[Lemon balm] causeth the mind and heart to become merry, and driveth away all troublesome cares and thoughts arising from melancholy . . . ." Culpeper also recommended lemon balm for "faintings and swoonings . . . to help digestion . . . open obstructions of the brain . . . [and] procure women's courses [menstruation]."

In North America, colonists had surprisingly little regard for the bees' favorite herb. They used lemon balm primarily to relieve menstrual cramps and to induce sweating, a traditional treatment for fever.

America's 19th-century Eclectic physicians, forerunners of today's naturopaths, also had few uses for lemon balm. Despite the herb's long history as a tranquilizer, they considered it a mild stimulant.

Contemporary herbalists tout lemon balm's traditional roles as a tranquilizer, digestive aid, and treatment for wounds and viral infections.

Therapeutic Uses

Culpeper was way off base claiming that lemon balm "open[s] obstructions in the brain," but many of the plant's other traditional uses have withstood scientific scrutiny. In addition, researchers have discovered a benefit the ancients ever imagined—that lemon balm has potent antiviral action.

WOUNDS. Lemon balm contains compounds (polyphenols) that help fight several infection-causing bacteria, among them *Streptococcus* and *Mycobacteria*. Lemon balm also contains eugenol, a natural anesthetic that helps relieve wound pain.

HERPES AND OTHER VIRAL INFECTIONS. Lemon balm has antiviral activity. Bulgarian researchers asked 66 people with recurrent herpes cold sores to apply a placebo skin cream or one continuing the herb (1 percent lemon balm extract). After applying the creams four times a day for 5 days, sores treated with lemon balm caused milder symptoms (redness, itching, burning) and healed significantly faster.

In a German study, 116 people with herpes lesions (cold sores or genital herpes) applied either a placebo cream or a cream containing 1 percent lemon balm extract. Subjects applied the creams two to four times a day for up to 10 days. By the second day, those using the lemon balm showed greater healing, and by the fifth, their sores were 50 percent more likely to have cleared. The researchers concluded: "Melissa was judged conclusively superior to the placebo by physician and patient alike." To be effective, however, lemon balm treatment must begin the moment sores erupt. In Germany, where herbal medicine is more mainstream than in the United States, lemon balm extract is an ingredient in herpes ointments. Can't find a lemon balm ointment? Compresses of a strong infusion should also help.

ANXIETY. Lemon balm won't "driveth away all troublesome cares," but a British study shows that it relieves anxiety. The researchers gave 24 volunteers mental challenges that produced stress. After treating them with lemon balm (600, 1200, and 1800 milligrams along with 120 milligrams of valerian), the participants were subjected to similar challenges. The 600 milligrams dose reduced their anxiety. (Oddly, the 1800 milligrams dose increased it.)

INSOMNIA. Animal studies have shown that several fragrant compounds in lemon balm oil have tranquilizing properties. This supports lemon balm's traditional role as a relaxant. In Germany, lemon balm is widely used as a tranquilizer and sedative. In one German study, a combination of lemon balm and valerian provided significant relief to 68 people with insomnia. In another report, the same herb combination proved as effective as the pharmaceutical tranquilizer/sedative triazolam (Halcion), but unlike the drug, it caused no morning "hangover." A third German study shows that this herb relieves insomnia in children. Commission E, the expert panel that evaluates herbal medicines for the German counterpart of the FDA, approves lemon balm as a treatment for insomnia.

HEART PALPITATIONS. These sudden episodes of rapid, pounding, fluttering heart beat can be scary. Iranian researchers gave a placebo or lemon balm (1,000 milligrams/day) top 71 adults, age 18 to 60, who'd complained of frequent palpitations for at least 3 months. After 2 weeks, the placebo group reported no relief, but those taking the herb saw their flutters reduced 37 percent.

ATTENTION DEFICIT/HYPERACTIVITY. German scientists assessed the behavior of 169 elementary school children labeled hyperactive by their physicians and families. Then the kids took a combination of lemon balm (320 milligrams/day) and valerian (page 473, 640 milligrams/day). After 7 weeks, both physicians and families agreed that the children's behavior had been significantly normalized.

DIGESTIVE UPSETS. German researchers have discovered that lemon balm relaxes the smooth muscle tissue of the digestive tract, supporting the herb's age-old reputation as a digestive aid. Many other herbs in the mint family, notably peppermint, are also traditional digestive aids. Commission E endorses lemon balm for treating indigestion.

WOMEN'S HEALTH. Herbs that relax the digestive tract may also calm another smooth muscle, the uterus. This explains lemon balm's traditional role in treating menstrual cramps.

Curiously, lemon balm has also been recommended as a uterine stimulant to promote menstruation. Until scientists clarify this, pregnant women should not take it.

Intriguing Possibility

Animal studies have shown that lemon balm interferes with the activity of thyroid-stimulating hormone, suggesting that it may prove useful as a treatment for an overactive thyroid gland (hyperthyroidism or Grave's disease).

Rx Recommendations

For a relaxing bath, tie a handful of balm into a cloth and run the bath water over it. In addition to the tranquilizing effect, you'll love the lemony aroma.

To treat wounds or herpes sores, make a hot compress using 2 teaspoons of leaves per cup of water. Boil for 10 minutes, strain, and apply with a clean cloth.

To treat a minor cut, crush some fresh balm leaves and apply them directly to the wound.

For a light, lemony-tasting infusion that helps soothe the stomach, relieve anxiety, or promote sleep, use 2 teaspoons of leaves per cup of water. Steep for 10 to 20 minutes, then strain. Drink up to 3 cups a day.

As a homemade tincture, take $\frac{1}{2}$ to $1\frac{1}{2}$ teaspoons up to three times a day.

When using commercial preparations, follow package directions.

Safety

Because lemon balm interferes with thyroid-stimulating hormone, it may aggravate problems associated with an underactive thyroid (hypothyroidism). There are no published reports of the herb having this effect, but anyone with hypothyroidism should consult a physician before ingesting lemon balm.

At high doses, lemon balm may aggravate anxiety. Do not exceed recommended amounts.

Pregnant and nursing women should not use lemon balm.

Do not give lemon balm to children under 2. In older children, adjust the recommended dose based on the child's weight. Give a 50-pound child one-third of the dose a 150-pound adult would take.

If you're over 65, start with a low dose, and increase only if necessary.

Inform health professionals of the herbs you use. Problematic herb-drug interactions are possible.

Lemon balm may cause allergic reactions or other unexpected side effects. If any develop, reduce your dose or stop taking it. For more on herb safety, see Chapter 2.

If symptoms get worse or persist longer than 2 weeks, consult a health professional promptly.

Gardening

Lemon balm is an erect, branching perennial that grows to 2 feet. It has the mint family's characteristic square stems and small, two-lipped white or yellow flowers that bloom in bunches throughout the summer. The above-ground parts die back each winter, but the root is perennial.

Lemon balm grows easily from seeds sown in spring or from cuttings or root divisions. Seeds germinate indoors or out and often do best when left uncovered. Simply keep them moist. Germination typically takes 3 to 4 weeks.

Lemon balm likes well-drained soil with a pH near neutral. Thin seedlings to 12-inch spacing. The herb prefers partial shade. It wilts in full sun and loses some aroma.

For medicinal use, the leaves should be harvested before the plant flowers. Cut the entire plant back to a few inches above the ground. Dry the leaves quickly, or they may turn black.

Lemon balm loses much of its fragrance when dried. After drying, powder the leaves, then store them in tightly sealed opaque containers to preserve its volatile oil.

LICORICE

Safe When Used Sensibly

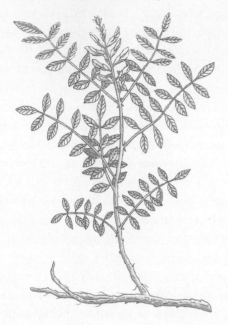

Family: Leguminosae; other members include beans and peas

Genus and species: *Glycyrrhiza glabra*

Also known as: No other names

Parts used: Rhizomes and roots

Licorice is both beneficial and controversial. Advocates note that it has been used around the world for millennia to treat coughs, colds, rashes, arthritis, ulcers, hepatitis, cirrhosis, and infections. Critics concede the herb's utility but insist that its "potentially life-threatening side effects" make it too dangerous to use.

In a few cases, enormous amounts of the concentrated licorice extracts used to flavor candies have caused harm. But for healthy adults who consume only recommended amounts, licorice's benefits greatly outweigh its risks.

Healing History

Licorice appears prominently in the first great Chinese herbal, the *Pen Tsao Ching* (*Classic of Herbs*) attributed to the mythical emperor-sage Shen Nung around 3000 BC. According to legend, the emperor tested dozens of herbs on himself and died after taking too much of a poison plant. Since Shen Nung, licorice has remained one of China's most popular healing herbs.

Licorice also has a long history in Western herbalism. Amid the treasures of King Tut's tomb, archeologists found a bundle of licorice sticks.

During the 3rd century BC, Hippocrates extolled licorice for coughs, asthma, and other respiratory complaints. He called it sweet root, in Greek, *glukos riza*, which evolved into the herb's genus, *Glycyrrhiza*.

The Romans changed *glycyrrhiza* to *liquiritia*, which evolved into "licorice." Noted 1st-century Roman naturalist Pliny recommended it as an expectorant and stomach soother. The Greek physician Dioscorides prescribed licorice juice for colds, sore throats, and chest and gastrointestinal complaints.

India's ancient Ayurvedic physicians extolled licorice as an expectorant, diuretic, and menstruation promoter.

The 12th-century medieval German abbess/herbalist Hildegard of Bingen prescribed the herb for stomach and heart problems. It was mentioned frequently in 14th- and 15th-century German and Italian herbals as a cough and respiratory remedy.

The 17th-century English herbalist Nicholas Culpeper described licorice as "a fine medicine . . . for those that have dry cough or hoarseness, wheezing or shortness of breath, phthisis [tuberculosis], heat of urine [burning], and griefs of the breast and lungs."

North American colonists found Native Americans drinking a tea brewed from American licorice as a cough remedy, laxative, earache treatment, and mask for the bitter flavor of other herbs.

America's 19th-century Eclectic physicians, forerunners of today's naturopaths, prescribed licorice for urinary problems, coughs, colds, and other "bronchial and pectoral [chest] affections."

Among American folk herbalists, licorice was considered a treatment for menstrual discomforts. Lydia E. Pinkham included it in her Vegetable Compound, the popular 19th-century patent medicine for "female hysteria," that era's term for menstrual and menopausal complaints.

Many cultures around the world have used licorice to treat a variety of cancers.

In contemporary Chinese medicine, licorice is known as "the great harmonizer." Its sweetness masks the bitter taste of many other medicinal herbs. Chinese physicians believe that in multi-herb formulas, licorice helps the other ingredients work together. It appears in a variety of formulas, including those for indigestion, asthma, depression, varicose veins, and inflammatory conditions.

Contemporary American herbalists recommend licorice for its soothing effects on the respiratory, urinary, and gastrointestinal tracts, especially as a treatment for ulcers. They also follow the Chinese example of using licorice to mask the bitter taste of other healing herbs.

A few herbalists believe that licorice has hormone-like action. They recommend it as a treatment for Addison's disease, adrenal gland insufficiency.

Therapeutic Uses

True to its Greek name, sweet root, licorice is 50 times sweeter than sugar. The herb contains a remarkable compound (glycyrrhetinic acid, GA), that has a broad range of healing powers. But a bitter battle has erupted over the sweet root's hazards.

COLDS, COUGHS, AND SORE THROATS. Several studies support licorice's traditional role as a cough remedy. Glycyrrhetinic acid is a cough suppressant. In Europe, licorice is a popular ingredient in cough and cold formulas. Commission E, the expert panel that evaluates herbal medicines for the German counterpart of the FDA, approves the herb as a cold and cough treatment.

ULCERS. In 1946, a Dutch pharmacist noticed that licorice candies and cough remedies were unusually popular with customers who had gastrointestinal ulcers. They claimed the herb provided better, longer-lasting relief than other ulcer medicines. Intrigued, the pharmacist published a report in a Dutch medical journal.

Soon after, the British medical journal *Lancet* and the *Journal of the American Medical Association* published studies showing that concentrated GA extracted from licorice healed ulcers in both animals and people. Unfortunately, it also causes swollen ankles, a classic sign of water retention (edema).

Edema is potentially serious. It can raise blood pressure, which can be dangerous for women who are pregnant or nursing and for anyone with diabetes, glaucoma, high blood pressure, heart disease, or a history of stroke.

By the late 1970s, mainstream medicine had developed an effective ulcer drug called cimetidine (Tagamet). Several studies compared licorice head-to-head against Tagamet. The pharmaceutical was more effective for stomach ulcers, but the two treatments were equally effective for duodenal (small intestine) ulcers—and licorice provided better protection against recurrences. However, water retention related to glycyrrhetinic acid continued to be a problem.

Eventually, researchers figured out why GA causes water retention. The chemical acts like the adrenal hormone aldosterone, which is involved in salt and water metabolism. Large amounts of aldosterone may cause a potentially serious condition (pseudoaldosteronism) whose symptoms include water retention, headache, lethargy, high blood pressure, and even heart failure.

Fortunately, scientists also discovered that they could retain licorice's ulcer-healing benefits but eliminate its hormonal side effects by removing 97 percent of its glycyrrhetinic acid. This led to the creation of a new semiherbal medicine, deglycyrrhizinated licorice (DGL).

European and British journals published research demonstrating DGL's antiulcer effectiveness and lack of serious side effects. In one 12-week study of 874 people with duodenal ulcers, published in the *Irish Medical Journal*, DGL healed ulcers faster than Tagamet.

American scientists who'd dismissed glycyrrhetinic acid as too hazardous, decided to take a second look. In the late 1970s, they conducted several studies, but unknowingly used improperly prepared DGL. It produced such poor results that the scientists deemed DGL to be totally ineffective against ulcers.

These unfortunate findings crushed any interest in licorice as an ulcer treatment in the United States. As it turned out, the improperly prepared DGL had released very little medicine (poor bio-availability).

In the late 1980s, researchers discovered that most ulcers are caused by bacteria and can be treated with antibiotics. As a result, DGL is of little interest to most American physicians, but it remains a popular ulcer remedy in Europe. Commission E endorses licorice for ulcer treatment.

People with ulcers who are interested in incorporating licorice into their treatment regimens should discuss the herb with their physicians.

CANKER SORES. Canker sores are painful mouth lesions that may last a week before clearing up. In one study, Indian researchers asked 20 people with canker sores to use a DGL mouthwash. Seventy-five percent experienced substantial relief after just one day, with complete healing by the third day.

HERPES. According to a study in *Microbiology and Immunology*, licorice stimulates production of interferon, the body's own antiviral compound. Herpes sores (genital herpes and cold sores) are caused by the herpes simplex virus. Some studies have shown that licorice inhibits its replication. Sprinkling some powdered licorice root on sores may speed their healing.

HEPATITIS. Chinese physicians have used licorice for centuries to treat liver problems including hepatitis, which may lead to liver cancer. Japanese researchers injected 453 people who had hepatitis C with a licorice preparation (100 milliliters a day for 8 weeks, then several times a week for 10 years). Within 15 years, 25 percent of the control group had developed liver cancer, but cancer developed in only 12 percent of those in the licorice group.

In a similar study, Indian researchers injected 18 hepatitis sufferers with a licorice preparation (40 milliliters a day for 30 days, then 100 milliliters three times a week for

8 weeks). In the non-injected control group, the survival rate was 31 percent, but among those treated with licorice, 72 percent.

The injectable licorice preparation used in these studies (Stronger Neo-Minophagen C) is not available in the United States. Nonetheless, the studies demonstrate that licorice is a potent antiviral. The herb provides liver protection in those with cirrhosis, and it has antiviral action against influenza viruses and HIV, the virus that causes AIDS.

People interested in licorice as a liver healer or HIV treatment should discuss it with their physicians.

OTHER INFECTIONS. Many laboratory studies have shown that licorice fights disease-causing bacteria (*Staphylococcus* and *Strepto-coccus*) and the fungus responsible for vaginal yeast infections (*Candida albicans*). Sprinkling some powdered licorice root on clean wounds may help prevent infection. *Streptococcus mutans* is a major cause of dental cavities. A study by UCLA researchers shows that it inhibits this bacteria. Rinsing the mouth with licorice tea might help prevent cavities.

MENOPAUSAL COMPLAINTS. A tip of the hat to Lydia Pinkham. In a pilot study, natu-ropathic researchers in Portland and Seattle gave 13 women complaining of hot flashes either a placebo or an herbal formula containing equal parts of licorice and four other herbs used to treat menopausal complaints: Chinese angelica (page 62), burdock (paged 117), motherwort (page 330), and wild yam root (1,500 milligrams three times a day). After 3 months, 6 percent of the placebo group reported significant relief from hot flashes, but in the herb group, 100 percent.

SORE THROAT. Surgery often requires intubation, sticking a tube down the throat to assist breathing. Austrian researchers asked 236 adults on their way to elective surgery requiring intubation to gargle pre-operatively with either sugar water or a licorice solution. After surgery, the herb group reported signifi-cantly less sore throat.

Intriguing Possibilities

ARTHRITIS. Licorice has anti-inflammatory properties. Animal studies suggest benefit against arthritis. If you'd like to try licorice for this purpose, discuss it with your physician.

CANCER. Licorice shows antitumor activity in experimental animals, probably because it stimulates the immune system.

Rx Recommendations

To prevent wound infection, first wash with soap and water, then sprinkle with powdered licorice.

To help soothe a cough or sore throat, add a pinch of sweet-tasting licorice to any herbal bev-erage tea.

For a decoction to treat canker sores, gently boil $\frac{1}{2}$ teaspoon of powdered herb per cup of water for 10 minutes, then strain. Drink up to 2 cups a day, holding the liquid in your mouth for a while so it washes over the sores.

As a homemade tincture, take $\frac{1}{2}$ to 1 tea-spoon up to twice a day.

When using commercial preparations, follow package directions.

Safety

In the United States, medical journals have been slow to pick up on licorice's benefits, but they've jumped all over its potential to cause pseudoaldosteronism. The problem is real, and some people should not take this herb. In moderation, however, most people can use it safely.

There have been no reports of licorice sticks or the powdered herb causing adverse reactions. All the problems, a few dozen reports in the world medical literature, have been caused by the highly concentrated licorice extracts used in some candies, laxatives, and tobacco products. The vast majority of these problems have resulted from overindulgence in licorice candies.

The *Journal of the American Medical Association* recounted the case of a man who ate 2 to 4 ounces of real licorice candies every day for 7 years. He developed weakness and hormone disturbances that required hospitalization. Another man ate more than 1 pound of licorice candy a day for 9 days. He, too, required hospital treatment. And a 15-year-old boy developed severely high blood pressure after eating more than 1 pound of licorice candy.

Clearly, consuming unusually large amounts of licorice can cause problems. For this reason, women who are pregnant or nursing and anyone with a history of diabetes, glaucoma, high blood pressure, stroke, or heart disease should be cautious about using the herb. It may raise blood pressure.

If you use licorice, familiarize yourself with its overdose symptoms: headache, facial puffiness, ankle swelling, weakness, and lethargy.

However, in the United States, most "licorice" candies are flavored with anise, not licorice. Real licorice is available in specialty shops.

Pregnant and nursing women should not use licorice.

Italian researchers have found that licorice reduces male sex hormone (androgen) levels in women. Androgens are responsible for libido.

Women interested in maintaining libido should use licorice cautiously.

Do not give licorice to children under 2. In older children, adjust the recommended dose based on the child's weight. Give a 50-pound child one-third of the dose a 150-pound adult would take.

If you're over 65, start with a low dose, and increase only if necessary.

Inform health professionals of the herbs you use. Problematic herb-drug interactions are possible.

Licorice may cause allergic reactions or other unexpected side effects. If any develop, reduce your dose or stop taking it. For more on herb safety, see Chapter 2.

If symptoms get worse or persist longer than 2 weeks, consult a health professional promptly.

Gardening

Licorice is an erect, hardy perennial that reaches 7 feet. Small, alternate, 1-inch-long leaflets and ½-inch purple midsummer flowers give the plant a graceful beauty.

Mature plants have long taproots that send out creeping horizontal rhizomes (stolons), which give rise to other shoots and more branching roots that create a tangled mass of underground growth. Licorice roots have brown bark and sweet, juicy, yellow pulp.

Hard freezes kill licorice. It grows best in warm, sunny climates or in greenhouses in pots 48 inches deep. Greenhouse licorice often requires artificial light.

Licorice is usually propagated from root cuttings containing eyes. Plant them vertically about an inch below the soil surface, with 18-inch spacing. Beds should be rich, well dug and well drained with added manure. Once established, this herb can become extremely invasive. Keep it contained.

Licorice requires little care. Expect slow growth the first year or two, then harvest rhizomes and roots during the fall of the third or fourth year. During harvest years, pinch back flowers. Flowering drains some of the roots' sweet sap.

Thick roots should be split to dry. Shade-dry roots for 6 months. Licorice root keeps well. Scientists who analyzed a sample from AD 756 found that even after more than 1,250 years, it still contained active compounds.

MACA

It Stimulates More Than Just the Imagination

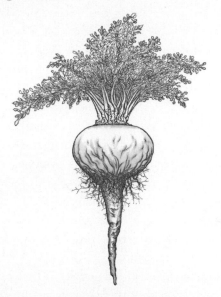

Family: Brassicaceae; other members include mustards, cabbage, and broccoli

Genus and species: *Lepidium meyenii*

Also known as: Peruvian ginseng

Parts used: Root

Maca is a perennial ground cover that produces matting, creeping stems, scalloped leaves, small white flowers, and a turnip-like tuber. It grows high in the Andes above 11,000 feet where few plants can survive the poor soil, freezing temperatures, and gale-force winds. Clearly, maca is a hardy herb. It makes livestock and people hardier, too—and possibly sexier.

Healing History

Before the Incas, ancient Andean shepherds ate maca's fleshy root as a vegetable and fed it to their livestock. They noticed that it made herds healthier and appeared to increase their fertility. As a result, maca gained a reputation as a nutritious food and sex stimulant.

The Incas domesticated maca 2,000 years ago and fed roots to their livestock. They also boiled dried tubers in water to make a sweet, aromatic porridge, *mazamorra*. In addition to nourishment, the Incas believed that maca boosted energy, elevated mood, prevented disease, enhanced memory, improved fertility, had laxative action, treated menstrual problems and menopausal complaints—and enhanced sex. Inca warriors ate maca before battle, believing it increased their stamina and ferocity. After conquering cities, Inca commanders forbid their men to eat it to minimize rapes of vanquished women.

When the Spanish conquered the Incas, they had trouble keeping their horses healthy and reproducing high in the Andes. Local people said, "Feed them maca." The health and fertility of the Spaniards' horses improved, and they embraced maca as a food and sex booster. They also required Andeans to supply them with several tons a year.

Maca's many healing actions resemble those of ginseng. Maca is botanically unrelated to ginseng, but the plant came to be called "Peruvian ginseng."

Therapeutic Uses

SEXUAL ENHANCEMENT. In traditional medical systems worldwide, plants that increased energy were believed to boost sexual energy as well. Supplement companies market the herb as a libido enhancer, and some research supports this.

❦ Animal studies show that maca significantly increases sperm production, copulation, and impregnation.

❦ Peruvian researchers gave adult men either a placebo or the herb (3 grams/day). After 8 weeks, maca had no effect on male sex hormones, but it increased sexual desire.

❦ Italian investigators gave 50 men suffering mild to moderate erectile dysfunction either a placebo or maca (1,200 milligrams powdered root twice a day). After 12 weeks, all participants reported firmer erections, but the maca group claimed significantly greater improvement.

❦ English researchers surveyed the libidos of eight bicycle racers and timed them on a 40 kilometer race course. Then the cyclists took either a daily placebo or maca. After 2 weeks of treatment, their race times improved and they reported more sexual desire.

❦ Australian scientists took blood from 14 older women and assessed their menopausal symptoms and sexual functioning. Then the women took either a placebo or maca (3,500 milligrams/day). After 6 weeks, the groups switched treatment (a cross-over study). Six weeks after that, the women were re-assessed. Before-and-after blood tests showed that maca had no effect on the hormones involved in menopause or sexuality. But while taking the herb, the women reported less menopausal anxiety and depression and enhanced sexual function.

❦ At Massachusetts General in Boston, researchers gave one of three treatments to 20 people suffering sexual dysfunctions induced by antidepressants (Prozac, Paxil, Zoloft): a placebo, low-dose maca (1,500 milligrams/day), or high-dose maca (3,000 milligrams/day). Compared with the placebo takers, both maca groups experienced increased desire. In addition, the high-dose group reported sexual enhancement.

❧ South Korean scientists analyzed 17 maca studies. "Our results provided limited evidence for the effectiveness of maca in improving sexual function."

"Limited" means "some." The case for maca as a sex stimulant is not yet compelling, but it looks like the herb tweaks libido and enhances lovemaking.

HOT FLASHES. The Incas were right about maca for women's health. Australian researchers gave menopausal women either a placebo or maca (1,000 milligrams twice a day). After 2 months, the herb provided significant relief of hot flashes.

Rx Recommendations

Human studies to date have used 2 to 3 grams/day in divided doses. Some sources recommend up to 5 grams/day. Follow package directions.

Safety

There have been no reports of significant side effects or toxicity. Maca has been used as a food for at least 2,000 years, which suggests safety.

Pregnant and nursing women should not use maca.

There is no reason to give maca to children.

If you're over 65, start with a low dose, and increase only if necessary.

Inform health professionals of the herbs you use. Problematic herb-drug interactions are possible.

Maca may cause allergic reactions or other unexpected side effects. If any develop, reduce your dose or stop taking it. For more on herb safety, see Chapter 2.

If symptoms get worse or persist longer than 2 weeks, consult a health professional promptly.

Gardening

Not grown in the United States.

MAITAKE

The "King of Mushrooms" for Many Reasons

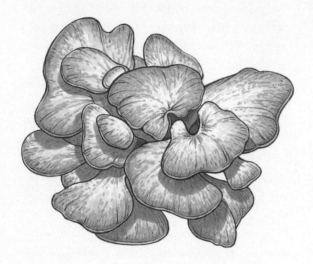

Family: Polyporaceae; other members include other mushrooms

Genus and species: *Grifola frondosa*

Also known as: King of mushrooms, sheep's head, ram's head, hen of the woods, dancing mushroom

Parts used: Whole fungus

Maitake mushrooms (pronounced my-TAH-kay) are native to Europe, northern Japan, and to the eastern United States from the Gulf Coast to Canada. They grow in temperate deciduous forests in clusters at the foot of trees, especially oaks. Clusters can weigh up to 100 pounds, hence the name king of mushrooms. Unlike many mushrooms, maitakes have no cap. Instead, the fruiting body has a frilly, wooly, feathery appear-ance that earned it such common names as sheep's head, ram's head, and hen of the woods. Maitake has also been called dancing mush-room. Some sources say that those who found the valuable delicacy danced for joy. Others say that in a breeze, the frilly fruiting bodies appear to dance. The Japanese have prized maitake mush-rooms as a culinary delicacy for centuries.

In medieval Japan, maitake mushrooms were worth their weight in silver. Hunters kept the mushroom's locations a secret, whispering their discoveries to their sons on their deathbeds. Regional lords offered it as tribute to the Shogun.

In 1979, Japanese mycologists figured out how to cultivate maitake commercially, making the mushroom much more available and cheaper.

Healing History

Traditional Japanese healers recommended maitake to treat high blood pressure and cancer.

A Chinese medical text (210 AD) recommend it to treat digestive upsets and hemorrhoids and to calm the nerves.

In the 1980s, Japanese scientists discovered that like shiitake and reishi mushrooms, mai-take is a potent immune stimulant. Since then, maitake has been the focus of a great deal of research.

Therapeutic Uses

Maitake research is still in its infancy. Only a few human trials have been published. But they confirm the many animal studies showing that maitake is a potent healer.

IMMUNE STIMULANT. Maitake activates several components of the immune system: T-cells, natural killer cells, and germ-devouring macrophages. It boosts production of interleukin-1. It's rich in beta-glucan, a compound that supports the body's defenses against cancer. And it increases synthesis of cytokines, which help the various components of the immune system coordinate their efforts.

CANCER. In laboratory experiments, maitake extract has inhibited the growth and reproduction of several cancer cell types. In animals, the mushroom has reduced the spread of metastatic cancers.

In a Chinese clinical trial, 63 people with various cancers were treated with radiation and chemotherapy. Some of them also received maitake (amount unspecified). In the maitake group, treatment was more successful. Japanese researchers have produced similar findings using a daily maitake dose of 4 to 6 grams/day.

WEIGHT CONTROL. Japanese researchers gave some animals high-fat, high-cholesterol feed, while others received the same feed with maitake added (5 to 20 percent of feed). As expected, the control animals gained weight, but the maitake group did not. By the end of the study, the control animals weighed 25 percent more than the maitake animals. Tokyo researchers told 30 overweight adults to continue eating as they had, but gave them maitake tablets, the equivalent of 7 ounces of the mushroom a day. Two months later, all of them had lost weight, ranging from 12 to 26 pounds.

HEPATITIS, LIVER PROTECTION. Chinese researchers treated 32 chronic hepatitis B sufferers with either standard medication or maitake. Liver enzymes returned to near normal in 57 percent of the drug group. But in the maitake group, the figure was 73 percent. In addition, in the weight control study just mentioned, the control animals also developed precursors of fatty liver disease. The maitake group did not.

VITAMIN D. Until recently, scientists believed that vitamin D could be obtained only from fortified milk, fish liver oils, or supplements, or by skin exposure to sunlight. In addition, maitake contains significant amounts of vitamin D, approximately 100 IU per 100 grams (roughly 25 IU/oz).

No wonder that like ginseng and eleuthero, maitake is considered an adaptogen, an herb that strengthens the entire body.

Intriguing Possibilities

Animal studies show that adding maitake extract to animal feed lowers their cholesterol, blood pressure, and blood sugar, suggesting possible use in treating diabetes and heart disease.

Laboratory studies at Washington State University hint that maitake may help treat malaria.

Rx Recommendations

Take 3 to 7 grams/day in capsules, tablets, or mixed into food. Increasingly, maitakes can be found dried in Asian and gourmet food stores.

Safety

No side effects reported. However, wild mushrooms may be poisonous. Mushroom hunters should be sure of what they've picked before eating.

Gardening

Maitake can be grown indoors from kits marketed by Fungi Perfecti. Visit www.fungi.com.

MARSHMALLOW

A Confection with Healing Roots

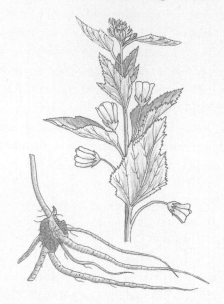

Family: Malvaceae; other members include cotton, hollyhock, and hibiscus

Genus and species: *Althaea officinalis*

Also known as: Althaea and cheeses

Parts used: Root

Yes, marshmallow is the plant that inspired the pillowy white confection toasted over campfires. But today's marshmallows contain none of their namesake herb and bear no resemblance to the marshmallow sweets of old.

It's a shame that so few people know marshmallow as anything other than a candy. The herb has a healing tradition that dates back some 2,500 years.

Healing History

Marshmallow was a food before it became a medicine. The Book of Job (30:4) refers to a plant whose name translates as mallow that was eaten during famines. And during the Middle Ages, when crops failed, people boiled marshmallow roots, then fried them with onions in butter. Today, backpacking guides suggest the plant for wilderness foragers.

Marshmallow's history as a healing herb goes back to Hippocrates, who prescribed a root decoction to treat bruises and blood loss from wounds. Four hundred years later, the Greek physician Dioscorides recommended marshmallow root poultices for insect bites and stings. He also prescribed a decoction for toothache and vomiting and as an antidote to poisons.

The Romans loved marshmallow. The Roman naturalist Pliny enthused, "Whosoever shall take a spoonful of the mallows shall that day be free from all diseases." This thinking led to the herb's genus name, *Althaea*, from the Greek *altho*, to cure.

Ancient India's Ayurvedic physicians used marshmallow to treat coughs and bronchitis.

Tenth-century Arab physicians applied marshmallow leaf poultices as a treatment for inflammation. Early European folk healers used marshmallow root both internally and externally to relieve toothache, sore throat, digestive upset, and urinary irritation.

Marshmallow was a special favorite of 17th-century English herbalist Nicholas Culpeper. "You may remember that not long since, there was a raging disease called the bloody flux . . . the College of Physicians not knowing what to make of it. My son was taken with [it] and . . . the only thing I gave him was mallows bruised and boiled in milk and drunk. In two days (the blessing of God be upon it), it cured him. And I here, to show my thankfulness to God, leave it to posterity."

Culpeper recommended marshmallow roots,

leaves, and seeds for their soothing action in treating "agues [fever] . . . torments of the belly . . . pleurisy, phthisis [tuberculosis], and other diseases of the chest . . . coughs, hoarseness . . . shortness of breath, wheezing, cramps . . . and swellings in women's breasts . . . and other offensive humors."

Colonists introduced marshmallow into North America, and by the mid-19th century, it was listed in the *U.S. Pharmacopoeia*, a standard drug reference. The Eclectic physicians of that time, forerunners of today's naturopaths, prescribed the herb externally for "wounds, bruises, burns, scalds, and swellings of every kind." They also recommended a root decoction internally for colds, hoarseness, diarrhea, gonorrhea, gastrointestinal problems, and "nearly every affection of the kidney and bladder."

Contemporary herbalists generally limit their recommendations to respiratory and gastrointestinal irritation. Some tout the herb for urinary complaints.

Thank the French for the spongy confection that bears the herb's name. Starting centuries ago, they peeled the root bark to expose its white pulp then boiled it to soften the texture and release the root's sweetness. Then they added sugar. The result: sweet, white, somewhat spongy sticks that over time evolved into today's campfire treat.

Therapeutic Uses

The spongy material in marshmallow roots is a fiber called mucilage. Mucilage absorbs water, swells like a sponge, and forms a soothing, protective gel.

WOUNDS. Applied topically, marshmallow mucilage gel helps soothe and protect cuts, scrapes, wounds, and burns.

RESPIRATORY PROBLEMS. Taken internally, marshmallow helps relieve stomach upset and the respiratory rawness of sore throat, cough, colds, flu, and bronchitis. Slovakian researchers used irritant chemicals to induce cough in animals then treated them with a variety of herbs considered cough suppressants. Marshmallow root worked best.

ACE inhibitors, a standard blood pressure medication, have an annoying side effect, cough. Iranian scientists gave 60 people with ACE inhibitor cough either a placebo or marshmallow (20 drops of tincture every 8 hours). After 4 weeks, the placebo group coughed just as much, but the herb group coughed significantly less.

Commission E, the expert panel that evaluates herbal medicines for the German counterpart of the FDA, approves marshmallow for treating coughs.

Intriguing Possibility

In one experiment, marshmallow improved the ability of white blood cells to devour disease microbes, a process called phagocytosis. This suggests that marshmallow's traditional role in treating wounds and gastrointestinal infections may have been therapeutic as well as soothing.

One animal study shows that marshmallow root reduces blood sugar levels, suggesting possible value in managing diabetes.

Rx Recommendations

For external use, chop the root very fine and add enough water to produce a gooey gel. Apply the gel directly to superficial wounds or sunburn. But if you have blistering sunburn or a wound that keeps bleeding despite bandaging, see a physician.

Prepare a sweet decoction to take advantage of marshmallow's soothing powers. Gently boil $\frac{1}{2}$ to 1 teaspoon of chopped or crushed root per cup of water for 10 to 15 minutes. Drink up to 3 cups a day.

When using commercial preparations, follow package directions.

Safety

The medical literature contains no reports of harm from marshmallow.

The safety of marshmallow has not been studied in pregnant and nursing women. They should ingest it cautiously, if at all.

Marshmallow may cause allergic reactions or other unexpected side effects. If any develop, reduce your dose or stop taking it. For more on herb safety, see Chapter 2.

If symptoms get worse or persist longer than 2 weeks, consult a health professional promptly.

Gardening

You can guess from its name where marshmallow grows—in marshes, bogs, and damp meadows and along stream banks. The plant is a downy, erect, 5-foot perennial with a long taproot. The stems are hairy and branching. They die back each autumn. The roundish, gray-green leaves, 1 to 3 inches long, are lobed, toothed, and covered with velvety hairs. Pink or white flowers bloom in summer. Flowers are up to 2 inches across and produce round fruits called cheeses, one of the herb's names.

In moist soil under full sun, marshmallow is a hardy plant that grows easily from seeds, cuttings, or root divisions. Seeds should be planted in spring, root divisions in autumn. Thin them to 2-foot spacing.

Do not harvest roots from plants less than 2 years old. In autumn, when the top growth has died back, dig out mature roots and remove the lateral rootlets. Wash, peel, and dry them whole or sliced.

MATÉ

The High-C Stimulant

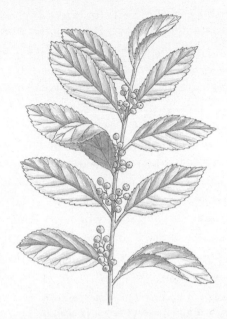

Family: Aquifoliaceae; other members include holly

Genus and species: *Ilex paraguayensis* or *I. paraguariensis*

Also known as: Yerba maté, Paraguay tea, and Jesuit tea

Parts used: Leaves

More than 300 years ago, Jesuit missionaries noticed that a group of South American Indians ate a virtually all-meat diet. Surprisingly however, they didn't develop "sailor's sickness" (scurvy), which decimated European mariners who ate similar diets at sea.

The Jesuits concluded that the Indians must be protected by the tea they drank out of cups made from calabash gourds. The missionaries dubbed it maté, from the Spanish for "gourd."

They began cultivating the holly-like shrub and using its leathery leaves to produce the bitter tea.

Maté (pronounced MAH-tay), also called yerba maté or Paraguay tea, was introduced into the United States in the 1970s as a coffee substitute. It contains caffeine and a rather large amount of vitamin C, which does, indeed, prevent scurvy.

Healing History

The Jesuits introduced maté to European colonists. Today, the herb is one of South America's most popular stimulants. In Argentina, Paraguay, and Uruguay, it's more popular than coffee or tea. More than 200 brands of maté are currently marketed in Argentina alone.

Argentinians consume 11 pounds of maté per capita annually. In Uruguay, that figure is 22 pounds. South American breads often have maté added. The herb is also an ingredient in a popular South American soft drink.

South Americans consider maté not only a pleasant stimulant but also an appetite suppressant, diuretic, and digestive aid. Argentinian cowboys (gauchos) sometimes live on just meat and maté, like the Indians of old.

Therapeutic Uses

A 6-ounce cup of maté contains about 50 milligrams of caffeine, comparable to a cup of tea or a can of cola. By comparison, a cup of instant coffee has about 65 milligrams of caffeine. A cup of brewed coffee has 100 to 150 milligrams.

FATIGUE. Maté is considerably less stimulating than a cup of brewed coffee, but it's still a stimulant. Commission E, the expert panel that evaluates herbal medicines for the German counterpart of the FDA, approves maté to treat fatigue.

COLDS. The Jesuits were right about maté preventing scurvy. The herb is fairly high in vitamin C, which also helps treat the common cold. Drinking maté when you have a cold gives you an extra dose of C.

PREMENSTRUAL SYNDROME (PMS). Diuretics help relieve the bloated feeling caused by premenstrual fluid retention. Women bothered by PMS might try maté during the uncomfortable days just before their periods.

Rx Recommendations

Maté has a distinctive odor that some find offensive. If you're okay with it, brew a pleasantly bitter infusion using 1 teaspoon of dried crushed herb per cup of boiling water steeped for 10 minutes. Add honey and lemon to taste. Drink up to 3 cups a day.

When using commercial preparations, follow package directions.

Safety

Caffeine is classically addictive. Large amounts may cause significant harm. Cup for cup, maté contains less caffeine than brewed coffee, but it still might cause problems. For a more detailed discussion of caffeine's safety, see page 165.

Maté also contains tannins, which have both pro- and anticancer action. A Uruguayan study in the *Journal of the National Cancer Institute* showed that heavy maté users have increased risk of esophageal cancer. The aver-

age Uruguayan consumes 22 pounds of the herb a year, so it's anyone's guess how much "heavy" users consume. Assuming this finding is correct, it has no real significance to Americans who drink maté tea only occasionally. Nevertheless, those with esophageal cancer should avoid it.

Pregnant and nursing women should not use maté.

Do not give maté to children under 2. In older children, adjust the recommended dose based on the child's weight. Give a 50-pound child one-third of the dose a 150-pound adult would take.

If you're over 65, start with a low dose, and increase only if necessary.

Inform health professionals of the herbs you use. Problematic herb-drug interactions are possible.

Maté may cause allergic reactions or other unexpected side effects. If any develop, reduce your dose or stop taking it. For more on herb safety, see Chapter 2.

If symptoms get worse or persist longer than 2 weeks, consult a health professional promptly.

Gardening

Maté is not cultivated in the United States. In South America, the plant grows wild near streams, but it is also extensively cultivated, especially in Argentina.

Maté is a perennial shrub with spineless, oval, toothed, leathery leaves. Its fruits (berries) are red, black, or yellow and about the size of black peppercorns.

MEADOWSWEET

Fragrant Herbal Aspirin

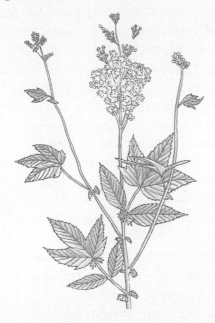

Family: Rosaceae; other members include rose, peach, almond, apple, and strawberry

Genus and species: *Filipendula ulmaria*, formerly *Spiraea ulmaria*

Also known as: Spiraea, bridewort, meadwort, dropwort, and queen-of-the-meadow

Parts used: Leaves and flowers

Consumers spend upward of $50 million a year on aspirin. But it's a rare aspirin user who knows that we owe the word "aspirin" to the beautiful, aromatic meadowsweet.

Healing History

During the Middle Ages, meadowsweet's delicate almond fragrance made it a popular air freshener, or "strewing herb." It was scattered around homes to minimize odors at a time when people rarely bathed and often shared living quarters with livestock. Early British herbalist John Gerard wrote, "The leaves and floures of Meadowsweet farre excelle all other strowing herbs for to decke up houses . . . for the smell thereof delighteth the senses." One fan of strewing meadowsweet was none other than Queen Elizabeth I, who had the flowers spread around her living quarters.

The herb's sweet aroma and lovely blossoms earned it a place in bridal bouquets, hence its name bridewort (wort is Old English for "plant"). Meadowsweet was also used to flavor mead, a fermented beverage made from honey and fruit juices, hence the name, meadwort.

Gerard documented meadowsweet's contributions to healing: "The floures boiled in wine and drunke do take away fits of ague [fever]. The distilled water of the floures dropped into the eies taketh away burning and itching thereof and cleareth the sight." Later, herbalists recommended meadowsweet to treat diarrhea, fevers, arthritis, "falling sickness" (epilepsy), and respiratory ailments.

Colonists introduced the herb into the Western Hemisphere. America's 19th-century Eclectic physicians, forerunners of today's naturopaths, considered meadowsweet "an excellent astringent . . . in diarrhea. [It] is less offensive to the stomach than other agents of its kind." They also prescribed it for menstrual cramps and vaginal discharge.

Contemporary herbalists recommend meadowsweet for colds and flu, nausea, heartburn, childhood diarrhea, and other digestive ailments, as well as for muscle aches and congestive heart failure.

From Salicin to Aspirin

In 1839, a German chemist discovered that meadowsweet flower buds contained salicin, a compound that had been isolated from white willow bark a decade earlier. Salicin has powerful pain-relieving (analgesic), fever-reducing, and anti-inflammatory action.

Unfortunately, salicin (and its close chemical relatives, notably salicylic acid) can also cause potentially serious side effects, including stomach upset, nausea, diarrhea, gastrointestinal bleeding, and ringing in the ears (tinnitus). In high doses, it may even cause respiratory paralysis and death.

Chemists began tinkering with salicin and salicylic acid, hoping to preserve the benefits while minimizing the hazards. In 1853, German chemists added a molecular acetyl group to a meadowsweet extract and synthesized acetylsalicylic acid.

But "acetylsalicylic acid" was a mouthful, so the scientists who created the compound combined the "a-" from acetyl with "-spirin," a variation of meadowsweet's former Latin name, *Spiraea*, to create *aspirin*.

The new compound provided greater relief from fever, pain, and inflammation than either salicin or salicylic acid. Unfortunately, it still had its predecessors' side effects, which disappointed its creators. They published news of aspirin's synthesis in an obscure German medical journal, and that was the end of the story—for 50 years.

In the 1890s, a German chemist, Felix Hoffman, became upset that his father's rheumatoid arthritis medication provided so little relief while causing so much stomach upset. Hoffman worked at the Fredrich Bayer pharmaceutical company. He began combing the journals for

leads to a better arthritis treatment. He came across the old report about aspirin and decided to make a batch himself. As the story goes, he gave some to his father, who pronounced it as effective as his prescribed medication, but with fewer side effects.

Hoffman had a tough time selling aspirin to his superiors at Bayer. Eventually, though, they saw its potential. In 1899, they introduced acetylsalicylic acid in Europe and North America under the brand name Aspirin.

Aspirin quickly became the household drug of choice for relief of pain, fever, and inflammation. Later, in one of the earliest U.S. trademark-protection battles, Bayer lost its trademark to the name Aspirin. The court ruled that the word had passed into general usage—and Aspirin with a capital "A" became aspirin with a lowercase "a." Ever since, the drug company has promoted its product as "Bayer Aspirin."

Therapeutic Uses

While meadowsweet gave us aspirin, the herb can't match all of the pharmaceutical's therapeutic effects. Still, its benefits are impressive.

PAIN, FEVER, AND INFLAMMATION. Meadowsweet does not pack aspirin's pain-relieving, fever-reducing, and anti-inflammatory punch. The herb contains only a small amount of salicylate, so even strong infusions may not have much effect. Tinctures provide more salicylate and greater relief.

On the other hand, meadowsweet is less likely to produce aspirin's major side effect, stomach upset. In fact, a few laboratory trials have shown that the herb *protects* laboratory animals from aspirin-induced stomach ulcers. This finding supports the Eclectics' observation that meadowsweet is gentle on the stomach. At least one animal study, however, suggests that meadowsweet increases the risk of ulcers when given with drugs that cause them.

If you'd rather take an herbal preparation than a pharmaceutical—especially if aspirin upsets your stomach—try meadowsweet for headache, arthritis, menstrual cramps, low-grade fever, and other types of pain and inflammation. And if you combine it with aspirin or another anti-inflammatory pain reliever—ibuprofen (Motrin) or naproxen (Aleve)—you may be able to reduce your dose of the pharmaceutical.

ARTHRITIS. Meadowsweet's aspirin-like effect can help treat the pain and inflammation of arthritis.

COLDS AND FLU. Because meadowsweet helps relieve pain, inflammation, and fever, Commission E, the expert panel that evaluates herbal medicines for the German counterpart of the FDA, approves the herb as a treatment for the common cold and flu.

DIARRHEA. Meadowsweet contains astringent tannins that can help relieve diarrhea. In addition, a European study showed the herb to be effective against *Shigella dysenteriae*, one bacterial cause of infectious diarrhea, lending credence to the herb's traditional use for this condition.

URINARY TRACT INFECTIONS. Meadowsweet is active against *Escherichia coli*, the bacteria most likely to cause urinary tract infections. One report calls the herb a urinary antiseptic.

Intriguing Possibilities

A great deal of research has shown that low-dose aspirin (one-half to one standard tablet a day) helps prevent the blood clots that trigger heart attack and most strokes. Meadowsweet's effect on heart disease and stroke has not been well researched, but animal studies show that it has anticoagulant (blood-thinning) properties, so it probably provides some cardiovascular protection.

Aspirin has also been shown to reduce the risk of digestive tract cancers, notably colon cancer. To date, no studies have linked meadowsweet to reduced risk of these conditions, but again, the herb probably offers similar benefits.

One study revealed that salicin reduces blood sugar (glucose), suggesting that meadowsweet may be valuable in managing diabetes.

Rx Recommendations

To prepare a pleasantly astringent infusion, use 1 to 2 teaspoons of dried, powdered herb per cup of boiling water. Steep for 10 minutes, then strain. Drink up to three cups a day.

As a homemade tincture, take $1/2$ to 1 teaspoon up to three times a day.

When using commercial preparations, follow package directions.

Safety

Aspirin is a well-documented asthma trigger. Research has shown that meadowsweet has the same effect. People with asthma or aspirin sensitivity should not use meadowsweet.

In children under age 16 who have fevers from colds, flu, or chickenpox, aspirin is associated with Reye's syndrome, a rare but potentially fatal condition. Meadowsweet has never been linked to Reye's syndrome, but it's closely related to aspirin so children who have fevers from those illnesses should not take it.

European animal studies suggest that meadowsweet may stimulate uterine contractions. The herb has no history of use as a menstruation promoter, but because aspirin has been associated with an increased risk of birth defects, women who are pregnant or trying to conceive should not ingest meadowsweet.

Pregnant and nursing women should not use meadowsweet.

Do not give meadowsweet to children under 2. In older children, adjust the recommended dose based on the child's weight. Give a 50-pound child one-third of the dose a 150-pound adult would take.

If you're over 65, start with a low dose, and increase only if necessary.

Inform health professionals of the herbs you use. Problematic herb-drug interactions are possible.

Meadowsweet may cause allergic reactions or other unexpected side effects. If any develop, reduce your dose or stop taking it. For more on herb safety, see Chapter 2.

If symptoms get worse or persist longer than 2 weeks, consult a health professional promptly.

Gardening

Meadowsweet is an eye-catching perennial with stems that usually grows to 2 feet, but under favorable conditions may reach 6 feet. It has elm-like leaves and large clusters of small, coiled white or pink flowers that bloom throughout summer and have a fragrant, sweet almond aroma. The flower clusters droop, hence the name dropwort. The plant stands taller and has more striking flowers than most other meadow plants, hence another of its names, queen-of-the-meadow.

Meadowsweet grows wild from Newfoundland to Ohio in marshes, along stream banks, and in moist forests and meadows. Propagate it from cuttings of its creeping underground perennial stem (rhizome).

Meadowsweet does best in rich, moist, well-drained soil under partial shade. Harvest the leaves and flowers when the plant is blooming.

MILK THISTLE
A Potent Liver Protector

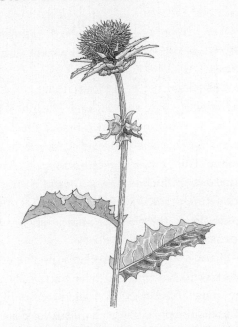

Family: Compositae; other members include daisy, dandelion, and marigold

Genus and species: *Silybum marianum*

Also known as: Silybum and holy thistle

Parts used: Seeds

Milk thistle has been used to treat liver conditions for more than 2,000 years. Modern science has confirmed what the ancients believed. Milk thistle is the single most important liver-protecting herb.

Healing History

Ancient herbalists may or may not have recognized the herb's value as a liver tonic. The 1st-century Roman naturalist Pliny wrote that its juice helped "carry off bile." But back then, "bile" included more body fluids than just the one produced by the liver, so it's not clear if Pliny specifically connected milk thistle to the liver.

But by the 17th-century, the connection was well established. British herbalist Nicholas Culpeper endorsed milk thistle as a treatment for jaundice, the yellowing of the skin and eyes caused by liver disease.

America's 19th-century Eclectic physicians, forerunners of today's naturopaths, prescribed milk thistle to treat liver conditions as well as varicose veins, menstrual complaints, and kidney problems.

Homeopaths use a microdose of the herb to treat liver disorders, gallstones, and varicose veins.

Therapeutic Uses

In 1968, German researchers isolated three liver-protective compounds from milk thistle seeds: silibinin, silidianin, and silicristin, collectively known as silymarin.

Silymarin benefits the liver in several ways. It binds tightly to the receptors on liver cell membranes that allow toxins in, thus locking them out. It's a powerful antioxidant, protecting liver cells from the biochemical process responsible for a great deal of harm. It spurs the repair of damaged liver cells. And it stimulates the immune system.

Medicine needs a good liver protector. Many conditions attack the liver, notably cirrhosis, mushroom poisoning, and hepatitis A, B, and C. Unfortunately, the pharmaceuticals prescribed to treat these conditions don't always work.

For hepatitis, doctors advise rest, antiviral medication, and refraining from ingesting anything that taxes the liver, for example, alcohol and many drugs. For mushroom poisoning, conventional treatment often fails, with fatal consequences. For cirrhosis, doctors can only offer relief from complications. Meanwhile, research has shown that milk thistle helps treat all of these conditions safely and effectively. Commission E, the expert panel that evaluates herbal medicines for the German counterpart of the FDA, approves milk thistle extract as a treatment for liver conditions.

HEPATITIS. Several European studies have shown that compared with hepatitis sufferers who did not receive silymarin, those who did recovered faster. In an Italian study, 20 people with hepatitis were given either a medically inactive placebo or silymarin. Those taking the herb showed greater normalization of liver function.

MUSHROOM POISONING. *Amanita* mushrooms are called "death caps" for good reason: They contain a potent liver poison. Every year, the news media report serious illnesses and occasional deaths among people who go wild mushroom hunting without being able to distinguish edible species from *Amanita*. Without treatment, the death rate from *Amanita* poisoning is around 50 percent. Standard medical treatment (activated charcoal) saves some lives, but the death rate is still around 35 percent. Milk thistle works better. In 2007, six members of a California family accidentally ate death caps and wound up in an emergency room. Treated with intravenous milk thistle, five (83 percent) survived.

Silymarin works by denying *Amanita*'s poison entry into liver cells. In one German study, 60 people who'd accidentally eaten death caps were treated with silymarin. None died. In another German study of 205 cases of *Amanita* poisoning, 189 received standard medical care and 16 received silymarin. In the standard-care

group, 24 percent died, but among those who took silymarin, none died.

In a multicenter European study, researchers analyzed 220 cases of *Amanita* poisoning treated with silymarin. The death rate was 13 percent, well below the rate associated with conventional medical treatment.

CIRRHOSIS. Several studies have determined that milk thistle helps stabilize liver function in people with cirrhosis. One study included 170 cases—91 caused by alcoholism, the rest from other causes—who took either a placebo or milk thistle extract (200 milligrams three times a day). Four years later, death claimed 31 of the placebo takers, but only 18 of those treated with milk thistle.

Scandinavian researchers recruited 97 heavy drinkers who had liver damage but not cirrhosis. Forty-seven took silymarin for 4 weeks. Compared with those taking placebos, the silymarin group showed significantly decreased levels of liver enzymes that had been abnormally high.

DRUG-INDUCED LIVER DAMAGE. Alcohol is not the only drug that harms the liver. With extended use of high doses, even such medicine-cabinet mainstays as acetaminophen (Tylenol) may cause liver damage. In one laboratory trial, silymarin protected animals given large liver-toxic doses of acetaminophen. In other studies, the compound has prevented the liver damage associated with antibiotics, antidepressants, and antipsychotic medications.

TOXIN-INDUCED LIVER DAMAGE. Silymarin also minimizes the damage associated with long-term exposure to several toxic industrial chemicals. In one study, workers with liver damage from toluene and xylene took 140 milligrams of silymarin three times a day. After a month, their abnormally high liver enzyme levels had droped to near normal.

DIABETES. Iraqi researchers gave one of three treatments to 59 diabetics who'd been taking a standard diabetes medication (glibenclamide, Glyburide). Some continued taking Glyburide. Others took the drug plus a placebo. And some took the drug plus milk thistle (200 milligrams/day). The herb reduced blood sugar the most.

Intriguing Possibilities

A Peruvian pilot study suggests that in lactating women, milk thistle increases milk production. Other research hints that silymarin lowers cholesterol and may reduce risk of complications from diabetes.

Rx Recommendations

Silymarin is fairly insoluble in water, so milk thistle infusions and decoctions don't supply clinically active amounts. German plant scientists have bred a high-silymarin variety of milk thistle that produces a standardized extract. A 200-milligrams dose of the extract contains 140 milligrams of silymarin. This dose, taken in tablets or capsules three or four times a day, has become standard in milk thistle research.

Look for a standardized extract containing 70 percent silymarin and use it according to package directions.

Safety

If you start to feel ill after eating wild mushrooms, call 911 or hurry to an emergency room.

A few reports suggest that milk thistle may cause stomach upset.

If you have liver disease, talk to your doctor about taking milk thistle.

Pregnant and nursing women should not use milk thistle.

Do not give milk thistle to children under 2. In older children, adjust the recommended dose based on the child's weight. Give a 50-pound child one-third of the dose a 150-pound adult would take.

If you're over 65, start with a low dose, and increase only if necessary.

Inform health professionals of the herbs you use. Problematic herb-drug interactions are possible.

Milk thistle may cause allergic reactions or other unexpected side effects. If any develop, reduce your dose or stop taking it. For more on herb safety, see Chapter 2.

If symptoms get worse or persist longer than 2 weeks, consult a health professional promptly.

Gardening

Native to Kashmir in India-Pakistan, milk thistle is a weedy plant that now grows throughout the temperate world. It typically reaches 5 to 10 feet and produces large, prickly leaves. When broken, the leaves and stems exude milky sap, hence the name milk thistle. The plant produces reddish purple flowers ringed with sharp spines. The flowers resemble miniature artichokes.

Like its close botanical relative, artichoke, milk thistle was once grown in Europe as a vegetable. Backpacking guides still suggest that wilderness foragers steam the prickly young leaves and stalks, which taste similar to spinach. Young leaves may also be eaten in salads.

MISTLETOE

A Christmas Kiss for Cancer Sufferers

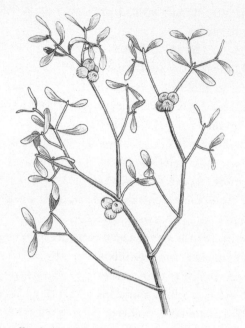

Family: Loranthaceae; all members are called mistletoe

Genus and species: *Viscum album* (European); *Phoradendron serotinum* or *P. tomentosum* (American)

Also known as: Viscum, *herbe de la croix,* and *lignum crucis*

Parts used: Leaves, fruits (berries), and young twigs

Mistletoe is best known for the sprigs under which people kiss at Christmas, a custom with an ironically gruesome origin. As a healing herb, mistletoe is also fraught with irony. One scientific authority calls it "gentle . . . [and] non-toxic." Others insist that "all parts of the plant should be regarded as toxic." The fact is, mistle-

toe's purported toxicity has been greatly over-stated. Europeans use it extensively—and safely—to treat cancer. Unfortunately, American oncologists have been slow to adopt this powerful healing herb.

Healing History

Mistletoe's association with kissing comes from Norse mythology. Balder, god of peace, was slain by an arrow made from mistletoe. When his parents, god-king Odin and goddess-queen Frigga, restored him to life, they gave the plant to the goddess of love and decreed that anyone who passed under it should receive a kiss.

Early Christians believed that during Jesus' time, mistletoe was a freestanding tree and that its wood was used to make the cross of the Crucifixion. God punished the plant by turning it into a parasite. This story gave mistletoe the name *lignum crucis* (wood of the cross) in Latin and *herbe de la croix* in French.

Hippocrates prescribed mistletoe for disorders of the spleen. Most other ancient physicians, particularly Dioscorides and Galen, advised using it only externally, foreshadowing the current controversy over its safety.

Roman soldiers reported that England's ancient Druid priests cut mistletoe from oak trees and used the plant in elaborate fertility rituals.

A French medical text from 1682 recommended mistletoe for "falling sickness" (epilepsy). Some herbals still prescribe it for convulsions (ironically, unusually high doses may cause convulsions).

Seventeenth-century English herbalist Nicholas Culpeper reiterated Hippocrates' recommendation, asserting that mistletoe "doth mollify hardness of the spleen, and helpeth old sores." He also advocated mistletoe for "falling sickness and apoplexy [stroke]," and advised wearing a sprig around the neck to "remedy witchcraft."

During the colonial period, several Native American tribes used American mistletoe to induce abortion and to stimulate contractions during childbirth.

America's 19th-century Eclectic physicians, forerunners of today's naturopaths, recommended both European and American mistletoe for epilepsy, typhoid fever, and dropsy (congestive heart failure). They also prescribed the herb for "hysterical" (gynecological) complaints: menstrual cramps, menstruation promotion, and treatment of postpartum hemorrhage. But the Eclectic text *King's American Dispensatory* (1898) warned that large amounts "possess toxic properties. Vomiting, catharsis, muscular spasms, coma, convulsions, and death have been reported from eating the leaves and berries."

Koreans use mistletoe tea to treat colds, muscle weakness, and arthritis. Chinese physicians prescribe the dried inner stems as a laxative, digestive aid, sedative, and uterine relaxant during pregnancy.

Over time, herbalists came to believe that European and American mistletoe had opposite effects. European mistletoe was reputed to reduce blood pressure and soothe the digestive tract, while the American variety was said to raise blood pressure and stimulate uterine and intestinal contractions.

Therapeutic Uses

Despite the traditional belief that European and American mistletoe have opposite actions, scientists have determined that the plants contain similar active constituents and have similar effects. Mistletoe has the ability to slow the pulse, stimulate gastrointestinal and uterine contractions, lower blood pressure, and treat cancer.

ENHANCED IMMUNITY. Studies from around the world show that mistletoe preparations, notably the Swiss mistletoe drug, Iscador, enhance immune function, boosting activity of several immune cells, macrophages, T-cells, and natural killer cells, and increasing production of cytokines, proteins that help regulate immune function. Injected preparations of mistletoe improve immune function in people with AIDS.

CANCER. Many European studies going back 30 years show that Iscador, which is administered by injection, enhances immune activity against various types of cancer, slowing tumor growth and sometimes reversing it. A sampling of recent studies:

- Swiss researchers analyzed six studies of surgery, radiation, and chemotherapy for breast cancer versus standard therapies plus Iscador. The Iscador groups survived significantly longer and reported better quality of life—improved feelings of well-being, increased appetite, reduced pain, and normalized sleep.

- German scientists gave 253 women with uterine endometrial cancer either standard therapies or those treatments plus Iscador. The Iscador group survived significantly longer and reported better quality of life.

- A different group of German researchers gave 148 women with ovarian cancer either standard therapies or those plus Iscador. For women with early, localized tumors, the herb provided no benefit. But among those with metastatic cancer—and most ovarian cancer is metastatic—Iscador showed significant benefit and those who used it reported significantly better quality of life.

🍀 Swiss researchers followed 320 people with pancreatic cancer. By the time they received Iscador most had advanced, metastatic (stage IV) disease. The 1-year survival rate for stage IV pancreatic cancer is around 10 percent, but among Iscador users 26 percent survived a year. For those with less advanced (stage III) disease, Iscador treatment doubled expected survival times.

🍀 German investigators analyzed 22 studies of Iscador chemotherapy from 1963 through 2008 that involved more than 10,000 cancer patients. Some trials showed no benefit, but overall, compared with those receiving standard care, those treated with Iscador survived significantly longer.

Distinguished German medical herbalist Rudolph Fritz Weiss, M.D., notes, "The great advantage offered by mistletoe extracts is that unlike [other chemotherapeutic] drugs, its . . . immunostimulant and tonic effects are nontoxic and well tolerated."

Commission E, the expert panel that evaluates herbal medicines for the German counterpart of the FDA, approves mistletoe as a complementary cancer therapy to be used in combination with mainstream treatments.

In the United States, mistletoe has not been seriously studied as a cancer treatment because of the herb's reputation as a poison. Ironically, many approved cancer chemotherapy drugs are also toxic. It's a shame American oncologists are not more interested in this herb.

BLOOD PRESSURE REGULATION. Mistletoe contains compounds that both raise and lower blood pressure, but overall, this herb reduces blood pressure. In Germany, where herbal medicine is considerably more mainstream than in the United States, mistletoe extract is an ingredient in many blood pressure medications. Dr. Weiss writes, "Anyone who treats hypertension [high blood pressure] will confirm that mistletoe by mouth has definite benefit . . . For a gentle antihypertensive drug that is well tolerated . . . and nontoxic in the usual dosage . . . mistletoe is the drug of choice."

High blood pressure is a serious condition that requires medical supervision. Use the herb only in consultation with your doctor.

Rx Recommendations

Take mistletoe only under the close supervision of a physician who has knowledge of herbs.

To treat high blood pressure, Dr. Weiss recommends a tea made from equal parts of mistletoe, hawthorn (page 263), and lemon balm (page 300). "Infuse 2 teaspoons of the mixture for 5 to 10 minutes," he writes. "Take 1 cup in the morning and 1 at night." Other herbalists recommend 1 cup a day of an infusion made with 1 teaspoon of freshly dried plant material steeped in 1 cup of boiling water for 10 minutes.

As a homemade tincture, the recommended dose for blood pressure control is five drops daily.

When using commercial preparations, follow package directions.

Safety

How toxic is mistletoe? The Eclectics reported coma, convulsions, and death from the ingestion of large doses of leaves and berries. Since then, there have been scattered reports of fatalities from consuming the berries or beverages made from them.

On the other hand, a review of more than 300 cases of mistletoe ingestion, published in *Annals of Emergency Medicine*, found no deaths associated with the herb. A majority of those who consumed the plant—typically its berries—developed no symptoms of poisoning.

In a 1996 review of 11 cases of mistletoe ingestion (amounts up to 20 berries), researchers affiliated with the Kentucky Regional Poison Control Center reported generally minor stomach upset, except in two infants who suffered more severe reactions. There were no deaths. The researchers concluded that ingesting mistletoe causes "infrequent symptoms, and in all but one case would not require direct medical supervision."

Based on these findings, it would appear that mistletoe's reputation for toxicity is largely undeserved. Nonetheless, keep the herb away from young children.

Mistletoe contains a compound, tyramine, that may stimulate uterine contractions. Pregnant women should not use this herb, except possibly at term and only under the supervision of a physician to induce labor.

Mistletoe's abortion-inducing dose is close to its toxic dose. It should never be used to terminate pregnancy.

People with heart disease or a history of stroke should not take mistletoe, as the herb may slow the heart rate.

Nursing women should not use mistletoe.

Do not give mistletoe to children under 2. In older children, give it only under a doctor's direction. Adjust the recommended dose based on the child's weight. Give a 50-pound child one-third of the dose a 150-pound adult would take.

If you're over 65, start with a low dose, and increase only if necessary.

Inform health professionals of the herbs you use. Problematic herb-drug interactions are possible.

Mistletoe may cause allergic reactions or other unexpected side effects. If any develop, reduce your dose or stop taking it. For more on herb safety, see Chapter 2.

If symptoms get worse or persist longer than 2 weeks, consult a health professional promptly.

Gardening

Mistletoe is a parasitic shrub that grows in trees, rooting into their bark. Both European and American mistletoe are branching, woody evergreens that live on a large number of trees. The European herb has thin, leathery, tongue-shaped 2-inch leaves. The American variety also has leathery leaves, but they are broader and up to 3 inches long. Both plants produce small, sticky white berries, which contain single seeds.

Mistletoe is well adapted to its aerial existence. Its sticky white berries attract birds, which carry them to perches in other trees. The birds eat some but drop others, which stick to the tree bark. Within a few days, the seeds inside newly "planted" mistletoe berries produce tiny roots that bore into the host tree and establish new plants.

Mistletoe is gathered from the wild, not cultivated, although some crafters of mistletoe Christmas products reportedly "plant" the sticky seeds by inserting them into the bark of host trees.

MOTHERWORT

For Lower Blood Pressure

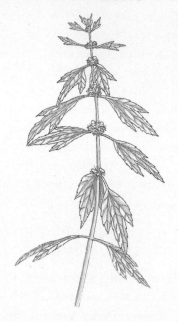

Family: Labiatae; other members include mints

Genus and species: *Leonurus cardiaca*

Also known as: Lion's tail and heartwort

Parts used: Leaves, flowers, and stems

"Wort" is Old English for "plant," but the name motherwort is somewhat misleading. The herb is more likely to prevent motherhood than promote it.

Also, despite one of the herb's popular names, lion's tail, motherwort won't strengthen the lionhearted. It's more apt to turn lions into lambs.

Healing History

The ancient Greeks and Romans used motherwort to treat both physical and emotional prob-lems of the heart—namely, palpitations and depression.

The ancient Chinese believed that motherwort promoted longevity. According to legend, a youth who had committed a minor crime was banished from his village to a remote valley with a spring surrounded by motherwort. Supposedly, he lived to be 300.

In Europe, motherwort first gained prominence as a treatment for cattle diseases. 16th-century British herbalist John Gerard called it "a remedy against certain diseases in cattell . . . and for that husbandmen much desire it." Gerard also recommended the herb for "infirmities of the heart."

Seventeenth-century English herbalist Nicholas Culpeper wrote, "There is no better herb to take melancholy vapors from the heart . . . and make a merry, cheerful soul." While Culpeper viewed motherwort primarily as an antidepressant, he also said, "It is . . . of much use in trembling of the heart [palpitations], and faintings, and swoonings, from whence it took the name cardiaca . . . .It took the name motherwort [because] it settles mothers' wombs . . . and is a wonderful help to women in their sore travail [labor] . . . .It also provoketh women's courses [menstruation]."

As the centuries passed, herbalists used motherwort in contradictory ways, both to relax the uterus during pregnancy and after childbirth and to stimulate menstruation and labor. Eventually, it came to be known as a uterine stimulant.

Colonists introduced motherwort into North America. The 19th-century Eclectic physicians, forerunners of today's naturopaths, recommended the herb as a menstruation promoter and expeller of afterbirth. They also prescribed it as a tranquilizer for "morbid nervous excitement, and all diseases with restlessness [and] disturbed sleep." The Eclectics did not consider motherwort a heart remedy.

Contemporary herbalists recommend motherwort as a tranquilizer, a women's health tonic, and a remedy for heart palpitations and delayed or suppressed menstruation.

Therapeutic Uses

Until recently, most scientists dismissed motherwort as useless. But the ancients who named the herb *cardiaca* may have been onto something.

HIGH BLOOD PRESSURE. Russian researchers measured the blood pressures of 50 people with high blood pressure (hypertension), before giving them motherwort (300 milligrams twice a day). After 28 days, 12 percent of the subjects did not respond, but 88 percent experienced blood pressure reductions.

HEART DISEASE. In China, laboratory studies have shown that motherwort helps relax heart cells. Other Chinese research suggests that it helps prevent the blood clots that trigger heart attack. These findings are preliminary, but combined with motherwort's ability to reduce blood pressure, they lend credence to the ancient view that motherwort is a heart tonic.

Commission E, the expert panel that evaluates herbal medicines for the German counterpart of the FDA, approves motherwort as a treatment for "nervous cardiac disorders."

If you have high blood pressure or heart disease and would like to incorporate motherwort into your treatment plan, do so only in consultation with your physician.

INSOMNIA AND ANXIETY. German studies suggest that motherwort has tranquilizing and mild sedative action. It may be effective in relieving insomnia and anxiety.

WOMEN'S HEALTH. Not many tranquilizers are also uterine stimulants, but motherwort contains a compound, leonurine, that encourages uterine contractions. This lends support to the herb's traditional role in childbirth and menstruation promotion.

Women who are trying to conceive or are pregnant should not take motherwort, except possibly at term and only under the supervision of a physician to help stimulate labor. For other women, the herb may help induce periods.

Rx Recommendations

To make a tranquilizing, uterine-stimulating, blood-pressure-lowering infusion, use 1 to 2 teaspoons of dried herb per cup of boiling water. Steep for 10 minutes, then strain. Drink up to 2 cups a day, a tablespoon at a time. Motherwort tastes very bitter. To improve flavor, add sugar, honey, and/or lemon, or mix it into an herbal beverage tea.

As a homemade tincture, take ½ to 1 teaspoon up to twice a day.

When using commercial preparations, follow package directions.

Safety

Because of motherwort's possible anticlotting effect, those with clotting disorders should not use it. This herb should also be avoided by people taking blood thinners (anticoagulants), including aspirin, garlic, willow bark, or vitamin E.

Some people develop rashes from contact with the plant.

Nursing women should not use motherwort.

Do not give motherwort to children under 2. In older children, adjust the recommended dose based on the child's weight. Give a 50-pound child one-third of the dose a 150-pound adult would take.

If you're over 65, start with a low dose, and increase only if necessary.

Inform health professionals of the herbs you use. Problematic herb-drug interactions are possible.

Motherwort may cause allergic reactions or other unexpected side effects. If any develop, reduce your dose or stop taking it. For more on herb safety, see Chapter 2.

If symptoms get worse or persist longer than 2 weeks, consult a health professional promptly.

Gardening

Motherwort's perennial root gives rise to stout, square stems tinged with red or violet that grow to 4 feet. The plant's lower leaves are sharply lobed, like maple leaves. Its upper leaves are narrow and toothed. It also produces whorls of small white, pink, or red flowers, which bloom in summer.

This herb grows so easily that it may become a pest. Plant seeds in spring and thin seedlings to 12-inch spacing. Motherwort prefers rich, moist, well-drained soil and full sun, but it tolerates less ideal conditions. Harvest the entire plant after flowers bloom.

MUIRA PUAMA

Herbal Viagra?

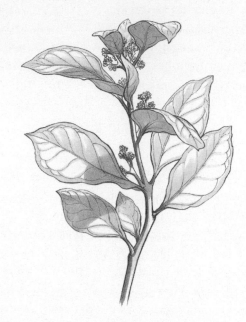

Family: Olacaceae; other members include various tropical trees

Genus and species: *Ptychopetalum olacoides*

Also known as: Marapuama, potency wood

Parts used: Root

Muira puama is a shrubby Amazonian tree that grows to 15 feet. In recent years, it has become popular as a male sex stimulant. Ironically, research to date suggests that it works better for women.

Healing History

For centuries, indigenous Amazonians considered muira puama a "nerve tonic," meaning a stimulant. They used its root to treat fatigue, depression, and the confusion that often develops during old age. All stimulants—among them, coffee and ginseng—have traditionally been considered sex stimulants. The same has been true for muira puama, hence the name potency wood.

Muira puama has also been used traditionally to treat indigestion, menstrual irregularity, and muscle aches.

Therapeutic Uses

Brazilian researchers have confirmed that muira puama is a noncaffeine stimulant.

SEX? Muira puama does not contain yohimbine, the erection-boosting compound in yohimbe bark (page 490). However, French researchers have demonstrated that it has sex-stimulating action. They surveyed 202 healthy women complaining of low libido on various aspects of their sexuality including frequency and intensity of sexual desire, erotic fantasies, intercourse, and orgasm, plus overall sexual satisfaction. Then the researchers gave the women a combination of muira puama and ginkgo (page 240). After 1 month, two-thirds reported significantly greater sexual desire, more frequent and more intense fantasies, more intercourse, and more orgasms that felt more intense. Brazilians can buy an over-the-counter product, Catuama, marketed as an energy-booster and sex stimulant. It contains muira puama plus caffeine, ginger, and a few other herbs.

ANTIOXIDANT. Antioxidant nutrients help prevent and reverse the cell damage at the root of heart disease, many cancers, and other degenerative conditions, for example, Alzhei-

mer's disease. Brazilian researchers have identified antioxidants in muira puama.

Intriguing Possibilities

Simulants have mild antidepressant action. In animal models of depression, Brazilian scientists have shown that muira puama is mood-elevating.

In addition to containing antioxidants, muira puama also inhibits the action of an enzyme (acetylcholinesterase) that plays an important role in learning and memory. Drugs used to treat Alzheimer's disease are acetylcholinesterase inhibitors. Muira puama has similar action. Animal studies show that the herb improves memory and learning. It's too soon to call muira puama a treatment for Alzheimer's, but one day it might be.

Rx Recommendations

The typical dose is 1 to 2 milliliters (about 1 teaspoon) of extract in water two to three times a day. Or follow package directions.

Safety

No significant side effects have been reported.

Pregnant and nursing women should not use muira puama.

Do not give this herb to children. If you're over 65, start with a low dose, and increase only if necessary.

Inform health professionals of the herbs you use. Problematic herb-drug interactions are possible.

Muira puama may cause allergic reactions or other unexpected side effects. If any develop, reduce your dose or stop taking it. For more on herb safety, see Chapter 2.

If symptoms get worse or persist longer than 2 weeks, consult a health professional promptly.

Gardening

Not grown in the United States.

MULLEIN

The Velvety Soother

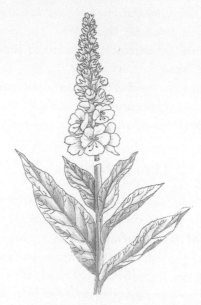

Family: Scrophulariaceae; other members include figwort, foxglove, and eyebright

Genus and species: *Verbascum thapsus*

Also known as: Candlewick plant, torches, velvet dock, flannel plant, feltwort, Aaron's rod, shepherd's staff, and lungwort

Parts used: Leaves, flowers, and roots

Mullein—the name rhymes with sullen—grows everywhere and is hard to miss. Despite this, however, few who encounter the velvet-leafed weed with its rod-like stem and striking yellow flowers appreciate its effectiveness as an herbal cough soother.

Healing History

When dried, mullein burns like a torch. Before the introduction of cotton, ancient cultures around the world used its leaves and stems as candle wicks, earning it the name candlewick plant. The dried stems and flowers were dipped in suet to make them burn longer, hence another of the herb's popular names, torches.

Ancient cultures also considered mullein a magical protector against witchcraft and evil spirits. Like other herbs used in magic, mullein has a long history as a healer. Its botanical family name, *Scrophulariaceae*, is derived from scrofula, an old term for chronically swollen lymph glands. Eventually, doctors identified scrofula as a form of tuberculosis.

The 1st-century Greek physician Dioscorides prescribed a decoction of mullein root in wine as a treatment for "fluxes of the belly" (diarrhea). During the Middle Ages, the French used the herb to treat malandre, an animal disease that causes boils on horses' necks. Malandre eventually became malen and finally, mullein.

Early on, the herb gained a reputation as a respiratory remedy, which endures to this day. In ancient India, Ayurvedic physicians prescribed mullein for cough. Seventeenth-century English herbalist Nicholas Culpeper wrote that gargling a mullein decoction "easeth toothache . . . and old cough." His contemporary, herbalist William Coles, wrote that farmers "give it their cattle against cough."

Colonists introduced mullein into North America, and Native Americans quickly adopted the herb for coughs, bronchitis, and asthma. The accepted way of using mullein in early America seems odd today: People smoked it.

America's 19th-century Eclectic physicians, forerunners of today's naturopaths, viewed mullein as a diuretic to treat water retention and as a stomach and respiratory soother, with mild pain-relieving and tranquilizing action. The Eclectic text *King's American Dispensatory* (1898) asserted, "Upon the upper portion of the respiratory tract, its influence is pronounced." The Eclectics recommended mullein for colds, coughs, asthma, and tonsillitis, as well as for diarrhea, hemorrhoids, and urinary tract infections.

During the late 19th and early 20th centuries, the *National Formulary*, the pharmacists' reference, listed mullein as a cough remedy. It was deleted in 1936 for lack of proof of effectiveness. Nonetheless, in his 1986 survey of folk medicine in Indiana, the late herb expert Varro E. Tyler, Ph.D., found mullein "a very popular Hoosier remedy for all types of respiratory complaints."

Contemporary herbalists recommend mullein as an internal treatment for coughs, colds, sore throat, and other respiratory complaints and as an external treatment (in compresses) for hemorrhoids.

Therapeutic Uses

In laboratory studies, at least, mullein inhibits the growth of the bacteria that cause tuberculosis, so perhaps it helped treat scrofula. Today, it's used mostly to soothe minor respiratory irritations.

COUGH AND SORE THROAT. Mullein contains a soluble fiber called mucilage that swells and turns into a slippery gel when it absorbs water. This accounts for its soothing action on the throat and skin. Distinguished German medical herbalist Rudolph Fritz Weiss, M.D., writes that mullein has a "well-founded reputation as a cough remedy." Commission E, the expert panel that evaluates herbal medicines for the German counterpart of the FDA, endorses mullein as a soothing treatment for colds.

HEMORRHOIDS. Its mucilage is not the only reason that mullein soothes hemorrhoids. The herb also contains astringent tannins, widely used to treat hemorrhoids and other skin conditions. One study showed that mullein also has anti-inflammatory properties.

DIARRHEA. The astringent tannins probably account for mullein's traditional role in treating diarrhea.

Intriguing Possibility

In a laboratory study, mullein infusion helped to combat the virus that causes genital herpes and cold sores. If you develop either of these conditions, you might apply a compress made from a strong mullein infusion.

Rx Recommendations

For an infusion to soothe cough, sore throat and diarrhea, use 1 to 2 teaspoons of dried leaves, flowers, or roots per cup of boiling water. Steep for 10 minutes, then strain. Drink up to 3 cups a day.

Mullein tastes bitter. Add sugar, honey, and/or lemon, or mix into an herbal beverage tea.

To help treat hemorrhoids, apply a compress made with a strong, cool infusion.

As a homemade tincture, take $\frac{1}{2}$ to 1 teaspoon up to three times a day.

When using commercial preparations, follow package directions.

Safety

Mullein seeds are toxic and may cause poisoning. There have been no reports of adverse effects from the herb's leaves, flowers, and roots.

Pregnant and nursing women should not use mullein.

Do not give mullein internally to children under 2. In older children, adjust the recommended dose based on the child's weight. Give a 50-pound child one-third of the dose a 150-pound adult would take.

If you're over 65, start with a low dose, and increase only if necessary.

Inform health professionals of the herbs you use. Problematic herb-drug interactions are possible.

Mullein may cause allergic reactions or other unexpected side effects. If any develop, reduce your dose or stop taking it. For more on herb safety, see Chapter 2.

If symptoms get worse or persist longer than 2 weeks, consult a health professional promptly.

Gardening

Mullein is a hardy biennial that grows almost anywhere in temperate climates. During its first year, the plant produces a rosette of 6- to 15-inch leaves that are greenish white, tongue-shaped, and hairy—hence its common names velvet dock, flannel plant, and feltwort. In its second year, mullein sends up a solitary, fibrous stem that reaches 3 to 6 feet, the source of common names such as Aaron's rod and shepherd's staff. In summer, a striking, cylindrical spike of small, dense, yellow, honey-scented flowers develops atop the stem.

Mullein grows easily from seed in light sandy soil under full sun, but it tolerates other conditions. Sow seeds in spring after the danger of frost has passed.

Harvest up to one-third of the leaves during the plant's first year and the rest the following year, before the flowers bloom. Pick the flowers as they open. Harvest the roots in autumn.

Mullein is a prolific self-sower. Many authorities recommend removing the flower heads before the seeds ripen to keep it under control.

MYRRH

A Thoroughly Modern Mouthwash—and Antiparasitic

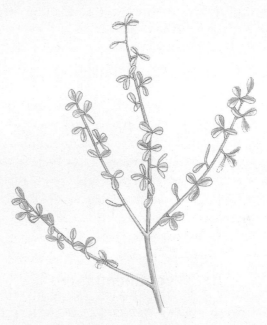

Family: Burseraceae; other members include balm of Gilead

Genus and species: *Commiphora abyssinica* or *C. myrrha*

Also known as: Balsamodendron

Part used: Gum resin from incisions in bark

In *Genesis*, Joseph's jealous brothers decide to sell him into slavery. But who would take him? The answer soon appeared: "And looking up, they saw a caravan of Ishmaelites coming from Gilead [Jordan], with their camels bearing gum, balm, and myrrh on their way to carry it down to Egypt" (*Genesis* 37:25). They sold Joseph to the Ishmaelites.

This is just the first of a dozen biblical references to myrrh, the hardened, tear-shaped nuggets of clear or reddish brown aromatic resin that exudes from incisions in the bark of a small Middle Eastern tree. Of course, the Bible's best-known mention of myrrh involves the three Magi offering the rare and costly herb to the newborn Jesus (*Matthew* 2:11).

Healing History

The world's oldest surviving medical text, the Ebers Papyrus (1500 BC), touts myrrh. The ancient Egyptians used it in embalming mixtures and as a treatment for wounds. From these humble beginnings, myrrh emerged in the Bible as an all-purpose aromatic for perfumes and insect repellents.

The Arabs called the herb *murr*, meaning "bitter." When the ancient Greeks adopted it, they attributed its teardrop shape to Myrrha, daughter of the Syrian king Thesis. Myrrha refused to worship Aphrodite, the goddess of love. Angered by this blasphemy, Aphrodite tricked Myrrha into committing incest with her father. When Thesis realized what he had done, he threatened to kill his daughter. To save her, the gods transformed her into a myrrh tree, whose teardrop resin recalls the girl's sorrow.

Hippocrates recommended myrrh to treat mouth sores. The Greeks also considered it an antidote to poisons.

As the centuries passed, myrrh became valued primarily as a mouthwash to treat bleeding gums, mouth ulcers, and sore throats. The 12th-century German abbess/herbalist Hildegard of Bingen prescribed a mixture of powdered myrrh and aloe for dental problems. Later herbalists recommended myrrh as an expectorant for colds and chest congestion.

By the Middle Ages, the belief that myrrh protected against poisons grew to encompass infectious disease. In 1665, when the Black Plague struck London, however, myrrh offered no benefit, and belief in its protective powers faded. But the powdered resin continued to be used to treat sores in the mouth and on the skin.

America's 19th-century Eclectic physicians, forerunners of today's naturopaths, considered myrrh an antiseptic for the external treatment of "indolent sores and gangrenous ulcers." They prescribed the herb internally for colds, laryngitis, asthma, bronchitis, indigestion, gonorrhea, sore throat, dental cavities, and bad breath. The Eclectics also cautioned that large doses of myrrh could have violent laxative action and cause sweating, nausea, vomiting, and accelerated heartbeat.

Contemporary herbalists recommend using powdered myrrh on well-washed wounds as an antiseptic. They also consider a gargle made from the herb to be effective against sore throats, colds, sore teeth and gums, coughs, asthma, and chest congestion.

Therapeutic Uses

Just as it has been for 1,000 years, today myrrh continues to be used for oral hygiene,

MOUTHWASH. Myrrh contains tannins, which have astringent action. Chinese researchers have identified other compounds in the herb that fight bacteria, and Indian scientists have discovered that it has anti-inflammatory action, all of which point to effectiveness as a mouthwash.

Myrrh tastes bitter but refreshing. It may help relieve the inflammation and destroy the bacteria involved in gingivitis, the early form of gum disease. Commission E, the expert panel that evaluates herbal medicines for the German counterpart of the FDA, approves myrrh as a treatment for mouth sores.

TOOTHPASTE. Myrrh is a common ingredient in European toothpastes. It's used to help fight the bacteria that cause tooth decay and gum disease. Indian researchers asked 30 people to brush with either Colgate toothpaste or a toothpaste containing myrrh. After brushing twice a day for a month, the Colgate group showed the same amount of dental plaque, but the myrrh users had significantly less.

PARASITES. Several veterinary studies show that myrrh kills intestinal parasites. These reports led to studies of the herb as a treatment for human schistosomiasis, a life-threatening, hard-to-treat parasite that infests some 150 million people in Asia and Africa. Egyptian researchers gave myrrh (600 milligrams/day for 6 days) to 67 people with schistosomiasis. Three months later, the researchers judged more than 90 percent cured. They called myrrh "safe and very effective." Another Egyptian study of 204 schistosomiasis sufferers also cured more than 90 percent. Side effects were mild and brief.

Intriguing Possibility

In an Italian study, treatment with myrrh appeared to raise the pain threshold of laboratory mice.

Myrrh may help prevent heart disease. Preliminary Indian studies suggest that the herb reduces cholesterol. It may also protect against the blood clots that trigger heart attack.

Rx Recommendations

To prepare a mouthwash, steep 1 teaspoon of powdered herb and 1 teaspoon of powdered boric acid in 1 pint of boiling water. Let stand for 30 minutes, then strain if you wish. Be sure the rinse is cool before using it. Do not swallow it.

For an infusion, use 1 teaspoon of powdered herb per cup of boiling water. Steep for 10 minutes, then strain if you wish. Drink up to 2 cups a day. Myrrh has an unpleasant, bitter taste. Add sugar, honey, and/or lemon, or mix into an herbal beverage tea.

If you return from travel to rural areas of Asia and Africa feeling ill and fatigued, consult a tropical medicine specialist. If you test positive for schistosomiasis, ask your doctor to try treating you with myrrh (600 milligrams/day).

As a homemade tincture, take $\frac{1}{4}$ to 1 teaspoon up to three times a day.

When using commercial preparations, follow package directions.

Safety

Myrrh has not been shown to stimulate uterine contractions, but its traditional use as a menstruation promoter should serve as a red flag to pregnant women. Nursing women should also avoid it.

Large doses of the herb may produce violent laxative action. They might also cause other symptoms described by the Eclectics: sweating, nausea, vomiting, and rapid heartbeat.

Do not give myrrh to children under 2. In older children, adjust the recommended dose based on the child's weight. Give a 50-pound child one-third of the dose a 150-pound adult would take.

If you're over 65, start with a low dose, and increase only if necessary.

Inform health professionals of the herbs you use. Problematic herb-drug interactions are possible.

Myrrh may cause allergic reactions or other unexpected side effects. If any develop, reduce your dose or stop taking it. For more on herb safety, see Chapter 2.

If symptoms get worse or persist longer than 2 weeks, consult a health professional promptly.

Gardening

Not grown in the United States. Myrrh is a large shrub or small tree that grows in the Middle East, Ethiopia, and Somalia. Pale yellow oil drips from cuts in its dull gray bark and hardens to form teardrop-shaped nuggets, which are powdered for medicinal purposes.

NEEM

The Indian Bug and Germ Killer

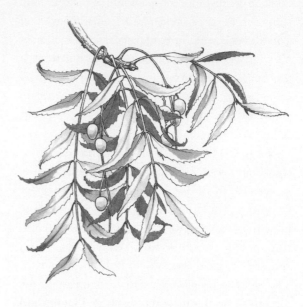

Family: Meliaceae; other members include mahogany

Genus and species: *Azadrichta indica*

Also known as: Margosa

Parts used: Leaf and bark extract

Recently, bugs infested one of my houseplants. I sprayed it with diluted neem oil. After two applications, the bugs were gone. Oil of neem is a widely marketed natural pesticide. But neem is far more than just an herbal bug killer. This Indian tree has been a mainstay of India's traditional Ayurvedic medicine for more than 1,000 years.

Healing History

The word neem comes from the Sanskrit *nimba*, meaning "bestower of good health." Its medical use dates back to India's ancient religious texts, the Vedas, which called the tree *sarva roga niva-rini*, "the one that cures all ailments." According to the Neem Foundation, based in Mumbai (Bombay), India, which promotes the tree's medical and commercial uses, neem is an ingredient in many traditional Ayurvedic medical formulas. Indians have used it for centuries to treat skin conditions: acne, eczema, psoriasis, warts, herpes, athlete's foot, chicken pox, and skin cancer.

Therapeutic Uses

The Vedic promise that neem "cures all ailments" is a stretch, but modern Indian researchers continue to gush over it. One extolled the tree as "omnipotent . . . a wonder tree because of its diverse utility." Diverse is right.

PESTICIDE. Many studies show that neem repels, kills, or disrupts reproduction of a large number of agricultural pests, among them, the boll weevil, which infests cotton, and the beetles that threaten Florida citrus groves. Neem may also help worldwide efforts to eradicate malaria. Though rare in the United States, malaria is the fourth leading cause of childhood death in the developing world, killing more than 700,000 people a year. Korean researchers have shown that at concentrations as low as one part per million, the neem constituent, azadirachtin, kills virtually 100 percent of the larvae of mosquitoes that transmit malaria. But unlike petrochemical pesticides, neem-based pesticides apparently carry no risk to nonpest animals.

DENTAL HEALTH. Neem extract kills the bacteria that cause plaque, tooth decay, and gum disease. Writing in the *International Dental Journal,* Indian researchers assessed the amount of dental plaque and gum inflammation in 48 volunteers and then asked them to use one of three products after breakfast and before bed: toothpaste containing neem extract, toothpaste with a pharmaceutical antiplaque ingredient, or a pharmaceutical mouthwash. After 6 weeks, the neem product was as effective as the pharmaceuticals.

ULCERS. Several studies show that neem reduces secretion of stomach acid and treats ulcers. One group of Indian researchers induced ulcers in animals and then gave them either neem leaf extract or an antiulcer drug, Zantac. The two were equally effective. Other Indian researchers measured stomach acid secretion in people with ulcers, and then gave them neem extract (30 milligrams twice a day). After 10 days, they showed a highly significant decrease in acid secretion. When the participants took 30 to 60 milligrams of bark extract twice a day for 10 weeks, their ulcers "almost completely healed" without significant side effects.

Intriguing Possibilities

Several animal studies show that neem leaf extract is spermicidal. But don't count on this herb as a reliable contraceptive.

In a laboratory study at Howard University in Washington, D.C., researchers exposed white blood cells to HIV, the virus that causes AIDS. They all became infected. Then they treated different white blood cells with neem leaf extract and subsequently exposed them to HIV. Only 25 percent became infected. Combine neem's anti-HIV and spermicidal actions, and the herb might be used by women intravaginally as a spermicide that helps prevent the spread of HIV.

Indian researchers recently tested the safety of such a spermicide in 20 women free of AIDS. The neem preparation caused some genital irritation, itching, and burning, but no medically worrisome side effects. The next step would be a larger study to test neem's effectiveness in the battle against AIDS transmission.

Rx Recommendations

Nurseries sell neem oil as a pesticide. Follow package directions.

Neem toothpaste and neem leaf and bark extracts are available at some health food stores. Or search "neem toothpaste" or "neem extract" on the Internet. Follow label directions.

Safety

It's fine to use toothpastes than contain neem—just be sure to spit it out. Neem oil is toxic. It has poisoned infants and children. Keep it away from children, and do not ingest it.

Pregnant and nursing women and children should not use neem.

If you're over 65, start with a low dose, and increase only if necessary.

Inform health professionals of the herbs you use. Problematic herb-drug interactions are possible.

Neem may cause allergic reactions or other unexpected side effects. If any develop, reduce your dose or stop taking it. For more on herb safety, see Chapter 2.

If symptoms get worse or persist longer than 2 weeks, consult a health professional promptly.

Gardening

Neem is a broad-leafed evergreen tree native to India that can grow to 100 feet with a trunk girth of 8 feet. It produces large, honey-scented flowers. It prefers tropical or subtropical conditions, but can survive temperatures that fall as low as 35°F for brief periods. It prefers rich soil, but can thrive in just about any soil that is not marshy or waterlogged. Indians have introduced it to Fiji, Africa, Australia, Latin America, and the American Southwest.

Neem trees also thrive indoors as potted plants. They do best in south-facing windows under full sun. Plant seeds in well-drained potting mix. Water regularly. Fertilize periodically.

NETTLE

Good News for Men with Enlarged Prostates

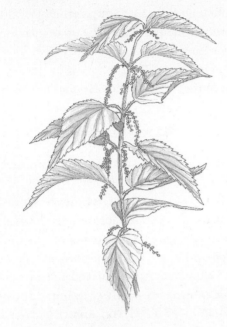

Family: Urticaceae; other members include other nettles

Genus and species: *Urtica dioica*

Also known as: Stinging nettle, common nettle, and greater nettle

Parts used: Leaves, stems, and roots

Nettle stings hurt, but this herb can also help men over 50 who have noncancerous prostate enlargement, medically known as benign prostatic hypertrophy (BPH).

Healing History

Around the third century BC, Hippocrates' Greek contemporaries prescribed nettle juice externally to treat snakebite and scorpion stings and internally as an antidote to plant poisons such as hemlock and henbane. (Nettle is not an antidote to these poisons.)

When in cold climates, Roman soldiers flailed themselves with nettle branches because the herb's sting warmed their skin. This practice, called urtication, evolved into a treatment for the joint stiffness of arthritis that is still in use today.

Early European herbalists touted nettle tea to combat cough and tuberculosis. Strange as it seems today, as a treatment for asthma, they recommended smoking the herb. Herbalists also prescribed nettle to cure scurvy and stop bleeding, particularly nosebleeds.

As time passed, nettle juice gained reputations for preventing scurvy and stimulating hair growth. It remained an ingredient in hair-growth nostrums well into the 19th century.

Seventeenth-century English herbalist Nicholas Culpeper endorsed all the nettle prescriptions that preceded him, then added one of his own: "The decoction of the leaves in wine is singularly good to provoke women's courses [menstruation]."

Native American women believed that drinking nettle tea during pregnancy strengthened the fetus and eased delivery. They also used the herb to stop uterine bleeding after childbirth, an application that early settlers adopted. Nursing mothers took nettle to increase milk production.

America's 19th-century Eclectic physicians, forerunners of today's naturopaths, recommended nettle primarily as a diuretic to treat urinary, bladder, and kidney problems. The Eclectic text *King's American Dispensatory* (1898) describes the herb as an excellent styptic (bleeding stopper) and treatment for infant diarrhea, hemorrhoids, and eczema.

Contemporary herbalists recommend nettle

mostly for treatment of BPH, but also as a diuretic.

Therapeutic Uses

BENIGN PROSTATE ENLARGEMENT.
Traditionally, doctors prescribed diuretics to treat BPH. In 1950, a German researcher tried nettle root, with some success—increased urine volume and less need to get up at night to urinate. But nettle was largely forgotten as a BPH treatment until the 1970s and did not become widely used in the United States until the 1990s.

Nettle works by inhibiting 5-alpha-reductase, an enzyme that plays a key role in the overgrowth of prostate tissue that's characteristic of BPH. (The pharmaceuticals used to treat BPH are also 5-alpha-reductase inhibitors.)

Iranian researchers gave 620 BPH sufferers either a placebo or nettle (120 milligrams/day). After 6 months, 16 percent of the placebo group reported benefits using standard measures of BPH. But in the nettle group, the figure was 81 percent.

In most studies, nettle has been paired with saw palmetto. Russian researchers gave 257 men with BPH either a placebo or a combination of nettle (120 milligrams twice a day) and saw palmetto (160 milligrams twice a day) for 6 months, then stopped treatment and followed the men for another year. Compared with the placebo group, urine flow in the herb group improved 19 percent, and overall BPH symptoms scores fell by half.

German researchers gave 140 BPH sufferers a standard dose of a popular pharmaceutical BPH treatment (Flomax) or a combination of nettle (120 milligrams twice a day) and saw palmetto (160 milligrams twice a day). After more than a year, both treatments showed the same benefit. The herb combination worked as well as the drug.

Commission E, the expert panel that evaluates herbal medicines for the German counterpart of the FDA, endorses nettle root preparations for mild to moderate BPH.

URINARY TRACT INFECTIONS.
As a diuretic, nettle can help flush the bladder of the bacteria that cause urinary tract infections (UTIs). Commission E approves nettle leaf preparations for the prevention of UTIs and kidney stones.

HIGH BLOOD PRESSURE.
In the United States, physicians prescribe pharmaceutical diuretics to treat high blood pressure. In Germany, where herbal medicine is more mainstream, doctors may prescribe nettle instead of drugs. According to noted German medical herbalist Rudolph Fritz Weiss, M.D., "Nettle juice is definitely useful [in] diuretic therapy. It has the advantage of being well tolerated and safe, as distinct from the [pharmaceutical] thiazides."

High blood pressure is a serious condition that requires professional care. If you'd like to include nettle in your overall treatment plan, discuss it with your physician.

CONGESTIVE HEART FAILURE.
Physicians may prescribe diuretics to treat the fluid retention associated with congestive heart failure. This condition demands professional care. If you'd like to include nettle in your treatment plan, talk to your physician.

PREMENSTRUAL SYNDROME (PMS).
Diuretics help relieve the bloating caused by premenstrual fluid buildup. Women bothered by

PMS may want to try taking nettle in the days before their periods.

HAY FEVER. A study at the National College of Naturopathic Medicine in Portland, Oregon, found that freeze-dried nettle (300 milligrams twice a day) provides significant relief from hay fever symptoms.

ARTHRITIS. German researchers assessed the pain of 40 people with various forms of arthritis, including osteoarthritis, rheumatoid arthritis, and gout. Then they gave 20 of them a standard dose of the prescription arthritis medication diclofenac (Voltaren, 200 milligrams/day). The rest took just 50 milligrams of the drug plus about 2 ounces of stewed nettle leaves. (Cooking removes the nettle hairs and their sting, making the leaves a vegetable similar to spinach.) After 2 weeks, both the drug-only group and the drug-nettle group reported about 70 percent improvement in their pain scores.

Diclofenac is a nonsteroidal anti-inflammatory drug (NSAID). NSAIDs may cause abdominal distress and gastrointestinal bleeding, which can become serious. Combining diclofenac with nettle provided equivalent pain relief while allowing a substantial decrease in the NSAID dose—meaning less risk of NSAID side effects.

SCURVY. Nettle is a good source of vitamin C. This validates the herb's traditional role in treating scurvy, caused by vitamin C deficiency.

Intriguing Possibility

Nettle has some antioxidant action, suggesting that it might help prevent and treat cancer. German researchers have discovered that nettle root extract impairs the growth of prostate cancer cells. In the future, this herb might treat not just BPH, but also prostate cancer.

Rx Recommendations

To prepare a pleasant-tasting diuretic infusion, use 1 to 2 teaspoons of dried herb per cup of boiling water. Steep for 10 minutes, then strain. Drink up to 3 cups a day.

As a tincture, use $\frac{1}{4}$ to 1 teaspoon up to twice a day.

To treat hay fever, look for freeze-dried nettle capsules in health food stores. If you can't find them, try an infusion or a tincture.

For arthritis, harvest nettle leaves (wearing gloves and protective clothing), then steam the leaves until they are wilted. If you don't have access to nettle leaves, try an infusion or a tincture.

To treat BPH, buy a commercial root preparation and follow package directions.

Safety

Nettle's main safety issue is its sting. The hairs that give the herb a downy appearance are actually hollow needles attached to sacs filled with irritant compounds. Brushing against the plant bends the hairs, squeezing the irritants onto the skin. The pain can last for 12 hours.

Herbal folklore is filled with remedies for nettle stings. One age-old recommendation is to rub the affected area with nettle juice. Rubbing with other herbs—notably peppermint—also reportedly helps. This makes some sense. The menthol in peppermint has some anesthetic action.

The most famous remedy for nettle stings is

dock, immortalized in this old British rhyme: "Nettle in, dock out / Dock rub nettle out." Non-herbal treatments include washing the affected skin with soap and water, applying topical hydrocortisone cream (such as Cort-Aid), and taking oral antihistamines.

Diuretics deplete the body of potassium, an essential nutrient. If you take nettle frequently, be sure to eat potassium-rich foods such as bananas and fresh vegetables.

Some weight-loss programs tout diuretics to eliminate water weight, but weight-loss experts advise against taking diuretics. Any pounds lost this way almost invariably return. The key to permanent weight control is a low-calorie, low-fat, high-fiber diet and regular, moderate exercise.

Nettle has been shown to stimulate uterine contractions in rabbits. For this reason and because of its diuretic action, pregnant women should not take the herb internally. Nursing women should also avoid diuretics.

Do not give nettle to children under 2. In older children, adjust the recommended dose based on the child's weight. Give a 50-pound child one-third of the dose a 150-pound adult would take.

If you're over 65, start with a low dose, and increase only if necessary.

Inform health professionals of the herbs you use. Problematic herb-drug interactions are possible.

Nettle may cause allergic reactions or other unexpected side effects. If any develop, reduce your dose or stop taking it. For more on herb safety, see Chapter 2.

If symptoms get worse or persist longer than 2 weeks, consult a health professional promptly.

Gardening

Nettle is only one of 500 species of *Urtica*, a name derived from the Latin *uro*, meaning "to burn." And burn they do. Just be thankful that the Javanese species, *U. urentissima*, doesn't grow in North America. Its burning sting may last a year.

Nettle's erect stem grows from a creeping underground rhizome. It has opposite, serrated, heart-shaped, dark green leaves. It is dioecious, meaning that male and female flowers grow on separate plants. If you harvest nettle, wear heavy gloves, a long-sleeved shirt, and long pants to avoid contact with the hairs and the irritants they transmit.

Nettle grows very easily from seeds or root divisions in just about any soil. Plant seeds in spring. Take root divisions in autumn after the leaves have died back.

Harvest the leaves (wearing gloves and protective clothing) before the plants flower in late spring or early summer. You may boil or steam young leaves like spinach and eat them as a vegetable. Boiling or drying eliminates the sting. The fresh tender shoots do not sting and may be used in salads.

PAPAYA

The Tropical Digestive Aid

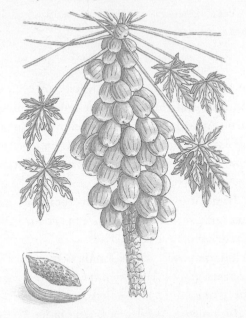

Family: Caricaceae; other members include custard apple

Genus and species: *Carica papaya*

Also known as: Pawpaw and melon tree

Parts used: Fruits, leaves, and latex

Cookbooks caution that gelatin (Jell-O) won't gel if you add pineapple. The same is true if you add papaya, only more so. Both fruits contain digestive enzymes that prevent the proteins in gelatin from solidifying. Those powerful enzymes are key to papaya's therapeutic powers.

Healing History

Centuries ago, the indigenous peoples of the Caribbean noticed that meat wrapped in papaya's broad leaves became more tender. Today, papaya extract is the active ingredient in most commercial meat tenderizers.

Caribbean peoples cut incisions into mature but unripe papayas, collected the milky fluid (latex), and applied it to their skin to treat psoriasis, ringworm, wounds, and infections. Caribbean women ate unripe papayas to trigger menstruation, abortion, and labor.

After Europeans introduced papaya into tropical Asia, it quickly became incorporated into local healing practices. Filipinos used a root decoction to treat hemorrhoids. The Javanese believed that eating papaya fruit prevented arthritis. The Japanese used the latex to treat digestive disorders. And throughout Asia, the leaves were applied to wounds.

Papaya played no role in traditional American herbal medicine. But since the 1980s, as tropical fruits have become more widely available in this country, papaya has grown in popularity—and the plant's leaves and latex are available in some specialty herb shops.

Contemporary herbalists recommend papaya fruit and leaf infusions to aid digestion, ease stomach upset, and eliminate intestinal worms. They also suggest applying the leaves and latex externally to wounds.

Therapeutic Uses

Papaya fruit, leaves, and latex contain several enzymes that account for the herb's action as a digestive aid and its ability to tenderize—that is, predigest—the protein in meats. The latex contains the most enzymes, followed by the leaves and then the fruit, but even fruit's enzymes enhance digestion. (Incidentally, one of those enzymes, papain, is the active ingredient in cleaning solutions for soft contact lenses.)

DIGESTIVE PROBLEMS. Of all papaya's enzymes, papain may be the most important. It's similar to the human digestive enzyme pepsin, which breaks down proteins. In fact, papain is sometimes called "vegetable pepsin." Papaya's other enzymes are similar to rennin, which breaks down milk proteins, and to pectase, which helps digest starches.

HERNIATED DISKS. In 1982, the FDA approved another papaya enzyme, chymopapain, as a treatment for herniated ("slipped") vertebral disks in the back. Injected directly into the affected area, chymopapain helps dissolve cellular debris.

Intriguing possibility

Animal research suggests that papaya may help prevent ulcers. Two groups of animals ingested large doses of ulcer-inducing aspirin and steroids after some had eaten papaya for 6 days. The papaya group developed significantly fewer ulcers, implying that people who take aspirin or steroids regularly might benefit by eating papaya.

Rx Recommendations

Papaya fruit is ripe when soft and tastes similar to cantaloupe. Have some with meals to stimulate digestion. Caribbean cuisines use the fruit liberally.

For a pleasant-tasting infusion to aid digestion, use 1 to 2 teaspoons of dried, powdered leaves per cup of boiling water. Steep for 10 minutes, then strain if you wish. Drink during or after meals, especially those high in protein (red meat and dairy products). Do not boil papaya leaves; boiling deactivates the papain.

When using commercial preparations, follow package directions.

Safety

Pregnant and nursing women and children may eat ripe papaya fruit but should avoid the latex and medicinal doses of the herb's leaves. Many cultures used papaya latex and leaves as a menstruation promoter and labor inducer.

Some allergic reactions, including asthma, have been reported. The latex may cause stomach inflammation (gastritis).

Inform health professionals of the herbs you use. Problematic herb-drug interactions are possible. For more on herb safety, see Chapter 2.

If symptoms get worse or persist longer than 2 weeks, consult a health professional promptly.

Gardening

Native to the Caribbean and now naturalized throughout the tropics, papaya trees reach 25 feet. The trunk is hollow, with spongy wood and fibrous, light-colored bark used to make rope. Its leaves are smooth, hand-shaped (palmate), and large, often 2 feet across.

The fruits are yellow-green, pear-shaped, mini-melons, hence the name melon tree, with tasty orange-yellow pulp. Papayas sold in the United States are typically the size of large potatoes, but in the tropics, they grow much larger and weigh up to 10 pounds.

PARSLEY

More Than Just a Garnish

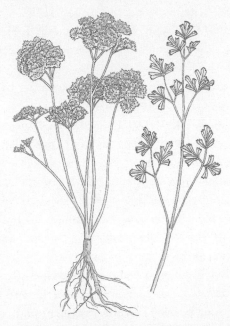

Family: Umbelliferae; other members include carrot, celery, fennel, dill, and angelica

Genus and species: *Petroselinum crispurn*, *P. hortense*, and *P. sativum*

Also known as: Rock selinon

Parts used: Leaves, fruits (seeds), and roots

Few herbs are more familiar than parsley. Recipes galore call for it and the lacy sprigs adorn many restaurant plates—often remaining uneaten. How unfortunate. Parsley is nutritious and an effective after-meal breath freshener, among other benefits.

Healing History

Parsley is one of the first herbs to appear in spring. For centuries, it has been used in the Seder, the ritual Jewish Passover meal, as a symbol of new beginnings.

The ancient Greeks saw this herb differently. In Greek mythology, parsley sprang from the blood of Opheltes, infant son of King Lycurgus of Nemea, who was killed by a serpent while his nanny directed thirsty soldiers to a spring. For centuries, Greek soldiers believed that any contact with parsley before battle signaled impending death. Because of its death association, the Greeks planted parsley on graves.

Eventually, parsley's association with death faded as it came to symbolize strength. Later Greeks crowned athletic victors with parsley wreaths.

But the shadow of bad luck clung to the herb well into the Middle Ages. Some Europeans considered parsley a "devil's herb," sure to bring disaster upon those who grew it—unless they planted it on Good Friday.

Parsley was not widely used in ancient medicine, but the Roman physician Galen prescribed it for "falling sickness" (epilepsy) and as a diuretic for water retention. The Romans also munched sprigs to freshen their breath—the beginnings of the parsley garnish on restaurant plates.

Medieval German abbess/herbalist Hildegard of Bingen prescribed parsley compresses for arthritis and parsley boiled in wine for chest and heart pain.

Seventeenth-century English herbalist Nicholas Culpeper reiterated Galen's recommendations and added to them, prescribing parsley to "provoke urine and women's courses [menstruation] . . . to expel wind . . . to break the stone [kidney stones] and ease the pains and torments thereof . . . and against cough." Culpeper also endorsed parsley compresses for inflamed eyes and black-and-blue marks, and suggested that the herb "fried with butter and applied to [the] breasts" relieved nipple soreness in nursing mothers.

Over the centuries, herbalists recommended topical applications of parsley to treat insect bites, wounds, and lice and internally to treat dysentery, gallstones, and some tumors.

From the 1850s through 1926, the *U.S. Pharmacopoeia*, a standard drug reference, recognized parsley as a laxative, a substitute for quinine in treating malaria, and a diuretic for kidney problems and the fluid accumulation of congestive heart failure.

America's 19th-century Eclectic physicians, forerunners of today's naturopaths, echoed the *U.S. Pharmacopoeia*. Their text, *King's American Dispensatory* (1898), chronicled the isolation of apiol from parsley oil and recommended it as a treatment for "menstrual derangements," although it also noted that high doses could cause "intoxication, giddiness, flashes of light, vertigo, and ringing in the ears [tinnitus]."

During the early 20th century, large doses of apiol were used to induce abortion, despite its considerable toxicity.

Contemporary herbalists recommend parsley in cooking as a rich source of vitamins A and C, calcium, and iron. They suggest the fresh herb as a breath freshener and an infusion or a tincture as a diuretic, digestive aid, and gas expeller.

Therapeutic Uses

Parsley roots, leaves, and fruits (seeds) all contain the plant's volatile oil, but seeds contain the highest concentrations.

Parsley oil contains the compounds apiol and myristicin, two significant diuretics that are also uterine stimulants and mild laxatives. Commission E, the expert panel that evaluates herbal medicines for the German counterpart of the FDA, approves parsley as a diuretic.

BAD BREATH. Parsley is unusually rich in the green plant pigment chlorophyll, which is the active ingredient in many breath fresheners, for example, Clorets. This supports the herb's ancient use as a breath freshener.

HIGH BLOOD PRESSURE. Physicians often prescribe diuretics to treat high blood pressure. A study in the *American Journal of Chinese Medicine* suggests that parsley's diuretic action helps control blood pressure. In Germany, where herbal medicine is more mainstream than in the United States, doctors often prescribe parsley seed tea for high blood pressure.

High blood pressure is a serious health problem that requires professional care. If you'd like to include parsley in your treatment plan, consult your physician.

CONGESTIVE HEART FAILURE. Physicians often prescribe diuretics to combat the fluid accumulation of congestive heart failure. This condition demands professional care. If you'd like to include parsley in your treatment regimen, talk to your physician.

PREMENSTRUAL SYNDROME (PMS). As a diuretic, parsley may help relieve the bloated feeling caused by premenstrual fluid buildup. Women bothered by PMS might eat more parsley before their periods. Try tabouli, the parsley-rich Mediterranean salad.

LABOR. Both apiol and myristicin are uterine stimulants. Russian physicians and midwives use a preparation, Supetin, to induce uterine contractions during labor. It contains 85 percent parsley juice.

ALLERGIES. A study published in the *Journal of Allergy and Clinical Immunology* shows that parsley inhibits the secretion of histamine, which triggers allergy symptoms. Parsley's apparent antihistamine action may help people with hay fever or hives.

FEVER. Parsley has never been proven effective against malaria, so the *U.S. Pharmacopoeia* was incorrect on that score. But apiol helps reduce fever (antipyretic). Don't count on parsley to replace aspirin, ibuprofen, or acetaminophen, but you might try it in addition to mainstream medications.

Intriguing Possibilities

Animal studies suggest that parsley reduces blood sugar levels, suggesting value in treating diabetes.

Parsley contains psoralen, a chemical that's best known for causing sun sensitivity. But psoralen shows promise in the treatment of one form of cancer, cutaneous T-cell lymphoma.

Rx Recommendations

To freshen breath, chew on a few sprigs of fresh parsley.

For a pleasant-tasting infusion, use 2 teaspoons of dried leaves or root or 1 teaspoon of crushed seeds per cup of boiling water. Steep for 10 minutes, then strain. Drink up to 3 cups a day.

As a homemade tincture, take ½ to 1 teaspoon up to three times a day.

When using commercial preparations, follow package directions.

Safety

Warning: Unless you are an experienced field botanist, *never* pick wild parsley. It closely resembles three potentially lethal plants: water hemlock, poison parsley (also known as poison hemlock), and fool's parsley (dog parsley or small hemlock).

Diuretics deplete the body of potassium, an essential nutrient. If you use medicinal preparations of parsley frequently, eat potassium-rich foods such as bananas and fresh vegetables.

Some weight-loss programs tout diuretics to eliminate water weight, but weight-management experts discourage this. Pounds lost with diuretics almost invariably return. The key to permanent weight control is a low-calorie, low-fat, high-fiber diet and regular moderate exercise.

Pregnant women may eat culinary amounts of parsley, but should avoid medicinal preparations, except possibly at term and under the supervision of a health professional, to help induce labor. Other women might try parsley tea to bring on their periods.

Nursing women should avoid diuretics, including medicinal amounts of parsley.

The psoralen in parsley has been known to cause skin rashes in agricultural workers who harvest large quantities. People with sensitive skin should be aware of this possible side effect.

The Eclectics were right about large doses of parsley oil causing headache, nausea, vertigo, giddiness, hives, and liver and kidney damage. But the medical literature contains no reports of problems from the herb itself, even when used in medicinal quantities.

Children may eat parsley sprigs. But do not give medicinal preparations of parsley to children under 2. In older children, adjust the recommended dose based on the child's weight. Give a 50-pound child one-third of the dose a 150-pound adult would take.

If you're over 65, start with a low dose, and increase only if necessary.

Inform health professionals of the herbs you use. Problematic herb-drug interactions are possible.

Parsley may cause allergic reactions or other unexpected side effects. If any develop, reduce your dose or stop taking it. For more on herb safety, see Chapter 2.

If symptoms get worse or persist longer than 2 weeks, consult a health professional promptly.

Gardening

Parsley is a small, bright green biennial that reaches 12 inches the first year and up to 3 feet the second year, when it flowers. The plant has a thick, carrot-like taproot and juicy stems terminating in feathery, deeply divided, curly or flat leaves, depending on variety. Its tiny yellow-green flowers develop on the umbrella-like canopy (umbels) characteristic of the Umbelliferae family.

Although it's a biennial, parsley should be cultivated as an annual. The seeds are slow to germinate, often requiring up to 6 weeks. Sow them any time from early spring to autumn. Parsley can be sown indoors and transplanted, but most authorities recommend outdoor planting with ¼ inch of soil cover.

Parsley grows best in moist, sandy, well-drained loam with a neutral pH. Thin seedlings to 8-inch spacing. Late-season planting is fine. Even as a seedling, the herb usually survives one or two frosts.

Harvest when plants have reached about 8 inches. Harvest the fruits when they appear full size and gray brown. Dig the roots during the autumn of the first year or the spring of the second.

PASSIONFLOWER

Relieves Tension and Insomnia

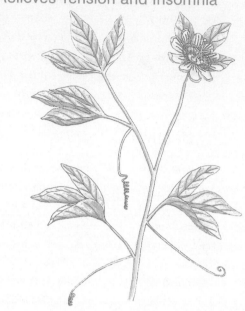

Family: Passifloraceae; other members include granadilla, sweet calabash, and Jamaican honeysuckle

Genus and species: *Passiflora incarnata*

Also known as: Maypop, apricot vine, and water lemon

Parts used: Leaves

Around 1560, two decades years after Francisco Pizarro brutally crushed the Incas' last rebellion and forced their conversion to Christianity, Dr. Nicolas Monardes of Seville apparently developed a guilty conscience for his countrymen's carnage. An avid botanist, he studied the plants sent back from the New World for some sign of divine approval of the Spanish conquest. He found it in a vine that had large, beautiful blossoms with parts that seemed to evoke the Passion of the Crucifixion.

To Dr. Monardes, the plant's three styles represented the three nails of the cross. Its ovary looked like a hammer. Its corona evoked the crown of thorns, and its 10 petals suggested the 10 true apostles (the original 12 minus Judas, the betrayer, and Peter, who denied Christ). Dr. Monardes christened the vine passionflower.

Healing History

The Incas brewed a tonic tea from passionflower. The herb's pleasant taste and its Christian symbolism quickly turned its leaves into a popular item in Europe, where it was used as a tranquilizer and mild sedative.

When colonists settled the American Gulf Coast, they found the area's Native Americans using a tea made from local passionflower to calm nervousness. They also applied the crushed leaves as poultices on cuts and bruises.

Southerners adopted passionflower as an ornamental and used it medicinally as a tranquilizer. In 1839, two Gulf Coast Eclectic physicians touted it in the *New Orleans Medical Journal* as a nonnarcotic sedative and digestive aid.

The Eclectics, forerunners of today's naturopaths, adopted passionflower as "an important remedy" for insomnia, restlessness, menstrual discomforts, diarrhea, epilepsy, and whooping cough. They also prescribed the leaf juice externally for burns, scalds, wounds, and toothache.

Contemporary herbalists recommend passionflower primarily as a tranquilizer and sedative. They also consider it a digestive aid and pain reliever.

From 1916 to 1936, passionflower was recognized as a tranquilizer and sedative in the *National Formulary*, the pharmacists' reference. But in 1978, the FDA banned the herb from sleep aids for lack of proven effectiveness.

Therapeutic Uses

If the FDA had kept up herbal research since the 1970s, the agency might have reconsidered its ban.

STRESS, ANXIETY, INSOMNIA. Passionflower contains several tranquilizing compounds—maltol, flavonoids, and passiflorine, which is chemically similar to morphine. The plant also contains stimulants (harmala compounds). Various researchers have concluded that the herb has complex activity in the central nervous system, with an overall mild tranquilizing-sedative effect despite the presence of stimulants.

Passionflower is clearly sedative in both animals and humans. French researchers gave 91 people with anxiety problems either a placebo or a preparation containing passionflower and several other herbs (including hawthorn and valerian). After 28 days, those taking the herb formula reported significantly less anxiety.

In Europe, passionflower is an ingredient in many tranquilizing and sedative preparations. It's nonnarcotic, so no need for a prescription, and no possibility of addiction. Commission E, the expert panel that evaluates herbal medicines for the German counterpart of the FDA, approves passionflower for nervousness and restlessness.

ATTENTION DEFICIT HYPERACTIVITY DISORDER (ADHD). German researchers gave 115 children with ADHD, age 6 to 12, a three-herb combination one to three times a day: St. John's wort (60 milligrams), valerian root

(28 milligrams), and passionflower (32 milli-grams). In consultation with the children's physicians, some took only the herb formula while others used the herbs along with pharmaceuticals. After 1 month, based on parental observations and physician evaluations, 87 percent of the children showed improvement. Those who took the herbs with one or more drugs fared no better than the kids who took only the herbs.

DIGESTIVE PROBLEMS. Passionflower relaxes the smooth muscle lining the digestive tract (antispasmodic), which lends credence to its traditional use as a digestive aid.

WOMEN'S HEALTH. Antispasmodics relax not only the digestive tract but also other smooth muscles, such as the uterus. Women might try it for menstrual discomforts.

WOUNDS. One study suggests that passionflower helps relieve pain, while two others show that it kills many disease-causing molds, fungi, and bacteria. These findings support the Native American and Eclectic use of passionflower as a wound treatment.

Intriguing Possibilities

In animal studies, passionflower's harmala compounds dilate (open) the coronary arteries. Blocked coronary arteries result in heart attack, so the herb may help prevent and treat heart disease.

Animals experimentally addicted to morphine experienced easier withdrawal when treated with passionflower.

Rx Recommendations

For first-aid in the garden, crush a few passionflower leaves and flowers and press into minor cuts until you can wash and bandage them.

For a pleasant-tasting infusion that may help you relax, calm down, or fall asleep, use 1 teaspoon of dried leaves per cup of boiling water. Steep for 10 to 15 minutes, then strain. For insomnia, drink a cup of tea before bed. For other conditions, drink up to 3 cups a day.

As a homemade tincture, take $\frac{1}{4}$ to 1 teaspoon up to three times a day.

When using commercial preparations, follow label directions.

Safety

Some sources warn that passionflower contains cyanide, a potent poison. This is a botanical error. Ornamental blue passionflower, *Passiflora caerulea*, contains the poison. The healing herb, *P. incarnata*, does not. Check labels to be sure you're buying *P. incarnata*.

The harmala compounds in passionflower are uterine stimulants. Whole passionflower has not been associated with miscarriage, but pregnant women would be prudent to stay away from an herb with such complex effects on the central nervous system. Nursing women should also avoid it.

Do not give passionflower to children under 2. In older children, adjust the recommended dose based on the child's weight. Give a 50-pound child one-third of the dose a 150-pound adult would take.

If you're over 65, start with a low dose, and increase only if necessary.

Inform health professionals of the herbs you use. Problematic herb-drug interactions are possible.

Passionflower may cause allergic reactions or other unexpected side effects. If any develop, reduce your dose or stop taking it. For more on herb safety, see Chapter 2.

If symptoms get worse or persist longer than 2 weeks, consult a health professional promptly.

Gardening

Passionflower has a perennial root with fast-growing, climbing, annual tendrils that may reach 30 feet. The leaves are dull green, 4 to 6 inches long, and deeply divided into three to five lobes with serrated edges. Its sweet-scented white flowers are 3 inches across and tinged with purple. They bloom in May, hence the name maypops, and produce egg-size yellow or orange edible fruits, the source of the names apricot vine and water lemon.

Passionflower grows easily from seeds, cuttings, or root runners divided in autumn. It prefers rich, slightly acidic, well-watered, well-drained loam in locations with plenty of light but shaded from strong, direct summer sun.

The perennial root is hardy but may not survive temperatures below 25°F. The vine tendrils need something to climb on, such as a fence or trellis.

Harvest leaves when plants bloom. If generously watered, the fruits are edible and sweet.

PAU D'ARCO
The Bark That Treats Yeast Infections

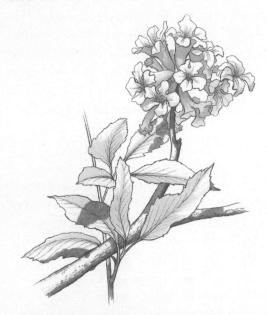

Family: Bignoniaceae; other members include jacaranda

Genus and species: *Tabebuia impetiginosa*

Also known as: lapacho, ipe, taheebo, trumpet tree

Parts used: Inner bark

The Incas used the wood of the South American tree they called *lapacho* to make bows for hunting. The Spanish adopted this use and called the tree pau d'arco, meaning "bow stick." The name stuck, and now it refers to various trees of the *Tabebuia* genus that grow in the mountains of Brazil, Argentina, Bolivia, Paraguay, and Peru. But pau d'arco does more than shoot arrows. It also helps treat vaginal yeast infections—and shows promise against cancer.

Healing History

A thousand years ago, the Incas considered pau d'arco indispensable for treating fever, sore throat, dysentery, snakebite, bladder and yeast infections, and even cancer. Early explorers noticed that while most nearby trees had fungus growing on them, pau d'arco did not. As a result, the tree began to be used to treat fungal infections.

Therapeutic Uses

YEAST INFECTION. Speaking of fungal infections, pau d'arco is effective against *Candida albicans*, the fungus that causes vaginal yeast infections. Writing in the *British Journal of Phytotherapy,* a Dutch researcher suggests soaking a tampon in strong pau d'arco infusion while also taking the herb orally.

ANTIBIOTIC. Since the 1950s, South American researchers have shown that pau d'arco's inner bark has antibacterial action. Researchers at the University of Rio de Janeiro discovered that it helps treat *Staph* infections that resist pharmaceutical antibiotics. Korean researchers at Seoul National University have found that it's also active against the bacteria that cause food poisoning, thus validating the herb's traditional use as a treatment for dysentery. Brazilian researchers have found that pau d'arco kills some tropical parasites, among them, the organism that causes Chagas' disease. Finally, pau d'arco has some antiviral activity, especially against herpes.

Intriguing Possibilities

Pau d'arco might possibly treat cancer. During the 1950s, Brazilian researchers discovered that it was effective against leukemia and other can-cers. During the 1960s, our own National Cancer Institute (NCI) studied lapachol, the pau d'arco constituent with the most pronounced antitumor activity. But the NCI obtained disappointing results and gave up on the plant.

The NCI was a bit hasty. Recent studies by Korean researchers have focused on another pau d'arco constituent, beta-lapachone. Laboratory studies show that this compound kills cancer cells in the lung, colon, and prostate. Pau d'arco is still years away from being used to treat cancer, but the Incas may have been on to something.

Rx Recommendations

Follow package directions, but when using tablets or capsules, the recommended dose is 1 to 4 grams/day in divided doses. To use pau d'arco to treat yeast infection, open a few capsules and make a strong infusion, immerse a tampon, and insert. Repeat every few hours while also taking the herb by mouth. When using a tincture, take 1 to 2 teaspoons three times a day. A tampon may also be immersed in tincture.

Safety

Large doses may cause nausea, vomiting, diarrhea, and dizziness.

Pau d'arco has anticoagulant action. Users might notice that they bruise more easily and that cuts take longer to clot. Those with clotting disorders and anyone taking anticoagulant drugs or about to have surgery should not use this herb.

Pregnant and nursing women should not use it.

Do not give pau d'arco to children under 2. In older children, adjust the recommended dose based on the child's weight. Give a 50-pound child one-third of the dose a 150-pound adult would take.

If you're over 65, start with a low dose, and increase only if necessary.

Inform health professionals of the herbs you use. Problematic herb-drug interactions are possible.

Pau d'arco may cause allergic reactions or other unexpected side effects. If any develop, reduce your dose or stop taking it. For more on herb safety, see Chapter 2.

If symptoms get worse or persist longer than 2 weeks, consult a health professional promptly.

Gardening

Pau d'arco grows in the Andes and in parts of Paraguay and Brazil. It is not grown in the United States. It takes 40 years for tree to mature enough to produce medicinally valuable bark. The bark is similar to cork and can be harvested without killing the tree. Trees can live 700 years. They produce trumpet-shaped violet flowers, hence the name trumpet tree.

PELARGONIUM

For Bronchitis, Colds, and Tonsillitis

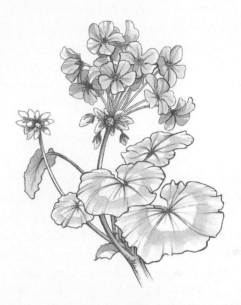

Family: Geraniaceae; other members include geranium

Genus and species: *Pelargonium sidoides*

Also known as: South African geranium, kalwerbossie, and rabassam

Parts used: Root juice

Native to the grasslands of southern Africa, *P. sidoides* is a low-growing perennial that produces velvety, heart-shaped, mildly aromatic leaves and distinctive dark, reddish purple (almost black) flowers in spring and summer. But this geranium is more than just a pretty plant. It's also a real healer.

Healing History

For centuries, the Zulu and other indigenous tribes of southern Africa used *Pelargonium sidoides* to treat respiratory conditions.

Therapeutic Uses

Pelargonium has immune-stimulating action. It activates germ-devouring natural killer cells and spurs production of interferon, which helps defend cells against infection.

COLDS. Ukrainian scientists gave 103 adult cold sufferers a placebo or *Pelargonium sidoides* (30 drops three times a day). In the pelargonium group, symptoms were only half as severe. After 10 days, 31 percent of the placebo group pronounced themselves cured. In the pelargonium group, the figure was 79 percent.

Another Ukrainian study involved 207 adults with initial cold symptoms who took a placebo or pelargonium (30 or 60 drops three times a day). On day 5, everyone rated their symptom severity. Compared with the placebo takers, both pelargonium groups reported symptoms only half as severe.

BRONCHITIS. In nonsmokers, bronchitis typically develops at the tail end of colds as a dry, hacking cough that can take weeks to resolve. Eventually, some people get fed up and see their doctors, who typically prescribe an antibiotic. Antibiotics treat bacterial bronchitis, but only rarely is cold-related bronchitis caused by bacteria. Before you call your doctor, try *P. sidoides*.

German researchers gave 468 adult bronchitis sufferers either a placebo or *P. sidoides* (30 drops of root juice three times a day). After 7 days, the herb provided significantly greater relief: "Treatment with pelargonium clearly reduced the severity of symptoms and allowed users to return to work 2 days faster."

Russian investigators gave 124 adult bronchitis sufferers either a placebo or pelargonium (30 drops three times a day). After 4 days, one-third of the placebo group reported improvement, but among those who took the herb, two-thirds said they felt better.

Other Russian scientists gave 220 children diagnosed with bronchitis either a placebo or pelargonium three times a day (10 drops age 1 to 6, 20 drops age 6 to 12, and 30 drops age 12 to 18). After 7 days, everyone felt better, but the herb group experienced faster, more complete recovery.

SINUS INFECTION. Doctors treat sinus infection with antibiotics, but sometimes the drugs don't work. Ukrainian researchers gave 104 people with sinus infections either a placebo or pelargonium (60 drops three times a day). After 21 days, those taking pelargonium reported residual symptoms only half as severe.

TONSILLITIS. Other Ukrainian researchers gave 143 children with tonsillitis either a placebo or *P. sidoides* (20 drops twice a day). After 6 days, the herb group reported significantly reduced symptoms.

Rx Recommendations

Most studies have used 30 drops three times a day. Or follow package directions.

Safety

Pelargonium has been a popular herbal medicine in German since the 1980s. No serious side effects have been reported, but stomach upset, and rarely, allergic reactions are possible.

Those with kidney or liver disease should avoid this herb.

Pregnant and nursing women should not use this herb.

Do not give this herb to children under 2. In

older children, adjust the recommended dose based on the child's weight. Give a 50-pound child one-third of the dose a 150-pound adult would take.

If you're over 65, start with a low dose, and increase only if necessary.

Inform health professionals of the herbs you use. Problematic herb-drug interactions are possible.

Pelargonium may cause allergic reactions or other unexpected side effects. If any develop, reduce your dose or stop taking it. For more on herb safety, see Chapter 2.

If symptoms get worse or persist longer than 2 weeks, consult a health professional promptly.

Gardening

Pelargonium sidoides can be grown indoors or out in temperate climates from seed or cuttings treated with rooting hormone. It grows to 6 to 12 inches. This herb prefers full sun, sandy or clay-loam soil, and generous watering in summer, less during winter. Once established, it's drought-tolerant. In spring, top dressing with fertilizer improves growth and flowers in summer. In winter, dead leaves and old flower stalks should be removed. Start outdoor plants in pots indoors, then transplant.

PENNYROYAL
A Good Herb with a Bad Reputation

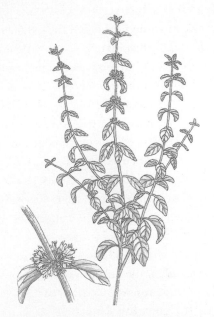

Family: Labiatae; other members include mints

Genus and species: *Mentha pulegium* (European); *Hedeoma pulegioides* (American)

Also known as: Pulegium, hedeoma, fleabane, tickweed, mosquito plant, and squawmint

Parts used: Leaves and flowers

Few healing herbs have a reputation as bad—or as undeserved—as pennyroyal. Critics charge that ingesting even small amounts can be fatal. While as little as 2 tablespoons of pennyroyal *oil* can cause death, the dried herb is not dangerous. Pennyroyal's highly aromatic leaves and flowers are a safe decongestant, cough remedy, and digestive aid.

Healing History

Pennyroyal became popular during the 1st century AD after the Roman naturalist Pliny noted that the aromatic plant repelled fleas (hence its name fleabane). When crushed and rubbed on the skin or strewn, pennyroyal repels other insects as well (hence the names tickweed and mosquito plant).

Pliny also touted pennyroyal as a cough remedy and digestive aid. He recommended hanging the plant in sickrooms in the belief that its fragrance promoted healing. The Greek physician Dioscorides agreed, adding that pennyroyal stimulates menstruation and helps expel the afterbirth.

During the early Middle Ages, pennyroyal was recommended for truly bizarre purposes. Physician-philosopher St. Albertus Magnus wrote that by covering drowning bees in the herb's warm ashes, "they shall recover their lyfe after a space of one houre."

During the 16th century, British herbalist John Gerard touted pennyroyal's ancient use as an expectorant: "Penny-royale taken with honey cleanseth the lungs and cleareth the breast from all gross and thick humors."

Seventeenth-century English herbalist Nicholas Culpeper recommended the herb for many other conditions: "Drunk with wine, it is of singular service to those stung or bit by any venomous beast . . . applied to the nostrils with vinegar, it is very reviving [for] fainting . . . being dried and burnt, it strengtheneth the gums, and is helpful for those troubled with the gout . . . being applied as a plaster, it taketh away carbuncles [boils]."

Colonists introduced European pennyroyal (*Mentha pulegium*) into North America but dis-covered that Native Americans were already using the American herb (*Hedeoma pulegioides*) for similar purposes—externally to dress wounds and repel insects and internally to treat colds, flu, coughs, and congestion and to stimulate menstruation and abortion. Folk healers also recommended aromatic pennyroyal garlands for headache and dizziness.

During the early 19th century, Thomsonian herbalists packed pennyroyal leaves into the nostrils to treat nosebleeds. After the Civil War, Eclectic physicians, forerunners of today's naturopaths, adopted the herb as a stimulant, fever treatment, digestive aid, and menstruation promoter. Their text *King's American Dispensatory* (1898) described the herb as "an excellent remedy for the common cold" and recommended it for arthritis, whooping cough (pertussis), "colic in children . . . and hysteria" (menstrual discomforts).

Around 1887, the Eclectics began using pennyroyal oil, which they considered more convenient than the raw herb. They also recognized its potential hazards. *King's Dispensatory* mentioned a case of pennyroyal poisoning caused by ingesting just 1 tablespoon.

From 1831 to 1916, the *U.S. Pharmacopoeia*, a standard drug reference, listed pennyroyal as a stimulant, digestive aid, and menstruation promoter. From 1916 to 1931, the book listed its oil as an intestinal irritant and abortion inducer.

Contemporary herbalists advise against ingesting pennyroyal oil because of its toxicity, but they recommend the whole herb externally as an insect repellent and treatment for cuts and burns. They also suggest taking the herb (not the oil) internally for colds, coughs, upset stomach, flatulence, anxiety, and menstruation promotion.

Therapeutic Uses

Despite their botanical differences, herbalists use European and American pennyroyal—and their oils—interchangeably. Pennyroyal oil contains pulegone, a compound that accounts for its ability to repel insects, promote menstruation, and induce abortion.

INSECT REPELLENT. Pliny was right. Pennyroyal oil helps repel flies, gnats, mosquitoes, fleas, and ticks. It is the active ingredient in most natural insect repellents. If you buy an herbal flea collar for your dog or cat, it's likely to contain pennyroyal oil.

CONGESTION AND COUGH. Pennyroyal is among the most aromatic mints. A strong, aromatic infusion can serve as a decongestant and expectorant.

DIGESTIVE PROBLEMS. Pennyroyal contains compounds similar to the stomach-soothing menthol in its botanical relative peppermint. While pennyroyal's stomach-settling action is weaker than peppermint's, the herb is still an effective digestive remedy.

Rx Recommendations

To repel insects, rub fresh, crushed plant material over your body, or mix pennyroyal tincture into a skin cream and apply.

To make an herbal flea collar, try hanging a pennyroyal garland or a bag of the herb from a regular collar. Do not apply pennyroyal oil to your pet's fur or skin. The animal may ingest a toxic dose from self-licking.

For an infusion to help treat coughs, congestion, or stomach upset, use 1 to 2 teaspoons of dried herb per cup of boiling water. Steep for 10 to 15 minutes, then strain. Drink up to two cups a day. Its aroma resembles spearmint's, but it's sharper and not as inviting. The taste is warm and pleasant, initially bitter with a cool finish.

As a homemade tincture, use $1/4$ to $1/2$ teaspoon up to twice a day.

When using commercial preparations, follow package directions.

Safety

Ever since pennyroyal's abortion-inducing oil was first distilled more than a century ago, the plant has been notorious because of its oil's toxicity. Pulegone does indeed stimulate uterine contractions. Unfortunately, the dose necessary for abortion is close to the lethal dose, a fact that many women learned the hard way. As little as $1/2$ teaspoon of pennyroyal oil can cause convulsions. Doses not much larger can be fatal.

The British journal *Lancet* cited a case of abortion-related pennyroyal oil poisoning as early as 1897. Since then, many similar reports have appeared. As recounted in the *Journal of the American Medical Association*, a pregnant 18-year-old woman died within 2 hours after taking 2 tablespoons of the oil, despite emergency treatment. Clearly, women wishing to terminate pregnancy should not use pennyroyal oil. In fact, no one should.

Although small amounts of pennyroyal oil can be fatal, the oil is a super-concentrated extract of the herb. Infusions made from dried pennyroyal leaves pose no hazard. University of Illinois pharmacognosist Norman Farnsworth, Ph.D., estimates that it would take 75 gallons of strong pennyroyal infusion to approach the potential toxicity of a fatal dose of pennyroyal oil.

Pregnant and nursing women should not use pennyroyal.

Do not give pennyroyal to children under 2. In older children, adjust the recommended dose based on the child's weight. Give a 50-pound child one-third of the dose a 150-pound adult would take.

If you're over 65, start with a low dose, and increase only if necessary.

Inform health care professionals of the herbs you use. Problematic herb-drug interactions are possible.

Pennyroyal may cause allergic reactions or other unexpected side effects. If any develop, reduce your dose or stop taking it. For more on herb safety, see Chapter 2.

If symptoms get worse or persist longer than 2 weeks, consult a health care professional promptly.

Gardening

The European herb is a perennial that spreads by underground runners. Its square stems grow to about 12 inches, and its opposite, oval leaves are smooth or slightly hairy. Tight whorls of small lilac flowers appear in midsummer. European pennyroyal may be propagated from root runner divisions in early spring or fall or by rooting stem cuttings during summer.

American pennyroyal is an annual with square stems that reach 15 inches. Its leaves resemble the European variety, but its summer-blooming flowers tend to be smaller and bluer. It must be grown from seeds sown in spring or fall. Cover them with ¼ inch of soil. Thin seedlings to 5-inch spacing.

Both plants do best in rich, well-watered, sandy, slightly acidic loam under full sun, though the European herb tolerates partial shade. It also needs room to spread. Its runners emerge after it flowers.

Harvest both plants' leaves and flowers when they are in full bloom. In fall, cut them back to a few inches above the ground and hang the herb to dry.

PEPPERMINT AND SPEARMINT

Marvelous Menthol

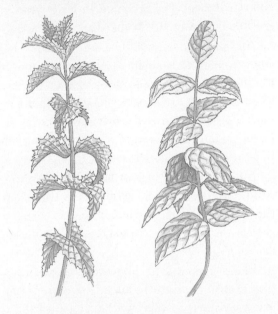

Family: Labiatae; other members include balm, basil, catnip, horehound, marjoram, and pennyroyal

Genus and species: *Mentha piperita* (peppermint); *M. spicata, M. viridis, M. aquatica, M. cardiaca* (spearmint)

Also known as: No other names, but there are hundreds of varieties of mint

Parts used: Leaves and flowers

Ever have an after-dinner mint? These candies evolved from the ancient custom of concluding feasts by chewing a sprig of mint to soothe the stomach. Modern research has shown the wisdom of this age-old practice and has verified several other therapeutic uses of peppermint and spearmint.

Both mints are popular in herbal medicine, and both have similar effects. But of the two, peppermint is generally regarded as tastier. It's more medicinally potent, too.

Spearmint was the original medicinal mint. Peppermint appeared later, a natural hybrid of spearmint species. Authorities aren't exactly sure which species combined to form the spicier mint or when it first appeared. All of the mints were considered one plant, mint, until 1696 when British botanist John Ray differentiated them.

Healing History

Mint was mentioned as a stomach soother in the Ebers Papyrus, the world's oldest surviving medical text. From Egypt, mint spread to Palestine, where it was accepted as payment for taxes. In *Luke* (11:39), Jesus scolds the Pharisees, "You pay tithes of mint and rue . . . but have no care for justice and the love of God."

From the Holy Land, mint spread to Greece and entered Greek mythology. It seems that Pluto, god of the dead, fell in love with the beautiful nymph Minthe. Pluto's goddess-wife, Persephone, became jealous and changed Minthe into mint. Pluto could not bring Minthe back to life, but he gave her plant a fragrant aroma. Minthe evolved into the mints' genus name, *Mentha*.

Greek and Roman homemakers added mint to milk to prevent spoilage and served the herb after meals as a digestive aid. The Roman naturalist Pliny wrote that mint "reanimates the spirit" and recommended hanging it in sickrooms to assist convalescence. The Greek physician Dioscorides considered mint "heating" and therefore a promoter of lust. Other Greek and Roman herbalists prescribed mint for everything from hiccups to leprosy.

Chinese and Ayurvedic physicians have used mint for centuries as a tonic and digestive aid and as a treatment for colds, coughs, and fevers.

Twelfth-century German abbess/herbalist Hildegard of Bingen recommended mint for digestion and gout.

Seventeenth-century English herbalist Nicholas Culpeper wrote, "[Mint] is very profitable to the stomach . . . especial to dissolve wind [and] help the colic . . . It is good to repress the milk in women's breasts . . . and a very powerful medicine to stay women's courses [stop menstrual flow]. It helpeth the biting of a mad dog . . . and is good to wash the heads of young children against all manner of breaking out, sores, and scabs. . . ."

Culpeper disagreed with Dioscorides on mint and sex, however. Instead of calling it a lust promoter, Culpeper considered it "an especial remedy for venereal [sexual] dreams and pollutions in the night [nocturnal emissions], being applied outwardly to the testicles."

Shortly after Culpeper's time, peppermint and spearmint were differentiated. Herbalists decided that the former was the better digestive aid, cough remedy, and treatment for colds and fever.

Colonists found Native Americans using American mints to treat coughs, chest congestion, and pneumonia. They introduced peppermint and spearmint, and the plants quickly went wild.

By the late late 19th century, the Eclectics, forerunners of today's naturopaths, prescribed peppermint for headache, coughs, bronchitis, stomach distress, and hysteria (menstrual discomforts). They also added it to laxatives to disguise their unpleasant taste and minimize intestinal cramping.

The Eclectics also valued spearmint but considered it "inferior to peppermint" except for its superior ability to treat fever.

Chemists distilled menthol from peppermint oil around 1880. The Eclectic text *King's American Dispensatory* (1898) touted menthol's "germicidal properties," and its "anesthetic power" when applied to wounds, burns, scalds, insect bites and stings, eczema, hives, and toothache. The Eclectics also used menthol vapors in inhalants and chest rubs to relieve asthma, hay fever, and morning sickness.

Contemporary herbalists recommend peppermint externally for itching and inflammations and internally as a digestive aid and treatment for menstrual cramps, motion sickness, morning sickness, colds, cough, flu, congestion, headache, heartburn, fever, and insomnia. Some herbalists consider peppermint and spearmint interchangeable, but most believe peppermint to be more potent. Herbalists also recommend these herbs for relaxing herbal baths.

Therapeutic Uses

Both spearmint and peppermint owe their healing value to their aromatic oils. Peppermint oil is mostly menthol. Spearmint oil contains a similar compound, carvone. These chemicals have similar properties, but as the herbalists of old believed, menthol is more potent and more widely used in herbal medicine.

DIGESTIVE PROBLEMS. Thumbs-up for after-dinner mints. Menthol and carvone soothe the smooth muscle lining the digestive tract, preventing muscle spasms (antispasmodics).

In Germany, where herbal medicine is more mainstream than in the United States, an over-the-counter digestive remedy, Enteroplant, has two active ingredients: peppermint oil (90 milli-grams/capsule) and caraway oil (50 milligrams/capsule). German researchers gave 45 people with chronic indigestion either a placebo or Enteroplant (one capsule three times a day with meals). After 4 weeks, the placebo group reported no change in abdominal distress, but 95 percent of the peppermint-caraway group reported significant improvement, with 63 percent declaring themselves pain-free.

In another German study, the scientists gave 118 adults with chronic indigestion either a standard pharmaceutical (ciapride, 10 milli-grams three times a day before meals) or Enteroplant before meals. Four weeks later, the herbal treatment produced slightly better results.

Commission E, the expert panel that evaluates herbal medicines for the German counterpart of the FDA, endorses peppermint for indigestion and abdominal distress.

NAUSEA. Cancer chemotherapy often causes nausea. Iranian researchers gave 200 cancer patients taking chemo one of four treatments: a standard pharmaceutical antinausea drug, the drug plus a placebo, the drug plus spearmint oil, or the drug plus peppermint oil. After several chemotherapy treatments, the two groups taking the mints reported fewer than half as many episodes of vomiting.

IRRITABLE BOWEL SYNDROME (IBS). This condition causes abdominal cramps, bloating, flatulence, diarrhea or constipation, and possibly heartburn and queasiness.

British scientists analyzed five studies of peppermint oil as a treatment for IBS. In three, the oil was enteric coated, meaning that the capsules passed intact through the very acidic stomach and released the oil in the intestine. In two, the capsules were uncoated and released

the oil in the stomach. The two studies that used noncoated capsules showed no benefit, but all studies employing enteric-coated capsules showed significant benefit. It appears that for peppermint oil to relieve IBS, the capsules must be coated.

University of Missouri researchers gave 50 children with IBS, age 8 to 17, either a placebo or enteric-coated peppermint oil (depending on their weight, either 94 milligrams or 187 milligrams three times a day). After 2 weeks, 43 percent of the placebo group reported improvement but in the peppermint group, 71 percent, a highly significant difference. None of the placebo takers said they felt "much better," 42 percent of the herb group did.

Danish researchers reviewed 16 trials of enteric-coated peppermint oil capsules (180–200 milligrams one to three times a day) to treat IBS. On average, 29 percent of placebo takers reported relief, but in the peppermint oil group, 58 percent. Compared with currently available drugs, the researchers called peppermint oil "the drug of first choice" for IBS.

PAIN. The Eclectics were right about menthol's "anesthetic power." It's an ingredient in many over-the-counter pain-relieving skin creams, including Absorbine and Bengay, and ointments marketed to soothe insect bites and stings and rashes caused by poison ivy, oak, and sumac. Throat lozenges such as Cepacol also contain menthol. Finally, some cigarettes contain menthol to numb the throat irritation smoking causes. Commission E approves peppermint oil as a treatment for muscle aches.

COLDS, CONGESTION. Menthol vapors help relieve nasal, sinus, and chest congestion. Menthol is an ingredient in Afrin Nasal Spray, Mentholatum, and Vicks VapoRub. Peppermint is an FDA-approved remedy for the common cold, primarily because of its decongestant action. Commission E also approves peppermint as a cold remedy.

COUGH. In addition to its decongestant action, menthol is an effective cough suppressant. English researchers instructed 20 volunteers to inhale a compound that triggers coughing. Five minutes beforehand, the participants received either one of two medically inactive placebos or menthol. The menthol significantly suppressed coughing. Menthol is an ingredient in Hall's, Luden's, Ricola, Robitussin, and Vicks Cough Drops.

HEADACHES. In two similar studies, German researchers gave tension headache sufferers either a placebo or various combinations of peppermint and eucalyptus oils that they rubbed on their foreheads and temples. The herb treatments produced greater relief. The mostly eucalyptus oil formula provided the most muscle relaxation, while the predominantly peppermint oil formula yielded the greatest headache relief. The researchers recommended herbal treatment instead of or in addition to over-the-counter pain relievers.

INFECTIONS. The Eclectics were onto something when they described menthol as germicidal. In laboratory studies, peppermint oil kills many types of bacteria and fungi, including *Candida ablicans*, which causes vaginal yeast infections, plus the herpes simplex virus, which causes cold sores and genital herpes. These findings validate peppermint's traditional roles in treating wounds and bronchitis.

WOMEN'S HEALTH. Antispasmodics soothe not only the smooth muscle lining in the digestive tract but also other smooth muscles, such as the uterus. Several herbals recommend peppermint as a treatment for morning sickness. *The Toxicology of Botanical Medicines*, however, suggests that medicinal concentrations of peppermint may promote menstruation and miscarriage.

LACTATION PROBLEMS. Breastfeeding often causes nipple pain and damage that forces new mothers to stop nursing before they or their doctors would like. In Iran, a traditional remedy for such problems is peppermint compresses. Iranian researchers asked 196 first-time mothers to use compresses of either expressed breast milk (EBM) or peppermint tea. In the EBM group, 27 percent developed nipple problems, but in the peppermint group, just 9 percent did.

ATHLETIC PERFORMANCE. Menthol is mildly stimulating. Iranian researchers tested the athletic prowess of 30 male athletes, average age 24, and then gave them either a drop of water under the tongue or a drop of water containing 50 microliters of peppermint oil. After 1 hour, the placebo group's performance remained about the same, but the peppermint group improved significantly.

Intriguing Possibility

An animal study suggests that pretreatment with peppermint protects the digestive tract from damage caused by radiation.

Rx Recommendations

For an anesthetic to treat wounds, burns, scalds, and herpes sores, apply a few drops of peppermint oil directly to the affected area.

For a decongestant, cough suppressant, or digestive infusion, use 1 to 2 teaspoons of dried peppermint or spearmint per cup of boiling water, steep for 10 minutes, and strain. Drink up to 3 cups a day. Peppermint has a sharper taste than spearmint, and it cools the mouth.

As a homemade tincture, take ¼ to 1 teaspoon up to three times a day.

When using commercial preparations, follow the package directions.

For an herbal bath, fill a cloth bag with a few handfuls of dried or fresh herb and let the water run over it.

Safety

As dried plant material, neither peppermint nor spearmint has been reported to cause problems, except for skin irritation in sensitive individuals.

Do not ingest these mints' oils. As little as a teaspoon (about 2 grams) may trigger heart rhythm disturbances (cardiac arrhythmias) or prove fatal.

Pregnant women who want to try peppermint for morning sickness should stick with dilute, beverage-tea concentrations rather than more potent medicinal infusions. Women with a history of miscarriage should not use this herb while pregnant.

You may give dilute peppermint or spearmint preparations cautiously to children under age 2, but youngsters may find the taste too pungent.

In older children, adjust the recommended dose based on the child's weight. Give a 50-pound child one-third of the dose a 150-pound adult would take.

If you're over 65, start with a low dose, and increase only if necessary.

Inform health care professionals of the herbs you use. Problematic herb-drug interactions are possible.

Peppermint may cause allergic reactions or other unexpected side effects. If any develop, reduce your dose or stop taking it. For more on herb safety, see Chapter 2.

If symptoms get worse or persist longer than 2 weeks, consult a health care professional promptly.

Gardening

Spearmint is a perennial that reaches 2 feet and spreads by underground runners. It has the mint family's characteristic square stems with wrinkled, lance-shaped, serrated, 2-inch leaves, and flower spikes with whorls of small white, pink, or lilac flowers that bloom in midsummer.

Peppermint looks like spearmint, but it grows somewhat taller, spreads by surface runners, has stems with a purplish cast, and has longer, less wrinkled leaves.

Mints crossbreed so easily that it's often impossible to tell what's sprouting from seed. To propagate true peppermint or spearmint, use root cuttings. Any piece of root with a joint (node) can produce a plant. Contain your mint bed or plant in containers. In rich, moist, well-drained soil, under full sun or partial shade, mints may become pests.

Frequent cutting encourages bushiness. Harvest leaves as they mature. Cut plants back to within a few inches of the ground after flowers appear. Most species become woody after a few years, so dig them out and plant new root cuttings.

POMEGRANATE

From Biblical Fruit to Modern Healer

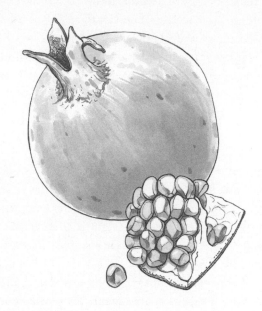

Family: Lythraceae; other members include myrtle

Genus and species: *Punica granatum*

Also known as: No other name

Parts used: Fruit juice

In the Bible, the Promised Land flows with milk, honey—and pomegranates. In addition, in an erotic double entendre in the Biblical *Song of Songs* (8:2), the bride invites the groom to "drink the juice of my pomegranate."

The name "pomegranate" derives from the Latin *pomum* (apple) and *granatus* (seeded). The generic name, *Punica*, refers to the Phoenicians, who cultivated the shrubby tree around the ancient Mediterranean and prized the sweet, tart juice contained in its seeds.

Native to the area from northern India to eastern Iran, pomegranate and its juice have been popular throughout the Middle East, Iran (Persia), and India since ancient times. But until recently, the only pomegranate product popular in the West was the syrup made from its reduced juice, grenadine. Now that's changing as tasty pomegranate juice has become a popular beverage, thanks to its richness in antioxidants.

Healing History

Middle Eastern folk herbalists used pomegranate juice to treat cuts, sore throat, diarrhea, and gum disease. Hippocrates, the father of medicine, recommended boiling the juice to treat fever.

Therapeutic Uses

Like all brightly colored fruits and vegetables, the pigments that give pomegranate juice its deep red color (punicalagins) are potent antioxidants that help prevent and heal the cell damage at the root of heart disease, most cancers, and many other conditions. However, pomegranate juice is among nature's richest sources of antioxidants, containing more than either tea or red wine.

ANTIOXIDANT. University of Florida researchers asked 11 adults to abstain from fruits, vegetables, and antioxidant supplements for 3 days to minimize the amounts of antioxidants in their bloodstreams. Then they consumed 800 milligrams of pomegranate extract. Subsequent blood samples showed a major jump in antioxidants.

HEART DISEASE. Noted heart disease researcher Dean Ornish, M.D., asked 45 people with heart disease and poor blood flow through their hearts to drink either a placebo beverage or pomegranate juice (1 cup a day). After 3 months, blood flow through the heart decreased in the placebo group, but increased significantly in those who drank the pomegranate juice, thus reducing risk of heart attack.

STROKE. Israeli researchers reported similar results in a study of pomegranate juice's effects on blood flow through the carotid artery, which carries blood into the brain. After 1 year, the placebo group's carotid arteries were showed 9 percent narrower. But the pomegranate juice drinkers' were 30 percent more open, meaning increased blood flow into the brain and significantly less risk of stroke.

BLOOD PRESSURE. High blood pressure is a major risk factor for heart attack and the leading risk factor for stroke. The Israeli study also showed that 1 year of daily pomegranate juice consumption reduced blood pressure 21 percent, adding to protection against heart attack and stroke.

DIABETES. Diabetes is a major risk factor for heart attack and stroke. In another study, the Israeli team asked people with Type 2 diabetes to drink pomegranate juice (2 cups a day). After 3 months, blood tests showed biochemical markers indicating improved blood flow and less risk of heart attack and stroke.

CANCER. Several laboratory and animal studies show that pomegranate juice and extract have antitumor properties. UCLA researchers gave pomegranate juice (8 ounces/day) to men with prostate cancer who'd been treated with treatment surgery, radiation, or hormones, but still had rising levels of prostate-specific antigen (PSA), suggesting residual cancer. Controls who did not drink the juice saw their PSA double in an average of 15 months. But in the pomegranate group, PSA doubling took 54 months.

Intriguing Possibilities

Several laboratory studies show that pomegranate juice and extract activate immune constitu-

ents that help prevent inflammatory diseases including arthritis and Crohn's disease. The herb also boosts immune response to bacterial infection. Researchers have not yet shown clear benefit in treating these diseases, but that's a good bet.

Animal studies show that pomegranate juice aids fetal brain development and protects against prenatal brain injury.

Rx Recommendations

Eat pomegranates in season. Drink 1 or 2 cups/day of commercial juice.

Safety

No side effects have been reported. Allergic reactions are possible.

Pomegranate juice is tart. Commercial brands add considerable sugar. Those who must watch sugar intake, for example, diabetics, should be careful.

Gardening

The Spanish brought pomegranates to California and Arizona during the 16th century. Now they're grown throughout the southwest United States. Pomegranates grow on small deciduous trees that look like woody, thorny shrubs. Mature trees reach 6 to 12 feet in full sun. They tolerate alkaline soil, drought, desert heat, and winter lows to about 15°F. Juicy fruits require adequate watering. But over-watering rots the roots. Buy plants in 5-gallon containers. The "Wonderful" variety is the most popular in the United States. Or try growing pomegranate from seed or 6-inch cuttings treated with rooting hormone planted vertically, with the dormant bud exposed.

PSYLLIUM

Metamucil Reduces Cholesterol

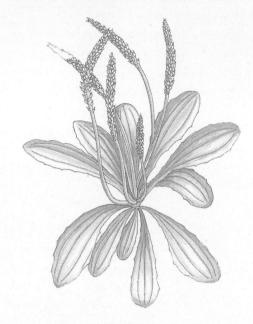

Family: Plantaginaceae; other members include about 250 *Plantago* species, including rib grass

Genus and species: *Plantago psyllium*

Also known as: Fleaseed, plantago, and plantain

Part used: Seeds

Mention psyllium (pronounced SILLY-um), and most people say, "Huh?" But mention the laxative, Metamucil, and everyone says, "Oh, yes."

Except for some sweetener, color, and flavoring, Metamucil *is* psyllium, the seeds of a hardy plant distributed worldwide. Psyllium is among the safest, gentlest laxatives.

In addition, modern research shows that psyllium seed has a remarkable ability to reduce cholesterol. This makes the herb beneficial in preventing heart disease and most strokes.

Healing History

Psyllium is often called plantain, but should not be confused with the other plantain (*Muca paradisiaca*), a palm-like tree that produces fruits similar to bananas.

For centuries, traditional Chinese and Ayurvedic physicians have used the seeds and leaves of several Asian *Plantago* species to treat diarrhea, hemorrhoids, constipation, urinary problems, and, more recently, high blood pressure.

Psyllium entered European folk medicine in the 16th century as a remedy for diarrhea and constipation. Seventeenth-century English herbalist Nicholas Culpeper recommended the seeds for inflammation, gout, hemorrhoids, and sore nipples (mastitis) in nursing mothers.

European physicians eventually adopted psyllium, but it was not widely used on this side of the Atlantic until after World War I.

Therapeutic Uses

About one-third of psyllium's seed coat is the soluble fiber, mucilage. When exposed to water, psyllium seeds swell to more than 10 times their original size and become gelatinous. The herb's mucilage accounts for its medicinal action.

CONSTIPATION. Psyllium's bulk-forming action increases stool volume. Larger stools press on the colon wall, triggering the wavelike contractions (peristalsis) that we recognize as "the urge." As stool gains bulk, it also becomes softer and easier to pass.

Israeli researchers gave 35 people with chronic constipation either a placebo or laxatives containing psyllium and aloe. After 2 weeks, the placebo group showed scant improvement. But those taking the psyllium-aloe combination reported softer stools, more frequent bowel movements, and less use of pharmaceutical laxatives.

Most Americans eat a low-fiber diet, with fewer fruits, vegetables, beans, and whole grains than nutrition authorities recommend. A low-fiber diet results in hard, dense stools that are often difficult and painful to pass. Psyllium's fiber content and water-absorbing action compensate to some extent for dietary fiber deficiency.

Today, psyllium is one of North America's most popular bulk-forming laxatives. It's the active ingredient in Metamucil, Fiberall, and several other products. Commission E, the expert panel that evaluates herbal medicines for the German counterpart of the FDA, endorses psyllium as a treatment for constipation and irritable bowel syndrome, which may involve either constipation or diarrhea.

HEMORRHOIDS. Because psyllium softens stool, it can bring some relief from the pain and bleeding of hemorrhoids, according to a report in *Diseases of the Colon and Rectum*. This supports Culpeper's recommendation. Commission E approves psyllium as a hemorrhoid treatment.

DIARRHEA. Psyllium absorbs excess fluid in the gut and helps restore normal bulk to stool. Commission E approves psyllium for the treatment of diarrhea.

HIGH CHOLESTEROL. Oat bran has garnered much of the publicity, but all high-fiber foods, notably psyllium, draw cholesterol from the bloodstream preventing it from narrowing artery walls and increasing risk of heart disease and stroke. Many studies show that as dietary fiber consumption increases, risk of elevated cholesterol decreases.

🍀 A study in *Archives of Internal Medicine* shows that a teaspoon of psyllium three times a day for 8 weeks produced significant decreases in cholesterol levels. The research-

ers concluded that many people with moderately elevated cholesterol may be able to cut it to healthy levels with psyllium alone, without cholesterol-lowering medication.

🍀 A similar study in the *Journal of the American Medical Association* finds that a teaspoon of psyllium a few times a day reduces total cholesterol by about 5 percent in 12 weeks. Heart disease experts say that for every 1 percent decrease in total cholesterol, heart attack risk drops 2 percent, so a 5 percent cholesterol reduction means a 10 percent drop in heart attack risk.

🍀 Mexican researchers placed 125 people with diabetes—all at high risk for heart attack—on a low-fat diet. In addition, the participants were given either a placebo or psyllium (about 2 teaspoons three times a day). After 3 months, those taking psyllium had significantly lower cholesterol levels.

In all of these trials, psyllium treatment caused no significant side effects, just some transient stomach upset, making the herb safer than prescription cholesterol medications. If you'd like to include psyllium in a cholesterol reduction program, consult your physician.

In 1997, the FDA hopped on the psyllium bandwagon. Any food that contains at least 1.7 grams of psyllium can make a label claim that it helps prevent heart disease. One is Kellogg's Bran Buds.

Intriguing Possibilities

One study shows that psyllium protects laboratory animals from intestinal damage by toxic food additives. The psyllium increased the bulk of the animals' stools, so the toxic chemicals had less direct contact with sensitive intestinal tissues and less opportunity to cause harm. Researchers believe that the same mechanism is the reason that a high-fiber diet is associated with reduced risk of colorectal cancer. The American Cancer Society recommends a high-fiber diet, for example, a few teaspoons of psyllium daily, to reduce risk of colon cancer.

Like other dietary fibers, psyllium reduces blood sugar (glucose) in laboratory animals, suggesting a possible role in human diabetes management.

Rx Recommendations

Most studies show that a teaspoon or two of psyllium three times a day, along with *plenty* of water or fruit juice, usually relieves constipation. Psyllium is odorless and almost tasteless, but it has a gritty texture that some people find unpleasant.

If you take a commercial preparation, follow the label directions.

Safety

Psyllium does not work by itself. It swells only in the presence of fluid. If you take psyllium without lots water or juice, there's a risk of a psyllium plug blocking your intestine. Drink at least one tall glass of water or juice whenever you take psyllium.

Inhaling dust from psyllium seeds may trigger allergic reaction. Severe allergic reactions are extremely rare, but if you develop breathing difficulties after ingesting psyllium, seek emergency help immediately.

Psyllium has no history as a menstruation promoter, but other *Plantago* species do. Although constipation is a common complaint during pregnancy, doctors discourage pregnant women from taking laxatives, even psyllium, and control constipation with high-fiber foods (fruits, vegetables, beans, and whole grains), fluids, and exercise.

Do not give psyllium to children under 2. In older children, adjust the recommended dose based on the child's weight. Give a 50-pound child one-third of the dose a 150-pound adult would take.

If you're over 65, start with a low dose, and increase only if necessary.

Inform health professionals of the herbs you use. Problematic herb-drug interactions are possible.

Psyllium may cause allergic reactions or other unexpected side effects. If any develop, reduce your dose or stop taking it. For more on herb safety, see Chapter 2.

If symptoms get worse or persist longer than 2 weeks, consult a health professional promptly.

Gardening

Psyllium is an annual that reaches 18 inches and produces inconspicuous white flowers in summer that soon give way to small brown seed pods.

Most psyllium used in the United States is imported from France. Psyllium is not a garden herb here. It looks like a weed, and if growers don't harvest seed pods before they break open, the wind scatters the seeds—a major problem considering that each pod contains up to 15,000 seeds that sprout quickly and grow aggressively.

PUMPKIN SEED

From Jack-o-Lanterns to Benign Prostate Enlargement

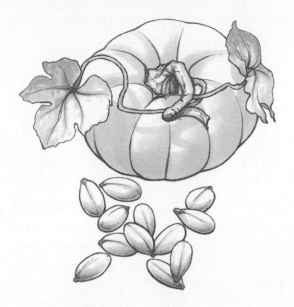

Family: Cucurbitaceae; other members include gourds

Genus and species: *Cucurbita pepo*

Also known as: Pepo; in Spanish, pepitas

Parts used: Seed, seed oil

Pumpkins are native to Central America. The oldest seeds, dated to 14,000 BC, were found in Mexico. But by Biblical times, pumpkins were grown throughout the world, from ancient China to ancient Rome, where Dioscorides, the father of botany, mentioned them as a food.

Our word, pumpkin, comes from the Greek *pepon*, meaning large melon. Large is right. Pumpkins can weigh more than 1,000 pounds.

Pumpkin pulp is very nutritious, particularly high in vitamin A. It can be cooked as a vegetable or made into soup, but it's most popular as a Thanksgiving pie filling.

Carved pumpkins, jack-o-lanterns (or jack o'lanterns), are central to Halloween. The custom originated in Britain and Ireland, which share a long tradition of carving lanterns from hollowed vegetables, particularly turnips, and placing candles inside for decorative use in winter. The term "jack-o-lantern" was coined in the 17th century and originally referred to a night watchman, the man (or jack) with the lantern.

Recent research shows that pumpkin seeds help prevent benign prostate enlargement.

Healing History

Once pumpkins were introduced into Europe, pumpkin seed oil became a culinary specialty in Eastern Europe and gained a folk reputation for treating the urinary symptoms associated with benign prostate enlargement: reduced flow, trouble starting and stopping, and night-time wakeups to urinate.

Pumpkin seeds and the seed oil have also been used in German and Eastern European folk medicine to treat intestinal parasites.

Therapeutic Uses

BENIGN PROSTATE ENLARGEMENT. Pumpkin seed oil contains constituents that arrest the overgrowth of prostate tissue (benign prostate hypertrophy or BPH). However, scientists remain unclear about the biochemical mechanism of this effect. Other herbs that help prevent BPH (saw palmetto, page 423, and pygeum, page 377) interfere with the action 5-alpha-reductase, an enzyme involved in spurring overgrowth of prostate tissue. But pumpkin seed oil is a very weak 5-alpha-reductase inhibitor. Whatever the mechanism, pumpkin seeds and their oil have been shown to reduce risk of BPH.

German researchers assessed BPH symptoms in 2,245 middle-aged men, then had them ingest pumpkin seed oil capsules (Prosta Fink Forte, 500 to 1,000 milligrams/day). After 3 months, the men's symptom scores decreased significantly.

Commission E, the German counterpart of the FDA, approves pumpkin seed for treatment of benign prostate enlargement.

KIDNEY STONES. Two Thai studies show that pumpkin seeds reduce risk of kidney stones.

Intriguing Possibilities

Pumpkin seed oil is rich in the tranquilizing amino acid tryptophan. Pumpkin seeds and their oil have been tested as treatments for insomnia and anxiety—so far inconclusively.

Rx Recommendations

For BPH prevention, Commission E recommends 10 grams of pumpkin seeds a day, about one-third of an ounce, or a handful. Or take 480 milligrams/day of seed oil in divided doses. Or follow package directions.

Safety

No significant side effects. Allergic reactions are possible.

Gardening

Pumpkins grow throughout most of North America. Plant in late spring when all danger of frost has passed and the soil has warmed. Plant seeds 1 inch deep in mounds, a half-dozen seeds per hill. Allow 5 feet between hills. Once established, thin plants to retain the best two or three per hill. Water and weed regularly. Harvest in October, retaining some stem. Pumpkins without stems do not keep well.

PURSLANE

Don't Pull This Tasty, Healing Weed

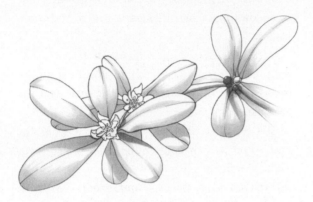

Family: Portulacaceae; other members include miner's lettuce

Genus and species: *Portulaca oleracea*

Also known as: Pigweed, hogweed, pusley

Parts used: Leaves, seeds

Healing History

Archeologists have unearthed purslane seeds at many prehistoric sites in the Middle East. The sour-salty-lemony herb has been used as a vegetable and salad green for at least 2,000 years. In the days before refrigeration, Europeans pickled purslane and ate it in winter when fresh vegetables were unavailable. From France to China, it's still eaten in salads. When steamed, it tastes like spinach.

The ancient Romans used purslane to treat dozens of conditions: headache, stomach distress, dysentery, and intestinal worms—so many that Pliny the Elder advised wearing the plant as an amulet to protect against evil. Dioscorides, a 1st-century Greek physician who traveled with Roman armies, considered purslane a cooling herb useful in treating "hot" conditions: fever, infections, and inflammation.

Arab physicians also used the plant to treat fever, diarrhea, and hemorrhoids and as a poultice on wounds and inflammations.

West Africans used this herb to treat sore, cramped muscles. The Zulus of southern Africa used it as an emetic.

Echoing Pliny, medieval Europeans considered purslane a protector against witchcraft. They strewed the leaves around sick beds to deter evil spirits.

Sixteenth-century English herbalist John Gerard noted that purslane "is much used in salads." A century later, his countryman Nicholas Culpeper wrote, "This herb, if placed under the tongue, assuages thirst. Applied to the gout, it easeth pains thereof."

Traditional Chinese physicians prescribed purslane in herbal blends to treat bee stings, diarrhea, and hemorrhoids.

Contemporary herbalists consider purslane more a food than medicine.

Therapeutic Uses

Purslane is one of the richest plant sources of antioxidant vitamins A (beta-carotene), C, and E and of alpha-linoleic acid (ALA, an omega-3 fatty acid), which helps prevent heart disease. The herb contains more beta-carotene than carrots.

HEART DISEASE. Harvard scientists

assessed dietary ALA intake among 76,283 women nurses, then followed them for 10 years. As ALA intake increased, deaths from heart attacks decreased. Compared with nurses who consumed little ALA, those who ate the most were 45 percent less likely to suffer a fatal heart attack.

Crete has one of the world's lowest rates of heart disease, and purslane is a popular vegetable there. French researchers assigned 606 adults either to the modestly low-fat, low-cholesterol regimen advocated by the American Heart Association or to the diet typical in Crete that included a good deal of purslane. After 2 years, blood tests showed that those on the Cretan diet had significantly lower risk of heart disease.

BLOOD PRESSURE. A diet high in plant foods helps control blood pressure. Israeli scientists gave 63 adult diabetics either a placebo or purslane (three 500 milligram capsules a day). After 3 months, those taking purslane showed lower blood pressure.

Iranian researchers assessed the blood pressure of 48 diabetic adults and then gave them either a daily cup of yogurt or yogurt with purslane seeds (10 grams, about one-third of an ounce). After 5 weeks, the groups switched treatments (a crossover trial). While taking purslane, participants' blood pressure declined significantly.

WEIGHT CONTROL. In the Iranian study just mentioned, participants lost weight while taking purslane—about a pound in 5 weeks.

CHOLESTEROL. Animal studies show that purslane lowers cholesterol. Iranian investigators gave obese adolescents either a placebo or purslane (500 milligrams of powdered seeds twice a day). After 1 month, the herb group showed significantly reduced LDLs, the bad cholesterol.

Scientists in Yemen gave 30 diabetics either a standard medication (Metformin) or purslane seeds (5 grams, around 2 tablespoons twice a day). After 3 months, the purslane group's cholesterol dropped significantly—and so did their weight.

DIABETES. In the Yemeni and Israeli studies just mentioned, participants' blood sugar (glucose) declined significantly, showing that purslane helps manage diabetes.

MUSCLE RELAXANT. Purslane is high in potassium, which helps relieve muscle spasms and cramping. Animal studies show that it relaxes cramped muscles. Nigerian researchers gave purslane to people complaining of muscle cramps and found that the herb reduced cramping by 50 percent—just as well as pharmaceutical muscle relaxants (such as Valium).

DIGESTIVE AID. Purslane contains mucilage, a soluble fiber that swells and becomes gummy on exposure to water. When placed in animal feed, the mucilage in purslane prevents diarrhea. Other mucilaginous herbs (psyllium, page 370) help prevent and treat both constipation and diarrhea.

INFLAMMATION. Dioscorides may have been right about purslane treating inflammation. Chinese researchers have discovered that the herb contains several anti-inflammatory compounds, among them: oleracimine and oleracone.

Intriguing Possibility

Animal studies show that purslane relieves pain and might help protect the liver from prolonged use of acetaminophen (Tylenol).

Rx Recommendations

Use fresh purslane and its seeds as a vegetable. Seeds should be crushed. Leaves may be steamed. Both can be incorporated into soups, stews, and casseroles. Or blend the leaves with olive oil for a tasty pesto. If you take capsules, most studies have used 500 milligrams three times a day.

Safety

Purslane has been eaten as a vegetable for millennia. There are no reports of significant harm.

However, animal studies suggest that large amounts may stimulate uterine contractions. Pregnant women should not use this herb except at term.

Gardening

Native to India but now grown in temperate locales worldwide, purslane is a dark green, broad-leaved, succulent annual that grows to 6 inches. It has reddish brown stems, alternate, fleshy, wedge-shaped leaves and clusters of yellow flowers that bloom in summer.

Most American gardeners consider purslane a weed and are more likely to pull it than cultivate it. What a waste of a tasty vegetable. Purslane prefers sandy soil and sun. Once established, it requires little water.

PYGEUM
African Plum Prevents Prostate Enlargement

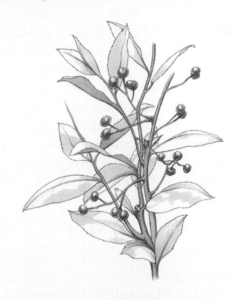

Family: Rosaceae; other members include rose, plum, cherry, pear, and apple

Genus and species: *Pygeum africanum* or *Prunus africana*

Also known as: African plum, African prune, African cherry, iron wood, red stinkwood

Parts used: Bark

Pygeum is an evergreen tree native to the mountains of sub-Saharan Africa and Madagascar. It grows to 80 feet and thrives at altitudes ranging from 3,000 to 10,000 feet. Pygeum timber, used for furniture and firewood, is remarkably hard, hence the name iron wood. When harvested, it has a pungent bitter-almond smell, hence the name stinkwood. Aged wood turns mahogany-colored and odorless. The fruits resemble plums, prunes, or cherries, hence some of the tree's other common names. Fruits are too bitter for human consumption, but are a favorite food of mountain gorillas.

Healing History

Southern Africans used pygeum bark to treat urinary problems, including "old man's disease," an archaic term for benign prostate enlargement. Eighteenth-century European explorers brought the bark to Europe, where it was slow to catch on. European herbalists and physicians began recommending it for prostate enlargement only in the 1960s. Today it is a popular treatment for the condition throughout Europe, particularly in France.

Therapeutic Uses

BENIGN PROSTATE ENLARGEMENT. Medically, this condition is known as benign prostate hypertrophy or BPH. Like saw palmetto (page 423), pygeum contains constituents that interfere with the action 5-alpha-reductase, an enzyme that encourages overgrowth of prostate tissue and causes BPH symptoms: reduced urine flow, trouble starting and stopping, and night-time wakeups to urinate.

Many studies have shown that pygeum reduces risk of BPH:

- In a German trial, 263 BPH sufferers were given either a placebo or pygeum (50 milligrams twice a day). After 2 months, one-third of the placebo group reported benefit, but among pygum users, two-thirds.

- Slovakian scientists assessed BPH symptoms in 85 men, then gave them pygeum (50 milligrams twice a day). After 2 months, their symptoms decreased significantly—and the benefit persisted for a month after stopping treatment.

- Researchers with the Minneapolis VA Hospital analyzed 18 studies of pygeum for BPH: "Pygeum provided a moderately large improvement in urologic symptoms and flow measures. [Compared with placebo takers], men using Pygeum were more than twice as likely to report improvement in symptoms. Peak flow increased 23 percent. Night-time wakeups to urinate decreased 19 percent."

Rx Recommendations

Studies have used 75 to 200 milligrams/day of bark extract. Most have used 100 milligrams/day in one dose, or two daily 50-milligram doses, morning and night.

Safety

Nausea and abdominal distress are possible.

Women and children have no need for pygeum and should not use it.

Inform health professionals of the herbs you use. Problematic herb-drug interactions are possible.

Pygeum may cause allergic reactions or other unexpected side effects. If any develop, reduce your dose or stop taking it. For more on herb safety, see Chapter 2.

If symptoms get worse, consult a health professional promptly.

Gardening

Not grown in the United States. Use of pygeum bark for BPH prevention has spurred unsustainable harvesting, leaving the tree endangered. However, it is now being cultivated commercially with bark harvested in a sustainable manner.

RASPBERRY

A Potent Antioxidant

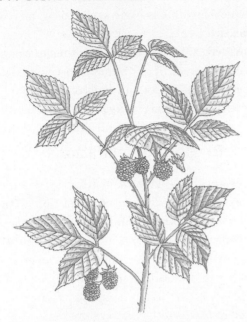

Family: Rosaceae; other members include rose, peach, almond, apple, and strawberry

Genus and species: *Rubus idaeus* and *R. strigosus*

Also known as: Hindberry and bramble

Parts used: Leaves and fruits

For more than 2,000 years, herbalists considered raspberry a minor healer, a footnote under blackberry. Since the 1940s, however, it has emerged from blackberry's shadow and virtually replaced it in herbal medicine—all because it has become *the* herb for pregnant women. The latest research also shows that raspberry fruits are very high in antioxidants, the nutrients that help prevent many degenerative diseases.

Healing History

The ancient Greeks, Chinese, Indians, and Native Americans hardly distinguished raspberry from blackberry. They used the leaves of the two bushes interchangeably, externally to treat wounds and in tea to treat diarrhea.

Seventeenth-century English herbalist Nicholas Culpeper recommended raspberry leaf as "very binding" (astringent) and good for "fevers, ulcers, putrid sores of the mouth and secret parts [genitals] . . . spitting blood [tuberculosis] . . . piles [hemorrhoids], stones of the kidney . . . and too much flowing of women's courses [heavy menstrual flow]."

America's 19th-century Eclectic physicians, forerunners of today's naturopaths, continued the long tradition of treating raspberry as a me-too after blackberry. The Eclectic text *King's American Dispensatory* (1898) recommended blackberry as being "of much service in dysentery . . . pleasant to the taste, mitigating suffering, and ultimately effecting a cure." Then it noted that raspberry helped, too.

Contemporary herbalists recommend raspberry to relieve diarrhea and to end nausea and vomiting, especially the morning sickness of pregnancy. One herbalist of the 1980s went so far as to call raspberry a "panacea during pregnancy . . . allaying morning sickness, preventing miscarriage, [and] erasing labor pains."

Nutritionists tout raspberries for their antioxidant content.

Therapeutic Uses

Raspberry is no panacea during pregnancy and won't erase labor pains. But science has confirmed its value for pregnant women.

PREGNANCY COMPLAINTS. Raspberry

emerged from blackberry's shadow in 1941, when an animal study published in the British medical journal *Lancet* showed that it contains a "uterine relaxant." Over the next 30 years, several other studies confirmed this finding. Today, physicians in England and Europe prescribe a number of raspberry preparations for morning sickness, uterine irritability, and threatened miscarriage. Many herbal pregnancy blends sold in the United States include it.

But does raspberry ease labor? Australian researchers asked 192 women pregnant with their first child to take either a placebo or raspberry (1.2 grams of leaf twice a day from 32 weeks gestation to delivery). The herb did not shorten the first stage of labor (contractions, cervical dilation). But it did shorten the second stage (pushing) and reduced the need for forceps delivery—30 percent in the control group, but only 19 percent among those taking the herb.

DIARRHEA. Raspberry leaves contain astringent tannins. This explains traditional use of raspberry leaf tea for diarrhea.

ANTIOXIDANT. Raspberries owe their red color to high levels of anthocyanoside pigments, compounds that are potent antioxidants. Antioxidants help prevent and reverse the harm to cells caused by highly reactive oxygen molecules called free radicals. Scientists now agree that free radical damage (oxidative damage) is the underlying cause of heart disease, many cancers, and other degenerative illnesses.

Antioxidants—among them, vitamins C and E, the mineral selenium, and anthocyanosides—are found in fruits and vegetables. Researchers at the Jean Mayer USDA Human Nutrition Research Center on Aging at Tufts University in Boston analyzed the antioxidant content of dozens of common plant foods. Those richest in antioxidants turned out to be the dark-colored fruits and berries that contain generous amounts of anthocyanosides, including raspberries, blackberries, blueberries, cherries, and red grapes.

CATARACTS. Cataracts are a major cause of vision impairment and blindness among older Americans. They develop when oxidative damage clouds the eye's normally clear lens. For reasons that remain unclear, anthocyanosides have unusually powerful effects on the eyes. In one Italian study, 50 people with early-stage cataracts were given extracts of bilberry, a fruit similar to raspberry, in combination with another antioxidant, vitamin E, three times a day. The treatment stopped cataract progression in 97 percent of participants. Raspberries and bilberries contain comparable amounts of anthocyanosides, so presumably raspberries have similar effects.

MACULAR DEGENERATION. The nerve-rich retina at the back of the eye plays a key role in central vision—what's in front of you. Macular degeneration involves deterioration of the macula, the most sensitive part of the retina—the part responsible for seeing the fine detail of what's in front of you.

In a European study, 31 people with various types of retinal eye problems, including macular degeneration, took bilberry extract. Those with macular degeneration experienced significant vision improvement. Again, raspberries presumably produce similar benefits.

DIABETIC RETINOPATHY. Diabetes damages all of the blood vessels in the body, including the tiny capillaries in the eye that nourish the retina. When these capillaries become debilitated, they leak blood into the eye, causing the blurred vision of retinopathy.

Bilberry's powerful antioxidants help strengthen retinal blood vessels, reducing blood leakage. In the European macular degeneration study mentioned above, people with diabetic retinopathy showed significant improvement when treated with bilberry. Raspberries probably produce similar benefits.

Intriguing Possibilities

One animal study shows that raspberry helps reduce blood sugar (glucose) levels, suggesting the herb's possible value in diabetes management.

Rx Recommendations

For a treat rich in antioxidants, enjoy raspberries. Whether fresh, frozen, canned, or in preserves, they supply generous amounts of anthocyanosides.

For a pleasantly astringent, sweet infusion to treat diarrhea or the discomforts of pregnancy, use 1 to 2 teaspoons of dried herb per cup of boiling water. Steep for 10 to 15 minutes and strain. Drink as needed.

As a homemade tincture, take $\frac{1}{2}$ to 1 teaspoon up to three times a day.

When using commercial preparations, follow package directions.

Safety

Standard medical advice warns pregnant women against taking any drugs during pregnancy because of the possibility of harming the fetus. Raspberry used medicinally is an exception to this rule, but consult your prenatal care provider.

Raspberry has been widely recommended as a uterine relaxant for decades, and there are no reports in the medical literature of any adverse effects on mothers or their babies. Women with a history of miscarriage may find it especially valuable.

You may use cool, dilute raspberry tea cautiously to treat infant diarrhea in consultation with the child's physician.

In older children, adjust the recommended dose based on the child's weight. Give a 50-pound child one-third of the dose a 150-pound adult would take.

If you're over 65, start with a low dose, and increase only if necessary.

Inform health professionals of the herbs you use. Problematic herb-drug interactions are possible.

Raspberry may cause allergic reactions or other unexpected side effects. If any develop, reduce your dose or stop taking it. For more on herb safety, see Chapter 2.

If symptoms get worse or persist longer than 2 weeks, consult a health professional promptly.

Gardening

Raspberry's perennial invasive roots produce a dense, spreading mass of thorny biennial stems that, under favorable conditions, grow quite long. The bush has serrated, lance-shaped leaves, small white summer-blooming flowers, and hanging clusters of tart red berries that become very sweet as they ripen.

Raspberry bushes grow so vigorously and invasively that they quickly become impenetrable pests. Rooting them out is quite difficult. Even when cleared, stray root fragments send up new shoots. If you grow raspberries, be sure they're well contained.

Plant ½-inch root cuttings in a few inches of soil. Raspberry grows best under full sun in loose, rich, well-drained soil amended with manure or compost.

Harvest leaves at any time. Mature fruits appear in summer. For ease of harvesting the berries, train the branches along supports, and prune mercilessly.

RED CLOVER

A Controversial Treatment for Menopausal Discomforts

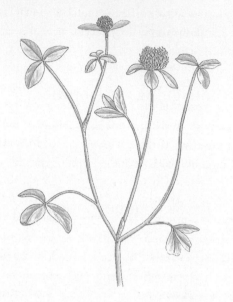

Family: Leguminosae; other members include beans and peas

Genus and species: *Trifolium pratense*

Also known as: Trifolium, purple clover, sweet clover, and cow clover

Parts used: Flowers

Red clover is one of the world's oldest agricultural crops, cultivated as livestock forage since prehistoric times. The small, ball-shaped flowers of the three-leafed herb have been used for almost as long in herbal healing. But despite millennia of medicinal use, this herb is still controversial.

Healing History

Because of its importance in early agriculture, red clover has a long history as a religious symbol. The ancient Greeks, Romans, and Celts of pre-Christian Ireland all revered it. Early Christians linked the plant to the Trinity, and some say red clover is the model for Ireland's symbol, the shamrock. It was also the model for the suit of clubs in playing cards.

During the Middle Ages, red clover was considered a charm against witchcraft. A more potent protector was the rare four-leaf clover, which represented the cross and the four aspects of happiness: health, wealth, excellent reputation, and a faithful lover. Today, children still search for four-leaf clovers.

Traditional Chinese physicians have long used red clover blossoms in expectorant herb blends. Russian folk healers recommended the herb for asthma. Other cultures have used it externally in salves for skin sores and eye problems and internally as a diuretic to treat water retention and as a sedative, anti-inflammatory, cough medicine, and cancer treatment.

America's 19th-century Eclectic physicians, forerunners of today's naturopaths, loved red clover. Their text *King's American Dispensatory* (1898) deemed the herb "one of the few remedies which favorably influences pertussis [whooping cough] . . . possess[ing] a peculiar soothing property." The Eclectics recommended red clover for coughs, bronchitis, and tuberculosis. But they waxed truly enthusiastic about the herb as a cancer treatment: "It unquestionably retards the growth of carcinomata."

During the late 19th and early 20th centuries, red clover was the major ingredient in many patent medicines known as Trifolium Compounds. The most popular, produced by the William S. Merrell Chemical Company of Cincinnati, combined red clover and several other herbs. Manufacturers claimed that Trifolium Compounds were whole-body tonics and treatments for skin diseases, syphilis, and scrofula (tuberculosis of the lymph nodes).

In 1912, the American Medical Association's Council on Pharmacy and Chemistry attacked Trifolium Compounds, saying, "We have no information to indicate they possess medicinal properties." Nonetheless, red clover remained in the *National Formulary*, the pharmacists' reference, as a treatment for skin diseases until 1946.

Red clover was also one of the herbs in ex—coal miner Harry Hoxsey's controversial alternative cancer treatment (page 31).

Contemporary herbalists recommend red clover externally as a treatment for eczema and psoriasis and internally to aid digestion, ease the discomforts of menopause, and relieve coughs, bronchitis, and whooping cough. Some continue to recommend it for cancer.

Therapeutic Uses

Red clover doesn't get much respect. The FDA says, "There is not sufficient reason to suspect it of any medicinal value." That's a bit of an overstatement. Many studies show that red clover produces benefit, especially for menopausal discomforts, but other studies dispute this.

MENOPAUSAL COMPLAINTS. Red clover contains plant compounds chemically similar to estrogen (phytoestrogens), among them, isoflavones similar to those found in soybean (page 439). Consumption of soy foods and soy isoflavone supplements have been shown to reduce menopausal hot flashes. The Australian red clover supplement, Promensil, available in the United States, contains similar isoflavones. If soy isoflavones reduce hot flashes, red clover isoflavones should, too. Or maybe not.

Several studies have shown that red clover relieves hot flashes:

♣ Australian researchers surveyed the menopausal complaints of 109 women, then gave them either a placebo or red clover (80 milligrams/day). Three months later, the herb group reported significantly fewer hot flashes. Then the groups switched treatments (a crossover trial). Again, after 90 days, the red clover group experienced significantly fewer hot flashes.

♣ Scientists in Ecuador gave 60 postmenopausal women either a placebo or red clover isoflavones (80 milligrams/day). After 90 days, "red clover isoflavone supplementation significantly decreased menopausal symptoms."

♣ Dutch researchers gave 30 women complaining of more than five hot flashes a day either a placebo or red clover isoflavones (80 milligrams/day). After 12 weeks, the herb group experienced a 44 percent reduction of hot flashes.

♣ Researchers in Gig Harbor, Washington, gave 25 women with menopausal complaints a red clover–based isoflavone supplement. After 12 weeks, they reported 46 percent fewer hot flashes.

Makers of red clover products tout these reports.

However, two analyses of multiple trials conclude that red clover is, at best, only marginally effective for menopausal complaints.

♣ British researchers analyzed five studies. They found "a marginally significant effect of red clover isoflavones for treating hot flashes.

Whether this effect is clinically relevant [makes a real difference] remains unclear."

♣ Scientists in New Zealand analyzed five studies. "There was no significant difference in frequency of hot flashes between red clover and placebo."

For menopausal complaints, the value of red clover, if any, remains controversial. If you'd like to try it, feel free—as long as there's no medical reason to limit your exposure to phytoestrogens. It might work for you. Or not.

HEART DISEASE AND STROKE. An Australian study of 27 postmenopausal women showed that red clover (40 milligrams/day) significantly improves arterial elasticity and health. This suggests that the herb may help prevent heart disease, the leading cause of death in postmenopausal women.

Intriguing Possibilities

INFECTIONS. One laboratory study shows that red clover is effective against several kinds of bacteria, including the type that causes tuberculosis. This finding lends some credence to the Eclectics' use of the herb in treating TB.

CHOLESTEROL. Several studies have investigated red clover's effects on cholesterol. Again, the results have been maddeningly inconsistent. Some show small decreases. Others show no effect.

CANCER. Researchers from the National Cancer Institute (NCI) felt compelled to investigate the antitumor properties of red clover after the Institute's own Jonathan Hartwell, Ph.D., published a monograph in the *Journal of Natural Products* in which he pointed out that 33 different cultures around the world had used red clover to treat cancer. Sure enough, NCI researchers confirmed that red clover contains four antitumor compounds, including daidzein and genistein, which are also isoflavone phytoestrogens.

In addition, red clover contains significant amounts of vitamin E. This vitamin is a potent antioxidant that helps prevent cancer and heart disease.

Red clover is no substitute for mainstream cancer treatment, but for those with cancers not aggravated by estrogen (non-estrogen-dependent tumors), red clover may hold some promise. Consult your physician about adding the herb to your treatment regimen.

BENIGN PROSTATE ENLARGEMENT (BPH) AND PROSTATE CANCER. Pilot studies suggest that red clover may help treat BPH and reduce risk of prostate cancer.

Rx Recommendations

For a pleasantly sweet infusion, use 1 to 3 teaspoons of dried flowers per cup of boiling water. Steep for 10 to 15 minutes, then strain. Drink up to 3 cups a day.

As a homemade tincture, use $\frac{1}{2}$ to $1\frac{1}{2}$ teaspoons up to three times a day.

When using commercial preparations, follow the package directions.

Safety

The medical literature contains no reports of harm from red clover. But because this herb is rich in phytoestrogens, some people should avoid it. Estrogens may accelerate the growth of estrogen-dependent breast and gynecological tumors. Estrogen also increases the risk of blood clots (thromboembolisms) and inflammation of blood vessels (thrombophlebitis). People who have a history of any of these disorders or of heart disease or stroke should use red clover cautiously, if at all. And women on estrogen-based birth control pills should consult their physicians before using this herb.

Pregnant and nursing women should not use red clover.

Do not give red clover to children under 2. In older children, adjust the recommended dose based on the child's weight. Give a 50-pound child one-third of the dose a 150-pound adult would take.

If you're over 65, start with a low dose, and increase only if necessary.

Inform health professionals of the herbs you use. Problematic herb-drug interactions are possible.

Red clover may cause allergic reactions or other unexpected side effects. If any develop, reduce your dose or stop taking it. For more on herb safety, see Chapter 2.

If symptoms get worse or persist longer than 2 weeks, consult a health professional promptly.

Gardening

Red clover is a three-leafed perennial that grows to 2 feet. Many tiny florets compose its fragrant, edible, red or purple, ball-shaped flowers.

Because it's a legume, red clover adds nitrogen to the soil, and its deep roots help break up compacted soil. Plant seeds in spring or fall. In sunny conditions, this herb thrives in a variety of moist, well-drained soils but does not grow well in sand or gravel. Harvest the flowers when the tops are in full bloom.

RED PEPPER

For Pain, It's Hot!

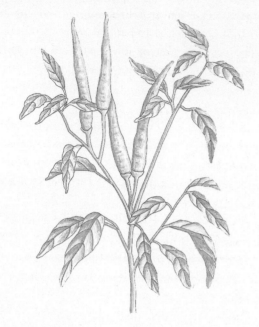

Family: Solanaceae; other members include potato, tomato, eggplant, and tobacco

Genus and species: *Capsicum annuum* and *C. frutescens* (green and red bell pepper, paprika, and pimiento are all milder varieties of *C. annuum*)

Also known as: Hot, African, Tabasco, Guinea, and bird pepper; Louisiana long (and short) pepper, cayenne chili pepper, and capsicum

Parts used: Fruits

Red pepper's fiery taste and crimson color make it one of the world's most noticeable and popular spices—and it's as hot in healing as it is on the tongue. Extracts of red pepper provide remarkably effective relief from certain types of severe, chronic pain. The herb also helps prevent and treat ulcers.

Red pepper has been discovered at Central American archeological sites dating to 7000 BC. The herb has been a culinary staple in Asia since ancient times. But European were unaware of it until Columbus returned with it from his first voyage to the New World.

Some call red pepper cayenne, a name derived from the Caribbean Indian word *kian*. Today, Cayenne is the capital of French Guiana. Ironically, only a tiny fraction of the U.S. red pepper supply comes from South America or the Caribbean. Most comes from India and Africa. Tabasco (Louisiana red pepper) grows along the Gulf Coast.

Because so little of this herb comes from around Cayenne, the American Spice Trade Association considers the name a misnomer and calls it red pepper.

Healing History

Seventeenth-century English herbalist Nicholas Culpeper wrote that immoderate use of red pepper "inflames the mouth and throat so extremely it is hard to endure," and "might prove dangerous to life." But he believed that small amounts "help digestion, provoke urine, relieve toothache, preserve the teeth from rottenness, comfort a cold stomach, expel the stone from the kidney, and take away dimness of sight."

Culpeper urged women to mix red pepper, gentian, and bay laurel oil in cotton and insert it vaginally to "bring down the courses" (menstruation). He warned, though, that "if [it] be put into the womb after delivery, it will make [the woman] barren forever."

During the 18th century, some mixed red pepper with snuff to boost the inhaled tobacco's kick. English herbalist Phillip Miller warned against this, saying that the combination caused "such violent fits of sneezing as to break the blood vessels in the head."

In India, the East Indies, Africa, Mexico, and the Caribbean, red pepper enjoys a long history as a digestive aid. This use never caught on among Europeans, who have traditionally believed that hot spices cause stomach ulcers.

The first North American to advocate red pepper in healing was Samuel Thomson, creator of Thomsonian herbal medicine, which enjoyed considerable popularity before the Civil War. Thomson believed most disease was caused by cold and cured by heat, so he prescribed "warming" herbs, among them red pepper.

After the Civil War, America's Eclectic physicians, forerunners of today's naturopaths, called red pepper capsicum and recommended it externally for arthritis and muscle soreness and internally as a digestive stimulant and treatment for colds, coughs, fever, diarrhea, constipation, nausea, and toothache. The Eclectics also advised placing the herb in socks to warm cold feet, a use echoed in some herbals today.

The Eclectics considered red pepper invaluable in the treatment of delirium tremens, the hallucinations and violent tremors that afflict advanced alcoholics: "Capsicum is the very best agent that can be used in delirium tremens. It enables the stomach to take and retain food. The best form is in a tea or strong beef soup. There is no danger of overdose as a [large] quantity may be swallowed with evident pleasure and without ill results."

American folk healers have also recommended dusting children's hands with powdered red pepper to stop thumb sucking and nail biting.

An estimated 25 percent of the world's population uses red pepper daily as a culinary spice. Some 2.5 million acres are planted with the herb.

Contemporary herbalists prescribe capsules of cayenne powder for colds and gastrointestinal and bowel problems, and as a digestive aid. They also recommend cayenne plasters for arthritis and muscle soreness.

Therapeutic Uses

Red pepper owes its heat and medicinal value to a compound found in its fruit, capsaicin. Research supports the herb's traditional uses as a digestive aid and pain reliever.

DIGESTIVE PROBLEMS. Red pepper stimulates secretion of saliva and stomach acids. Saliva contains enzymes that initiate the breakdown of carbohydrates, while stomach (gastric) secretions contain acids and enzymes that do the same.

In cultures with bland cuisines, such as the traditional American meat-and-potatoes diet, many people mistakenly believe that highly spiced foods damage the stomach and contribute to ulcers. In a study in the *Journal of the American Medical Association*, researchers used tiny video cameras to examine volunteers' stomach linings after both bland meals and meals liberally spiced with jalapeño peppers. The researchers found no difference in stomach condition, concluding, "Ingestion of highly spiced meals by normal individuals is not associated with [gastrointestinal] damage.

Some evidence suggests that red pepper helps *prevent* ulcers by inhibiting growth of *Helicobacter pylori*, the bacteria that cause them.

DIARRHEA. In addition to its action against *H. pylori*, red pepper helps combat other bacteria, lending credence to traditional claims t infectious diarrhea.

AIN. For centuries, herbalists
rubbing red pepper into the
at muscle and joint pain (counter-
irritant). The body can pay attention to only so
many pain signals at once. The minor superficial pain caused by counterirritants such as red
pepper reduces the nervous system's ability to
alert the brain to deeper, more severe pain.

More recently, red pepper has been shown to
possess direct pain-relieving properties for certain kinds of chronic pain. For reasons still
unexplained, capsaicin interferes with the
action of substance P, the compound in peripheral nerves that sends pain signals to the brain.
Since the 1980s, dozens of studies have shown
capsaicin to be remarkably effective at relieving
many types of pain.

The FDA has approved capsaicin for use in
many over the-counter pain-relieving creams,
including Arthricare, Capzasin, Dencorub, Icy
Hot Arthritis Therapy, Pain-X, and Zostrix.

OSTEOARTHRITIS. The most common
type of arthritis, it causes joint pain and stiffness for more than 27 million Americans, 14 percent of adults over 25 and 34 percent of those
over 65.

At the Veterans Affairs Hospital in Miami,
researchers asked 113 people with osteoarthritis
to treat their stiff, painful joints four times a
day with either a placebo ointment or one containing capsaicin. After 12 weeks, the capsaicin
users reported significantly greater relief.

At Rush-Presbyterian–St. Luke's Medical
Center in Chicago, a similar 9-week study of 59
people with osteoarthritis produced similar
results applying capsaicin cream twice a day.

FIBROMYALGIA. Fibromyalgia causes
muscle pain and tenderness. At the Medical College of Wisconsin in Milwaukee, 45 fibromyalgia
sufferers rubbed their painful or tender spots
four times a day with salves containing either a
placebo or capsaicin. After a month, those using
the herb reported significantly less pain and
tenderness.

PSORIASIS. In some cases, the red, scaly
patches caused by psoriasis become very itchy
(pruritic). At the University of Michigan, 197
people with pruritic psoriasis treated their skin
with creams containing either a placebo or capsaicin. After 6 weeks, the capsaicin group
reported significantly greater relief.

SHINGLES. Capsaicin ointment is the most
effective known treatment for the pain of shingles
(herpes zoster), an adult disease caused by the
same virus that produces chickenpox in children.
The virus remains dormant in the body until
later in life when it inexplicably reappears in
some people as shingles, causing a rash on one
side of the body that progresses from red bumps
to blisters to crusty pox resembling chickenpox.

In healthy adults, shingles clears up by itself
within 3 weeks. But some people—typically the
elderly or those with other illnesses—develop
severe, chronic pain, a condition that doctors
call post-herpetic neuralgia. But thanks to capsaicin, they suffer less.

DIABETIC NEUROPATHY. A common
complication of diabetes, diabetic neuropathy
causes pain in the arms, hands, legs, feet, and
possibly elsewhere. Researchers at several U.S.
medical centers instructed people with diabetic
neuropathy to apply creams containing either a
placebo or capsaicin four times a day. After
8 weeks, the capsaicin group reported significantly less pain, improved sleep, and greater ability to work, walk, and enjoy recreational activities.

CLUSTER HEADACHES. Capsaicin helps

relieve cluster headaches, which cause extremely severe pain on one side of the head. At the University of Florence in Italy, researchers had 16 cluster headache sufferers apply a capsaicin preparation inside their nostrils on the affected side for several days. Eleven of the participants (69 percent) experienced complete relief.

In another study, people with cluster headaches rubbed a capsaicin preparation inside their nostrils and outside of their noses. Within 5 days, 75 percent reported less pain and fewer headaches. They also reported burning nostrils and runny noses, but these side effects subsided within a week.

SELF-DEFENSE. Capsaicin is the active ingredient in many self-defense sprays, aptly known as pepper sprays. When directed into an assailant's eyes, pepper spray causes pain and temporary blindness that lasts up to 30 minutes, but does not damage the eye.

Intriguing Possibility

Red pepper may help cut cholesterol and prevent heart disease, according to Indian and U.S. researchers. While it's too early to endorse red pepper for these conditions, the common kitchen spice may someday aid heart health.

Rx Recommendations

Season food with red pepper to taste, but err on the side of caution. A little too much can set your mouth afire. If this occurs, the best treatment is milk. Casein, a protein in milk, pulls capsaicin off the taste buds.

For an infusion to aid digestion and help prevent or treat ulcers, use $\frac{1}{4}$ to $\frac{1}{2}$ teaspoon per cup of boiling water. Drink it after meals.

For external application to help treat pain, mix $\frac{1}{4}$ to $\frac{1}{2}$ teaspoon into a cup of warm vegetable oil and rub it on the affected area.

When using a commercial capsaicin ointment, follow label directions.

Safety

Chopping red peppers may burn the fingertips, a condition dubbed "Hunan hand," first identified in a cook preparing a Hunan Chinese recipe that called for chopping a mound of the fiery fruits. He wound up in an emergency room with severe hand pain.

Red pepper does not wash off the hands easily. Vinegar removes it best. Even with careful washing, the pungent herb may remain on the fingertips for hours and cause severe pain if contaminated fingers touch the eyes. Consider wearing rubber gloves when handling red peppers.

Red pepper has not been linked to menstruation promotion since the 17th century, but some research suggests that its stems and leaves—not the powdered fruits—stimulate uterine contractions in animals. Pregnant women or those trying to conceive should stick to the powdered fruits.

Do not give red pepper to children under 2. In older children, adjust the recommended dose based on the child's weight. Give a 50-pound child one-third of the dose a 150-pound adult would take.

If you're over 65, start with a low dose, and increase only if necessary.

Inform health professionals of the herbs you use. Problematic herb-drug interactions are possible.

Red pepper may cause allergic reactions or

other unexpected side effects. If any develop, reduce your dose or stop taking it. For more on herb safety, see Chapter 2.

If symptoms get worse or persist longer than 2 weeks, consult a health professional promptly.

Gardening

Red pepper is a shrubby, tropical perennial with shiny, pendulous, leathery fruits. It grows best in tropical or subtropical areas but also prospers in south-facing windows and greenhouses. The fruits' boxy shape is the source of the plant's genus name, *Capsicum*, from the Latin *capsa*, meaning box.

In southern states, seeds may be sown after the danger of frost has passed. Farther north, sow seeds indoors in flats 8 weeks before the final frost date, then transplant. Space seedlings 12 inches apart.

Red pepper prefers rich, well-watered, sandy soil and full sun, but it tolerates some shade. When harvesting the ripened fruit, be careful to leave some stem, or the peppers may spoil. Hang red peppers in a warm, dry place to dry, which takes several weeks.

REISHI

"Mushroom of Immortality" Is a Stretch—But Not by Much

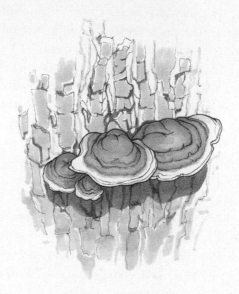

Family: Polyporaceae; other members include other mushrooms

Genus and species: *Ganoderma lucidum*

Also known as: Spirit plant, *ling zhi*. mushroom of immortality, *mannentake*

Parts used: Powdered mushroom

Reishi is a hard, woody fungus that grows on tree stumps and decaying wood in Asia, Europe, and North America. Its cap is so shiny it looks lacquered. Unlike other mushrooms, reishi caps come in six colors: blue, red, yellow, white, black, and purple.

Traditional Japanese hung dried reishi at their front doors to repel evil. When they married, Japanese women carried a reishi mushroom into their new home for good luck.

Healing History

Extolled in Chinese medical texts since the 1st century AD, Chinese physicians prescribe reishi to promote longevity, strengthen life force (*qi*), and treat fatigue, respiratory conditions, and liver ailments. Reishi's Chinese name, *ling zhi*, means "spirit plant" and reflects its connection to *qi*. Its connection to longevity earned it the name "mushroom of immortality." Users don't live forever, but this mushroom is so medically potent, it certainly might extend longevity.

Therapeutic Uses

Like ginseng (page 246) and eleuthero (page 200), herbalists consider reishi an adaptogen that strengthens the whole body.

IMMUNE ENHANCEMENT. Chinese researchers have shown that reishi activates many components of the immune system, among them: B-cells, T-cells, natural killer cells, and interleukins.

ANTIOXIDANT. Antioxidants prevent and help reverse the cell damage at the root of heart disease, cancer, and many other conditions associated with aging. Chinese scientists have found that reishi possesses "substantial antioxidant activity."

HEART DISEASE AND STROKE. Researchers in the United States, Switzerland, and China have discovered that reishi lowers cholesterol and blood pressure, both of which reduce risk of heart disease and stroke. Chinese scientists have found that it also helps prevents the internal blood clots that trigger heart attacks and most strokes.

CANCER. Laboratory studies show that reishi increases production of the body's own cancer-fighter, tumor necrosis factor. Animal studies around the world have shown that reishi helps prevent cancers of the lung, colon, breast, and prostate. In addition to its antioxidant and immune-boosting action, both of which help prevent and treat cancer, reishi also prevents new blood vessels from forming to feed growing tumors (angiogenesis inhibition), as a result, starving them. In China and Japan, physicians often prescribe resihi to supplement mainstream cancer therapies.

DIABETES. Reishi lowers blood sugar, suggesting that it helps manage diabetes. Diabetes is a major risk factor for heart disease, so reishi's effects on blood sugar also help prevent heart attack.

KIDNEY AND LIVER PROTECTION. Taiwanese researchers have discovered that reishi's antioxidant action protects the kidneys and liver from chemical damage.

BACTERIAL INFECTION. Korean researchers tested reishi against common bacteria by adding it to antibiotics. Compared with antibiotics alone, combined treatment killed significantly more bacteria.

HERPES. Japanese researchers asked 15 people with recurrent herpes (genital herpes and cold sores) how long their sores typically lasted—about 9 days. Then they gave them an herb mixture that was mostly reishi. Subsequent outbreaks cleared up in an average of 4 days, a highly significant difference.

Intriguing Possibilities

Preliminary studies suggest that reishi may help treat cirrhosis.

Rx Recommendations

Most sources suggest 500 to 2,000 milligrams of powdered mushroom twice a day. Follow package directions or your practitioner's.

Safety

Reishi may cause dizziness, stomach upset, skin irritation, diarrhea or constipation and can interfere with blood clotting. Side effects typically subside after 3 to 6 months of steady use.

Pregnant and nursing women should not use reishi.

Do not give reishi to children under 2. In older children, adjust the recommended dose based on the child's weight. Give a 50-pound child one0third of the dose a 150-pound adult would take.

If you're over 65, start with a low dose, and increase only if necessary.

Inform health professionals of the herbs you use. Problematic herb-drug interactions are possible.

Reishi may cause allergic reactions or other unexpected side effects. If any develop, reduce your dose or stop taking it. For more on herb safety, see Chapter 2.

If symptoms get worse or persist longer than 2 weeks, consult a health professional promptly.

Gardening

Reishi is an Asian mushroom, but it grows in woodsy areas of North America on tree stumps or decaying wood, typically plum or oak. Reishi grows very slowly, hence its Japanese name *mannentake,* which means 10,000-year-old mushroom. Commercial cultivation began in Asia in the 1980s. Those with patience can grow it indoors from kits marketed by Fungi Perfecti, www.fungi.com, or Mycosource, www.mycosource.com. Reishi tastes very bitter. Don't eat it as a food.

RHODIOLA

Russia's Secret Cold War Adaptogen

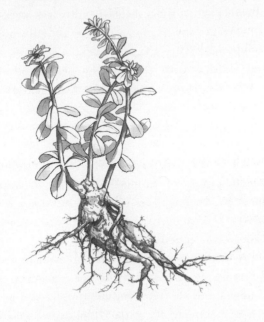

Family: Crassulaceae; other members include jade plant

Genus and species: *Rhodiola rosea*

Also known as: Golden root, rose root, arctic root

Parts used: Root

Rhodiola is a perennial that grows to 30 inches, produces bushy yellow flowers, and has a thick, gold-pink rhizome, hence the names golden and rose root. It thrives in some of the harshest conditions on earth—high in arctic mountains from Scandinavia to Siberia. It also helps people thrive despite physical challenges, such as fatigue and many illnesses.

For centuries, rhodiola enjoyed a folk reputation in Russia as a whole-body strengthener. After World War II, Russian researchers Nikolai Lazarev and Israel Brekhman investigated it. They coined the term "adaptogen" to describe plants such as rhodiola and ginseng that strengthen the body by providing a large number of health benefits. They also discovered the adaptogenic benefits of eleuthero (Siberian ginseng, page 200).

But the Soviet military kept rhodiola secret. During the Cold War, they were convinced that the herb could provide a competitive edge to Russian soldiers and Olympic athletes. During the 1970s while fighting in Afghanistan, one Soviet soldier, Zahir Ramazanov, drank a great deal of rhodiola tea. It boosted his endurance, quickened his hiking, and helped him recover faster from several illnesses.

In the 1990s, Ramazanov moved to New York and began importing rhodiola and translating then newly declassified Russian research about its many adaptogenic benefits. Eventually the herb came to the attention of Richard Brown, M.D., a Columbia University psychiatrist. At the time, his wife, Patricia Gerbarg, M.D., was in a bad way, debilitated by a case of Lyme disease that had gone undiagnosed for years. Standard therapies weren't helping. She tried rhodiola. Ten days later, she felt better. After a few months, she felt cured. Since the mid-1990s, Ramazanov, Brown, and Gerbarg have been instrumental in popularizing rhodiola.

Healing History

For a plant kept secret for so long, rhodiola has a long history in herbal medicine. Since ancient times, folk healers in Scandinavia and Russia have used it has been to treat a broad range of conditions. The Vikings used it to increase their strength and endurance.

Dioscorides, the Greek physician who traveled with Roman legions mentioned it in his classic book *De Materia Medica* (77 AD).

In traditional Tibetan medicine, rhodiola has been revered for centuries. Elsewhere in Asia, it was used to treat colds and flu. During the early 19th century, French physicians prescribed rhodiola as a "brain tonic." From 1725 well into the 1960s, Swedish, Norwegian, Russian, France, German, and Icelandic medical journals touted rhodiola, but at the time, American researchers had little interest in medicinal herbs, and rhodiola remained largely unknown in the United States until the 1990s.

Therapeutic Uses

STAMINA. In animal studies, rhodiola improves endurance substantially. Belgian researchers gave competitive cyclists either a placebo or rhodiola (200 milligrams). An hour later, the herb group showed significantly greater aerobic capacity.

Russian scientists gave 161 military cadets either a placebo or rhodiola. The herb produced "a pronounced antifatigue effect."

Swedish investigators gave 60 adults either a placebo or rhodiola (576 milligrams of extract a day). After 4 weeks, the herb group experienced significantly less fatigue, increased ability to concentrate, and decreased blood levels of the stress hormone, cortisol.

English researchers reviewed 11 rigorous clinical trials that involved 503 subjects. Their conclusion: Rhodiola increases blood oxygenation, reducing fatigue and increasing strength and stamina.

STRESS. Chinese researchers measured standard biomarkers of stress in laboratory animals, then gave some rhodiola while subjecting all the animals to loud noises. Untreated animals showed clear signs of emotional stress. The rhodiola group showed significantly less stress.

German investigators assessed the burnout symptoms of 101 anxious, exhausted, stressed out adults, and then gave them rhodiola (200 milligrams twice a day). A month later, they reported significantly more energy, less anxiety, and greater ability to concentrate. The main side effect: upset stomach.

COGNITIVE ABILITY. In maze studies, rhodiola improves animals' learning speed and memory. In hospitals, medical mistakes are most likely to occur late at night when physicians feel fatigued and drowsy.

Armenian researchers gave 56 medical residents on overnight duty either a placebo or rhodiola and shortly after, administered a battery of mental acuity tests. The herb group fared significantly better.

A similar Russian experiment tested rhodiola in students preparing for exams. Those who took the herb showed significantly less mental fatigue.

German scientists gave 20 middle-aged adults several memory tests and then gave them rhodiola (200 milligrams). An hour later, retesting showed improved memory.

HEART DISEASE AND STROKE. High blood pressure is a key risk factor for heart attack and the leading risk factor for stroke. A Chinese study shows that rhodiola lowers it.

Heart rhythm disturbances (arrhythmias) are potentially serious. A Russian study shows that rhodiola produces "a pronounced anti-arrhythmic effect."

DEPRESSION. Scandinavian researchers gave 89 depression sufferers either a placebo or rhodiola (340 milligrams/day). After 6 weeks, standard mood tests showed significant improvement in the herb group.

INSOMNIA. The depression study just mentioned also showed that rhodiola improved the quality of users' sleep.

LIVER PROTECTION. Korean researchers fed laboratory animals a compound that injures the liver. They also gave some animals rhodiola. The animals given rhodiola suffered significantly less liver damage.

CANCER PREVENTION AND TREATMENT. Russian studies show that rhodiola reduces risk of cancer-causing DNA mutations. The herb also helps treat cancer. Russian researchers gave it to people with bladder cancer, a disease that typically recurs. Compared with untreated bladder cancer sufferers, those who took rhodiola experienced significantly fewer recurrences.

Intriguing Possibilities

Pilot research suggests that rhodiola may help normalize irregular menstrual periods.

Rx Recommendations

Take 5 to 10 drops of tincture two to three times a day, 15 to 30 minutes before eating, or 200–450 milligrams/day of extract. Or follow package directions.

Safety

Caffeine-like jitters are possible. People with bipolar disorder should not use rhodiola.

Pregnant and nursing women should not use this herb.

Do not give rhodiola to children under 2. In older children, adjust the recommended dose based on the child's weight. Give a 50-pound child one-third of the dose a 150-pound adult would take.

If you're over 65, start with a low dose, and increase only if necessary.

Inform health professionals of the herbs you use. Problematic herb-drug interactions are possible.

Rhodiola may cause allergic reactions or other unexpected side effects. If any develop, reduce your dose or stop taking it. For more on herb safety, see Chapter 2.

If symptoms get worse or persist longer than 2 weeks, consult a health professional promptly.

Gardening

Not grown in the United States, except Alaska. Interested in growing? Contact the Alberta (Canada) Rhodiola Rosea Growers Organization, www.arrgo.ca.

RHUBARB

More Than Pie Filling

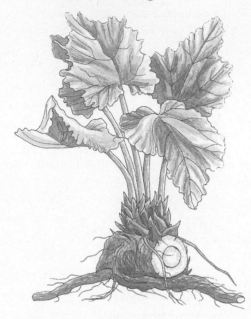

Family: Polygonaceae; other members include buckwheat

Genus and species: *Rheum officinale* and *R. palmatum* (Garden rhubarb, *R. rhaponticurn*, has similar but less powerful action)

Also known as: Rheum, or Chinese, Himalayan, Turkish, or medicinal rhubarb

Parts used: Roots

Rhubarb is an odd plant. Its roots are medicinal. Its stems make tasty pies. And its leaves are poisonous.

Healing History

Chinese physicians have used rhubarb root since ancient times. They prescribed it externally as a treatment for cuts and burns, and internally in small amounts to treat dysentery. They also discovered that large amounts have powerful laxative action and promote menstruation. During the 13th century, Marco Polo's journal mentioned rhubarb's medicinal use in Asia.

Over the centuries, Indian, Russian, and European herbalists discovered that their own native rhubarb species have similar though less powerful effects.

Seventeenth-century English herbalist Nicholas Culpeper endorsed rhubarb's laxative action: "This herb purges downward." He also recommended it externally as "a most effectual remedy to heal scabs and running sores." In addition, Culpeper claimed that rhubarb "heals jaundice . . . provokes urine . . . is very effectual for reins [gonorrhea] . . . and helps gout, sciatica . . . toothache . . . the stone [kidney stones] . . . and dimness of sight."

Later herbalists repudiated most of Culpeper's recommendations, prescribing small doses of rhubarb root for diarrhea and larger doses as a laxative.

America's 19th-century Eclectic physicians, forerunners of today's naturopaths, used rhubarb primarily to treat diarrhea and dysentery. The Eclectic text *King's American Dispensatory* (1898) noted the herb's effectiveness for constipation but said "it sometimes produces griping [cramping]." The Eclectics also considered the herb helpful in treating "hepatic derangement" (liver problems) and delirium tremens.

Bacterial dysentery was a common—and often fatal—disease in British East Africa between World Wars I and II. In 1921, Nairobi-based physician R. W. Burkitt wrote in the British medical journal *Lancet* that he'd treated it with rhubarb almost exclusively for 3 years: "I know of no remedy that has such a magical effect. No one who has ever used rhubarb would dream of using anything else . . . in this dreadful tropical scourge."

Contemporary herbalists are divided on rhubarb. Some recommend low doses for diarrhea and large doses for constipation. Others simply recommend it as a laxative.

Therapeutic Uses

The ancient Chinese were right about rhubarb's dual effects.

DIARRHEA. Small amounts of rhubarb help relieve diarrhea.

CONSTIPATION. Larger amounts have powerful laxative action. Rhubarb contains anthraquinones, compounds similar to those found in other laxative herbs: buckthorn (page 115), cascara sagrada (page 134), and senna (page 430).

For constipation, anthraquinone laxatives should be used only as a last resort. First, eat more fresh fruits and vegetables, drink more water, and get more exercise. If that doesn't work, try a bulk-forming laxative such as psyllium (see page 370). If you still need help, try cascara sagrada, generally regarded as the gentlest anthraquinone. Finally, if you still have difficulty, try rhubarb, buckthorn, or senna in consultation with your physician.

Commission E, the expert panel that evaluates herbal medicines for the German counterpart of the FDA, endorses rhubarb root as a laxative.

MENOPAUSAL UPSETS. German researchers gave 112 menopausal women either a placebo or rhubarb (4 milligrams/day). Twelve weeks later, the herb group reported significantly fewer hot flashes and other discomforts.

WOMEN'S HEALTH. Some animal studies suggest that rhubarb stimulates uterine contractions, lending some credence to the herb's use in China as a menstruation promoter. Women who are pregnant or trying to conceive should avoid rhubarb. Other women might try it to start their periods.

Intriguing Possibility

Chinese researchers report that rhubarb root helps prevent the progression of kidney failure.

Rx Recommendations

For diarrhea, make a decoction by gently boiling $\frac{1}{2}$ teaspoon of powdered root per cup of water for 10 minutes, then strain if you wish. Take 1 tablespoon at a time periodically, up to 1 cup a day. Rhubarb tastes bitter and unpleasant. Add honey, sugar, and/or lemon.

For constipation, make a decoction by boiling 1 to 2 teaspoons of powdered root per cup of water for 10 minutes, then strain if you wish. Take 1 tablespoon at a time, up to one cup a day.

If you're using a homemade tincture, take $\frac{1}{4}$ teaspoon daily for diarrhea and $\frac{1}{2}$ to 1 teaspoon daily for constipation.

When using commercial preparations, follow package directions.

Safety

Rhubarb may turn urine bright yellow or red. This is harmless.

Rhubarb stems may be used in pie fillings, but the plant's leaf blades contain oxalic acid, which is poisonous. Ingesting the leaves can cause burning in the mouth and throat, nausea, vomiting, weakness, and other symptoms. Deaths have occurred.

Because of rhubarb's powerful action, laxative amounts should not be used by people with chronic intestinal problems such as ulcers or colitis.

Do not use laxative amounts of rhubarb for more than 2 weeks. Over time, it causes lazy bowel syndrome, inability to defecate without chemical stimulation.

Pregnant and nursing women should not use anthraquinone laxatives.

Do not give rhubarb to children for medicinal purposes.

If you're over 65, start with a low dose, and increase only if necessary.

Inform health professionals of the herbs you use. Problematic herb-drug interactions are possible.

Rhubarb may cause allergic reactions or other unexpected side effects. If any develop, reduce your dose or stop taking it. For more on herb safety, see Chapter 2.

If symptoms get worse or persist longer than 2 weeks, consult a health professional promptly.

Gardening

The medicinal species are not garden herbs. Medicinal rhubarb is a large, leafy perennial that reaches 10 feet. Its root is thick and branching, brown on the outside and yellow inside. Its round, hollow stems are jointed and terminate in branching spikes of numerous small flowers.

Garden rhubarb reaches only 3 feet. It has purple stems and thick roots—reddish outside and yellow inside. Garden rhubarb is a less potent herbal healer. If you use it medicinally, start with the amounts recommended above, but be prepared to use more.

Garden rhubarb requires a dormant period in winter and does not do well in the South, where winters are warm. Sow seeds or root cuttings 4 feet apart in late spring in deeply dug, well-watered beds under full sun or partial shade. Add compost and mulch in winter. Harvest stems for pies the second year and roots the fourth.

ROOIBOS

The South African Antioxidant

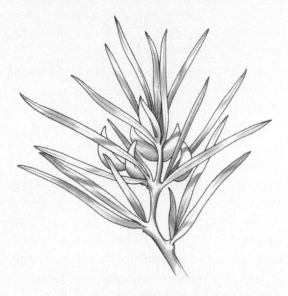

Family: Fabaceae; other members include peas, lentils, green beans

Genus and species: *Aspalathus linearis*

Also known as: Red tea, red bush tea, and in Dutch, rooibosch

Parts used: Stems and leaves (needles)

South Africa's draconian system of racial segregation, apartheid, ended in 1994, and so did the worldwide boycott of South African exports. By the millennium, one South African product had become popular in the United States—red-colored, pleasant-tasting rooibos (ROY-bus) tea. Rooibos also shows considerable potential in healing.

Healing History

The indigenous peoples of South Africa loved red bush tea so much that they climbed the rugged mountains near the Cape of Good Hope to collect the stems and needle-like leaves of the rooibos shrub. They drank it as a beverage and used it medicinally to treat allergies, indigestion, and colic.

Dutch colonists (Afrikaners) adopted the plant as a cheap alternative to black tea, an expensive import.

Commercial cultivation began in the mountains west of Cape Town in the 1930s. Export to England began during World War II, when the English had trouble obtaining black tea.

South Africa's white minority imposed apartheid in 1948, and by the 1960s, the world began boycotting the country's exports, including rooibos. Apartheid ended in 1994, and rooibos exports resumed and soared. In 2000, the estimated 600 growers harvested 4,000 tons. Today the figure is 14,000 tons, and rooibos is available at Starbucks.

Rooibos teas vary in color from pale to deep red. As the ratio of leaves/needles to stems increases, the color darkens. Most rooibos teas use leaves that have been oxidized, but in one variety, green rooibos, the leaves remain unoxidized.

Therapeutic Uses

Rooibos is high in antioxidants, compounds that help prevent and reverse the cell damage at the root of heart disease, cancer, and many other conditions associated with aging. As this book goes to press, rooibos research is in its infancy—mostly laboratory and animal studies with only a few human (clinical) trials. But rooibos seems destined to become a useful healing herb.

CHOLESTEROL. South African scientists

assessed 40 adults' blood levels of antioxidants and cholesterol and then instructed them to drink 6 cups of rooibos tea a day. After 6 weeks, their antioxidant levels increased significantly. Their LDL (bad) cholesterol fell and their HDL (good) cholesterol increased.

WRINKLES. Thai researchers assessed facial wrinkles in older adults and then asked them to apply a skin cream with added tea (page 449) and rooibos daily. After 28 days, the herbal skin cream reduced wrinkling by 10 percent.

Intriguing Possibilities

IMMUNE FUNCTION. Laboratory and animal studies show that rooibos strengthens the immune system.

INFLAMMATION. Laboratory and animal studies show that the herb has anti-inflammatory action.

DIABETES. South African animal studies suggest that rooibos helps control diabetes.

ULCERS. Bulgarian scientists have shown that rooibos impairs the ability of *Helicobacter pylori* bacteria to cause ulcers.

FERTILITY. Animal trials show that rooibos increases sperm motility (forward motion).

OSTEOPOROSIS. Canadian investigators have shown that rooibos spurs the activity of the cells that build new bone (osteoblasts).

LIVER PROTECTION. Slovakian researchers exposed animals to compounds that cause liver damage. Simultaneous administration of rooibos tea significantly reduced risk of liver damage—and helped heal animals whose livers had been damaged. Several other studies have confirmed the herb's liver-protective action.

Rx Recommendations

For a pleasant-tasting, noncaffeinated infusion, use 1 to 2 teaspoons of herb per cup of boiling water. When using commercial preparations, follow package directions.

To fight wrinkles, mix a strong rooibos infusion with skin cream.

Safety

For centuries, South Africans have used rooibos with no reports of problems. But in 2013, Brown University doctors diagnosed liver damage in a 52-year-old man who drank a great deal of rooibos tea. After stopping rooibos, his liver healed. In 2015, Israeli investigators discovered liver-damaging compounds (pyrrolizidine alkaloids) in some samples of rooibos tea.

As was the case with kava (page 285), the rapid, soaring popularity of rooibos—production tripling since 2000—has apparently resulted in some adulteration with plant material that contains pyrrolizidines. It's not clear how much of a problem this is. At this writing, reports of liver damage are rare, and several animal studies show that rooibos *protects* the liver. Still, if you have liver disease or are pregnant or nursing, don't use this herb.

If you're over 65, start with a low dose, and increase only if necessary.

Inform health professionals of the herbs you use. Problematic herb-drug interactions are possible.

Rooibos may cause allergic reactions or other unexpected side effects. If any develop, reduce your dose or stop taking it. For more on herb safety, see Chapter 2.

If symptoms get worse or persist longer than 2 weeks, consult a health professional promptly.

Gardening

Rooibos is a bushy shrub that grows to 6 feet. Native to the mountains on the west coast of southern South Africa, it grows in a symbiotic relationship with the area's unique soil microorganisms. Attempts to grow it elsewhere—Australia, China, the United States—have largely failed. The U.S. supply is imported.

ROSE
A Rose Is a Rose Is a Medicine

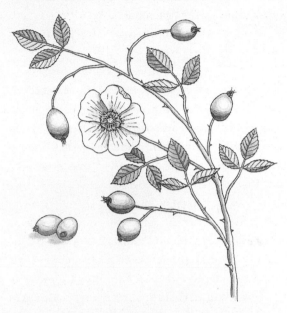

Family: Rosaceae; other members include peach, apple, almond, and strawberry

Genus and species: *Rosa canina*, *R. rugosa*, and *R. centifolia*

Also known as: Hipberry

Parts used: Fruits (hips) and petals

Prized since the dawn of history, the rose is the queen of flowers. In herbal healing, however, this plant becomes noteworthy only after the velvety petals have fallen away, revealing its cherry-size fruits, or "hips."

Rose hips contain vitamin C, but authorities disagree on how much. Some herbalists call rose hips one of the best natural sources of vitamin C. Scientific sources scoff at this claim, asserting that it would take more than a dozen cups of rose hip tea to help treat colds and flu.

While herbalists have generally overstated the herb's vitamins C content, it still helps treat colds and flu—and heart disease.

Healing History

Roses were a favorite of the ancient Egyptians, who used the fragrant petals as air fresheners and rose water as a perfume. During the 1st century AD, when Marc Antony wooed Cleopatra, legend has it the Egyptian queen ordered the floors of her palace covered knee deep in rose petals to welcome her lover.

In Greece, Hippocrates recommended rose flowers mixed with oil for diseases of the uterus. India's traditional Ayurvedic physicians have long considered rose petals cooling and astringent, leading to their application as poultices to treat skin wounds and inflammations. The Ayurvedics also used rose petals and rose water as laxatives.

Western herbalists mirrored the Ayurvedics. The 12th-century German abbess/herbalist Hildegard of Bingen recommended rose hip tea as the initial treatment for just about every illness.

Seventeenth-century English herbalist Nicholas Culpeper called the herb "binding and restringent [astringent]." He wrote that it "strengthens the stomach, prevents vomiting, stops tickling coughs . . . [is] good against all kinds of fluxes [diarrhea] . . . [and is] of great service in consumptions [tuberculosis]."

As the centuries passed, European herbalists recommended dried rose petal tea for headache, dizziness, mouth sores, and menstrual cramps.

Americans have always loved roses. The flowers were among the first planted around the White House, which now boasts an enormous rose garden. However, American herbalists considered the rose only a minor healer. The 19th-century Eclectic physicians, forerunners of today's naturopaths, did not use rose petals at all. They beat the hips into a pulp and used it as a base for making pills that contained other medicines.

Roses almost disappeared from early 20th-century herbals. Then came the discovery of vitamin C in the 1930s and the finding that rose hips contain it.

Contemporary herbalists are almost unanimous in their praise of rose hips as a source of vitamin C. One bestselling herbal claims, "Rose hips are rich in vitamin C, richer by far ounce for ounce than oranges. Some people say we should make rose hip tea a part of our daily diet."

Because of rose hips' vitamin C content, herbalists tout them for colds and flu. Some also recommend the herb as a mild laxative.

Therapeutic Uses

There's nothing wrong with making rose hips a part of your daily diet, but don't count on them—or the prepackaged teas containing them—to supply all the vitamin C you need. This is especially true if you're using the vitamin to treat the common cold and flu.

While rose hips contain a significant amount of vitamin C, the drying process destroys from 45 to 90 percent of it, and infusions extract only about 40 percent of what's left. That still leaves a fair amount of vitamin C, but it's considerably less than most herbals promise.

Many companies that manufacture vitamin C supplements claim their products are made from rose hips. In fact, no supplement contains vitamin C exclusively from rose hips. Commercial "rose hip" preparations combine the hips with ascorbic acid from other sources.

COLDS AND FLU. The weight of scientific evidence shows that vitamin C is of only marginal benefit in cold prevention. But once you feel a cold coming on, the nutrient helps reduce the severity and duration of the illness—provided you take at least 2,000 milligrams/day from the moment you feel the tell-tale scratchy throat until you feel well again.

It's not easy to obtain 2,000 milligrams of vitamin C exclusively from rose hips, but there's no harm in combining the herb with other sources.

Another argument in favor of rose hip infusions is that hot liquids help relieve the sore throat, nasal congestion, and cough associated with colds. They also warm the throat, which helps impair viral replication (cold viruses reproduce best at around 95°F).

HEART DISEASE AND STROKE. Swedish researchers recruited 331 obese, diabetic adults whose condition put them at high risk for heart attack and stroke. Half took a daily placebo, half powdered rose hips (40 grams/day, about 4 ounces). After 6 weeks, the placebo group showed no change in heart disease risk factors, but the herb group's blood pressure and cholesterol both dropped, meaning less risk of heart attack and stroke.

OSTEOARTHRITIS. This is the most common type of arthritis, caused by wear and tear. Scandinavian researchers analyzed three rigorous studies of rose hips for osteoarthritis of the knee, involving 306 people, average age 66, who took a daily placebo or rose hips (various doses). Tests before and after treatment showed that the herb significantly reduced pain and stiffness.

MOUTH SORES. Commission E, the expert panel that evaluates herbal medicines for the German counterpart of the FDA, approves rose petal infusion for one of its many traditional uses: treating canker sores.

Rx Recommendations

For a pleasant-tasting, mildly astringent infusion that may help treat colds, flu, and canker sores, use 2 to 3 teaspoons of dried chopped hips or dried powdered petals per cup of boiling water. Steep for 10 minutes and strain if you wish. Drink as needed.

As a homemade tincture, use ½ to 1 teaspoon as needed.

When using commercial preparations, follow package directions.

Safety

High doses of vitamin C may cause diarrhea. If that occurs, reduce your intake.

High doses of vitamin C may also strain the kidneys. This is not a problem for people with healthy kidneys, but those with kidney disease should consult their physicians before using large amounts of rose hips.

Do not give rose hips to children under 2. In older children, adjust the recommended dose based on the child's weight. Give a 50-pound child one-third of the dose a 150-pound adult would take.

If you're over 65, start with a low dose, and increase only if necessary.

Inform health professionals of the herbs you use. Problematic herb-drug interactions are possible.

Rose hips may cause allergic reactions or

other unexpected side effects. If any develop, reduce your dose or stop taking it. For more on herb safety, see Chapter 2.

If symptoms get worse or persist longer than 2 weeks, consult a health professional promptly.

Gardening

Roses have been bred for every climate. "Old roses" are generally more fragrant than newer hybrids, but they have less showy, faster-wilting flowers. Consult a nursery for the varieties best suited to your conditions and desires. Enjoy the flowers, then, when the petals fall, harvest, dry, and powder the hips.

ROSEMARY

The Tasty Natural Preservative

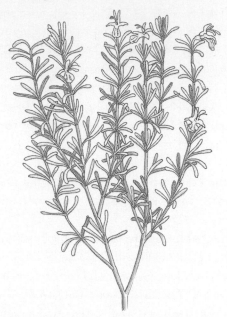

Family: Labiatae; other members include mints

Genus and species: *Rosmarinus officinalis* and *R. prostratus*

Also known as: Rosemarine and *incensier* (French)

Parts used: Leaves

Thousands of years before refrigeration, ancient people noticed that wrapping meats in crushed rosemary leaves deterred rotting and imparted a fresh fragrance and pleasing flavor. To this day, the herb remains a favorite herb for meat dishes.

Rosemary's ability to preserve food also led to the belief that it helped preserve memory. Greek students wore rosemary garlands to assist their powers of recall. As the centuries passed, the herb was incorporated into wedding ceremonies as a symbol of spousal fidelity and into funerals to help survivors to remember the dead. In Hamlet, Ophelia gives Hamlet a sprig, saying, "There's rosemary . . . for remembrance."

Healing History

The ancients used rosemary as they used all aromatic, preservative herbs—for respiratory and gastrointestinal problems. Traditional Chinese physicians mixed it with ginger as a treatment for headache, indigestion, insomnia, and malaria.

During the Middle Ages, rosemary's association with weddings evolved into use as a love charm. If a young person tapped another with a rosemary twig containing an open blossom, the couple would supposedly fall in love.

Placed under a pillow, the aromatic herb was believed to prevent bad dreams. Planted around a home, it was reputed to repel witches. By the 16th century, planting rosemary near front doors became a bone of contention in England. The belief arose that this signified a household where the woman ruled. Some men ripped out rosemary plants as evidence that they, not their wives, ruled the roost.

In 1235, Queen Elizabeth of Hungary became paralyzed. According to legend, a hermit soaked a pound of rosemary in a gallon of wine for several days, then rubbed it on her limbs, curing her. Rosemary-wine combinations became known as Queen of Hungary's Water and for centuries were used externally to treat gout, dandruff, baldness, and skin problems. As the centuries passed, pennyroyal and marjoram were incorporated into what became known as Hungary Water.

The French hung rosemary around sickrooms and in hospitals as a kind of healing incense, calling it *incensier*. As recently as World War II, French nurses burned a mixture of rosemary leaves and juniper berries in hospital rooms as an antiseptic.

Colonists brought rosemary to North America. An early medical guide, *The American New Dispensatory*, recommended the herb's leaves and flowers and Hungary Water for use "in nervous and menstrual affections, for strokes, paralysis, and dizziness."

Oddly, those great proponents of botanical medicine, the Eclectics, forerunners of today's naturopaths, had little use for rosemary. Their text *King's American Dispensatory* (1898) called the herb a digestive aid and menstruation promoter but declared that it was "seldom used except as a perfume."

Central American folk healers use rosemary oil as an insect repellent and menstruation promoter.

Contemporary American herbalists say that rosemary stimulates the circulatory, digestive, and nervous systems. They recommend it as a treatment for headache, indigestion, and depression and as a gargle for bad breath. They also advocate its external use for muscle aches and in baths for relaxation.

Therapeutic Uses

Rosemary may not guarantee marital fidelity, A's on exams, or vivid memories of the departed—but the ancients were right about the herb's ability to preserve meats.

FOOD POISONING. Meats spoil in part because their fats oxidize and turn rancid. Rosemary oil contains compounds that are potent antioxidants. In fact, rosemary's preservative power compares favorably with the commercial food preservatives BHA and BHT. Rosemary's preservative action may help prevent food poisoning on your next picnic. Mix the crushed leaves generously into hamburger meat and tuna, pasta, and potato salads.

INFECTIONS. The same compounds that retard spoilage also inhibit the action of many microorganisms that cause infection. For minor cuts in the garden, press fresh, crushed rosemary leaves into wounds on the way to washing and bandaging them.

COGNITIVE FUNCTION. The "herb of remembrance" helps preserve memory and cognitive function. Dementia drugs inhibit the action of an enzyme, acetylcholinesterase. Several compounds in rosemary oil (and sage, page 411) are acetylcholinesterase inhibitors.

University of Miami scientists gave 40 adults a battery of cognitive function tests, then exposed them to rosemary oil vapor for 3 minutes. Subsequent testing showed brain wave changes associated with learning and better memory. An similar English trial produced the same findings.

Researchers at the Maryland University of Integrated Health gave 28 cognitively healthy adults, age 65 to 90, either a placebo or one of four doses of rosemary in tomato juice (750 milligrams, 1500 milligrams, 3000 milligrams, or 6000 milligrams). For 5 weeks, each participant took each treatment with week-long no-treatment washout periods in between. After each dose, participants completed standard mental acuity tests at 1 hour, 2.5 hours, and 6 hours. The lowest dose of rosemary (750 milligrams) significantly improved recall. But higher doses impaired it. If you're concerned about your memory, use just a pinch of rosemary, no more.

DIGESTIVE PROBLEMS. Like most culinary herbs, rosemary helps relax the digestive tract (antispasmodic), validating ancient use of the herb as a digestive aid. Commission E, the expert panel that evaluates herbal medicines for the German counterpart of the FDA, approves rosemary as a treatment for indigestion.

CONGESTION. Like other aromatic herbs, rosemary may help relieve nasal and chest congestion caused by colds, flu, and allergies.

WOMEN'S HEALTH. Antispasmodics soothe not only the digestive tract but other smooth muscles as well, for instance, the uterus. Theoretically antispasmodic, rosemary should calm the uterus, but Italian researchers have discovered that it does exactly the opposite. Pregnant women should steer clear of medicinal preparations of rosemary. Other women might try the herb to bring on their periods.

Intriguing Possibilities

Antioxidants help prevent cancer. The high levels in rosemary spurred Pennsylvania State University researchers to add powdered leaves to laboratory animal feed. Then all the animals were injected with carcinogenic chemicals. Compared with the animals eating plain food, those consuming rosemary were significantly less likely to develop cancer.

Rosemary contains a COX-2 pain-relieving compound, carnosol. A pilot study at New York Presbyterian Medical Center hints that the herb may soothe pain.

Rx Recommendations

For a pleasantly aromatic infusion to settle the stomach or clear a stuffy nose, use 1 teaspoon of crushed herb per cup of boiling water. Steep for 10 to 15 minutes, then strain. Drink up to 3 cups a day.

As a homemade tincture, use ¼ to ½ teaspoon up to three times a day.

When using commercial preparations, follow package directions.

Safety

In culinary amounts, rosemary poses no hazards. But even small amounts of rosemary oil may cause stomach, kidney, and intestinal irritation. Larger doses may cause poisoning. Do not ingest more than a drop or two of concentrated rosemary oil.

Pregnant and nursing women should not use medicinal preparations of rosemary or its oil.

Do not give rosemary to children under 2. In older children, adjust the recommended dose based on the child's weight. Give a 50-pound child one-third of the dose a 150-pound adult would take.

If you're over 65, start with a low dose, and increase only if necessary.

Inform health professionals of the herbs you use. Problematic herb-drug interactions are possible.

Rosemary may cause allergic reactions or other unexpected side effects. If any develop, reduce your dose or stop taking it. For more on herb safety, see Chapter 2.

If symptoms get worse or persist longer than 2 weeks, consult a health professional promptly.

Gardening

Rosemary is a woody, pine-scented, evergreen perennial with needlelike leaves. It reaches 3 feet in the United States and produces small, pale blue flowers in summer. Creeping rosemary (*Rosmarinus prostratus*) is widely used in the western United States as a ground cover and cascade over garden walls.

Rosemary can be grown from seeds, but germination is problematic and seedlings develop slowly. Most herb growers start with cuttings. If you sow seeds, plant them in the spring, 6 inches apart. Plant cuttings in sandy soil, leaving only one-third of each twig showing.

Rosemary prefers light, sandy, well-drained soil and full sun. Overwatering may cause root rot. If you live where temperatures dip below zero, mulch plants each autumn or grow the herb in pots, bring them indoors in winter, and keep them in a south-facing window.

Cut twigs and strip the leaves any time after the plants have become established.

SAFFRON

The New Herbal Antidepressant

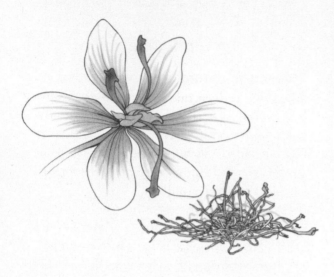

Family: Iridaceae

Genus and species: *Crocus sativus*

Also known as: Saffron crocus, autumn crocus, zafran

Part used: The flower's stigmas ("threads")

Saffron is worth more than its weight in gold. It takes some 200,000 dried stigmas from 75,000 flowers to produce just 1 pound. As every cook knows, saffron is among the world's most expensive spices, often sold in fractions of a gram. But given the high cost of many pharmaceutical antidepressants, it just might be a bargain.

Healing History

Our word, saffron, comes from the Arabic, *safran*, meaning yellow, a reference to the flower's threads. The plant is unknown in the wild. Greek mythology holds that a god bewitched wild crocus, transforming it into saffron. Archeologists explain that ancient humans created saffron by selectively breeding other *Crocus* species for longer, more numerous threads.

Yellow pigments from saffron-precursor plants have been discovered in prehistoric Iranian sites dated to 45,000 BC. The Sumerians were among the first to use it medicinally, around 3000 BC, notably for "melancholy" (depression). They also used the threads in dyes, perfumes, and ritual offerings to their gods.

Alexander the Great added saffron threads to his baths, believing that the costly spice healed battle wounds. Egypt's Queen Cleopatra adopted saffron baths to enhance lovemaking.

The Romans introduced saffron into southern Europe. It arrived in Britain around 1350. The town of Saffron Walden in southeast England was the British center of cultivation. The Arabs introduced it into Spain, where it became a key ingredient in paella. By the early 19th century, competition from Spain had ended English saffron farming.

Medieval Europeans used the herb (ineffectively) to treat the Black Plague. The Chinese used it to treat depression. India's Ayurvedic physicians prescribed it as a whole-body strengthener (tonic).

Seventeenth-century English herbalist Nicholas Culpeper prescribed saffron for measles, smallpox, and "hysterical depression" (mood swings of premenstrual syndrome, menstruation, and menopause). But he warned that more than a pinch might cause sedation.

Colonists introduced saffron into the Western Hemisphere. It was particularly popular among the Pennsylvania Dutch, who still grow it in eastern Pennsylvania.

During saffron's 2,700 years of documented history, various cultures have used it to treat dozens of conditions, including acne, fever, asthma, depression, wounds, menstrual cramps, and urinary tract infections. Contemporary herbalists rarely recommend saffron because of its high cost. But they may change their minds, given saffron's antidepressant action.

Therapeutic Uses

Saffron contains several pharmacologically active compounds: safranal, crocetin, and picro-crocin. Most studies come from Iran, the world's leading producer.

DEPRESSION. Traditional Persian physicians prescribed saffron for depression. Iranian researchers gave 30 adults with mild-to-moderate depression either a pharmaceutical antidepressant (imipramine, Tofranil) or saffron (30 milligrams/day). After 6 weeks, both treatments showed equivalent mood elevation.

Another Iranian team repeated this study in 40 depressed adults, comparing a different pharmaceutical (fluoxetine, Prozac) and saffron (30 milligrams/day). After 6 weeks, the herb worked as well as the drug.

A third Iranian team gave 40 depressed adults either Prozac or saffron (15 milligrams twice a day). After 8 weeks, both treatments provided the same benefit.

PREMENSTRUAL SYNDROME. PMS may cause mood swings that include feeling blue. Iranian investigators gave 50 women with premenstrual distress either a placebo or saffron (15 milligrams twice a day). After four menstrual cycles, the saffron group showed significant mood normalization.

ALZHEIMER'S DISEASE. Laboratory and animal studies suggest that saffron might help slow progressive dementia. Iranian researchers gave 54 people with mild-to-moderate Alzheimer's either a standard pharmaceutical (donepezil, Aricept) or saffron (15 milligrams/day for 4 weeks, then 30 milligrams/day for 18 weeks). After 22 weeks, both treatments provided the same benefits.

MACULAR DEGENERATION. Antioxidants help prevent this common cause of older adult vision impairment, and saffron is high in antioxidants. Italian researchers tested the vision of 29 people with early MD, then gave them saffron (20 milligrams/day). After 3 months, all of them showed significantly improved vision.

ERECTILE DYSFUNCTION. Iranian investigators assessed the erections of 20 men complaining of erection difficulties and then gave them saffron (200 milligrams/day). After 10 days, standard tests of erection showed statistically significant improvement.

Intriguing Possibilities

Laboratory studies suggest that saffron's crocetin has cancer-preventive value.

Rx Recommendations

Because of its high price, saffron adulteration has been a problem for centuries. Common adulterants include safflower (*Carthamus tinctorius*, "Portuguese saffron") and/or turmeric (*Cucuma longa*, page 464). It's difficult to tell the difference between real and adulterated or counterfeit saffron, but here are some clues: Saffron threads are uniformly dark red. Threads colored differently may be counterfeit. Pour a few drops of cold water on a thread or two. With real saffron, it takes a while for the water to begin to turn pale yellow. When adulterated, the water changes color immediately.

If you take saffron for depression, premenstrual syndrome, Alzheimer's, or macular degeneration, most studies have used 30 milligrams/day, or for erectile dysfunction, 200 milligrams/day.

Safety

Saffron has been used for thousands of years with few reports of problems. However, large amounts may cause dizziness, anxiety, sedation, nausea, headache, and dry mouth. Very large amounts—more than 5 grams—can be toxic, even fatal.

Culinary amounts of saffron are safe during pregnancy and nursing, but larger amounts may stimulate uterine contractions. Pregnant and nursing women should limit their consumption.

Do not give medicinal amounts of saffron to children.

If you're over 65, start with a low dose, and increase only if necessary.

Inform health professionals of the herbs you use. Problematic herb-drug interactions are possible.

Saffron may cause allergic reactions or other unexpected side effects. If any develop, reduce your dose or stop taking it. For more on herb safety, see Chapter 2.

If symptoms get worse or persist longer than 2 weeks, consult a health professional promptly.

Gardening

Saffron is a perennial that grows to 12 inches. Its beautiful flowers bloom in autumn. Saffron thrives in hot, dry areas of the Mediterranean and Middle East under full sun. It prefers well-watered, well-drained clay soils with plenty of compost or manure. Seeds are sterile. Propagate plants by dividing bulbs. Almost all the world's saffron grows from Spain to India. Iran grows 90 percent of the world crop.

SAGE

An Herb for the Wise

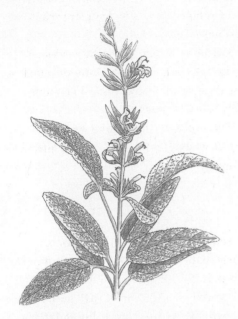

Family: Labiatae; other members include mints

Genus and species: *Salvia officinalis*

Also known as: Garden, meadow, Spanish, Greek, and Dalmatian sage

Parts used: Leaves

Close your eyes and imagine Thanksgiving turkey stuffing. Smell that warm, rich aroma? Chances are, it's sage.

Thousands of years before the Pilgrims stuffed the first Thanksgiving turkey, herbalists worldwide celebrated the healing powers of this aromatic herb. The genus name for sage, *Salvia*, comes from the Latin word meaning "to heal."

Throughout history, sage has been used so extensively that it gained a reputation as a panacea, prompting the late herb expert Varro E. Tyler, Ph.D., to write, "If one consults enough herbals . . . every sickness known to humanity will be listed as being cured by sage." Sage is no cure-all, but it's an antiperspirant, preservative, wound treatment, and digestive aid. It might even help treat dementia.

Healing History

The ancient Greeks and Romans used sage as a meat preservative. They also believed that like another powerful preservative, rosemary, it could enhance memory.

But sage gained a much broader medicinal reputation. The Roman naturalist Pliny prescribed it for snakebite, epilepsy, intestinal worms, chest ailments, and menstruation promotion. The Greek physician Dioscorides considered sage a diuretic and menstruation promoter and recommended its leaves as bandages.

Around the 10th century, Arab physicians believed that sage extended longevity to near-immortality. After the Crusades, Europeans embraced this belief. Students at the medieval medical school in Salerno, Italy, recited, "Why should a man die who grows sage in his garden?" The same thought evolved into a medieval English proverb: "He that would live foraye [forever] / Must eat sage in May."

The French called the herb *toute bonne*, meaning "all's well," and had their own adage: "Sage helps the nerves, and by its powerful might / Palsy is cured and fever put to flight." Charlemagne ordered sage grown in the medicinal herb gardens on his imperial farms.

In Chaucer's *Canterbury Tales*, "The Knight's Tale" echoed the ancient use of sage as a treatment for wounds: "To use on . . . wounds and broken arms . . . sage they drank. . . ."

Around the year 1000, an Icelandic herbal recommended sage for bladder infections and kidney stones. The twelfth-century German abbess/herbalist Hildegard of Bingen prescribed sage for headache and gastrointestinal and respiratory ailments, from the common cold to tuberculosis.

During the 16th century, Dutch explorers introduced sage to the Chinese, who prized the herb so highly that they gladly traded 3 pounds of tea for a pound of the new European healer. Chinese physicians used sage to treat insomnia, depression, gastrointestinal distress, mental illness, menstrual complaints, and nipple inflammation (mastitis) in nursing mothers.

India's traditional Ayurvedic physicians used Indian sage similarly. They also prescribed it for hemorrhoids, gonorrhea, vaginitis, and eye disorders.

Sixteenth-century British herbalist John Gerard called sage "singularly good for the head and brain. It quickeneth the senses and memory, strengtheneth the sinews, restoreth health to those that have palsy, and taketh away shaky trembling of the members."

During the 17th century, English herbalist Nicholas Culpeper seconded Gerard, and recommended sage "boiled in water or wine to wash sore mouths and throats, cankers, or the secret parts [genitals]. It will preserve faculty and memory."

Colonists introduced sage into North America, where folk healers employed it to treat insomnia, epilepsy, measles, seasickness, and intestinal worms.

America's 19th-century Eclectic physicians, forerunners of today's naturopaths, used sage primarily to treat fever. They also prescribed sage poultices for arthritis and the tea as "a valuable anaphrodisiac [sexual depressant] to check excessive venereal desires . . . used in connection with moral . . . and other aids, if necessary."

As late as the 1920s, U.S. medical texts recommended sage tea as a gargle for sore throat and sage leaf poultices for sprains and swellings.

Modern herbalists recommend sage as an external treatment for wounds and insect bites; as a gargle for bleeding gums, sore throat, laryngitis, and tonsillitis; and as an infusion to reduce perspiration, terminate milk production, and relieve dizziness, depression, menstrual irregularity, and intestinal upsets.

Therapeutic Uses

The name *toute bonne* overstates sage's healing potential, but the herb's aromatic oil has therapeutic value, notably one unique action that sets sage apart from all other healing herbs—it's an antiperspirant.

EXCESSIVE PERSPIRATION. Several studies show that sage cuts perspiration by as much as 50 percent, with the maximum effect occurring 2 hours after ingestion. This explains sage's traditional uses against fever, which causes profuse sweating, and for arresting lactation.

Today, Germans can buy a sage-based antiperspirant (Salysat). Commission E, the expert panel that evaluates herbal medicines for the German counterpart of the FDA, approves sage infusion for treatment of excessive perspiration.

WOUNDS. In laboratory studies, sage oil kills several infection-causing bacteria. This lends credence to the herb's age-old use in treating wounds. Unlike Dioscorides, today's physicians would not recommend bandaging wounds with sage leaves, but you can use fresh leaves as garden first-aid for minor wounds.

FOOD POISONING. Meats spoil in part

because their fats turn rancid (oxidize). Like rosemary, sage contains powerful antioxidants that preserve food almost as well as the commercial preservatives BHA and BHT. Sage's preservative action may help prevent food poisoning on your next picnic. Mix it generously into hamburger meat and tuna, pasta, and potato salads.

COGNITIVE FUNCTION. Like rosemary, sage contains acetylcholinesterase inhibitors, key ingredients in dementia medications. British researchers gave cognitive function tests to 44 healthy young adults, then gave them either a placebo or sage oil (50 microliters). When retested, the sage group showed some improvement.

HEART DISEASE. Iranian researchers gave 67 overweight older adults newly diagnosed with high cholesterol either a placebo or sage leaf extract (500 milligrams three times a day). After 2 months their total cholesterol dropped 20 percent. Experts estimate that for every 1 percent decrease in cholesterol, heart attack risk drops 2 percent. If this study is valid, sage cut participants' risk of heart attack 40 percent.

DIGESTIVE PROBLEMS. Like most culinary spices, sage helps relax the smooth muscle lining the digestive tract (antispasmodic). This supports the herb's traditional role as a gastrointestinal soother. Commission E approves sage for indigestion.

SORE THROAT. Sage contains astringent tannins that account for its traditional use in treating canker sores, bleeding gums, and sore throat. In Germany, where herbal healing is more mainstream than in the United States, physicians recommend a hot sage gargle for sore throat and tonsillitis.

MENOPAUSAL COMPLAINTS. Sage's antiperspirant action persuaded Swiss researchers to investigate it for relief of hot flashes, which cause sweating. They recruited 69 menopausal women who reported at least five hot flashes a day. All the women took sage extract (280 milligrams/day). After 2 months, their hot flashes decreased significantly, from an average of 9.3 a day to just 3.8.

TRANQUILIZER. English researchers assessed the stress levels of 30 adults and then gave them a series of treatments: a placebo or sage (300 milligrams/day or 600 milligrams/day) with week-long washout periods in between. At 1 and 4 hours after each treatment, the scientists re-examined subjects' stress levels. Both doses of sage significantly reduced anxiety, elevated mood, and increased contentment.

MENSTRUATION PROMOTION. As an antispasmodic, sage should theoretically calm the uterus. Some studies suggest, however, that sage oil may stimulate it instead, which explains its traditional role in menstruation promotion. Pregnant women should not take medicinal doses of sage, but other women might try it to trigger their periods.

Intriguing Possibilities

John Gerard may have been prescient when he wrote that sage "quickeneth memory." A pilot study in Iran suggests that the herb (60 drops of tincture/day for 4 months) slows the progression of Alzheimer's disease.

One German study hints that sage reduces blood sugar (glucose). Diabetes is a serious condition requiring professional care. If you'd like to include sage in your management plan, consult your physician.

Rx Recommendations

For garden first-aid, press fresh leaves into cuts or scrapes until you can wash and bandage them.

For an infusion, use 1 to 2 teaspoons of dried leaves per cup of boiling water. Steep for 10 minutes, then strain. Drink up to 3 cups a day. The infusion may also be used as a gargle. Sage tastes warm, pleasantly aromatic, and somewhat pungent.

As a homemade tincture, take ½ to 1 teaspoon up to three times a day. This may help reduce wetness if you perspire a lot.

When using commercial preparations, follow the package directions.

Safety

In rare instances, ingestion of sage tea may cause inflammation of the lips and mouth.

Concentrated sage oil is toxic and should not be ingested.

Sage contains fairly high levels of a toxic compound (thujone), large amounts of which causes a variety of symptoms possibly including convulsions. Some sources call sage potentially toxic. However, the heat involved in brewing sage infusion eliminates much of the thujone, so the risk is negligible. But with tinctures, ingest only the recommended amount.

Pregnant and nursing women should not use sage beyond culinary amounts.

Do not give sage to children under 2. In older children, adjust the recommended dose based on the child's weight. Give a 50-pound child one-third of the dose a 150-pound adult would take.

If you're over 65, start with a low dose, and increase only if necessary.

Inform health professionals of the herbs you use. Problematic herb-drug interactions are possible.

Sage may cause allergic reactions or other unexpected side effects. If any develop, reduce your dose or stop taking it. For more on herb safety, see Chapter 2.

If symptoms get worse or persist longer than 2 weeks, consult a health professional promptly.

Note: When smoked, one species of sage, *Salvia divinorum*, has intoxicant/hallucinogenic action. It has become a recreational drug. At this writing, *S. divinorum*, is legal in most states. It's available on the Internet.

Gardening

Sage is a perennial, branching, evergreen shrub that reaches about 3 feet. It has square, woolly, woody stems near its base, but it's herbaceous near plant tops. Its 2-inch leaves are oval, velvety, and gray green, with long stalks. Depending on the species, sage's small, summer-blooming flowers are pink, white, blue, or purple.

Sage is not related to the West's sagebrush, so named because of its vaguely sage-like aroma.

Sage may be propagated from seeds or cuttings. Germination takes a few weeks. Sow seeds ½ inch deep in spring. It takes about 2 years to grow good-size plants from seeds. Most authorities recommend planting cuttings.

Sage grows well in most soils, but requires good drainage and full sun. Water well until plants have become established, after which they require less water. The plants become woody and less productive after a few years. Replace them. If your winter temperatures fall below zero, mulch sage each fall.

Harvest leaves before flower buds open by cutting plants back to four inches above ground. Discard stems and leaf stalks. Store dried leaves in airtight containers.

ST. JOHN'S WORT

The Premier Herbal Antidepressant

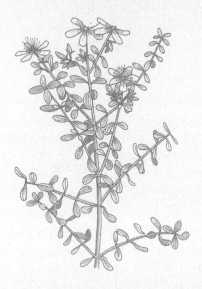

Family: Hypericaceae; other members include rose of Sharon

Genus and species: *Hypericum perforatum*

Also known as: Hypericum

Parts used: Leaves and flowers

St. John's wort has been used in herbal healing for more than 2,000 years, mostly as a treatment for wounds. Today, the herb is more popular than ever. Why? In the 1980s, scientists discovered that it's an antidepressant—and as potent as prescription pharmaceuticals. Before the herb gained fame as an antidepressant, annual sales worldwide totaled $10 million. Now they top $500 million.

Healing History

"Wort" is Old English for "plant." The leaves and flowers of St. John's wort contain glands that,

when pinched, release a red oil. Early Christians named the plant in honor of John the Baptist, because they believed it released its blood-red oil on August 29, the anniversary of the saint's beheading.

In the 1st century AD, the Roman naturalist Pliny prescribed St. John's wort steeped in wine as a cure for the bites of poisonous snakes. The Greek physician Dioscorides recommended it externally for burns and internally as a diuretic, menstruation promoter, and treatment for sciatica and recurring fevers (malaria).

The Greeks and Romans also believed that St. John's wort protected against witches' spells. Christians adopted this pagan belief, burning the herb in bonfires on St. John's Eve, June 23, to purify the air, drive away evil spirits, and ensure healthy crops, This poem from 1400 captured how people back then viewed this herb:

St. John's wort doth charm all witches away
If gathered at midnight on the saint's holy day.
Any devils and witches have no power to harm
Those that gather the plant for a charm.
Rub the lintels with that red juicy flower;
No thunder nor tempest will then have the power
To hurt or hinder your house; and bind
Round your neck a charm of a similar kind.

Under the Doctrine of Signatures, the medieval belief that an herb's physical appearance revealed its healing value, red plants were believed to treat bleeding wounds. "The juicy red flower" of St. John's wort was no exception. During the 16th century, herbalist John Gerard recommended it as a "most precious remedy for deepe wounds," and wrote that the herb "provoketh urine and is right good against stone in the bladder."

In 1618, the first *London Pharmacopoeia*

advised chopping St. John's wort flowers, immersing them in oil, and placing the mixture in the sun for 3 weeks. The resulting tincture was a standard treatment for wounds and bruises for several hundred years.

Seventeenth-century English herbalist Nicholas Culpeper called St. John's wort "a singular wound herb; boiled in wine and drank, it healeth inward hurts or bruises; made into an ointment, it opens obstructions, dissolves swellings, and closes up the lips of wounds. . . . [It] helpeth all manner of vomiting and spitting blood [tuberculosis]."

Early colonists introduced St. John's wort into North America, but they found Native Americans using the American variety in much same way Europeans used the Old World plant—as a tonic and treatment for diarrhea, fever, snakebite, wounds, and skin problems.

Nineteenth-century botanical medicine authority Charles Millspaugh, M.D., touted St. John's wort's value as a wound treatment during the Civil War: "Lacerations of parts rich in nerves yield nicely to this drug." Dr. Millspaugh was a homeopath at a time when homeopathy was as popular as mainstream ("regular") medicine. He railed against conventional medicine's dismissal of the herb: "Any homeopath of at least 3 months practice can attest to its merits." Homeopaths prescribed St. John's wort for wounds, asthma, bites, sciatica, diarrhea, hemorrhoids, and some types of paralysis.

America's 19th-century Eclectic physicians, forerunners of today's naturopaths, also considered St. John's wort an effective wound healer and tetanus preventive. They advocated the whole herb as a treatment for "hysteria" (menstrual discomforts) because of its "undoubted power over the nervous system."

Contemporary herbalists recommend St. John's wort enthusiastically as an antidepressant. Some also tout it for viral illnesses, notably herpes and HIV.

Therapeutic Uses

St. John's wort contains hypericin, an antidepressant, and antiviral and immune-boosting compounds (flavonoids), which explain its action against viral, bacterial, and fungal infections.

DEPRESSION. During the 1980s, German researchers discovered that hypericin interferes with monoamine oxidase (MAO). MAO inhibitors are an important class of antidepressants. In German pilot studies, people with mild to moderate depression obtained significant relief from St. John's wort—mood elevation, improved self-esteem, greater interest in life, increased appetite, and more normal sleep patterns.

Herbalists began recommending the herb for depression, but it did not rocket to prominence until 1996, when German researchers published a meta-analysis of clinical trials in the *British Medical Journal* (now *BMJ*). Meta-analysis is a statistical technique that allows the results of small studies to be combined as if they'd been one large trial. One large study is more compelling than several small ones.

The meta-analysis included 23 trials involving 1,757 adults with mild to moderate depression. The researchers found that placebos improved mood in 22 percent of users, but among those who took St. John's wort, 55 percent.

Since then, dozens of studies have confirmed that St. John's wort is an effective antidepressant. In 1999, University of Hawaii researchers conducted another meta-analysis of six rigorous trials conducted since the earlier report. Again,

St. John's wort provided significant benefit.

How beneficial is it? About as effective as the most popular class of pharmaceutical anti-depressants, the selective serotonin reuptake inhibitors (SSRIs), including Prozac, Paxil, and Zoloft.

❧ German researchers gave 161 people with mild to moderate depression either Prozac (fluoxetine) or St. John's wort (400 milli-grams twice a day). After 6 weeks, 72 Prozac users and 71 percent of those taking the herb experienced significant mood elevation—but the herb caused fewer side effects.

❧ Harvard researchers conducted a similar trial, comparing Prozac and St. John's wort in 135 people with mild to moderate depres-sion. In this study, "St. John's wort was sig-nificantly more effective than Prozac."

❧ German scientists gave 251 clinically depressed adults either Paxil (paroxetine) or St. John's wort (300 milligrams three times a day). After 6 weeks, the Paxil group improved 45 percent on standard mood scales. But the St. John's wort group improved 57 percent with fewer side effects. The researchers con-cluded that St. John's wort "is at least as effective as Paxil and is better tolerated."

❧ Researchers at St. John's Episcopal Hospital in New York City gave 30 depressed adults either Zoloft or St. John's wort (900 milli-grams/day). After 6 weeks, 40 percent of the Zoloft group showed significant improve-ment. But in the herb group, the figure was 47 percent. The scientists noted that St. John's wort "is at least as effective" as Zoloft.

❧ Iranian researchers analyzed 13 rigorous tri-als of St. John's wort versus SSRI antide-

pressants (Prozac, Paxil, Zoloft, etc.). Their conclusion: The herb works as well as the drugs with fewer side effects.

❧ Finally, German researchers analyzed 29 trials that compared St. John's wort to place-bos and to pharmaceutical antidepressants. Their conclusion: For mild to moderate depression, St. John's wort "is similarly effec-tive to standard antidepressants."

Australian researchers analyzed the cost-effectiveness of St. John's wort versus two widely prescribed pharmaceutical antidepressants (Zoloft and Effexor). Over 12 months of daily use, Zoloft cost $199 more, Effexor, $469 more.

St. John's wort works best for mild to moder-ate depression, but at least one study suggests that it also relieves severe depression.

The herb also helps prevent depression recur-rences. German researchers gave either a pla-cebo or St. John's wort to 703 adults, age 18 to 65, who'd suffered several episodes of major depression. After 18 months, those taking the herb were significantly less likely to have suf-fered another recurrence.

Like pharmaceutical antidepressants, St. John's wort requires some patience. According to German medical herbalist Rudolph Fritz Weiss, M.D., the benefit "does not develop quickly . . . [It may take] 2 or 3 months."

Commission E, the expert panel that evalu-ates herbal medicines for the German counter-part of the FDA, approves St. John's wort as a treatment for depression.

SEASONAL AFFECTIVE DISORDER (SAD). SAD is winter depression caused by short day length and little exposure to sunlight. British researchers gave 301 SAD sufferers either stan-dard therapy (exposure to ultra-bright light) or light therapy plus St. John's wort. Both treatments produced significant mood elevation. But those who also took the herb reported significantly more restful and refreshing sleep.

MENOPAUSAL COMPLAINTS. In addition to hot flashes, many menopausal women suffer mood swings and depression. Korean researchers gave 77 menopausal women either a placebo or a combination of black cohosh and St. John's wort. Black cohosh relieves hot flashes (page 97) but does not treat the psychological challenges of menopause. After 3 months, the herb group reported fewer hot flashes and less depression. Several similar German and Canadian studies showed similar results.

INFECTIONS. Hypericin is active against several bacteria and many viruses: influenza, herpes, polio, hepatitis C, and HIV, the virus that causes AIDS.

Hypericin's "dramatic" activity against HIV, discovered in 1988 by researchers at New York University and the Weizmann Institute in Israel, sent many AIDS sufferers rushing to health food stores for the herb. Some reported benefits, including improved immune function.

Unfortunately, enthusiasm for hypericin has waned, since the introduction of today's AIDS drugs (protease inhibitors). Ironically, people taking protease inhibitors should avoid St. John's wort. The herb interferes with the action of these drugs.

WOUNDS. Several studies support St. John's wort's traditional use as a wound treatment. Hypericin and other antibiotic and anti-inflammatory compounds in the herb's red oil help prevent infection and speed healing. A German study showed that compared with conventional treatment, a St. John's wort ointment (not available in the United States) substantially reduced the healing time of burns—with less scarring. Commission E approves topical application of St. John's wort preparations for treatment of minor wounds and burns.

RESTLESS LEG SYNDROME. This maddening neurological annoyance involves jumpy, twitchy legs in bed that interfere with sleep. Brazilian researchers gave St. John's wort (300 milligrams/day 2 hours before bed) to 21 people with chronic restless legs. Ten days later, 81 percent reported quieter legs and improved sleep.

Rx Recommendations

To treat depression, most studies have used 300 milligrams three times a day Follow label directions.

To heal wounds, apply crushed leaves and flowers to the affected area after you have cleaned it with soap and water. Or apply a tincture.

For treatment of AIDS, consult a physician.

Safety

In livestock fed large amounts of St. John's wort, the hypericin concentrates near the skin and causes sun sensitivity (photosensitization) and blistering sunburn. Laboratory animals injected with large doses of hypericin have died after exposure to sunlight.

As a result, in 1977, the FDA declared St. John's wort "unsafe." The agency mistakenly presumed that humans would suffer the same problem. But no. Millions of people have used St. John's wort to treat depression, but reports of photosensitization are rare. On the other hand, if you have fair, sensitive skin or have experienced photosensitivity when using other medications, take extra precautions in the sun.

Initially, researchers called hypericin an antidepressant because it appeared to be an MAO inhibitor. People who take pharmaceutical MAO inhibitors must refrain from eating a large number of foods to avoid unpleasant side effects. Many people taking St. John's wort did not observe these food restrictions but did not develop MAO side effects. German researchers have discovered why: Although hypericin resembles an MAO inhibitor, it is more complicated chemically and more similar to an SSRI, the Prozac family of antidepressants. No food restrictions are necessary.

St. John's wort reduces blood levels of birth control pills around 15 percent, suggesting that the herb may interfere with oral contraceptives. Women wishing to avoid pregnancy should not use the herb while taking birth control pills.

AIDS patients report that the herb is relatively nontoxic, but some have experienced sun sensitivity, drowsiness, nausea, and diarrhea.

St. John's wort oil may irritate sensitive skin.

Do not take St. John's wort in combination with any other antidepressant medication without consulting your physician. Likewise, don't take the herb if you take protease inhibitors.

Also, do not use St. John's wort if you take cyclosporine to control organ transplant rejection. The herb may interfere with the drug.

Pregnant and nursing women should not use St. John's wort unless advised to do so by a physician, for example, for post-partum depression.

Do not give St. John's wort to children under 2. In older children, adjust the recommended dose based on the child's weight. Give a 50-pound child one-third of the dose a 150-pound adult would take.

If you're over 65, start with a low dose, and increase only if necessary.

Inform health professionals of the herbs you use. Problematic herb-drug interactions are possible.

St. John's wort may cause allergic reactions or other unexpected side effects. If any develop, reduce your dose or stop taking it. For more on herb safety, see Chapter 2.

If symptoms get worse or persist longer than 2 weeks, consult a health professional promptly.

Gardening

St. John's wort is a woody, invasively spreading perennial that reaches 2 feet and smells like turpentine. Its leaves are dotted with glands that produce the red oil. Its striking star-shaped flowers bloom bright yellow in summer. They also contain the leaf oil and turn red when pinched.

The herb is best propagated from root divisions in spring or fall. It grows in almost any well-drained soil under full sun or partial shade. Contain it to control spreading.

Although it's a perennial, St. John's wort is not particularly long-lived. Replant it every few years. Harvest the leaves and flowers as the plants bloom. Dry them and store in airtight containers.

SARSAPARILLA

A Sex-Linked Reputation

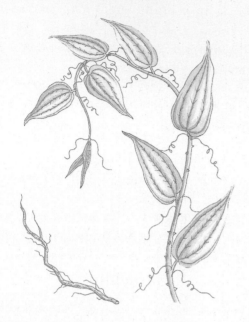

Family: Liliaceae; other members include lily, tulip, garlic, and onion

Genus and species: *Smilax officinalis*, *S. febrifuga*, and other *Smilax* species

Also known as: Mexican, Vera Cruz, Honduran, Jamaican, American, and Ecuadoran sarsaparilla

Parts used: Rhizomes and roots

In old Western movies, cowboys who didn't want whiskey told saloonkeepers, "Give me a sarsaparilla." Chances are the bartender gave him a bottle of Ayer's Sarsaparilla, a popular 19th-century soft drink. But cowboys who ordered sarsaparilla were usually thinking about more than refreshment. The herb was among the most widely used treatments for syphilis, and men often ordered it after visiting brothels.

Sarsaparilla does not treat syphilis, but modern studies suggest this herb does have some intriguing benefits.

Healing History

The ancient Greeks and Romans considered European sarsaparilla an antidote to poisons. But European herbalists largely ignored it until the 16th century, when Spanish explorers discovered the Caribbean species, a prickly (*zarza*) vine (*parra*) that was small (*illa*). That description evolved into "sarsaparilla."

Caribbean Indians and Native Americans used sarsaparilla to treat skin conditions and urinary complaints. They also considered it a tonic for preserving youthful vigor, both physical and sexual.

In 1494, an epidemic of unusually virulent syphilis swept Europe, killing thousands. Europeans considered the disease an import from the New World, and that's where they looked for herbs to treat it. They focused on sarsaparilla.

The conquistadors began shipping Mexican sarsaparilla back to Spain around 1530, and by 1600, it was widely used throughout Europe as a strengthening tonic and treatment for syphilis. Sarsaparilla and syphilis have been entwined ever since.

Sarsaparilla enjoyed a meteoric rise in popularity. Seventeenth-century English herbalist Nicholas Culpeper called it the treatment of choice for "the French disease," the English term for syphilis. Echoing the ancients, he wrote, "If the juice of the berries be given to a new-born child, it shall never be hurt by poison." Culpeper also recommended sarsaparilla for eye problems, head colds, gas pains, pimples, and "all manner of aches in the sinews or joints."

By 1800, many physicians denounced sarsaparilla as completely ineffective against syphilis, but their words fell on deaf ears. Nineteenth-century records indicate that Britain imported 150,000 pounds a year, much of it for the treatment of the infection.

Syphilis was quite prevalent in 19th-century America. Physicians treat it with patent medicines euphemistically known as "blood purifiers," chief among them, Ayer's Sarsaparilla, marketed for blood purification and "disorders of the liver, stomach, and kidneys, as well as tuberculosis, tumors, rheumatism, female weakness, sterility, and pimples."

The U.S. Pharmacopoeia, a standard drug reference, listed sarsaparilla as a syphilis treatment from 1820 to 1882. But after the Civil War, the antisarsaparilla bandwagon gained momentum, and by the 20th century, most physicians had dismissed it as worthless.

Therapeutic Uses

Sarsaparilla is a minor medicinal herb, but it's far from useless. It contains saponin compounds that are diuretic. This property explains the herb's long association with the genitals. In addition, sarsaparilla binds certain toxins produced by bacteria (endotoxins) and speeds their elimination, which ironically makes it a blood purifier, though not in the historical sense.

HIGH BLOOD PRESSURE. Physicians often prescribe diuretics for high blood pressure. High blood pressure is a serious condition that requires professional care. If you'd like to include sarsaparilla in your treatment plan, consult your physician.

Diuretics deplete the body of potassium, an essential nutrient. If you use sarsaparilla frequently, be sure to eat potassium-rich foods such as bananas and vegetables.

CONGESTIVE HEART FAILURE. Physicians also prescribe diuretics to combat the fluid accumulation of congestive heart failure. If you'd like to include sarsaparilla in your treatment regimen, talk to your physician.

PREMENSTRUAL SYNDROME (PMS). Sarsaparilla's diuretic action may benefit women bothered by premenstrual fluid retention.

Intriguing Possibilities

Preliminary studies from around the world suggest that sarsaparilla helps treat psoriasis and leprosy. Some animal studies indicate that the herb may have liver-protective effects.

Medicinal Myths

Sarsaparilla contains a compound, sarsapogenin, that can be chemically converted to the male sex hormone testosterone. Some writers have claimed that sarsaparilla contains testosterone. It does not, and ingesting the herb does not raise testosterone levels.

Sarsaparilla has also enjoyed some popularity among bodybuilders who believe that it contains anabolic steroids, chemical relatives of testosterone that some body builders take (usually against medical advice) to increase muscle mass. Sarsaparilla contains no anabolic steroids.

Rx Recommendations

For a diuretic decoction, use 1 to 2 teaspoons of powdered root per cup of water. Bring to a boil, simmer for 10 to 15 minutes, then strain. Drink up to 3 cups a day. Sarsaparilla tastes initially sweetish, then unpleasant.

As a homemade tincture, take ¼ to ½ teaspoon up to three times a day.

When using commercial preparations, follow the package directions.

Safety

Sarsaparilla causes no significant side effects.

Some weight-loss programs tout diuretics to eliminate water weight, but weight-loss experts advise against taking diuretics. Any pounds lost with help from diuretics almost invariably return. The key to permanent weight control is a low-calorie, low-fat, high-fiber diet and regular exercise.

Ingesting large amounts of sarsaparilla's saponins may cause a transient burning sensation in the mouth and throat as well as stomach and intestinal irritation.

Pregnant and nursing women should not use sarsaparilla.

Do not give sarsaparilla to children under 2. In older children, adjust the recommended dose based on the child's weight. Give a 50-pound child one-third of the dose a 150-pound adult would take.

If you're over 65, start with a low dose, and increase only if necessary.

Inform health professionals of the herbs you use. Problematic herb-drug interactions are possible.

Sarsaparilla may cause allergic reactions or other unexpected side effects. If any develop, reduce your dose or stop taking it. For more on herb safety, see Chapter 2.

If symptoms get worse or persist longer than 2 weeks, consult a health professional promptly.

Gardening

Sarsaparilla is not a garden herb in the United States. It's a perennial, climbing, woody, prickly stemmed vine with pointed, generally oval-shaped leaves. Its small green, yellow, or bronze flowers are dioecious—plants are either male or female. The medicinal parts are the rhizome and roots.

SAW PALMETTO

The Top Choice for Prostate Enlargement

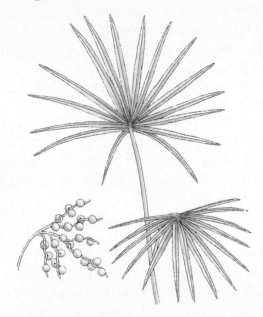

Family: Palmae; other members include the various palms

Genus and species: *Serenoa repens*

Also known as: Sabal and American dwarf palm

Part used: Fruits (berries)

Saw palmetto is a small palm tree native to Florida and the Gulf Coast that produces a brownish fruit. Centuries ago, Native Americans discovered that its fruits ("berries") have diuretic action and used them to treat urinary problems. Today, saw palmetto is the premier herbal treatment for benign prostate enlargement (medically, "benign prostatic hypertrophy" or BPH).

Healing History

Native Americans harvested the plant's leaves for mattress stuffing, thatched roofing, and for woven hats and baskets. During the 19th century, physicians throughout the South recommended berry preparations to treat coughs and bronchitis.

However, saw palmetto was used primarily for two other purposes—to enlarge women's breasts, and to treat BPH. *King's American Dispensatory* (1898), the standard text for Eclectic physicians, the forerunners of today's naturopaths, declared: "Continued use is said to slowly and surely cause the mammary glands to enlarge. Paradoxically, it also reduces hypertrophy of the prostate. [Saw palmetto] has been lauded as 'the old man's friend,' giving relief to the many annoyances commonly attributed to the enlarged prostate. It is reputed to strengthen the sexual appetite and restore sexual activity after exhaustive excesses."

By the early 20th century, doctors abandoned saw palmetto as they switched from herbs to pharmaceuticals. Fortunately, European researchers remained interested in the plant. During the 1960s, they discovered that the Eclectics were right. Saw palmetto fruits contain fatty acids (sitosterols) that help prevent and treat BPH.

Therapeutic Uses

Saw palmetto is no aphrodisiac nor does it enlarge women's breasts. But since the 1990s, the herb's berry extract has become a widely used treatment for BPH.

BENIGN PROSTATE ENLARGEMENT. In men over 40, testosterone declines while levels of other hormones increase, notably prolactin. This boosts the male sex hormone dihydrotestosterone, which spurs overgrowth of prostate tissue, causing BPH. An enzyme (5-alpha-reductase) converts testosterone to dihydrotestosterone. Pharmaceutical BPH treatments interfere with 5-alpha-reductase. Saw palmetto has the same biochemical action, thanks to its sitosterol compounds.

Many studies have shown that saw palmetto shrinks enlarged prostates and relieves BPH symptoms: the need to urinate immediately (urgency), difficulty getting started (hesitancy), decreased flow, difficulty finishing (dribbling), and most annoying, the need to get up at night to urinate (nocturia).

♣ European researchers gave 1,098 BPH sufferers either a standard drug (Proscar, finasteride) or the herb (160 milligrams twice a day). After 26 weeks, both treatments were comparably effective. Proscar decreased BPH symptoms by 39 percent, compared with 37 percent for saw palmetto. Urine flow improved 30 percent in the men taking the drug, 25 percent in the herb users. But saw palmetto caused fewer side effects, namely, less risk of erection problems and libido loss.

♣ Turkish researchers gave 60 men with BPH one of three treatments: a pharmaceutical (Flomax, tamsulosin), saw palmetto (320 milligrams/day) or a combination of the two. The herb worked as well as the drug, and the combination provided no additional benefit.

♣ Researchers at the Veterans Affairs hospital in Minneapolis analyzed 21 studies involving a total of 3,319 men and lasting up to 48 weeks. Their conclusion: Saw palmetto relieves BPH.

Occasionally, studies show no benefit, for example, a 2006 report published in the *New England Journal of Medicine*. But the weight of the evidence favors the herb. Commission E, the expert panel that evaluates herbal medicines for the German counterpart of the FDA, approves saw palmetto as a treatment for BPH. Most American men take prescription medications to treat BPH, but in Europe, saw palmetto is more popular.

Note: Neither saw palmetto nor pharmaceutical treatments cure BPH. They reduce prostate size and relieve symptoms. But over time, continued enlargement may necessitate surgery.

Intriguing Possibilities

Swiss researchers assessed the prostate symptoms and sexual function of 69 older men and then gave them saw palmetto (320 milligrams/day). After 9 weeks, as expected, their prostate symptoms improved. But unexpectedly, so did their libidos and erection firmness. If other trials confirm these sexual benefits, saw palmetto may become even more popular.

Chinese physicians prescribe an herbal formula—saw palmetto and other herbs—to treat prostate cancer. At the University of California, San Francisco, Medical Center, researchers gave the Chinese formula to 61 men with advanced prostate cancer whose tumors no longer responded to mainstream medication. Levels of prostate-specific antigen, a standard indicator of tumor activity, declined by 50 percent in three-quarters of the men. It's too early to call saw palmetto a treatment for prostate cancer, but that day may come.

Rx Recommendations

Most studies have used 320 milligrams of a standardized extract a day, split into two or three doses. Unfortunately, however, the more daily doses, the less likely people are to take their medicine as directed.

Researchers in Brussels, Belgium, conducted a yearlong study of 132 men with enlarged prostates to compare two different saw palmetto regimens: 160 milligrams twice daily versus 320 milligrams once a day. Both produced the same improvement.

To use saw palmetto, look for a standardized extract and take 320 milligrams a day.

Safety

If saw palmetto causes side effects, they're usually mild—stomach upset and headache. Allergic reactions are also possible.

There is no reason for children, pregnant, or nursing women to use saw palmetto.

Because saw palmetto has hormonal action, men with hormone disorders should consult a physician before taking it.

If you already take another BPH medication, do not take saw palmetto without consulting your physician.

If you are having trouble urinating or if you pass blood in your urine, talk to your doctor.

Gardening

Saw palmetto grows easily to about 10 feet in sandy soil. It's used as an ornamental in the Southeast. The plant produces edible brown-black fruits (berries).

SCHISANDRA
Five Tastes for Healing

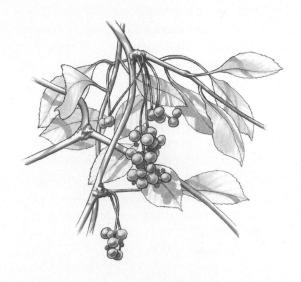

Family: Schisandraceae; other members include magnolia vine

Genus and species: *Schisandra chinensis*

Also known as: Schizandra, five-taste berry, *wu-wei-zi* (Chinese), *gomishi, hoku-gomishi* (Japanese)

Parts used: Dried berries

Schisandra is a woody, deciduous vine native to northeastern and north central China. It grows to 20 feet, producing clusters of small, bright red fruits (berries). Its Chinese name, *wu-wei-zi*, means five-taste berry. Taste is important in Chinese medicinal herbs, and shisandra is unusual because it incorporates all five: sweet, sour, bitter, salty, and spicy (pungent).

Healing History

As an herb with multiple tastes, schisandra often balances the components of multi-herb Chinese medicinal formulas. In addition, practitioners of Chinese medicine use it to treat fatigue, insomnia, night sweats, and respiratory problems including cough, asthma, and shortness of breath.

Therapeutic Uses

Few human studies of schisandra's effects have been conducted, so scientists aren't sure how it works. Most studies have used cell cultures or animals. Nonetheless, results have been intriguing.

ADAPTOGEN. Schisandra is most widely used as an adaptogen, an herb that strengthens the whole body, counteracts fatigue, and improves overall health and well-being. However, it is not as potent as other adaptogenic herbs ginseng, eleuthero, or rhodiola.

LIVER DISEASE. When animals consume chemicals that cause liver damage, schisandra spurs regeneration of liver cells. Indonesian researchers gave schisandra extract (HpPro, an analog of natural schisandra C, 7.5 milligrams three times a day) to 56 adults with cirrhosis, acute hepatitis, or chronic hepatitis. After 1 month, 12 of the 14 with cirrhosis showed improved liver function with four showing complete normalization, and everyone with hepatitis experienced normalization of liver enzymes, the standard measure of liver health.

Intriguing Possibilities

ALLERGIES AND ASTHMA. Korean researchers have discovered that schisandra inhibits the release of mast cells and pro-inflammatory compounds in the respiratory tract. Mast cells and inflammatory compounds play key roles in triggering allergies and asthma attacks, supporting the herb's traditional use to treat respiratory problems.

INSOMNIA. Some studies suggest that schisandra counteracts the stimulant action of caffeine. If confirmed, this finding would validate the traditional practice of using it to treat insomnia.

CANCER. Laboratory studies show that schisandra kills cancer cells. It's too soon to call it a cancer treatment, but one day it might be.

MEMORY. In animal studies, schisandra improves memory and learning.

ALZHEIMER'S DISEASE. Animal studies show that schisandra reduces the neurological damage caused by amyloid-beta peptide, a protein involved in the development of Alzheimer's.

Rx Recommendations

Take 1.5 to 6 grams of dried berries/day (1 to 4 teaspoons), or take 500 milligrams to 2 grams/day of extract.

Safety

Few side effects have been reported, but heartburn, stomach upset, loss of appetite, rashes, and hives are possible.

Pregnant and nursing women should not use schisandra.

Do not give this herb to children under 2. In older children, adjust the recommended dose based on the child's weight. Give a 50-pound child one-third of the dose a 150-pound adult would take.

If you're over 65, start with a low dose, and increase only if necessary.

Inform health professionals of the herbs you use. Problematic herb-drug interactions are possible.

Schisandra may cause allergic reactions or other unexpected side effects. If any develop, reduce your dose or stop taking it. For more on herb safety, see Chapter 2.

If symptoms get worse or persist longer than 2 weeks, consult a health professional promptly.

Gardening

Schisandra thrives in most soils. It likes shade and grows best up shaded walls. Chinese growers plant seeds in spring. The vine flowers from April to May. Flowers are an inch in diameter. Fruits (berries) should be harvested in autumn and sun-dried. This herb may also be propagated from cuttings of shoots taken in late summer.

SCULLCAP

An All-American Tranquilizer

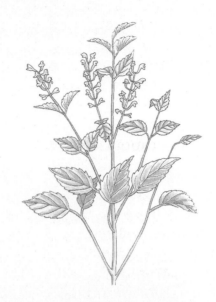

Family: Labiatae; other members include mints

Genus and species: *Scutellaria lateriflora*

Also known as: Skullcap, Virginia scullcap, Quaker bonnet, hoodwort, helmet flower

Parts used: Leaves

For an herb reputed to have calming effects, scullcap has caused considerable agitation. One respected herbalist calls the blue-flowered North American native "the most widely relevant tranquilizer." But skeptics have dismissed it as "nearly worthless and essentially inactive." The truth is, scullcap's traditional use as a tranquilizer has scientific support.

Healing History

For centuries, Chinese physicians have used Asian scullcap (*Scutellaria baicalensis*) as a tranquilizer-sedative and to treat many other conditions.

Writing in 1892, medical herbalist Charles F. Millspaugh, M.D., recounted the herb's odd history of use in the United States: "The first introduction of this plant into medicine was the experiments of Dr. Vandesveer [of Roysfield, New Jersey], in 1772, who claimed it curative and prophylactic [preventive] in hydrophobia [rabies], his reported cases being 1,400. This seems a large number to fall to one physician. His son after him claimed to cure 40 cases more in 3 years. [But] its worthiness was greatly doubted, and the plant much railed against. Many regulars [orthodox physicians] and empirics [folk herbalists] used the remedy with success, while many others wrote essays against it. . . . The plant has also proved itself a useful nervine [tranquilizer], antispasmodic [digestive aid], and tonic in wakefulness, convulsions, and delirium tremens."

America's 19th-century Eclectic physicians, forerunners of today's naturopaths, recommended scullcap primarily as a tranquilizer-sedative for insomnia and nervousness and as a treatment for "intermittent fever" (malaria), convulsions, and the delirium tremens of advanced alcoholism.

Nineteenth-century patent medicine makers used scullcap extensively in tonics for "female weakness" (menstrual discomforts).

Scullcap entered the *U.S. Pharmacopoeia*, a standard drug reference, as a tranquilizer in 1863 and remained there until 1916, when it moved to the *National Formulary*, the pharmacists' reference. It stayed there until 1947.

Contemporary herbalists recommend scullcap as a tranquilizer for insomnia, nervous tension, premenstrual syndrome, and drug and alcohol withdrawal. Some say the herb treats fever and convulsions.

Asian scullcap is one of the most widely used plants in Chinese medicine. Practitioners prescribe it for fever, viral infections (including flu and hepatitis), bacterial infections (strep throat and sinus infection), and high blood pressure.

Therapeutic Uses

American scientists are almost unanimous in their condemnation of scullcap. They've never gotten over those old, wild claims that it treats rabies. They should.

INSOMNIA, STRESS, AND ANXIETY. British researchers advertised for people struggling with anxiety, stress, mood swings, and/or irritability. They gave 31 adult respondents standard mood tests and then either a placebo or freeze-dried skullcap leaves (350 milligrams three times a day) for 2 weeks. Then the groups switched treatments (a crossover trial) for another 2 weeks. Scullcap provided significant relief from stress, anxiety, and insomnia—without causing fatigue or other side effects.

European and Russian studies have lent support to scullcap's traditional role as a tranquilizer. European physicians generally accept it as a tranquilizer and sedative. The herb is an ingredient in many European over-the-counter sleep preparations.

Intriguing Possibilities

Japanese researchers have discovered that Asian scullcap has anti-inflammatory properties.

Two Japanese animal studies suggest that

scullcap increases levels of "good" cholesterol (high-density lipoprotein, or HDL). As HDL levels increase, the risk of heart attack decreases. These findings suggest a role in human heart disease prevention.

Chinese physicians claim to have treated hepatitis successfully with the herb. It's too early to tout scullcap for this potentially serious liver disease, but it deserves further research.

Rx Recommendations

For a tranquilizing infusion, use 1 to 2 teaspoons of dried herb per cup of boiling water. Steep for 10 to 15 minutes, then strain. Drink up to 3 cups a day. Scullcap tastes bitter; adding honey, sugar, and lemon or mixing it with an herbal beverage blend will improve the flavor.

When using commercial preparations, follow package directions.

Safety

There are no reports of toxicity from scullcap infusions, but unusually large amounts of tincture may cause confusion, giddiness, twitching, and possibly convulsions.

Pregnant and nursing women should not use scullcap.

Do not give scullcap to children under 2. In older children, adjust the recommended dose based on the child's weight. Give a 50-pound child one-third of the dose a 150-pound adult would take.

If you're over 65, start with a low dose, and increase only if necessary.

Inform health professionals of the herbs you use. Problematic herb-drug interactions are possible.

Scullcap may cause allergic reactions or other unexpected side effects. If any develop, reduce your dose or stop taking it. For more on herb safety, see Chapter 2.

If symptoms get worse or persist longer than 2 weeks, consult a health professional promptly.

Gardening

Many scullcap species grow in Europe, but the American herb is the one used in herbal healing. Sometimes called Virginia scullcap, it grows throughout the United States and southern Canada.

The plant is a 2-foot, slender, branching, square-stemmed perennial with opposite, serrated leaves. The flowers have two lips. The upper lip includes an elongated cap-like appendage, the source of most of the herb's popular names: Quaker bonnet, hoodwort, and helmet flower.

Scullcap may be propagated from seeds or root divisions planted in early spring. Thin seedlings to 6-inch spacing. It grows in any well-drained soil under full sun and requires little care. Although it is a perennial, scullcap rarely lives longer than 3 years. Harvest the leaves in midsummer.

SENNA

A Powerful Laxative

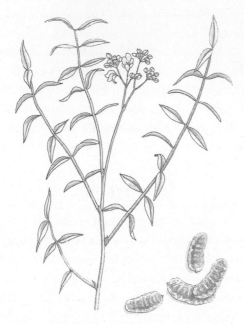

Family: Caesalpinaceae; other members
include brazilwood

Genus and species: *Cassia senna,*
C. acutifolia (Alexandrian and Khartoum),
C. angustifolia (Indian or Tinnevelly),
and *C. marilandica* (American)

Also known as: Cassia

Parts used: Leaflets and seed pods

Senna is a powerful laxative—so powerful, in
fact, that many authorities call it a cathartic.
Arab physicians first wrote of its bowel-
stimulating action in the 9th century, but their
descriptions imply centuries of traditional use
from the Middle East to India. Senna arrived in
Europe before the Crusades and has played a
prominent role in herbal healing ever since.

Both senna and cinnamon come from trees
with peelable bark, in Arabic, *quetsiah*, meaning
"to cut." *Quetsiah* evolved into senna's genus
name, *Cassia*. Today, both senna and cinnamon
may be called cassia, but the two have very different actions and should not be confused.

Healing History

Most traditional herbalists recommended senna
only as a laxative. But 17th-century English
herbalist Nicholas Culpeper, who came close to
prescribing every herb for every ill, could not
resist claiming that senna "cleanses the stomach, purges melancholy and phlegm from the
head, brain, lungs, heart, liver, and spleen,
cleansing those parts of evil humour; strengthens the senses, procures mirth, purifies the
blood [treats venereal disease], and is also good
in chronic agues [fevers]."

Native Americans recognized the laxative
action of the American form of senna but used
the herb primarily to treat fever. The 19th-
century Eclectics, forerunners of today's naturopaths, were influenced by Native American
medicine and called senna "very useful in all
forms of febrile [fever-producing] diseases in
which laxative action is desired."

Contemporary herbalists tout senna's laxative action but warn of its terrible taste and side
effects, primarily intestinal cramping.

Therapeutic Uses

Senna does not treat fever, nor does it "purge
melancholy and procure mirth." Quite the contrary. If you're not careful with this herb, you
may regret using it.

CONSTIPATION. Like aloe, buckthorn,
and cascara sagrada, senna contains anthraqui-

none compounds that stimulate the colon. The herb is an ingredient in many over-the-counter laxatives, including Correctol, Ex-Lax, Fletcher's Castoria, and Perdiem.

Senna and the other anthraquinone laxatives should be considered last resorts for constipation. First, increase your fruit, vegetable, and bran intake, drink more fluids, and get more exercise. If that doesn't work, try the bulk-forming laxative psyllium (see page 370). If that's not successful, try a gentler anthraquinone, cascara sagrada (see page 134). Finally, if you still need relief, try senna in consultation with your physician.

Commission E, the expert panel that evaluates herbal medicines for the German counterpart of the FDA, approves senna as a laxative.

COLONOSCOPY PREPARATION. Italian gastroenterologists performed colonoscopies on 383 older adults who used one of two preparations, either 4 liters of a laxative fluid or senna (24 tablets totaling 288 milligrams the afternoon and late evening prior). The senna group had cleaner colons and reported fewer discomforts.

Rx Recommendations

Because of senna's disgusting taste, herbalists discourage using the plant material and recommend over-the-counter products containing it. Follow package directions.

Those game enough to try the unprocessed herb can brew an infusion from 1 to 2 teaspoons of dried leaves per cup of boiling water. Steep for 10 minutes, then strain. Drink up to 1 cup a day in the morning or before bed for no more than a few days.

Senna tastes horrible. To make it more palatable, add sugar, honey, and lemon and/or mix it with taste-masking herbs such as anise, fennel, peppermint, chamomile, ginger, coriander, cardamom, and licorice.

Some sources say the pods have milder action than the leaves. Steep four pods in a cup of warm water for 6 to 12 hours. Drink up to 1 cup a day in the morning or before bed for no more than a few days.

As a tincture, use $\frac{1}{2}$ to 1 teaspoon in the morning or before bed for no more than a few days.

Safety

Those with gastrointestinal conditions—ulcers, colitis, or hemorrhoids—should not use senna.

Do not take senna for more than 2 weeks. Over time, it causes lazy bowel syndrome, an inability to have bowel movements without chemical stimulation.

Large amounts of senna cause diarrhea, nausea, and severe cramps with possible dehydration. Long-term use may cause enlargement of the fingertips (clubbing). An article in *Lancet* described this effect in a woman who had taken up to 40 senna laxative tablets a day for 15 years. Her fingers returned to normal when she stopped using the herb.

Senna leaves may cause a skin rash in people who are sensitive to the plant.

If you're over 65, start with a low dose, and increase only if necessary.

Pregnant and nursing women should also avoid this herb.

Inform health professionals of the herbs you use. Problematic herb-drug interactions are possible.

Senna may cause allergic reactions or other unexpected side effects. If any develop, reduce your dose or stop taking it. For more on herb safety, see Chapter 2.

If symptoms get worse or persist longer than 2 weeks, consult a health professional promptly.

Gardening

Native to Egypt and Sudan, it's a small, woody shrub that reaches 3 feet and has branching stems, pointed leaves, and seeds encased in a leathery pod. Most of the senna used in herbal medicine is grown in far southern India. One species grows in the eastern United States, but it is not a garden herb.

SHEPHERD'S PURSE
Stop Bleeding Naturally

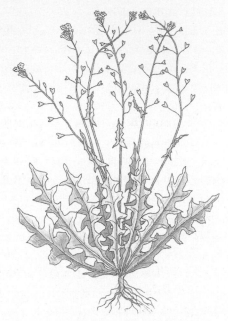

Family: Cruciferae; other members include cabbage, broccoli, and cauliflower

Genus and species: *Capsella bursa-pastoris*

Also known as: Lady's purse, rattle pouches, and rattle weed

Parts used: Leaves and flowers

Shepherds never get much respect. In the ancient world, theirs was a humble calling. And in the Old West, cattle ranchers condescended to "sheep herders." So perhaps we should not be surprised that the herb named for shepherds has shared a similar fate.

More than 300 years ago, Nicholas Culpeper wrote, "Few plants possess greater virtues than this, and yet it is utterly disregarded." No one is interested, some authorities say, because shepherd's purse is a common weed that's medically worthless. But the few scientific studies conducted to date have revealed some intriguing possibilities for treating bleeding and inducing labor.

Healing History

Ancient Greek and Roman physicians recommended shepherd's purse seeds as a laxative. But herbalists largely ignored it until the 16th century, when an Italian physician promoted it to stop bleeding, particularly to eliminate blood in urine. Some physicians adopted the plant, but most continued to dismiss it.

The Pilgrims introduced shepherd's purse into North America, where it quickly became a weed. Folk herbalists used it to stop bleeding, but physicians called it useless.

America's 19th-century Eclectic physicians, forerunners of today's naturopaths, prescribed shepherd's purse to stop bleeding. Their text *King's American Dispensatory* (1898) explained the age-old controversy over its effectiveness by observing that "the fresh herb is decidedly more active than the dried." *King's* called shepherd's purse effective for treating bloody urine, stopping excessive menstrual flow, and relieving diarrhea, dysentery, and bleeding hemorrhoids.

During World War I, when other coagulants were in short supply, wounded soldiers drank shepherd's purse tea.

Contemporary herbalists recommend the internal use of dried—not fresh—shepherd's purse for bloody urine, nosebleeds, heavy menstrual flow, and bleeding after childbirth. They also support the herb's external use as an astringent styptic for wounds and hemorrhoids.

Therapeutic Uses

Shepherd's purse is a minor herbal healer, but it may help some women with heavy menstrual flow or pregnant women waiting to go into labor—if they can stomach its taste.

BLEEDING. Shepherd's purse contains compounds that accelerate blood clotting, according to the British scientific journal *Nature*. German medical herbalist Rudolph Fritz Weiss, M.D., writes that the herb "definitely has haemostatic [blood-stopping] properties . . . [but they are] not very great."

First-aid experts recommend treating bleeding with sustained pressure on the wound. Blood in phlegm, urine, or stool requires prompt professional treatment.

Although shepherd's purse is no substitute for standard medical care, people with ulcers, colitis, Crohn's disease, or bleeding disorders or women with heavy menstrual flow might try it in consultation with their physicians.

Commission E, the expert panel that evaluates herbal medicines for the German counterpart of the FDA, approves shepherd's purse as a treatment for persistent nosebleeds and menorrhagia (heavy menstrual flow).

LABOR INDUCTION. Shepherd's purse contains compounds that stimulate uterine contractions like the drug oxytocin (Pitocin) given at term to trigger labor.

WOUNDS. Shepherd's purse has mild anti-inflammatory and astringent action, lending some support to its traditional role as a treatment for wounds and hemorrhoids.

Rx Recommendations

To stop bleeding or to hasten labor, use 1 teaspoon of dried herb per cup of boiling water. Steep for 10 minutes, then strain. Drink up to 2 cups a day. Shepherd's purse has a biting, unpleasant taste. To make it more palatable, add sugar, honey, and/or lemon or mix with an herbal beverage blend.

As a homemade tincture, use $\frac{1}{4}$ to $\frac{1}{2}$ teaspoon up to twice a day.

When using commercial preparations, follow package directions.

To use shepherd's purse externally on wounds or hemorrhoids, soak a clean cloth in either an infusion or a tincture.

Safety

Those with heart disease or a history of stroke or mini-strokes (TIAs) should not use shepherd's purse. It's pro-clotting action may cause the internal blood clots that trigger heart attacks or strokes.

Anyone anyone taking anticoagulant (blood-thinning) medication, including low-dose aspirin, should not use shepherd's purse.

The medical literature contains no reports of harm from this herb.

Pregnant women should not use shepherd's purse, except at term and in consultation with their physicians. Nursing women and those trying to conceive should not use shepherd's purse.

Do not give shepherd's purse to children under 2. In older children, adjust the recommended dose based on the child's weight. Give a 50-pound child one-third of the dose a 150-pound adult would take.

If you're over 65, start with a low dose, and increase only if necessary.

Inform health professionals of the herbs you use. Problematic herb-drug interactions are possible.

Shepherd's purse may cause allergic reactions or other unexpected side effects. If any develop, reduce your dose or stop taking it. For more on herb safety, see Chapter 2.

If symptoms get worse or persist longer than 2 weeks, consult a health professional promptly.

Gardening

Shepherd's purse is a foul-smelling annual that reaches 18 inches. Its slender stem rises from a rosette of deeply toothed leaves similar to dandelion. The stem bears a few small leaves and terminates in small white flowers. The fruits are wedge-shaped seed pods containing literally thousands of yellow seeds, hence the herb's common names: lady's purse, rattle pouches, and rattle weed.

Shepherd's purse grows easily from seeds planted in spring under full sun. It prefers well-drained sandy loam but tolerates most North American soils.

If unchecked, shepherd's purse can become a garden and lawn pest. To avoid this, clip the seed pods before they open. The young leaves have a peppery taste and may be added to soups and stews or eaten like spinach. Harvest the leaves as the flowers open.

SHIITAKE

This Tasty Mushroom Boosts
Immune Function

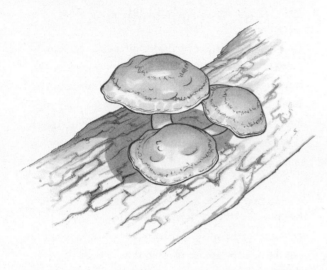

Family: Polyporaceae; other members include
other mushrooms

Genus and species: *Lentinula edodes*

Also known as: Chinese black mushroom,
fragrant mushroom

Parts used: Stem and cap, and cultured
mycelial extract

The English word, shiitake (shih-TAH-kay),
comes from the Japanese for "mushroom of the
shii tree," on whose decaying logs it grows in
China, Japan, Korea, and Southeast Asia. Shiitakes are prominent in those cuisines and may
be called Chinese black mushrooms because of
their dark color, or fragrant mushrooms because
of their distinctive aroma. Historians say the
Emperor of Japan first ate wild shiitakes in 199

AD. Cultivation began around 1000. Their first
documented medicinal use dates from around
1400. Today, shiitake mushrooms are Japan's
leading agricultural export.

Healing History

Traditional Japanese herbalists used shiitakes to
treat fatigue, muscle aches, intestinal parasites,
poor circulation, and heart disease. Traditional
Chinese physicians use the mushroom to treat
colds, flu, weakness, fatigue, liver problems, and
to invigorate *qi* (pronounced chi), life energy.

Therapeutic Uses

Shiitakes' medicinal benefits came West in 1974
when *Mushrooms as Health Foods* by Japanese
mycologist Kisaku Mori first appeared in
English. Shiitakes contain two medicinal
constituents—lentinan in the cap, and *Lentinula
edodes* mycelial extract (LEM) in the underground root-like part that's not eaten.

IMMUNE ENHANCEMENT. Laboratory
and animal studies show that lentinan and LEM
activate many components of the immune system:
natural killer cells, T-helper cells, interleukin-1
and -2, and germ-devouring white blood cells
(macrophages). These actions help treat all manner of illness, particularly viral infections and
cancer.

HEPATITIS. Shiitake's immune-boosting
action helps treat chronic hepatitis B, an infection that can lead to liver failure and/or cancer.
Chinese researchers gave lentinan to 44 people
with chronic hepatitis B. Two months later, their
immune systems were more active, and the
researchers noted "therapeutic effectiveness."

GENITAL WARTS. Chinese scientists

treated 36 genital wart sufferers with either laser therapy or laser plus lentinan (12.5 milligrams twice a day). After 2 months, 47 percent of the laser-only group experienced recurrences. But in the laser-lentinan group, just 11 percent.

HIV/AIDS. University of California researchers gave lentinan to 98 people with AIDS. Their immune function improved. Japanese researchers gave LEM to people with AIDS (9 grams/day) After 2 years, symptoms subsided in every one of them.

CANCER. Laboratory studies show that lentinan inhibits reproduction of various cancer cells and boosts immune function. Tumor shrinkage has been documented in animals with cancer fed lentinan. Japanese researchers gave standard care or that plus lentinan to people with advanced cancers. After 10 days, the lentinan group showed improved immune function and survived longer.

Another Japanese team gave standard chemotherapy with or without lentinan to people with advanced stomach cancer. In the standard care group, none survived a year, but in the lentinan group, half did.

Other Japanese scientists gave men with advanced prostate cancer either standard hormone and chemotherapy or that plus lentinan. In the standard-care group, 29 percent survived 5 years; in the lentinan group, 43 percent.

CHOLESTEROL. Japanese scientists encouraged 90 women with high cholesterol to add shiitakes to their diets (0.3 to 3 ounces/day). In just 7 days, their total cholesterol fell 7 to 14 percent. Every 1 percent drop in cholesterol reduces heart attack risk 2 percent, so a steady diet of shiitakes might cut heart attack risk by up to 28 percent.

VITAMIN D. Shiitake is one of the few plant sources of vitamin D.

Intriguing Possibility

A pilot study hints that shiitake may help treat tuberculosis.

Rx Recommendations

Enjoy shiitakes in any recipe that calls for mushrooms. They cost more than button mushrooms, but taste better. Fresh and dried shiitakes can be found at health food stores and some supermarkets. In studies showing health benefits, users consumed at least eight whole mushrooms a day, or took LEM in doses of 9 to 25 grams/day.

Safety

In healthy people, side effects are uncommon, but stomach upset is possible. In those with AIDS or cancer, more side effects have been reported, including fever, allergic reactions, and back and leg pain.

Pregnant and nursing women should not consumer more than typical food amounts.

Do not give shiitake to children under 2. In older children, the mushroom may be eaten as a food.

Shiitakes may cause allergic reactions or other unexpected side effects. If any develop, reduce your dose or stop taking it. For more on herb safety, see Chapter 2.

If symptoms get worse or persist longer than 2 weeks, consult a health professional promptly.

Gardening

Shiitake mushrooms can be grown indoors from kits marketed by Fungi Perfecti. Visit www.fungi.com.

SLIPPERY ELM

An Early American Favorite

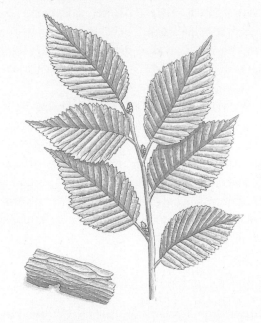

Family: Ulmaceae; other members include the elms

Genus and species: *Ulmus rubra* and *U. fulva*

Also known as: Red elm and Indian elm

Part used: Inner bark

During the 18th and 19th centuries, Americans loved slippery elm. Great elm forests covered the East, and even in cities, the versatile bark was always close at hand. It became the nation's leading home remedy for anything in need of soothing.

Soaked in water and wrapped around meats, slippery elm bark retarded spoilage in the days before refrigeration. Coarsely ground and mixed with water, it turned into a spongy gel that was molded into bandages and coatings for unpleasant-tasting medicines. Ground and mixed with water or milk, slippery elm bark turned into a soothing, nutritious porridge similar to oatmeal that fed infants and children and was used to treat sore throats, coughs, colds, and gastrointestinal ailments. Most home medicine cabinets contained slippery elm sore throat lozenges.

The herb is still listed in the *National Formulary*, the pharmacists' reference, and health food stores and some pharmacies still sell slippery elm throat lozenges. But America's once-great elm forests have been decimated by Dutch elm disease, and as a result, both our landscapes and our herbal healing heritage are poorer.

Healing History

The 1st-century Greek physician Dioscorides prescribed soaking in a European elm bath to speed the healing of broken bones. His prescription survived 1,500 years.

During the 17th century, English herbalist Nicholas Culpeper wrote, "The decoction being bathed in, heals broken bones . . . [and] is excellent [for] places . . . burnt with fire. The leaves bruised, applied, and being bound thereon with its own bark heal wounds." Culpeper also claimed that elm root decoction restored hair on bald scalps.

Colonists found the Native Americans using American slippery elm bark as a food and treatment for wounds, sore throats, coughs, inflamed nipples (mastitis), and many other ailments. The colonists adopted these uses and developed more, including applying slippery elm poultices to treat boils.

Native American women inserted slippery elm sticks to induce abortion, and white women adopted the practice, which caused many deaths from uterine infection and hemorrhage. As a result, several state legislatures passed laws forbidding the sale of slippery elm bark in pieces longer than 1½ inches.

America's early 19th-century Thomsonian herbalists recommended slippery elm tea as a laxative gentle enough for children. Thomsonian midwives lubricated their hands with the slippery bark before performing internal examinations.

By the Civil War, slippery elm was being used to treat syphilis, gonorrhea, and hemorrhoids. America's 19th-century Eclectic physicians, forerunners of today's naturopaths, loved the herb and suggested that "a tablespoon of the powder boiled in milk affords a nourishing diet for infants newly weaned, preventing the bowel complaints to which they are subject. Some physicians consider the constant use of it, during and after the 7th month of gestation, as advantageous in facilitating an easy delivery."

Contemporary herbalists recommend slippery elm bark externally to cover wounds and soothe skin problems and internally as a tea to treat sore throats and coughs as well as diarrhea, ulcers, colitis, and other gastrointestinal complaints.

Therapeutic Uses

Even the FDA, usually critical of herbal medicines, calls slippery elm "an excellent demulcent" (soothing agent). The herb's bark is rich in a soluble fiber called mucilage that swells and becomes spongy and gelatinous when mixed with water.

WOUNDS. When applied to thoroughly washed wounds, slippery elm bark mucilage dries to form an herbal bandage.

COUGHS, SORE THROATS, AND DIGESTIVE PROBLEMS. Slippery elm decoction helps soothe the throat and digestive tract. Besides providing mucilage, the herb stimulates production of digestive tract mucus, also a soother.

WOMEN'S HEALTH. Slippery elm decoction has a long history of use by pregnant women, and the medical literature contains no reports of problems. The active constituent, mucilage, should not harm the fetus. If you have a history of problematic pregnancy, however, consult your physician before trying slippery elm preparations.

Medical Myth

Slippery elm has never been shown to speed the healing of broken bones.

Rx Recommendations

For a poultice to bandage washed wounds, stir enough water into powdered bark to make a paste and apply to the affected area.

For a soothing decoction, use 1 to 3 teaspoons of powdered herb per cup of water. Blend a little water in with the powder first to prevent lumpiness. Bring to a boil and simmer for 15 minutes, then strain. Drink up to 3 cups a day. Slippery elm has a mild aroma and a maple flavor.

When using commercial preparations, follow package directions.

You may give slippery elm cautiously to children under age 2.

Safety

Allergic reactions are possible. Otherwise, the medical literature contains no reports of slippery elm causing harm.

Gardening

Slippery elm is a stately tree that reaches 60 feet. Its trunk bark is brown, but its branch bark is whitish. Its leaves are broad, rough, hairy, and toothed. Check local nurseries to see if this tree can be grown in your area.

SOYBEAN

FDA-Approved for Cholesterol Control

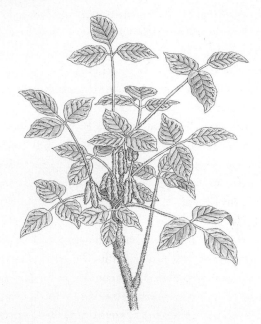

Family: Leguminosae; other members include beans and peas

Genus and species: *Glycine max*

Also known as: Soya

Parts used: Beans

Soybeans rank as the United States' fourth leading legal agricultural product, surpassed only by cattle, dairy products, and corn. An astonishing 70 million acres of American farmland are planted with soybeans, largely for cattle feed and export to Asia. The U.S. soybean crop accounts for almost half of the world production and generates more than $15 billion a year in revenue. Soybean is the source of tofu, made by coagulating soy milk and pressing the curds into blocks.

Healing History

The Chinese cultivated soybeans as early as 1200 BC, that country's second most important crop after rice. Soybeans served as a key source of protein for a culture that was largely vegetarian. The Chinese developed tofu around 200 BC.

The Japanese adopted soybeans and tofu enthusiastically. During the 18th century, soybeans were introduced into Europe, but they didn't arrive in the United States until Chinese immigrants brought them in the 1880s. Soybeans quickly became a major U.S. crop, raised almost entirely as cattle feed and for export to Asia.

Some Americans began eating tofu in the late 1960s, but through the 1980s, it was the food Americans loved to hate. The water-packed, spongy white blocks, resembling pressed cottage cheese, were the butt of countless put-downs on late-night TV.

But during the 1990s, public opinion began to shift. Tofu and other soy foods have still not become national favorites, but the jokes have largely ceased, for two reasons. First, soy foods, particularly soy-based textured vegetable protein, have become more familiar. Many supermarket items now contain soy protein, including soy dogs (a substitute for beef and pork franks), soy burgers (a substitute for hamburgers), and soy crumbles (a substitute for chopped meat).

Second, studies have now shown that the isoflavones in tofu and other soy foods offer a remarkable number of health benefits—so many that the FDA allows soy products to carry a health claim on their labels. (However, soy sauce does *not* contain appreciable amounts isoflavones.)

Therapeutic Uses

The key isoflavones in soybeans are genistein and daidzein. The chart shows how the various soy foods stack up for isoflavone content.

SOY PRODUCT	PORTION	ISOFLAVONES (MG)
Raw soybeans	½ cup (34 g)	176
Roasted soybeans	½ cup (30 g)	167
Tempeh	4 oz. (19 g)	61
Soy protein	1 oz. (26 g)	57
Soy flour	¼ cup (8 g)	44
Tofu	4 oz. (18 g)	38
Textured soy protein	¼ cup (18 g)	28
Soy milk	8 oz. (10 g)	20

Soy and soy products have a remarkable number of health benefits.

HIGH CHOLESTEROL. A few studies have shown that soy has little or no effect on cholesterol, but the great majority of trials show that it reduces cholesterol significantly and with it, risk of heart attack and most strokes.

❧ Wake Forest University researchers placed 156 men and women with high cholesterol on the diet recommended by the American Heart Association. In addition, the study participants were given one of five supplement drinks: a placebo or four beverages containing varying amounts of soy isoflavones. After 9 weeks, those who received the placebo showed no reduction in cholesterol, but all of those who received the soy drinks showed reductions, with cholesterol steadily declining as isoflavone content increased.

❧ Researchers at the Veterans Affairs Medical Center in Lexington, Kentucky, analyzed 38 studies of soy protein's effect on cholesterol. They found that soy lowered cholesterol significantly. Study participants who consumed 47 grams (1.7 ounces) of soy protein a day saw their total cholesterol decline considerably. The researchers concluded that substituting soy protein for animal protein significantly decreases cholesterol.

❧ English researchers analyzed 39 studies of soy's effects on cholesterol. The herb reduced cholesterol significantly.

In 1999, the FDA ruled that the labels of foods containing at least 6.25 grams of soy protein per serving may state that they reduce cholesterol and the risk of heart disease.

Commission E, the expert panel that evaluates herbal medicines for the German counterpart of the FDA, approves soy foods as a treatment for elevated cholesterol.

HOT FLASHES. At menopause, women produce less estrogen and many suffer menopausal discomforts, notably, hot flashes. Soy isoflavones are plant estrogens (phytoestrogens). They're similar to the human hormone, but chemically weaker. Soy phytoestrogens are strong enough to prevent and relieve hot flashes but not so strong that they cause estrogen's downsides, stimulation of breast tumors. In fact, mounting evidence suggests that soy foods help prevent breast cancer (see below).

❧ Italian researchers gave 104 women suffering severe hot flashes either a placebo or soy isoflavones (76 milligrams/day). After 1 month, the women taking the soy reported significantly fewer hot flashes.

❧ Harvard researchers gave 147 menopausal women either a placebo or a soy supplement. After 12 weeks, the soy group reported a 52 percent decreased in hot flashes.

❧ Dutch, British, and Harvard researchers analyzed 10 rigorous studies of soy for hot flashes. Seven showed significant benefit.

BLOOD PRESSURE. As people eat fewer animal foods and more plant foods, including beans, blood pressure decreases.

❧ Chinese researchers gave 302 adults with high blood pressure either biscuits without soy or biscuits contained about 2 ounces of soy protein. After 12 weeks, the soy group showed significantly lower blood pressure. English researchers analyzed nine studies, and concluded that soy "significantly reduces blood pressure."

❧ Other Chinese scientists analyzed 11 rigorous trials of soy for blood pressure control (1 to 2 ounces a day). Their conclusion: Soy foods reduce blood pressure. They also discovered why some studies don't show this—subjects' ages. Soy reduces blood pressure much better in those under 40 than over that age.

BREAST CANCER. Many studies have shown that compared with Americans, Asian women are substantially less likely to develop breast cancer. Epidemiologists once believed that Asian women's lower-fat diet accounted for the difference. Now, they believe that it's not only less fat, but more soy.

Human estrogen stimulates the growth of breast tumors. Weaker soy phytoestrogens attach to estrogen receptors on breast cells, effectively locking out the body's own estrogen and reducing its tumor-stimulating effect. In laboratory studies, breast cancer cells exposed to soy isoflavones had their growth reduced by 30 percent.

🍀 Australian researchers conducted diet surveys of 144 women newly diagnosed with breast cancer and 144 similar women who were cancer-free. After accounting for other known risk factors (family history, alcohol consumption, breast density), the cancer-free women consumed significantly more soy isoflavones.

🍀 University of Arkansas analyzed 14 soy-breast cancer studies and concluded that compared with women who consume little or no soy, those who eat it a few times a week have 22 percent less risk of breast cancer.

🍀 University of Southern California scientists reviewed 28 studies of dietary soy and breast cancer risk. Their conclusion: Soy modestly reduces risk. Compared with women who eat little or no soy, those who consume 2 ounces of tofu a day or 8 ounces of soy milk have 12 percent lower breast cancer risk.

🍀 Soy also reduces risk of breast cancer recurrence. Vanderbilt University researchers studied 5,041 breast cancer survivors age 20 to 75. As their soy consumption increased, their risk of recurrence decreased. Compared with survivors who ate the least soy, those who ate the most were 32 percent less likely to experience a recurrence and 29 percent less likely to die of the disease. And the After Breast Cancer Pooling Project, a 7-year study of 18,314 survivors by American and Chinese researchers, showed that a high-soy diet reduced risk of recurrence by 25 percent.

OTHER CANCERS. The Arkansas researchers also analyzed 15 studies of soy and colon cancer and six studies of soy and prostate cancer. They found that a high-soy diet reduces risk of colon cancer by 30 percent and prostate cancer by 34 percent.

OSTEOPOROSIS. Estrogen replacement reduces risk of osteoporosis, suggesting that soy might do the same. Thirty-one clinical trials have been published on the effects of soy foods on bone mineral density. Twenty-two (71 percent) show that the herb increases bone density. One of them, a study of 24,403 postmenopausal women followed for 4.5 years, shows that a high-soy diet reduces risk of fractures.

Researchers at the University of Illinois gave groups of postmenopausal women 40 grams of protein a day. In one group, the protein came from nonsoy sources (meat and dairy products). In another group, the protein included moderate levels of soy isoflavones, and in a third group, the protein included high levels of soy isoflavones. After 6 months, the women consuming the nonsoy protein showed bone loss, while those eating the most soy isoflavones showed significantly increased bone mineral density.

Intriguing Possibilities

A Chinese study suggests that a high-soy diet may reduce risk of ovarian cancer, and an Australian report hints that soy reduces risk of prostate cancer.

Oklahoma State University researchers have shown that 1.5 ounces of soy protein a day helps relieve osteoarthritis.

And an Australian study hints that as soy consumption increase, memory improves.

LEGUME	GENISTEIN (PPM)	DAIDZEIN (PPM)	TOTAL (PPM)
Soybeans	24	38	62
Black beans	45	0	45
Pinto beans	22	23	45
Lima beans	40	0	40
Kidney beans	29	3	31
Red lentils	25	5	30
Fava beans	20	5	25
Great Northern	17	7	24
Black-eyed peas	23	0	23
Mung beans	22	0	22

Rx Recommendations

If you get your soy from foods, most experts recommend consuming about 5 ounces of tofu (about 1.5 servings) containing approximately 50 to 70 grams of soy protein weekly. If you have any of the conditions that may be prevented by soy, feel free to eat more.

Soy isoflavones are also available as supplements. Follow the label directions.

Because soybeans are such a major crop in the United States, the soy trade organizations have had the financial resources to fund the studies showing its benefits. These results have not been duplicated for other beans, but according to research at the USDA, all edible beans contain isoflavones.

Soy contains the most isoflavones per serving, but it wouldn't take too many dishes made with other beans (burritos, baked beans, bean soups, or salads) to consume significant amounts of isoflavones. The chart shows how various legumes compare in terms of isoflavone content.

Safety

Estrogen counteracts the effects of male sex hormones. Phytoestrogens have similar action. Men with suppressed male sex hormones often have low sperm counts, so Harvard researchers investigated the effects, if any, of dietary soy on the sperm counts of 99 men at an infertility clinic. Those who ate the most soy had the lowest sperm counts. Men in couples trying to get pregnant should limit or avoid soy.

Soy is safe for the vast majority of people, but allergies and other sensitivities are possible.

Gardening

Soybean is an annual that grows from 1 to 5 feet tall. Fine hairs cover its stems, leaves, and bean pods, giving the plant a fuzzy appearance and feel. The pods contain up to four seeds (beans).

Soybean is not a garden herb, but if you grow peas, you might grow soybeans. The beans can be roasted and eaten.

STEVIA

100 Times Sweeter Than Sugar—
and More

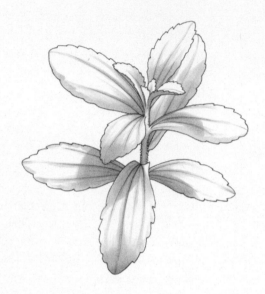

Family: Compositae; other members include
daisy, dandelion, and marigold

Genus and species: *Stevia rebaudiana
bertoni*

Also known as: Sweet herb, sugar leaf, yerba
dulce

Parts used: Leaves

Healing History

Stevia is native to Paraguay, Bolivia, and Brazil, where, for centuries, the indigenous Guarani
tribes called it *ka'a he'e* (sweet herb) and used it
to sweeten beverage teas and bitter medicinal
preparations. But scientists overlooked stevia
until 1899 when the Swiss botanist Moisés

Bertoni first described it—and appended his
name to the plant's species identity.

In 1931, French researchers isolated the
leaves' sweet compounds, stevioside and rebaudioside A, which, per unit weight, are more than
100 times sweeter than table sugar (sucrose).
One teaspoon of powdered stevia equals 3 cups
of sugar.

During the 1970s, other nonsugar sweeten-
ers (cyclamate and saccharin) were identified
as possible carcinogens. Looking for a safer
alternative, Japanese scientists focused on stevia and popularized the herb in Japan, where
today it accounts for 40 percent of the sweetener market.

During the 1980s, American tea companies
(Lipton and Celestial Seasonings) experimented
with adding stevia to their products. But in
1988, the Food and Drug Administration
received an anonymous complaint and with no
explanation banned stevia as an "unsafe food
additive" in 1991. Stevia supporters suspected
the complaint came from the maker of Nutra-
Sweet (aspartame), a controversial artificial
sweetener with its own safety issues that was
competing for the $1 billion a year nonsugar
sweetener market.

The American Herbal Products Association
and many herbally inclined pharmacists (phar-
macognosists) lobbied the FDA to reconsider.
The agency rescinded its ban in 2008.

Stevia is now available under brand names
including Truvia, PureVia, and Rebiana. Commercial stevia products are not the powdered
leaf. The sweet compounds (glycosides) must be
extracted by steeping the leaves in hot water
and then chemically extracting them from the
syrup. The resulting raw stevia is dried and processed into a powder.

Therapeutic Uses

Instead of spooning the familiar while granules into your coffee or tea, try a pinch of stevia. But this herb is more than just a sweetener.

DIABETES. Americans consume a surprisingly large amount of sugar. According to a 2014 report in the American Medical Association's journal *JAMA Internal Medicine*, average adult consumption increased from 16 percent of daily calories to 18 percent from 1988 to 2004. However, by 2010, consumption decreased to 15 percent due to publicity about sugar's association with obesity, diabetes, and heart disease. Simply substituting stevia for sugar whenever possible helps reduce the risk of developing these conditions.

In addition, studies in diabetic animals show that stevia helps control blood sugar. It does the same in humans. Danish investigators measured the blood sugar of 12 diabetics and then fed them a meal containing either sugar or stevia (1 gram). Four hours later, those who consumed the stevia showed much lower blood sugar.

Iranian scientists gave 62 diabetic adults a typical Iranian diet that included sugar or the same diet with a nonsucrose sweetener made from stevia and sorbitol. After 6 weeks, the two groups switched menus for another 6 weeks. While eating the stevia-sweetened diet, participants' blood insulin levels decreased significantly.

BLOOD PRESSURE. Animal studies show that stevia opens (dilates) the arteries, which lowers blood pressure. Taiwanese researchers gave 106 people with high blood pressure either a placebo or stevia (250 milligrams) three times a day. After 3 months, the stevia group showed significantly lower blood pressure.

Another Taiwan team gave 174 people with high blood pressure either a placebo or stevia (500 milligrams) three times a day. Two years later, the stevia group showed significantly lower blood pressure.

HEART DISEASE AND CANCER PREVENTION. Stevia is high in antioxidants, compounds that help prevent the cell damage at the root of heart disease and cancer.

Intriguing Possibilities

Animal studies show that stevia stimulates the immune system, helps prevent stroke, and has anti-inflammatory, antibacterial, and antifungal action.

Rx Recommendations

Stevia contains two sweet compounds, stevioside and rebaudioside A. Stevioside has a bitter licorice aftertaste. If you find it unpleasant, look for products that specify Rebaudioside A (rebA), which leaves no aftertaste. Follow package directions.

Stevia cannot be used as a substitute for sugar in baking.

Safety

When consumed in typical culinary amounts, there is no evidence that stevia causes harm.

However, the Internet contains accusations that the processing used to turn stevia leaf into stevia powder uses "toxic chemicals." Yes and no. The process involves steeping the leaves in hot water and then extracting the stevioside and rebaudioside using food grade alcohol or methanol. Now, ingesting pure methanol is toxic to humans, but there is no evidence that the use of the chemical in stevia processing poses any danger. Only a tiny, nontoxic amount, if any, remains in the final product. Medical literature contains no reports of stevia causing harm to either animals or people. Stevia has been a major sweetener in Japan since the 1970s, and tens of millions of Japanese have used it for almost 50 years with no reports of significant harm. Meanwhile, overuse of sugar has been linked to increased risk of obesity, diabetes, and heart disease—all major public health threats. If you're nervous about stevia, don't use it. But compared with sugar, this herb's benefits far outweigh its risks.

Allergic reactions or other unexpected effects are possible. If any develop, reduce the amount you use or stop taking it.

Pregnant and nursing women should not use this herb.

Inform health professionals of the herbs you use. Problematic herb-drug interactions are possible. For more on herb safety, see Chapter 2.

If symptoms get worse or persist longer than 2 weeks, consult a health professional promptly.

Gardening

Stevia is a spindly, multibranched perennial shrub that grows to 3 feet in subtropical, rainy locales. It prefers 12-inch spacing and well-drained sandy loam, but tolerates most soil types. Most of the world's crop grows in South and Central America, Japan, Israel, Thailand, and China. Growers harvest the leaves as the plants flower. Stevia is not a garden herb in the United States, but it may be grown in Florida and Southern California.

TARRAGON

Good for an Aching Tooth

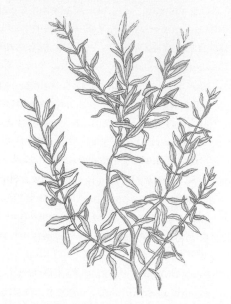

Family: Compositae; other members include daisy, dandelion, and marigold

Genus and species: *Artemisia dracunculus*

Also known as: French or Russian tarragon, estragon, and dragon herb

Parts used: Leaves

Tarragon is best known as the main seasoning in bearnaise sauce. Like all aromatic herbs, it also has a long history in herbal healing.

But unlike most other aromatics, tarragon fell from healing fashion in the 17th century. Only recently has the herb been rediscovered as an oral anesthetic with some potential for treating diabetes and preventing varicose veins.

Healing History

The ancient Greeks discovered that chewing tarragon numbs the mouth and used it to treat toothache. They also decided that its anesthetic power and its wide-ranging root runners meant that it could help relieve the discomforts of traveling. The 1st-century Roman naturalist Pliny wrote that tarragon prevented fatigue on long journeys. During the Middle Ages, pilgrims placed tarragon sprigs in their shoes.

Oddly enough for an herb that numbs the mouth, around the 10th century, Arab physicians recommended tarragon as an appetite stimulant.

Under the Doctrine of Signatures, the medieval belief that an herb's appearance revealed its medicinal value, tarragon's serpentine roots were considered a sign that it could cure snakebite. Over the centuries, the belief expanded to include the bites of rabid dogs. But by the 17th century, this belief had faded. Nicholas Culpeper, who recommended dozens of herbs for the bites of "venomous creatures," did not mention tarragon in this regard. In fact, he hardly mentioned it at all.

After Culpeper, herbalists virtually abandoned tarragon because it loses most of its aromatic healing oil as it dries. Even America's 19th-century Eclectic physicians, forerunners of today's naturopaths, prized medicinal herbs but had no use for tarragon.

Few contemporary herbalists value tarragon except in French cooking. Those who do recognize it reiterate its traditional uses as a diuretic, appetite stimulant, digestive aid, and toothache treatment.

Therapeutic Uses

Tarragon is no wonder herb, but it deserves a place in herbal healing. Its active component is its oil, but drying largely destroys it. Either fresh or frozen leaves or generous amounts of dried leaves must be used.

TOOTHACHE. Tarragon oil contains the same anesthetic compound, eugenol, as clove oil. This supports its age-old use for toothache. Tarragon provides only temporary relief of oral pain, however. If toothache persists, consult a dentist.

INFECTIONS. Like many culinary herbs, tarragon oil fights disease-causing bacteria in laboratory studies. You can use fresh leaves as garden first-aid for minor wounds.

Intriguing Possibilities

Animal studies by Rutgers University researchers show that tarragon lowers blood sugar, suggesting that it might help manage diabetes.

Tarragon oil contains rutin, a compound that strengthens blood vessel walls. Herbalists often recommend other herbs rich in rutin, notably violet and onion, for the treatment of varicose veins in the legs. These herbs may also help hemorrhoids, which are varicose veins in the anal area.

An animal study published in the *Journal of the National Cancer* Institute suggests that rutin has some antitumor activity.

Rx Recommendations

For temporary relief of oral pain, chew fresh leaves as needed.

For garden first-aid, apply fresh, crushed leaves to a cut or scrape until you can wash and bandage it.

For a pleasant, licorice-flavored infusion that may help prevent varicose veins and hemorrhoids, use 1 to 2 teaspoons of fresh or frozen herb per cup of boiling water. Steep for 10 to 15 minutes, then strain. Drink up to 3 cups a day.

As a homemade tincture, use $1/2$ to 1 teaspoon up to three times a day.

When using commercial preparations, follow package directions.

Safety

Large amounts of estragole, a compound in tarragon, produce tumors in mice. Tarragon has never been associated with human cancers, but until its effects are clarified, people with a history of cancer should probably not use the herb in medicinal amounts.

Otherwise, the medical literature contains no reports of tarragon causing harm.

Pregnant and nursing women should not use medicinal amounts of tarragon.

Do not give tarragon to children under 2. In older children, adjust the recommended dose based on the child's weight. Give a 50-pound child one-third of the dose a 150-pound adult would take.

If you're over 65, start with a low dose, and increase only if necessary.

Inform health professionals of the herbs you use. Problematic herb-drug interactions are possible.

Tarragon may cause allergic reactions or other unexpected side effects. If any develop, reduce your dose or stop taking it. For more on herb safety, see Chapter 2.

If symptoms get worse or persist longer than 2 weeks, consult a health professional promptly.

Gardening

Tarragon comes in two varieties, Russian and French. The former has less oil—and therefore, less flavor and medicinal value—so mentions of tarragon almost always refer to the French plant.

Russian tarragon may be grown from seeds, but the more desirable French variety must be propagated from cuttings or root divisions. Divide the roots in spring and plant 1-inch pieces of their tips, or take cuttings in summer. Thin plants to 2-foot spacing.

French tarragon is a perennial with creeping, serpentine roots and stems that reach 2 feet. Its leaves look like a larger version of rosemary.

Tarragon grows best in rich, well-drained soil under full sun. Make sure the roots do not become waterlogged. If your winter temperatures drop below the teens, mulch well each fall. Divide tarragon roots every few years to retain plants' vigor.

Tarragon leaves bruise easily. Harvest them carefully in early summer. Because it loses medicinal value when dried, freeze the fresh herb or preserve it in vinegar.

TEA

A Longer, Healthier Life in Every Cup

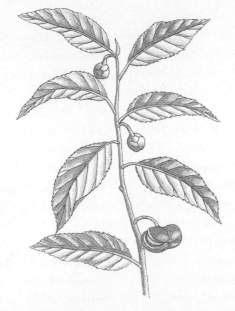

Family: Theaceae; other members include camellia

Genus and species: *Camellia sinensis*

Also known as: White, green, oolong, and black tea

Parts used: Leaves

Tea is the world's second most popular beverage after water. Worldwide sales total more than $10 billion a year.

Until the 1970s, most Americans drank it only as an alternative to coffee. But that's changed, in part because the research on tea's many health benefits has become more widely known. The fact is, drinking a few cups of tea every day—especially green tea—substantially reduces the risk of a remarkably large number of serious conditions, notably heart disease and cancer. In 2015, Americans consumed 80 billion cups of tea, more than 3.6 billion gallons.

First, let's clear up some confusion: Many people use the term "tea" to describe any herbal beverage made by steeping plant material in boiled water: chamomile tea, mint tea. This works colloquially, but in herbal medicine, it becomes confusing. Using the colloquial definition, coffee is a tea because it's a hot-water extract of plant material. Technically, however, hot-water extracts are not teas, but "infusions." In herbal medicine, "tea" is an infusion made with tea leaves (*Camellia sinensis*).

Few traditional herbals mention tea. In fact, many people don't even consider tea an herb. They typically ask, "Would you like coffee, tea, or herb tea?" Of course, coffee and tea are both herbs, so all of three choices are herb teas. However, in common parlance, "herb tea" typically means a noncaffeinated herbal beverage.

There are four basic types of tea: white, green, oolong, and black. They all begin as leaves of *Camellia sinensis*. Soon after harvesting, unless dried, the leaves wilt and oxidize, turning progressively darker as their chlorophyll breaks down and combines with oxygen in the air. Chemically, this is *oxidation*, but the tea industry calls it *fermentation*.

- White tea is picked and dried immediately, unwilted and unoxidized.
- Green tea is wilted but unoxidized.
- Oolong tea is wilted and partially oxidized.
- Black tea is wilted and fully oxidized.

Black tea accounts for 85 percent of American tea consumption, most of it consumed iced. Green tea accounts for about 14 percent. White and oolong account for the remaining 1 percent.

In addition, many teas have been named for the locale where the leaves were grown, for example, Darjeeling, a region of West Bengal, India, or Pu'er, named for a city in Yunnan province, China.

Teas have also been named for other reasons.

- The Chinese called black tea *pek-ho*. The British heard the term as "pekoe," which came to mean any black tea. The English considered tea so divine that they gave it the name "tea" from the Greek *thea*, meaning "goddess."

- English Breakfast is a blend of various black teas.

- Earl Grey is named for the second Earl Grey, a British prime minister in the 1830s who reputedly received a gift of black tea flavored with oil of bergamont, an orange-like citrus fruit. Traditionally, Earl Grey meant citrus-flavored black tea. But today Earl Grey white, green, and oolong teas are also available.

- Lapsang souchong is a smoked black tea originally from the Wuyi region of Fujian province, China. Today other teas are also smoked.

- Chai is an Indian combination of tea (usually black) with a blend of spices: cardamom, cinnamon, clove, and pepper.

Note: African red bush tea, sometimes called red tea, is not tea. It's rooibos (*Aspalathus linearis*, page 399), a plant native to South Africa.

Note: Tea tree is not tea. It's an Australian herb (*Melaleuca alterniflora,* page 458) whose oil is a powerful topical antiseptic.

A Brief History of Tea

Legend has it that 5,000 years ago, the mythical Chinese emperor Shen Nung asked a servant for a cup of boiled water. A few leaves from a nearby tree accidentally fell into it, giving the water a golden color and pleasant flavor. Shen Nung pronounced it refreshing. The Chinese have savored tea ever since.

As time passed, tea spread throughout Asia. It became particularly popular in Japan, where its preparation was elevated to an art form, the Japanese tea ceremony.

The first European to mention tea was Portuguese Jesuit Father Jasper de Cruz, who visited China in 1560. But it was Dutch traders who first brought tea to Europe, where it became an immediate hit—but only with the wealthy because tea was rare, coveted, and costly.

Tea arrived in England in 1652. By then, increased importation from China had reduced the price to the point where all but the poor could afford a few cups a day. Tea quickly replaced ale as England's national beverage.

In 1618, the Chinese ambassador to Russia presented czar Alexis with a gift of tea. The herb quickly became popular throughout Russia. So did the Tibetan method of brewing it in a large pot, which the Russians transformed into the samovar.

Around 1800 in England, Anna, the Duchess of Bedford, began serving tea with a light snack in the late afternoon. She invented "tea time."

Tea arrived in the Western Hemisphere in 1650 when Peter Stuyvesant introduced it to New Amsterdam, later New York. But it did not catch on until around 1700 when importation increased and the price dropped. By 1720, tea was a beloved staple in colonial America.

From 1754 to 1763, during what we call the French and Indian War, England fought the French for control of North America. It was an expensive war, and because it safeguarded the colonies, England decided that her American colonists should pay for it through taxes, including a tax on tea. The colonists hated the tea tax and boycotted English tea, buying smuggled Dutch tea instead. Then on December 16, 1773, Samuel Adams, John Hancock, and other disgruntled colonists stormed a British merchant ship and threw hundreds of pounds of tea into Boston harbor—the Boston Tea Party. In retaliation, the British closed the port of Boston and sent troops to occupy the city. One could argue that Americans' love of tea sparked the American Revolution.

Despite the Boston Tea Party, by the 19th century, Americans preferred coffee. But tea remained popular. In 1904, one tea merchant, Richard Blechynden, planned to give away cups of hot tea at the St. Louis World's Fair. But a heat wave struck and no one wanted his hot beverage. Blechynden served his tea over ice—the birth of iced tea. It was the hit of the Fair and quickly became a national craze.

In 1908, tea merchant Thomas Sullivan packaged individual cup-size portions of tea in porous paper wrappers. The idea went nowhere until some restaurants began serving tea "in the bag" to save waiters the time of handling loose tea. Tea bags have been with us ever since.

For most of the 20th century "tea" meant Lipton orange pekoe. But starting in the 1970s, as Americans developed a taste for exotic coffees, they also became more interested in other teas: green, white, oolong, Pu-er, Darjeeling, etc. Today, tea is more popular than ever in the United States, thanks, ironically, to coffee shops like Starbucks that also serve tea.

Healing History

Tea has been used in Chinese medicine for 3,000 years to treat headache, diarrhea, dysentery, colds, coughs, asthma, and other respiratory problems. The Chinese also view tea as a grease cutter and recommend drinking it with fatty meals.

Seventeenth-century English herbalist Nicholas Culpeper called tea "more used for pleasure than as a medicine," but suggested it as a digestive aid and "for all inward decays." He also recommended it for "violent headaches and sickness occasioned by inebriation." But he warned that tea should be avoided by those with "weak nerves."

America's 19th-century Eclectic physicians, forerunners of today's naturopaths, called tea "a harmless and refreshing beverage . . . unless taken very strong or in large quantities." They called it "very agreeable to the invalid," and recommended it for fever, colds, muscle aches, headache, and stomach distress. But they warned that its stimulant action might interfere with sleep.

In the 1930s, Maude Gieve, a prominent

Different Teas, Different Amounts of Caffeine

Tea leaves contain caffeine. But as the leaves dry, wilt, and oxidize, they lose water and become more compressed—and the caffeine they contain becomes more concentrated. As a result, white tea contains the least caffeine (less than 30 milligrams per 5-ounce cup). Green tea contains more (about 30 milligrams). Oolong has even more (around 50 milligrams). And black tea contains the most (about 100 milligrams per cup).

British herbalist, noted "tea is rarely used as a medicine, but the infusion is useful to relieve headaches."

Until the 1990s, tea was a minor player in U.S. herbal medicine. Americans drank it primarily as a mildly stimulating beverage, but also to treat diarrhea and colds and other respiratory problems. However, since the 1990s, tea has become a major herbal healer. It's remarkably rich in antioxidants and as a result, substantially reduces risk of heart disease, stroke, all major cancers, diabetes, osteoporosis, rheumatoid arthritis, dementia, and other several conditions.

Therapeutic Uses

Tea contains three compounds—caffeine, theobromine, and theophylline—that account for its stimulant action.

STIMULANT. Cup for cup, tea has about half the caffeine of brewed coffee. But if you drink 2 cups of tea, you don't get the same buzz as 1 cup of coffee. The reason is that tea also contains a compound (L-theanine) that has tranquilizing action. The Chinese say that tea produces "relaxed alertness."

COLDS, ASTHMA. Like coffee, the stimulants in tea open the bronchial tubes (bronchodilator). This action helps treat the chest congestions of colds and may help control asthma.

PAIN RELIEF. The combination of caffeine and pain relievers relieves headache better than pain relievers by themselves. Wash down aspirin, ibuprofen (Motrin), acetaminophen (Tylenol), or naproxen (Aleve) with a cup of tea, and the pain reliever works better. For more on this, see Coffee, page 165.

ANTIOXIDANT. Beyond its stimulant action, tea contains powerfully antioxidant polyphenols that, over the past 25 years, have rocketed this herb into medicinal prominence. Antioxidants help prevent and repair the cell damage at the root of heart disease, most strokes and cancers, and many other degenerative conditions associated with aging.

In traditional Chinese medicine, tea is considered a "grease cutter" that prevents diseases associated with fatty foods, for example, heart disease and cancer. In the 1980s, Japanese researchers discovered potent antioxidants in tea, notably epigallocatechin-3-gallate (EGCG), thus validating traditional Chinese medicine's claim.

However, the oxidation process that turns tea from white to green to oolong to black

Brewing the Perfect Cup of Tea

Don't boil the water. Or if it boils, allow it to cool a bit before pouring it over tea. The optimal steeping temperature for oolong and black teas is 175°F; for white and green teas, 140°F.

Tea strength depends on the amount of leaves used and steeping time. The amount typically recommended is 3 grams of leaf per cup, or about a rounded teaspoon. Steeping time is a matter of personal preference, but most experts recommend 2 to 3 minutes for green tea; longer for oolong and black teas. If you enjoy strong tea, leave the leaves in the water as you drink.

destroys some of the EGCG along the way. As a result, white and green teas have greater antioxidant content than oolong teas, which contain more antioxidants than black teas. In laboratory studies, black tea has been shown to have only around 10 percent of green tea's antioxidant punch. Black teas still contain significant amounts of antioxidants, which is why they reduce risk of heart disease and stroke—see below. But black teas have not shown much power to reduce cancer risk. For cancer prevention, green tea is the way to go because it's much more easily available than white tea, and it retains most of its EGCG. (Currently scientists can't explain why black tea reduces risk of heart disease and stroke, but not cancer.)

HEART DISEASE. In the West, tea began its transformation from a beverage into a health food in 1993, when Dutch researchers published a study in the prestigious British medical journal, *Lancet*. They studied the effects of various dietary antioxidants on risk of heart attack among residents of the Dutch city Zutphen. Men who consumed the most fruits and vegetables—all rich in antioxidants—had the lowest risk of heart attack. But tea was also very protective, a finding that surprised Western scientists and sent them scurrying to the earlier Japanese ECGC research.

How do tea's antioxidants reduce risk of heart disease? They lower cholesterol and blood pressure. They improve arterial health. And they reduce atherosclerosis, the formation of the fatty, cholesterol-rich deposits in the arteries that clog them, and in heart attacks, they block the coronary arteries.

Since then, dozens of studies have shown that tea—both black and green—helps prevent heart disease.

* In a different Dutch study, researchers followed 4,807 men for 5 years. Compared with those who drank no tea, men who drank a cup or two a day had 43 percent fewer heart attacks—and 70 percent fewer heart attack deaths.

* Saudi Arabian scientists surveyed 3,430 adults aged 30 to 70. As tea consumption increased, their risk of heart disease decreased significantly.

* Harvard researchers surveyed 340 people who had suffered heart attacks and a similar number of healthy controls. Drinking more than 1 cup of tea a day reduced heart attack risk 44 percent.

If tea really helps the heart, it should exhibit a "dose-response" effect—as tea consumption increases, heart disease risk should decline. That is the case. In the Harvard study, moderate tea drinkers were 31 percent less likely to suffer heart attack. The figure for heavy tea drinkers was 39 percent. The Saudi study also showed a dose-response effect.

Warning: If you drink tea for heart benefits, don't add milk. A German study suggests that milk neutralizes the ECGC, counteracting tea's heart-helping actions.

STROKE. Most strokes (ischemic strokes) are biologically similar to heart attacks. But instead of blocking one of the coronary arteries, ischemic strokes block arteries in the brain. Antioxidants reduce risk of ischemic stroke. Dutch researchers followed 552 men for 15 years. Compared with those who drank less than 2 cups of tea a day, men who drank more than 4 cups saw their stroke risk plummet 69 percent.

CANCER. Animal studies starting in the 1980s showed that green tea reduces risk of cancer. The first study to find the same benefit in humans was published in 1988. For that study, researchers in Kyushu, Japan, compared the diets and lifestyles of 139 people with stomach cancer and 2,852 people who were cancer-free. After accounting for other variables, the researchers determined that as green tea consumption increased, stomach cancer risk decreased significantly.

Since then, an occasional report has shown no cancer-protective benefits for green tea, but these few negative findings are vastly outnumbered by dozens of trials showing that as green tea consumption increases, risk of *all major cancers* decreases: lung, colon, breast, prostate, ovarian, esophageal, pancreatic, malignant melanoma, and stomach cancers, plus leukemia.

❦ Lung cancer. Japanese scientists compared the green tea consumption of 333 Okinawans with lung cancer and 666 who were cancer-free. Among women, tea drinking reduced cancer risk from 23 to 62 percent, with increasing amounts of tea producing greater risk reductions. Among men, risk reductions ranged from 15 to 43 percent.

❦ Breast cancer. Another group of University of Minnesota scientists analyzed 13 studies of green tea's effect on breast cancer risk. Compared with women who did not drink it, those who drank the most green tea had 22 percent less risk of breast cancer.

❦ Colon cancer. University of Minnesota researchers analyzed 25 studies of tea's impact on risk of colon cancer. Black tea had no effect. But compared with those who drank no green tea, regular green tea drinkers were significantly less likely to develop colon cancer.

❦ Prostate cancer. Australian researchers surveyed green tea drinking among 130 men with prostate cancer and 274 men who were cancer-free. Among those with cancer, 55 percent drank green tea. Among those free of prostate cancer, the figure was 80 percent. And as green tea consumption increased, cancer risk decreased.

❦ Ovarian cancer. Swedish scientists followed 61,057 women for 15 years. Compared with those who drank tea (green or black) less than once a month, women who drank more than 2 cups a day were 46 percent less likely to develop ovarian cancer.

Colorado State University scientists analyzed four large, rigorous studies of green tea's effect on ovarian cancer risk. A daily cup or two cut risk about 34 percent.

❦ Esophageal cancer. Chinese researchers compared green tea consumption among 902 people aged 30 to 74 who had esophageal cancer and 1,552 people who were cancer-free. For women, regular green tea drinking cut cancer risk 50 percent. For men who did not smoke or drink alcohol, green tea cut esophageal cancer risk 57 percent.

❦ Pancreatic cancer. Columbia University scientists documented green tea consumption among 451 Chinese in Shanghai with pancreatic cancer and 1,552 healthy controls. Regular green tea drinking reduced pancreative cancer risk 47 percent.

❦ Malignant melanoma. Italian researchers tracked tea drinking in 542 people with malignant melanoma and 538 healthy matched controls. Compared with those who did not drink tea, those who drank the most had 29 percent less risk of melanoma.

❧ Stomach cancer. Chinese scientists surveyed green tea drinking in 711 people with stomach cancer and 711 healthy matched controls. Compared with nondrinkers, those who drank green tea regularly had 29 percent less risk of stomach cancer.

❧ Liver cancer. Japanese investigators followed 41,761 older adults for 9 years. As their green tea consumption increased, their risk of liver cancer decreased. Compared with those who drank little green tea, men who consumed 5 or more daily cups had 37 percent less risk of liver cancer, and women who drank 5 cups a day or more showed 50 percent less risk.

❧ All digestive system cancers. These include malignancies of the esophagus, stomach, pancreas, liver, intestine, colon, and rectum. Shanghai researchers followed 69,310 older adults for 11 years. Compared with those who drank little tea, a few cups a day reduced risk of all digestive tract cancers 17 percent.

❧ Leukemia. Harvard researchers assessed green tea consumption in 252 leukemia sufferers and 637 healthy controls. As tea consumption increased, leukemia risk decreased.

❧ Bladder cancer. Chinese researchers analyzed 17 studies of tea's effect on bladder cancer risk in Asians. Black tea showed no protective value, but a daily cup or two of green tea reduced bladder cancer risk 19 percent.

Green tea shows a clear dose-response effect for cancer prevention. Consider breast cancer: Australian researchers categorized green tea consumption in 2,018 Chinese women as low, moderate, or high. Low intake reduced breast cancer risk, 13 percent; moderate, 32 percent; high, 41 percent. A study at the University of Southern California showed a similar dose-response effect.

Of course, some green tea drinkers still develop cancer. If green tea has cancer-preventive benefits, then compared with those who do not drink it, we would expect green tea drinkers to develop cancer later in life. That's precisely what Japanese researchers showed in a study correlating tea drinking in Japan with people's age at cancer diagnosis. Compared with Japanese who drank less than 3 cups of green tea a day, women who drank 10 or more developed all cancers an average of 9 years later. The figure for men was 3 years later.

If tea protects against cancer, we would also expect milder cancers in those who drink it. Another Japanese study confirms this. Compared with Japanese breast cancer sufferers who drank little or no green tea, those who regularly drank 8 to 10 cups a day had milder cases at diagnosis (fewer positive lymph nodes), a greater likelihood of estrogen-positive disease (improved prognosis), less risk of metastasis (spread), less risk of recurrence, and a better rate of survival.

Finally if tea protects against cancer, we would expect tea drinkers to have less chance of recurrence. Again, this is the case. Japanese researchers analyzed the breast cancers of 472 women. Those who drank the most green tea had the least likelihood of recurrences.

DIABETES. Japanese researchers followed 17,413 adults aged 40 to 65 for 5 years. Compared with those who drank less than 1 cup of green tea per week, participants who drank 6 or more daily cups were 33 percent less likely to develop Type-2 diabetes. Another Japanese researcher team documented similar findings using oolong tea.

FLU. Green tea has immune-stimulating action. At the start of flu season, Japanese researchers gave 200 adults either a daily placebo or green tea extract (the equivalent of drinking 3 cups a day). By the end of that flu season, 13 percent of the placebo group had developed flu, but in the green tea group, just 4 percent. A similar study by another Japanese team showed similar findings.

WEIGHT CONTROL. Caffeine increases basal metabolic rate, the rate at which the body burns calories while at rest. Several studies show that in physician-supervised weight-loss programs, coffee drinking modestly increases weight loss (see Coffee, page 165). French and Japanese studies show that tea also contributes to weight loss.

COGNITIVE FUNCTION. The risk factors for heart disease and stroke—high cholesterol, high blood pressure, sedentary lifestyle, high-fat diet, smoking, and diabetes—also increase risk for dementia. Tea helps prevent heart disease, so researchers have begun to study its impact on cognition. Animal studies suggest that tea's antioxidant constituents improve cognition.

In addition, Japanese researchers surveyed 1,003 elderly Japanese about their tea consumption and then gave them cognitive function tests. As green tea drinking increased, cognitive impairment decreased. One cup a day cut cognitive impairment in half.

Chinese scientists surveyed both tea and coffee consumption in 716 adults over 55. Compared with those who consumed little tea, those who drank the most scored significantly higher on mental acuity tests. High coffee consumption had no effect on cognition.

OSTEOPOROSIS. Fluoride plays a role in bone strength, and tea contains it. Japanese researchers surveyed the diets and lifestyles of 632 women and then tested their bone mineral density (BMD), a measure of bone strength. Compared with those who drank green tea infrequently, women who drank it regularly had significantly greater BMD. Studies in Australia and Iran agree that habitual tea drinking improves BMD and reduces risk of osteoporosis.

RHEUMATOID ARTHRITIS (RA). University of Alabama researchers followed 31,336 women aged 55 to 69 for 9 years. Initially, none had RA, but by the end, 158 had been diagnosed. They drank significantly less tea than those who remained RA-free. In fact, drinking more than 3 cups of tea a day reduced RA risk 61 percent.

ECZEMA. In addition to its potent antioxidant action, the EGCG in tea is also anti-inflammatory. Several studies have shown that it helps manage eczema. In one trial, Japanese scientists asked 118 people with severe eczema to add 3 daily cups of oolong tea to their treatment regimens. After 1 month, 63 percent showed "moderate to marked improvement."

DIARRHEA. Tea contains astringent tannins, whose binding action helps manage diarrhea. Tea is one component of the BRATT diet, a popular home remedy for diarrhea: bananas, rice, applesauce, tea, and toast.

TOOTH DECAY. Tea is a good source of decay-preventive fluoride. Both green and black teas contain more fluoride than fluoridated water. The tannins in tea may also help fight the bacteria that cause tooth decay. A Japanese study shows that tea inhibits the bacteria that cause tooth decay and produce dental plaque.

CONCEPTION. Caffeine interferes with conception (see Coffee, page 165). Tea contains caffeine and might be expected to do that same. But a study of 210 women enrolled in the Kaiser-Permanente health maintenance program in Oakland, California, shows that a daily cup of tea *increases* women's chances of pregnancy. The reason(s) for this remain unclear.

WRINKLES. Thai researchers assessed facial wrinkles in older adults and then asked them to apply a skin cream with added tea and rooibos (page 399) daily. After 28 days, the herbal skin cream reduced wrinkling 10 percent.

DEATH FROM ALL CAUSES. With tea reducing the risk of so many serious conditions, Japanese researchers wondered if it might be literally a life-saver. They followed 40,530 healthy Japanese adults for 11 years. Drinking tea decreased risk of death from *all causes*. Compared with those drinking less than 1 cup a day, people who drank tea regularly had reduced risk of death, with greater tea consumption corresponding to greater benefit. Drinking 5 or more cups a day cut death risk 12 percent in men and 23 percent in women.

Intriguing Possibilities

In a pilot study in Japan, people treated their genital warts with either an ordinary skin cream or the cream infused with green tea extract. In the tea group, the warts cleared up significantly faster.

A Chinese report claims that tea helps treat hepatitis. Hepatitis is a serious disease that requires professional care, but during convalescence, tea does no harm, and it may do some good.

Green tea contains anti-inflammatory compounds (polyphenols). British dermatologists exposed 16 fair-skinned adults to sunlight until they began to develop sunburn. Then participants took a daily green tea extract (540 milligrams). After 12 weeks, it took significantly more sun exposure to cause burning.

Japanese researchers have shown that green tea contains compounds with antihistamine action, so the herb may help manage hay fever and hives.

And an Egyptian study suggests that a few daily cups of green tea may shrink uterine fibroids, possibly allowing women to avoid surgery.

Rx Recommendations

Green tea is the variety with the most beneficial health effects. If you're used to the rich, full-bodied flavor of black tea, green tea may taste thin and watery at first. But over time, you may come to appreciate its delicate flavor.

How strong must green tea be to maximize its health benefits? University of Hawaii researchers steeped green tea for 3, 5, and 10 minutes, then ran laboratory tests to determine each brew's antioxidant content. They all packed about the same antioxidant punch. Apparently, the antioxidant compounds in green tea are released quickly, and steeping longer than 3 minutes does not appreciably increase them.

For a pleasantly bitter infusion, use 1 tea bag or 1 to 2 teaspoons of dried herb per cup of boiling water. Steep for 10 to 15 minutes and strain if you use loose tea.

In many of the studies showing that tea reduces risk of cancer and heart disease, participants drank more than 5 cups a day. That might expose you to more caffeine than you can comfortably tolerate. Decaffeinated tea retains its antioxidants.

Safety

Caffeine is a classically addictive drug that causes nervousness, restlessness, insomnia, and many other possible problems (see Coffee, page 165).

Caffeine has been linked to an increased risk of birth defects. Pregnant women should not consume it.

Large amounts of tea may cause gastrointestinal upset.

Do not give tea to children under 2. Young children may drink weak tea. Kids over 12 can drink adult-strength tea.

Inform health professionals of the herbs you use. Problematic herb-drug interactions are possible.

Tea may cause allergic reactions or other unexpected side effects. If any develop, reduce your dose or stop taking it. For more on herb safety, see Chapter 2.

If symptoms get worse or persist longer than 2 weeks, consult a health professional promptly.

Gardening

Tea is not grown in the United States. It's native to southwest China and northeast India. Tea leaves grow on a subtropical evergreen tree that can reach 30 feet. But growers prune it into a waist-high bush for easy leaf harvesting. China and India each produce about one-quarter of the world's supply, with most of the rest grown in Sri Lanka, Kenya, Turkey, Indonesia, and Vietnam.

TEA TREE

The Antiseptic from Down Under

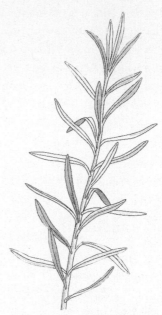

Family: Myrtaceae; other members include eucalyptus, myrtle, and clove

Genus and species: *Melaleuca alternifolia*

Also known as: Tea tree oil and Australian tea tree

Parts used: Leaf oil

Don't confuse tea tree (*Melaleuca alternifolia*) with tea (*Camellia sinensis,* page 449). Tea tree doesn't boast as much healing power as tea, but it still has some impressive therapeutic benefits.

Healing History

When the English explorer Captain James Cook first arrived in Australia in 1777, he found the indigenous people treating skin infections with crushed tea tree leaves. White colonists adopted the plant and used its leaves to make a tea-like beverage, hence the name tea tree. They also used the leaves to flavor beer. Australian physicians eventually introduced tea tree's medicinal benefits to Europe and the United States.

During the 1920s, surgeons and dentists began using tea tree oil as an antiseptic. During World War II, field doctors used it to disinfect wounds.

Today, tea tree oil is an ingredient in some antiseptic soaps, creams, acne products, deodorants, toothpastes, mouthwashes, and antifungal creams and vaginal suppositories.

Therapeutic Uses

Modern science has confirmed that the oil liberated by crushing tea tree leaves is a powerful antiseptic.

WOUNDS. An Australian study showed that tea tree oil kills many microorganisms that cause infection: yeast fungus (*Candida albicans*) and several bacteria—*Escherichia coli, Staphylococcus aureus,* and *Pseudomonas aeruginosa.* Another Australian study showed that even drug-resistant *Staphylococcus* bacteria may succumb to tea tree oil treatment.

SCABIES, HEAD LICE. Australians use tea tree oil to treat scabies, head lice, and insect bites and stings.

ATHLETE'S FOOT. Australian researchers gave athlete's foot sufferers a medically inactive placebo cream; a cream containing a pharmaceutical (tolnaftate, used in Desenex and Tinactin), or a cream containing 10 percent tea tree oil. The herb was as effective as tolnaftate.

ACNE. At Royal Prince Alfred Hospital in Australia, researchers gave 124 people with mild to moderate acne either an over-the-counter 5 percent benzoyl peroxide lotion or a tea tree oil lotion. The benzoyl peroxide lotion worked faster, but by the study's conclusion, both treatments were equally effective—and tea tree oil caused less skin irritation.

FUNGAL TOENAIL INFECTION. Stubborn, hard-to-treat fungal toenail infections discolor and thicken toenails. At the University of Rochester School of Medicine, researchers had 117 people with fungal toenail infections apply either a standard pharmaceutical (1 percent clotrimazole) or tea tree oil (100 percent) twice a day for 6 months. Sixty percent of those in both group experienced improvement.

YEAST INFECTION. Tea tree oil's activity against the yeast fungus has led to its use in treating vaginal yeast infections.

Intriguing Possibilities

Added to baths or vaporizers, tea tree oil may help speed recovery from respiratory infections.

Rx Recommendations

Use a cotton ball or cotton swab to apply 100 percent tea tree oil to affected skin or toenails twice a day.

For vaginal yeast infection, place a few drops of tea tree oil on a tampon. Leave it inserted for 24 hours, then remove. If continued treatment is necessary, use a new tampon.

Safety

Do not ingest tea tree oil. Swallowing as little as a few teaspoons can be fatal.

Anyone may use tea tree oil topically, including pregnant or nursing women, children, and the elderly. For those with sensitive skin (children and people with fair complexions), dilute the oil in vegetable oil before applying.

A report in the *New England Journal of Medicine* describes three boys who developed enlarged breasts (gynecomastia) after applying tea tree oil to their skin. Their breasts returned to normal when the oil was discontinued. Evidently, tea tree oil has estrogenic action that in rare cases causes breast tissue overgrowth. Oddly, however, there are no reports of women using tea tree oil for breast augmentation.

Pregnant and nursing women may use tea tree oil topically in consultation with their physicians.

Inform health professionals of the herbs you use. Problematic herb-drug interactions are possible.

Tea tree oil may cause allergic reactions or other unexpected side effects. If any develop, reduce your dose or stop taking it. For more on herb safety, see Chapter 2.

If symptoms get worse or persist longer than 2 weeks, consult a health professional promptly.

Gardening

Native to the swampy lowlands of New South Wales, Australia, tea tree is an evergreen that can reach 40 feet. It has narrow, needlelike leaves that when crushed, release the plant's antiseptic, aromatic oil. Its white flowers bloom in summer. The tree is not grown in the United States.

THYME
The Power Behind Listerine

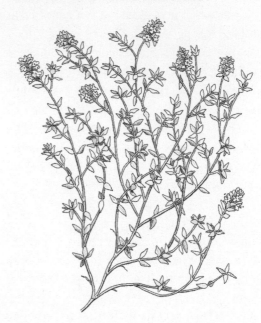

Family: Labiatae; other members include mints

Genus and species: *Thymus vulgaris* and *T. serpyllum*

Also known as: Common or garden thyme (*T. vulgaris*); wild thyme, creeping thyme, mother thyme, and mother of thyme (*T. serpyllum*)

Parts used: Leaves and flowers

Parsley, sage, rosemary, and . . . Listerine? Or Vicks VapoRub? Thyme is commonly found in kitchen spice racks, but without realizing it, millions of Americans also stock the herb's oil in their medicine cabinets. Thyme's inclusion in mouthwashes and decongestants is no coincidence. This herb boasts a long history of use as an antiseptic, cough remedy, and digestive aid.

Healing History

In ancient Rome, priests sprinkled thyme on sacrificial animals to make them more acceptable to the gods.

Both the Roman poet, Virgil, and his naturalist countryman, Pliny, mention thyme as a meat preservative. Like so many other aromatic herbs, thyme was introduced into cooking as an offshoot of its food-preserving action. The Romans also used it medicinally as a cough remedy, digestive aid, and treatment for intestinal worms.

The emperor Charlemagne ordered thyme grown in all of his imperial gardens as a culinary herb and medicine. The 12th-century German abbess/herbalist Hildegard of Bingen considered it the herb of choice for skin problems, anticipating its later use as an antiseptic.

During the Middle Ages, thyme became linked to courage. It was fashionable for noblewomen to embroider sprigs of thyme on scarves and give them to favorite knights departing for the Crusades.

As the centuries passed, thyme was used as an antiseptic during plagues. Those troubled by "melancholia" (depression) were advised to sleep on thyme-stuffed pillows.

Medieval anatomists named the lymph gland in the chest the thymus because it reminded them of thyme's flower.

Sixteenth-century British herbalist John Gerard recommended thyme for leprosy and to "cure sciatica . . . pains in the head . . . [and] falling sickness [epilepsy]."

During the 17th century, Nicholas Culpeper called thyme "excellent for nervous disorders . . . headaches . . . and a certain remedy for that troublesome complaint, the nightmare." He claimed that the herb "provokes the terms [menstruation], gives safe and speedy delivery to women in travail [labor], and brings away the after-birth." Culpeper also recommended thyme as "a noble strengthener of the lungs . . . an excellent remedy for shortness of breath. . . . It purges the body of phlegm . . . comforts the stomach much and expels wind."

By the late 17th century, apothecary shops were selling thyme oil as a topical antiseptic under the name "oil of origanum." In 1719, German chemist Caspar Neumann extracted thyme oil's active constituent, which he called "camphor of thyme." In 1853, French chemist M. Lallemand named it thymol.

From the mid-19th century through World War I, thymol enjoyed great popularity as an antiseptic. America's Eclectic physicians, forerunners of today's naturopaths, extolled it in their textbook *King's American Dispensatory* (1898): "Thymol is considered by many to be superior to carbolic acid [the antiseptic made famous by Joseph Lister, father of antiseptic surgery]. It prevents putrefaction and arrests it when it has commenced. . . . Dissolved in water, it forms an invaluable disinfectant [for] sick rooms." The Eclectics also prescribed thyme infusion for headache, gastrointestinal upsets, and "hysteria" (menstrual cramps) and as a menstruation promoter.

World War I caused a thymol crisis. Most of the world's supply was distilled in Germany. When the British and French declared war on Germany, they had to scramble to overcome a terrible shortage of the suddenly vital battlefield antiseptic.

Although thymol has since been replaced by more potent antiseptics, it remains an ingredient in several mouthwashes, including Listerine.

Contemporary herbalists recommend thyme externally for disinfecting wounds and internally for indigestion, sore throats, laryngitis, coughs, and nervousness.

Therapeutic Uses

Thyme's aromatic oil contains two medicinal compounds, thymol and carvacol. Both have preservative, antibacterial, and antifungal properties. They also have expectorant action and aid digestion.

INFECTIONS. In laboratory studies, thyme fights several disease-causing bacteria and fungi, supporting the herb's traditional role as an antiseptic. Infusions of the dried herb are nowhere near as powerful as the oil or distilled thymol, but you can use fresh leaves as garden first-aid for minor wounds.

COUGHS. German researchers have lent support to thyme's traditional role as a phlegm loosener (expectorant). In Germany, where herbal medicine is considerably more mainstream than in the United States, thyme preparations are frequently prescribed to relax the respiratory tract and treat coughs, whooping cough, and emphysema.

German medical herbalist Rudolph Fritz Weiss, M.D., writes, "Thyme is to the trachea [windpipe] and the bronchi what peppermint [page 363] is to the stomach and intestines." Commission E, the expert panel that evaluates herbal medicines for the German counterpart of the FDA, approves thyme as a treatment for cold-related coughs, bronchitis, and whooping cough.

DIGESTIVE PROBLEMS. Thymol and carvacol relax the smooth muscle tissue of the gastrointestinal tract, making thyme an anti-spasmodic. The action of these chemical constituents lends support to its traditional role as a digestive aid.

WOMEN'S HEALTH. Antispasmodics relax not only the digestive tract but also other smooth muscles, such as the uterus. Tincture of thyme may help relieve menstrual cramps, lending credence to the Eclectic physicians' use of this herb. Hoswever, in large amounts, thyme oil and thymol appear to be uterine stimulants.

Intriguing Possibility

In a laboratory study, Israeli scientists have found that thyme infusion inhibits the growth of *Helicobacter pylori*, the bacteria that causes most ulcers. It's too early to call thyme an ulcer treatment, but if you have ulcers, try drinking thyme tea.

Rx Recommendations

For garden accidents, crush fresh leaves into minor wounds until you can wash and bandage them. After you have thoroughly washed them, apply a few drops of thyme tincture as an antiseptic.

For an infusion to help settle the stomach, soothe a cough, or possibly help relieve menstrual symptoms, use 2 teaspoons of dried herb per cup of boiling water. Steep for 10 minutes, then strain. Drink up to 3 cups a day. Thyme tastes pleasantly aromatic, with a faint clovelike aftertaste.

As a homemade tincture, take ½ to 1 teaspoon up to three times a day.

When using commercial preparations, follow package directions.

Safety

Use the herb, not its oil. Even a few teaspoons of thyme oil can be toxic, causing headache, nausea, vomiting, weakness, thyroid impairment, and heart and respiratory depression.

One animal study showed that thyme suppresses thyroid activity. People with thyroid conditions should consult their physicians before taking medicinal doses.

Pregnant women may use thyme as a culinary spice, but should avoid large amounts and not ingest the oil. Nursing women should also avoid thyme oil.

Do not give medicinal preparations of thyme to children under 2. In older children, adjust the recommended dose based on the child's weight. Give a 50-pound child one-third of the dose a 150-pound adult would take.

If you're over 65, start with a low dose, and increase only if necessary.

Inform health professionals of the herbs you use. Problematic herb-drug interactions are possible.

Thyme and thyme oil may cause a rash in sensitive individuals. It may also cause allergic reactions or other unexpected side effects. If any develop, reduce your dose or stop taking it. For more on herb safety, see Chapter 2.

If symptoms get worse or persist longer than 2 weeks, consult a health professional promptly.

Gardening

Thyme is an aromatic, perennial, many-branched, ground-cover shrub that reaches about 12 inches. It has small, opposite, virtually stalkless leaves and lilac or pink flowers that bloom in midsummer.

This hardy herb can be propagated from seeds, cuttings, or root divisions. Seeds require a temperature around 70°F to germinate and often do best started indoors. For cuttings, snip 3-inch pieces from stems with new growth and place them in wet sand. Roots should appear in about 2 weeks.

Spring is the best time for root divisions. Uproot plants carefully, preserving as much of their root balls as possible. Divide them in half or thirds and replant the divisions 12 inches apart in moist soil.

Once established, thyme requires little care. It prefers well-drained, slightly dry soil. Wetting thyme leaves during watering reduces their fragrance.

Clumps tend to become woody after a few years. To prevent this, divide roots periodically.

Thyme survives frost, but in areas with cold winters, use mulch. Thyme may be killed if winter temperatures drop below 10°F.

Harvest the leaves and flowers just before the flowers bloom. Dry and store them in airtight containers to preserve the herb's oil.

TURMERIC (CURCUMIN)

Yellow Curry Is a Powerful Healer

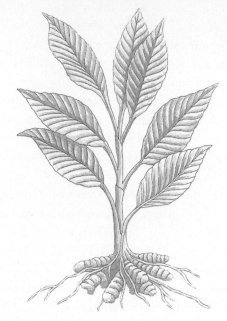

Family: Zingiberaceae; other members include ginger

Genus and species: *Curcuma longa*

Also known as: Curcuma

Parts used: Rhizomes and roots

Turmeric is a relatively recent addition to American spice racks, but for millennia, it's been a mainstay in Indian curries. The culinary herb is turmeric, but in herbal medicine, it's usually called curcumin, the name of the pigment that gives the rhizome its yellow color.

To date, curcumin has been studied in more than 1,500 laboratory and animal studies and several hundred human (clinical) trials. They show that this herb is a medicinal powerhouse that stimulates the immune system, is subtly pain-relieving, and reduces risk of heart disease, cancer, dementia, ulcers, colitis, arthritis, cataracts, scabies, liver damage, food poisoning, and irritable bowel syndrome. And because turmeric has been a food for thousands of years, it's not necessary to wait for definitive evidence to incorporate it—and more curry dishes—into your diet. Alternatively, you might take a curcumin supplement.

Healing History

In Indian cuisine, "curry" means any multi-spice blend. But in the United States most curry comes prepackaged with a yellow-gold color because it contains turmeric. This herb also holds a place of honor in India's traditional Ayurvedic medicine as a whole-body strengthener (tonic), digestive aid, and treatment for fever, infections, dysentery, arthritis, and jaundice and other liver problems.

Traditional Chinese physicians prescribed turmeric to treat liver and gallbladder problems, stop bleeding, and relieve chest congestion and menstrual discomforts.

The ancient Greeks were aware of turmeric, but unlike its close botanical relative, ginger, it never caught on in the West as either a culinary or a medicinal herb. It was only used to make orange-yellow dyes.

During the 1870s, chemists noticed that turmeric's orange-yellow root powder turned reddish brown when exposed to alkaline chemicals. This discovery led to the development of "turmeric paper," thin strips of tissue brushed with a decoction of turmeric, then dried. During the late 19th century, turmeric paper was used in laboratories around the world to test for alkalinity. Eventually, it was replaced by litmus paper, which continues to be used today.

American's botanically oriented 19th-century Eclectic physicians, forerunners of today's naturopaths, used turmeric paper but had little use for the herb itself, except to add color to medicinal ointments.

During the 1930s, Maude Grieve's influential *Modern Herbal* said that turmeric was "once a treatment for jaundice," then dismissed it as "seldom used in medicine except as a coloring."

Unlike their Eclectic predecessors, today's naturopaths extol turmeric for its many benefits, particularly as an anti-inflammatory. "Turmeric is one of nature's most potent anti-inflammatory agents," says Joseph Pizzorno, N.D., coauthor of *The Textbook of Natural Medicine* and former president of Bastyr University, the naturopathic medical school near Seattle. Naturopaths also recommend turmeric for the prevention and treatment of degenerative conditions, notably cancer and heart disease.

Therapeutic Uses

Curcumin has a remarkable number of healing actions.

IMMUNE ENHANCEMENT. Indian researchers tested the immune function of laboratory animals, then fed them a curcumin-enriched diet for 5 weeks. Subsequent retesting showed significant improvement in immune function.

FOOD POISONING. Because it stimulates the immune system, curcumin is effective against a number of disease-causing microorganisms, including *Salmonella* bacteria, a frequent cause of food poisoning (also called gastroenteritis or stomach flu).

ANTIOXIDANT. Cucumin is a very rich source of antioxidants that help prevent and reverse the cell damage (oxidative damage) at the root of heart disease, cancer, and many other conditions associated with aging. Spanish researchers assessed antioxidant activity in the blood of 18 men, then gave them turmeric (20 milligrams/day, a very low dose). Six weeks later, their antioxidant activity increased significantly.

CANCER. Curcumin helps prevent cancer in two ways. Its immune-boosting action has a cancer-preventive effect, and its high antioxidant content helps prevent the cell damage that sets the biochemical stage for cancer. Many laboratory and animal studies show that curcumin has anticancer activity. Reports published in journals such as *Cancer Letters, Cancer Research,* and *Carcinogenesis* show that curcumin inhibits the growth of many cancers, among them colon cancer and lymphoma.

Indian researchers tested smokers' urine for compounds that cause genetic mutations (mutagens), a marker for cancer-causing biochemical changes. Then participants took 1.5 grams of turmeric (about a teaspoon) for 30 days. Even though they didn't change their smoking habits, the number of mutagens in their urine decreased significantly.

❧ Colon cancer. University of Michigan researchers biopsied colon lesions in 41 people who had precancerous colon polyps. Then they took curcumin daily (either 2 grams or 4 grams). After a month, the 2-grams group showed no change in colon lesions, but in the 4-grams group 40 percent of colon lesions healed.

❧ Pancreatic cancer. Researchers at M.D. Anderson Cancer Center in Houston gave curcumin (8 grams/day) to 21 adults with advanced pancreatic cancer. One showed significant tumor regression. Now, this 5 percent response rate is may not sound like much, but advanced pancreatic cancer is very difficult to treat, so this finding is noteworthy.

🍀 Chemotherapy side effects. Italian investigators asked 80 people receiving cancer chemotherapy to record all their side effects and then gave them either a placebo or curcumin (500 milligrams/day). Two months later, the herb group reported significantly less nausea, vomiting, fatigue, and mental fuzziness.

HEART DISEASE. Turmeric's close botanical relative, ginger, reduces cholesterol, lowers blood pressure, and helps prevent the blood clots that trigger heart attacks and most strokes. Animal studies show that curcumin offers similar benefits.

In a pilot study, Indian researchers measured the cholesterol levels of 10 adults, then asked them to take curcumin (500 milligrams/day). After 10 days, their cholesterol levels had fallen significantly.

TYPE-2 DIABETES. A diet high in antioxidants helps prevent diabetes. Thai scientists gave 240 people with prediabetes markers either a daily placebo or turmeric. After 9 months, 16 percent of the placebo group progressed to diabetes, but in the turmeric group, only 1 percent did.

Chinese scientists gave 100 Type-2 diabetics either a placebo or curcumin (300 milligrams/day). After 3 months, the herb group showed significantly improved blood sugar levels.

Diabetes causes its many complications because, like Coke spilled on a movie theater floor, chronically high blood sugar gums up the body's tiny capillaries (microangiopathy). Italian researchers measured the capillary blood flow of 50 long-term diabetics, then gave half of them a placebo, while the other half took curcumin (1 gram/day). After 4 weeks, the placebo group showed no change in capillary blood flow, but in the curcumin group, blood flow improved and microangiopathy decreased.

COGNITIVE FUNCTION. Oxidative damage plays a key role in age-related loss of mental acuity and development of dementia. Antioxidants help prevent cognitive impairment, and curcumin is a powerful antioxidant. Researchers in Singapore surveyed the curry/curcumin consumption of 1,010 elderly Asians and then gave them a battery of cognitive function tests. Compared with those who ate curry/curcumin rarely, those who enjoyed them frequently had significantly better cognitive function, with function improving as curcumin intake increased.

Ohio State University researchers gave 34 healthy older adults either a placebo or turmeric (500 milligrams/day). After 4 weeks, the herb group showed significantly reduced blood levels of beta-amyloid, which contributes to Alzheimer's disease.

DEPRESSION. Australian scientists gave 56 people with major depression either a placebo or curcumin (500 milligrams twice a day). After 2 months, the curcumin group showed significant mood elevation.

CATARACTS. Cataracts are caused by oxidative damage to the lens of the eye, the type of damage that antioxidants help prevent. In one study, animals were fed a diet enriched with either corn oil or turmeric for 14 days, then exposed to conditions that produce cataracts. The animals fed turmeric developed significantly fewer cataracts.

OSTEOARTHRITIS (OA). This is what people mean when they as "arthritis," joint pain and stiffness caused by long-term wear and tear or injury. OA often responds to aspirin, ibuprofen (Motrin), or naproxen (Aleve), all nonsteroidal anti-inflammatory drugs (NSAIDs). Doctors also prescribe more powerful prescription NSAIDs. Unfortunately, NSAIDs often cause potentially severe stomach distress. Curcumin is a natural member of a non-NSAID class of anti-inflammatory agents, COX-2 inhibitors, that relieve pain with little risk of risk of stomach upset.

Belgian researchers assessed the OA symptoms of 861 older adults, average age 64, and then, in addition to any OA medication they took, gave them curcumin (84 milligrams twice a day or 162 milligrams three times a day with added emulsifier to aid absorption). After 6 months, both doses of curcumin produced significant relief. OA symptoms scores dropped by half, and most participants cut back on their drugs.

Italian investigators told 50 older adults with OA of the knee to continue taking their medication, but half the group also took curcumin (200 milligrams/day). Three months later, the herb group reported significantly less pain and stiffness.

Thai scientists gave either ibuprofen (Motrin) or turmeric (500 milligrams three times a day) to 367 adults with X-ray-confirmed osteoarthritis of the knee. After 4 weeks, both treatments produced the same benefits. Curcumin was as effective as ibuprofen—without possible stomach upset.

RHEUMATOID ARTHRITIS (RA). Indian researchers gave 45 RA sufferers one of three treatments: a standard pharmaceutical (diclofenac, 50 milligrams/day), curcumin (50 milligrams/day), or both. Curcumin relieved RA symptoms *better* than diclofenac and caused no side effects.

Several Indian studies have tested curcumin as a treatment for osteoarthritis and rheumatoid arthritis—with positive results. Indian researchers gave 45 rheumatoid arthritis sufferers either a standard NSAID, curcumin (500 milligrams/day), or both. All treatments helped, but curcumin provided the most pain relief without causing significant abdominal distress.

LIVER DAMAGE. Animal studies suggest that turmeric protects the liver from the damaging effects of many toxic compounds, including alcohol, aflatoxin, carbon tetrachloride, and the drugs used to treat tuberculosis.

Indian researchers gave 508 people in treatment for tuberculosis either standard medications or those drugs plus curcumin (1 gram twice a day) and guduchi (another Indian arthritis herb, 1 gram twice a day). In the drugs-only group, 14 percent developed signs of liver damage. But in the herb group, the figure was less than 1 percent. These findings lend credence to the herb's traditional use in liver ailments.

If you regularly drink alcohol and/or take certain pharmaceuticals, including acetaminophen (Tylenol), you may be at risk for liver damage. Curcumin might help protect your liver.

ULCERATIVE COLITIS. Japanese gastroenterologists gave either standard drugs or the drugs plus curcumin (1 gram twice a day) to 45 people who'd been treated for ulcerative colitis. After 6 months, 21 percent of the drugs-only group relapsed. But among those who took curcumin, the figure was only 5 percent.

ULCERS. Thai scientists gave 45 ulcer

sufferers large amounts of curcumin (600 milligrams five times a day). Within 2 weeks, many reported symptom improvement. After 12 weeks, 76 percent said they felt better.

IRRITABLE BOWEL SYNDROME. British researchers surveyed the symptoms of 207 people with irritable bowel syndrome, then gave them turmeric (1 gram twice a day). After 8 weeks, their symptom scores improved significantly.

INDIGESTION. Turmeric stimulates the flow of bile, which helps digest fats. This validates the herb's traditional role as a digestive aid. Commission E, the expert panel that evaluates herbal medicines for the German counterpart of the FDA, approves turmeric for indigestion.

PSORIASIS. Iranian researchers used standard scales to assess the psoriasis severity of 40 adults and then instructed them to apply either a placebo cream or one containing turmeric (0.5 percent curcumin twice a day). After 9 weeks, the herb treatment reduced lesion severity by 15 percent, a statistically significant benefit.

SCABIES. In an Indian study, 814 people infested with the tiny, itchy mites were treated with a combination of curcumin and another Indian herb, neem (page 340). Almost all study participants (97 percent) reported their scabies gone in 3 to 15 days. Turmeric treatment was cheaper than standard medical scabicides and caused no adverse reactions.

Intriguing Possibilities

Delayed-onset muscle soreness (DOMS) develops 12 to 48 hours after exercising beyond one's conditioning level. Turmeric is a COX-2 pain reliever. Spanish researchers gave 20 athletes either a placebo or curcumin (400 mg/day), and then supervised as they exercised beyond their typical workouts. The herb group developed less DOMS.

Columbia University investigators gave curcumin (360 milligrams four times a day) to five people with inflammatory bowel disease (Crohn's). After 3 months, four of the five improved, with symptoms scores declining up to 44 percent.

In laboratory studies, curcumin shows potent action against disease-causing protozoa, lending credence to its traditional use in treating amoebic dysentery. One of the world's most pernicious protozoa is the one-celled animal that causes malaria. Indian researchers infected mice with the disease and then gave them curcumin. After herb treatment, blood levels of the protozoa dropped 80 percent.

At the cellular level, curcumin inhibits the cascade of biochemical reactions involved in cystic fibrosis (CF). Studies of laboratory animals bred to develop CF suggest that curcumin extends their lives. It's too early to call the herb a treatment for CF, but in the future, it might be. Meanwhile, for those with CF, there's no harm in eating turmeric-rich curries and taking curcumin supplements.

Indian animal studies suggest that curcumin might have a mood-elevating effect.

Other laboratory and animal studies suggest that turmeric lowers blood sugar and may help prevent gallstones and Parkinson's disease.

Medicinal Myth

The Chinese used turmeric to stimulate menstruation. To date, no research has shown that the herb has any effect on the uterus.

Rx Recommendations

For a stomach-soothing infusion, use 1 teaspoon of turmeric powder per cup of warm milk. Drink up to 3 cups a day. Turmeric tastes pleasantly aromatic, but in large amounts, it becomes bitter.

Or buy curcumin supplements. Dr. Pizzorno recommends 400 milligrams of curcumin three times a day. Or follow package directions.

To make a curcumin salve, mix powdered herb into any skin lotion.

Safety

Unusually large amounts of turmeric may cause stomach upset.

Inform health professionals of the herbs you use. Problematic herb-drug interactions are possible.

Turmeric and curcumin may cause allergic reactions or other unexpected side effects. If any develop, reduce your dose or stop taking it. For more on herb safety, see Chapter 2.

If symptoms get worse or persist longer than 2 weeks, consult a health professional.

Gardening

Turmeric is not a garden herb in North America. Grown from India to Indonesia, it's a perennial with a pulpy, orange, tuberous rhizome (underground stem) that grows to 2 feet in length. The aerial parts, which reach 3 feet, include large, lily-like leaves, a thick, squat, central flower spike, and funnel-shaped yellow flowers.

UVA-URSI
The Urinary Antiseptic

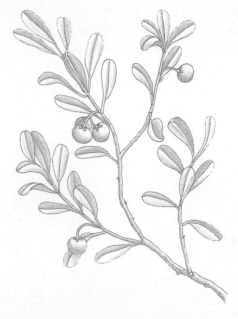

Family: Ericaceae; other members include azalea, blueberry, and cranberry

Genus and species: *Arctostaphylos uva-ursi*

Also known as: Bearberry, bear's grape, upland cranberry, and arbutus

Parts used: Leaves

Ancient Mediterranean bears must have loved the bright red, mealy, currant-size berries of this delicate, branching, perennial ground cover. Both this herb's Greek genus name, *Arctostaphylos*, and its Latin species name, *uva-ursi*, mean bear's berry. The plant is often called bearberry in English. It's the leaves, however, not the berries, that are medicinal.

Uva-ursi has been used as a diuretic and urinary antiseptic for more than 1,000 years by cultures as widely separated as the Chinese and

Native Americans. Today, it is an ingredient in many herbal diuretics and weight-loss formulas. Even the late herbal conservative Varro E. Tyler, Ph.D., described uva-ursi as "a modestly effective urinary antiseptic and diuretic."

However, uva-ursi may not be effective if it's taken in combination with certain foods, information that some herbals fail to mention.

Healing History

The Roman physician Galen used uva-ursi's astringent leaves to treat wounds and stop bleeding, but the herb was largely ignored by Western herbalists until the 13th century. Then, Marco Polo reported that Chinese physicians prescribed it as a diuretic to treat kidney and urinary problems. Polo's famous travelogue popularized uva-ursi in Europe for urinary and kidney complaints.

Uva-ursi's association with the kidney was strengthened by the medieval Doctrine of Signatures, the once widely held belief that plants' physical appearance revealed their healing virtues. The herb grows in rocky, gravelly places, and at the time, kidney stones were called "gravel."

North American colonists found Native Americans using uva-ursi for urinary problems. Some tribes also mixed its leathery leaves with tobacco to created the smoking mixture, kinnikinnik.

Uva-ursi entered the *U.S. Pharmacopoeia*, a standard drug reference, as a urinary antiseptic in 1820 and remained there until 1936. Chemists isolated the herb's major active compound, arbutin, in 1852.

America's 19th-century Eclectics, forerunners of today's naturopaths, recommended uva-ursi for diarrhea, dysentery, gonorrhea, bed-wetting, and "chronic affections of the kidneys and urinary passages."

Today, homeopaths recommend a microdose of uva-ursi for incontinence, blood in the urine, and kidney and urinary tract infections.

Contemporary herbalists continue to recommend uva-ursi for kidney and urinary problems.

Therapeutic Uses

Compounds in the urinary tract transform uva-ursi's active constituent, arbutin, into an antimicrobial antiseptic, hydroquinone. In addition, the herb contains several other diuretic compounds (including ursolic acid), powerful astringents (tannins), and allantoin, a chemical that helps promote the growth of healthy new cells.

URINARY TRACT INFECTION. The diuretic compounds in uva-ursi support its age-old use for urinary tract infections (UTIs) and other urinary ailments. The herb is notably effective against *Escherichia coli*, the most frequent cause of UTIs. Some herbalists report that uva-ursi has cured UTIs that were unresponsive to pharmaceutical antibiotics, even though pharmaceutical antibiotics are generally more effective.

For mild urinary symptoms, try uva-ursi as herbal first-aid. For urinary problems that require professional care, use the herb in addition to standard therapies. Commission E, the expert panel that evaluates herbal medicines for the German counterpart of the FDA, approves uva-ursi for urinary tract ailments.

However, there's an important catch to using uva-ursi. To receive the greatest antiseptic benefit, the urine must be alkaline. This means that those who take the herb should avoid acidic foods and supplements: sauerkraut, citrus fruits and their juices, and vitamin C. In addition, cut down on high-protein foods—meats, poultry, fish, and dairy. Proteins are composed of amino acids that turn the urine acidic.

PREMENSTRUAL SYNDROME. Diuretics may provide relief from the premenstrual bloating that bothers many women.

HIGH BLOOD PRESSURE. Physicians often prescribe diuretics to treat high blood pressure. High blood pressure is a serious condition that requires professional care. If you would like to include uva-ursi in your treatment plan, consult your physician.

CONGESTIVE HEART FAILURE. Congestive heart failure involves serious heart fatigue that impairs the heart's ability to pump blood. Physicians often prescribe diuretics to treat it, so urva-ursi may help. However, congestive heart failure requires professional care. If you would like to include uva-ursi in your treatment plan, talk to your physician.

WOUNDS. When applied topically, uva-ursi's allantoin may help spur wound healing. Allantoin is the active ingredient in Derma-Heal, an over-the-counter skin cream.

DIARRHEA. The astringent tannins in uva-ursi are binding and help relieve diarrhea.

Intriguing Possibility

In animal studies, uva-ursi has shown action against hepatitis. It's too early to call it therapeutic, but it may help.

Rx Recommendations

To treat minor wounds, apply fresh, crushed leaves to cuts and scrapes after thoroughly washing them with soap and water. You might also dip a clean cloth in a decoction and apply the compress to the affected area.

To minimize the unpleasantly astringent taste of this high-tannin herb, soak the leaves in cold water overnight. Then, to prepare a decoction for relief from urinary symptoms or diarrhea, simmer 1 teaspoon per cup of boiling water for 10 minutes, then strain. Drink up to 3 cups a day.

As a homemade tincture, use $\frac{1}{4}$ to 1 teaspoon up to three times a day.

When using commercial preparations, follow package directions.

Safety

Uva-ursi often turns urine a dark green. This is harmless and no cause for alarm.

Diuretics deplete the body of potassium, an essential nutrient. If you use uva-ursi regularly, be sure to eat more potassium-rich foods such as bananas and fresh vegetables.

Pregnant and nursing women should not take diuretics, including uva-ursi. Uva-ursi also stimulates uterine contractions in animal studies, making it even more off-limits to women who are pregnant or trying to conceive.

Herbal weight-loss formulas typically contain diuretics, among them uva-ursi. Diuretics boost urine production and temporarily eliminate some water weight. But pounds lost with help from diuretics almost invariably return, and weight-loss experts advise against using diuretics. The keys to permanent weight control include a low-calorie, low-fat, high-fiber diet and regular moderate exercise.

The astringent tannins uva-ursi help treat diarrhea. The main medical hazard of diarrhea is dehydration, and as uva-ursi is a diuretic, this herb may increase dehydration. If you use uva-ursi to treat diarrhea, be sure to drink plenty of water and other nonalcoholic fluids.

Uva-ursi has such high levels of tannins that it has been used to tan leather. Large doses of tannins may cause stomach upset.

Tannins also have both pro- and anticancer action. Some authorities warn against their use, but tannins' role in human cancers, if any, remains unclear. That said, people who have a history of cancer should either add milk, which neutralizes tannins, or not use large amounts of uva-ursi.

Do not give uva-ursi to children under 2. In older children, adjust the recommended dose based on the child's weight. Give a 50-pound child one-third of the dose a 150-pound adult would take.

If you're over 65, start with a low dose, and increase only if necessary.

Inform health professionals of the herbs you use. Problematic herb-drug interactions are possible.

Uva-ursi may cause allergic reactions or other unexpected side effects. If any develop, reduce your dose or stop taking it. For more on herb safety, see Chapter 2.

If symptoms get worse or persist longer than 2 weeks, consult a health professional promptly.

Gardening

Uva-ursi grows throughout the temperate world. It has a long, fibrous root; woody stems and branches; 1-inch-long, leathery, evergreen, paddle-shaped leaves; and tiny white flowers tinged with red. The plant rarely grows taller than a few inches and prefers a dry, rocky, or sandy habitat.

Propagate uva-ursi from cuttings. Be patient. The plant takes an unusually long time to root. It's more convenient simply to buy small plants from a specialty herb nursery.

Uva-ursi prefers poor, gravelly, acidic soil, under full sun or partial shade. Keep your uva-ursi patch well weeded until the plants have become established. It does not transplant well. Once established, uva-ursi spreads to become a hearty, attractive ground cover.

Harvest leaves in autumn before the first frost. Their leathery texture make them difficult to air-dry. Spread them in a single layer on a cookie sheet and dry them in the oven.

VALERIAN

You're Getting Sleepy. . . .

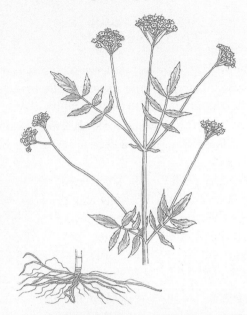

Family: Valerianaceae; other members include spikenard and Jacob's ladder

Genus and species: *Valeriana officinalis*

Also known as: Garden valerian, phu, and all-heal

Parts used: Rhizomes and roots

Back in the 13th century, the elders of Hamelin, Germany, decided to rid their town of rats. They hired an itinerant flute player, one Pied Piper, whose music attracted the rodents, allowing him to lead them out of town. But when the Pied Piper returned for his fee, the elders of Hamelin refused to pay him. In revenge, he used his flute to charm Hamelin's children away forever.

In modern versions of this story, the Pied Piper's powers are entirely musical, but early German folklore also credits him with being an accomplished herbalist. In addition to his hypnotic flute playing, the Pied Piper charmed both the rats and the children with hypnotic valerian root.

Valerian can, indeed, charm rats—and cats. The herb contains chemicals similar to those in catnip.

Healing History

Valerian has such a disagreeable odor that ancient Greek and Roman authorities, including Dioscorides, Pliny, and Galen all turned up their noses. The term *Valeriana* first appeared around the 10th century, derived from the Latin *valere*, to be strong—as in smell.

Dioscorides recommended valerian as a diuretic and antidote to poisons. Pliny considered it a pain reliever. Galen prescribed it as a decongestant and sleep aid.

By the time the plant's name became valerian, early European herbalists considered it a panacea and also called it all-heal. The 12th-century German abbess/herbalist Hildegard of Bingen recommended the herb as a tranquilizer and sleep aid about 100 years before the mythological Pied Piper used it as a hypnotic.

During the late 1500s, valerian's popularity grew after an Italian physician claimed that the herb had cured him of epilepsy. In 1597, British herbalist John Gerard wrote that in Scotland "no broth or physic [medicine] . . . be worth anything" if it did not include valerian. Gerard recommended the herb enthusiastically for chest congestion, convulsions, bruises, and falls.

Seventeenth-century English herbalist Nicholas Culpeper added several of his own recommendations: "The decoction of the root . . . is of special virtue against the plague. . . . [It] provokes women's courses [menstruation] . . . is singularly good for those troubled with cough . . . is excellent [for] any sores, hurts, or wounds. . . ." Later, European herbalists considered the herb a digestive aid and treatment for "hysteria" (menstrual discomforts).

Early colonists discovered several Native American tribes using the pulverized roots of American valerian to treat wounds. This use intrigued Samuel Thomson, the founder of Thomsonian herbal medicine, which was popular before the Civil War. Thomson called valerian "the best nervine [tranquilizer] known."

Valerian entered the *U.S. Pharmacopoeia*, a standard drug reference, as a tranquilizer in 1820 and remained there until 1942. It was listed in the *National Formulary*, the pharmacists' guide, until 1950.

America's 19th-century Eclectic physicians, forerunners of today's naturopaths, prescribed valerian as a "calmative . . . for epilepsy . . . mild spasmodic affections . . . [and] hypochondria." But the Eclectic text *King's American Dispensatory* (1898) warned against large doses because they caused "restlessness, agitation, giddiness, nausea, and visual illusions."

During World War I, Europeans afflicted with "overwrought nerves" from artillery bombardment often found some relief by taking valerian.

Contemporary herbalists generally agree with David Hoffmann's *Holistic Herbal*, which deems valerian "one of the most useful relaxing herbs." Today's herbalists recommend it for nervousness, anxiety, insomnia, headache, and intestinal cramps.

In Germany, where herbal medicine is considerably more mainstream than in the United States, valerian is the active ingredient in more than 100 over-the-counter tranquilizers and sleep aids. Some are specially formulated for children, echoing the Pied Piper.

Therapeutic Uses

All parts of valerian contain valepotriates, compounds with sedative properties. The highest concentration is found in the roots.

INSOMNIA. Many studies have found valerian to be an effective sedative.

❀ German researchers gave 128 people with insomnia either medically inactive placebos or valerian root (400 milligrams/day). Those who took the herb showed significant improvement in sleep quality without morning grogginess or other significant side effects.

❀ Another German team gave 68 adults with chronic insomnia either a placebo or a sleep aid containing valerian (320 milligrams) and lemon balm (160 milligrams), another herbal tranquilizer (page 300). Those taking the herbal formula fell asleep significantly faster, enjoyed significantly longer periods of sleep, and reported significantly greater overall feelings of well-being. The herbal preparation caused no morning hangover.

❀ Swiss researchers repeated this study using a slightly different formula: 360 milligrams of valerian and 240 milligrams of lemon balm once a day, 30 minutes before bedtime. Once again, those who took the herbal combination reported significantly better sleep quality with no side effects.

❀ A third German study used standard physiological tests to measure the depth of sleep in 14 elderly people with insomnia. Compared with those who took placebos, the study participants who took valerian passed more quickly from light stage 1 sleep into deeper sleep. Other studies have reported similar results.

🍀 Another German trial tested valerian in 918 children with insomnia. Eighty-one percent showed significant improvement in sleep duration and quality.

🍀 Finally, an Australian analysis of 16 rigorous trials showed that valerian reliably improves sleep, particularly by reducing the time it takes to fall asleep.

Commission E, the expert panel that evaluates herbal medications for the German counterpart of the FDA, endorses valerian for sleep problems.

Some researchers have compared valerian with benzodiazepines such as diazepam (Valium) and triazolam (Halcion). But valerian is a milder and safer.

🍀 The benzodiazepines can cause dependence and addiction. Regular users may develop a tolerance and require increasing amounts to obtain the desired effect. When the drug is stopped, they may develop withdrawal symptoms, including restlessness, insomnia, headache, nausea, and vomiting. Although a psychological dependence may develop, valerian is not addictive and discontinuation rarely produces withdrawal symptoms, though anxiety is possible.

🍀 The benzodiazepines' sedative effects increase substantially with simultaneous use of alcohol or barbiturates. The combination is often used in suicide attempts. Valerian's sedative effect increases less with alcohol or barbiturates.

🍀 The benzodiazepines often cause morning grogginess. Unusually large amounts of valerian may cause morning grogginess, but recommended amounts rarely do.

🍀 Children born to women who used Valium while pregnant are at increased risk for cleft palate. Valerian has not been linked to birth defects.

RESSTLESS LEG SYNDROME. This condition causes leg twitching that interferes with sleep. University of Pennsylvania researchers assessed the sleep quality of 37 adults complaining of restless leg and then gave them either a placebo or valerian (800 milligrams an hour before bed). After 8 weeks, the valerian group reported significantly better sleep.

CORONARY ARTERY BYPASS SURGERY. This common procedure involves transplanting pieces of leg artery into the heart to detour around arterial blockages. However, half of those who have bypass surgery experience postsurgical mental fuzziness and memory lapses. Iranian researchers assessed the mental acuity of 61 people about to have bypasses and then gave them either a placebo or valerian (530 milligrams) the day before surgery and for 60 days after. The herb group experienced significantly fewer cognitive problems.

Intriguing Possibilities

Animal studies suggest that valerian has anticonvulsant effects, lending some credence to its traditional use in treating epilepsy.

Animal studies also show that valerian reduces blood pressure. Animal findings don't always apply to people, but if you have high blood pressure and want to incorporate valerian into your treatment plan, consult your physician.

Finally, laboratory studies hint that valerian may help control cancer.

Rx Recommendations

As a sleep aid, buy a commercial valerian root extract or tincture and follow the label directions. Herbalists discourage using valerian infusions because they taste terrible.

Safety

Unusually large amounts of valerian may cause headache, giddiness, blurred vision, restlessness, nausea, and morning grogginess.

In 1998, a report in the *Journal of the American Medical Association* generated headlines by suggesting that withdrawal from valerian might have contributed to serious complications in a man hospitalized for congestive heart failure. It's possible—but this man was taking almost a dozen pharmaceutical drugs, had undergone two invasive procedures (lung biopsy and cardiac catheterization) under anesthesia, and had taken up to 2 grams of valerian a day for several years, many times the recommended dose.

The Duke University physicians who reported the case concluded: "Valerian root may be associated with serious withdrawal symptoms following abrupt discontinuation." Given this man's precarious medical situation, this seems extremely unlikely for healthy people who take valerian in at recommended dosage.

Harm from valerian overdose is unlikely. The journal *Veterinary and Human Toxicology* reported the case of a woman who tried to commit suicide by taking 40 capsules of valerian root extract, each containing 470 milligrams of root

extract. She experienced fatigue, abdominal cramps, chest tightness, light-headedness, dilated pupils, and hand tremors, all of which cleared up without medical treatment in 24 hours. Medical tests, including liver function tests, were all normal.

Pregnant and nursing women should not use valerian.

Do not give valerian to children under 2. In older children, adjust the recommended dose based on the child's weight. Give a 50-pound child one-third of the dose a 150-pound adult would take.

If you're over 65, start with a low dose, and increase only if necessary.

Inform health professionals of the herbs you use. Problematic herb-drug interactions are possible.

Valerian may cause allergic reactions or other unexpected side effects. If any develop, reduce your dose or stop taking it. For more on herb safety, see Chapter 2.

If symptoms get worse or persist longer than 2 weeks, consult a health professional promptly.

Gardening

Valerian is a hardy fernlike perennial that reaches about 5 feet. Its medicinal roots appear as long, cylindrical fibers issuing from its rhizome. Its stem is erect, grooved, and hollow. Tiny white, pink, or lavender flowers develop in umbrella-like clusters and bloom from late spring through summer. When dried, valerian roots have an unpleasant odor, once described by American herbalist Michael Moore as "the smell of dirty socks."

Valerian may be propagated from seeds or root divisions. Seeds have limited viability.

When viable, they germinate in about 20 days. Roots may be divided in spring or fall. Thin plants to 12-inch spacing. Valerian grows in many soils but does best in rich, moist, well-drained loam under full sun or partial shade. Once established, the plants self-sow and spread by root runners. Older plants become weedy and overcrowded and lose vitality. Thin them when harvesting their roots.

Valerian has an effect on cats similar to that of catnip. Intoxicated felines have been known to destroy plants. Use chicken-wire fencing if necessary. Harvest roots in the fall of their second year and split thick roots to speed drying.

VERVAIN

A Joy of a Healer

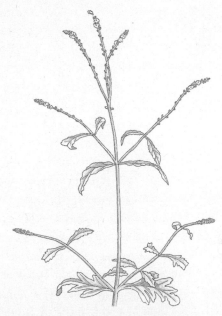

Family: Verbenaceae; other members include teak and many other tropical trees and shrubs

Genus and species: *Verbena officinalis* (European); *V. hastata* (American)

Also known as: Simpler's joy, blue vervain, verbena, herb-of-the-cross, enchanter's herb, and Indian hyssop

Parts used: Leaves, flowers, and roots

During the Middle Ages, healing herbs were often called "simples," and herbalists "simplers." Vervain was prescribed so frequently for so many conditions that it became known as simpler's joy.

The name has some basis in fact. The top medical complaint is pain, and like aspirin or ibuprofen, vervain relieves minor pain and inflammation.

Healing History

In Egyptian mythology, as Isis, goddess of fertility, grieved for her murdered brother-husband, Osiris, vervain grew from her tears. A thousand years later, vervain entered Christian mythology as the herb pressed into Christ's wounds to stanch his bleeding, hence its name herb-of-the-cross.

Hippocrates recommended vervain for fever and plague. The court physician to Roman emperor Theodosius the Great prescribed it for tumors of the throat (goiters). He advised cutting a vervain root into two pieces, tying one around the patient's throat, and hanging the other over a fire. As the heat and smoke shriveled the hanging root, the tumor was supposed to shrink.

The Romans spread vervain throughout Europe, where it became especially popular among the Druids of pre-Christian England. They used the herb in magic spells, hence its name enchanter's herb.

The 12th-century German abbess/herbalist Hildegard of Bingen prescribed a decoction of vervain and vermouth for "toxic blood [infections], toothache, [and] discharges from the brain to the teeth."

Our word vervain comes from the Celtic fer-faen, from fer, to drive away, and faen, a stone. This refers to the herb's traditional use for treating kidney stones.

During the Middle Ages, vervain became a popular acne remedy. People who had pimples stood outside at night holding a handful of the herb wrapped in a cloth. When a shooting star passed, they rubbed the cloth over their pimples and the blemishes were supposed to disappear.

From a remedy for acne, vervain evolved into a treatment for other skin problems. Seventeenth-century herbalist Nicholas Culpeper wrote, "The leaves bruised, or the juice mixed with vinegar, does wonderfully cleanse the skin, and take away morphew [dandruff]." Culpeper recommended vervain to treat jaundice, gout, cough, wheezing, bleeding gums, shortness of breath, fever, plague, gravel (kidney stones), and dropsy (congestive heart failure). He also said that "used with hog grease, it helps with swellings and pains of the secret parts [genitals]."

Colonists introduced European vervain into North America, and it quickly went wild. They also found Native Americans using the American species, also known as Indian hyssop, to treat fever and gastrointestinal complaints and to clear cloudy urine.

During the Revolutionary War, military physicians relied on vervain to relieve pain, loosen bronchial mucus, and induce vomiting. More than a century later, the Eclectics, forerunners of today's naturopaths, recommended it as a treatment for fever, colds, coughs, intestinal worms, menstrual irregularity, and bruises, and as a tonic during convalescence.

Contemporary herbalists recommend vervain as a tranquilizer, expectorant, menstruation promoter, and treatment for headache, fever, depression, seizures, wounds, dental cavities, and gum disease.

Therapeutic Uses

PAIN AND INFLAMMATION. Chemically, vervain is quite different from aspirin, but German and Japanese studies suggest that it has similar effects, combining mild pain relief with some anti-inflammatory action. These findings support vervain's traditional use in treating headache, toothache, wounds, and kidney stones.

Medicinal Myth

Vervain has never been shown to treat dandruff, induce vomiting, promote menstruation, or expel kidney stones. Its primary benefit is its ability to provide mild pain relief.

Rx Recommendations

For a very bitter infusion to help treat headache, mild arthritis, and other minor pains, use 2 teaspoons of dried herb per cup of boiling water. Steep for 10 to 15 minutes, then strain. Drink up to 3 cups a day. Mask vervain's bitterness with sugar, honey, and lemon or mix the herb with an herbal beverage tea.

As a homemade tincture, use ½ to 1 teaspoon up to three times a day.

When using commercial preparations, follow package directions.

Safety

European animal studies show that vervain depresses heart rate, constricts the bronchial passages, and stimulates the intestines and uterus. Because it may slow heart rate, it should not be used by anyone with congestive heart failure or a history of heart disease. The possibility of bronchial constriction may cause problems for people with asthma and other respiratory conditions. Intestinal stimulation may aggravate chronic gastrointestinal conditions, such as colitis or Crohn's disease.

Because of vervain's potential stimulating effect on the uterus, pregnant women should steer clear, except possibly at term and under the supervision of a physician to help induce labor.

Nursing women should not use vervain.

Do not give vervain to children under 2. In older children, adjust the recommended dose based on the child's weight. Give a 50-pound child one-third of the dose a 150-pound adult would take.

If you're over 65, start with a low dose, and increase only if necessary.

Inform health professionals of the herbs you use. Problematic herb-drug interactions are possible.

Vervain may cause allergic reactions or other unexpected side effects. If any develop, reduce your dose or stop taking it. For more on herb safety, see Chapter 2.

If symptoms get worse or persist longer than 2 weeks, consult a health professional promptly.

Gardening

Vervain is a 3-foot perennial with thin, erect, stiff stems. Its opposite leaves are oblong and toothed near the ground and lance-shaped and deeply lobed higher up. The plant develops slender flower spikes that bear small blue or lilac flowers from early summer through mid-fall. The herb's bluish flowers gave it the name blue vervain.

Vervain grows easily from seeds planted in spring after the danger of frost has passed. For a perennial, this herb is short-lived, but it self-sows. Vervain prefers rich, moist loam under full sun. Harvest the leaves and flowers as the plants flower.

WHITE WILLOW

Herbal Aspirin

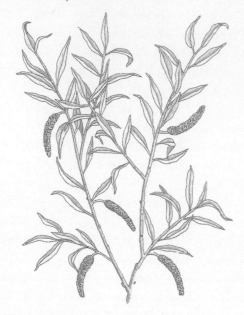

Family: Salicaceae; other members include
poplar

Genus and species: *Salix alba*

Also known as: Salicin willow

Part used: Bark

Chemists originally created aspirin from salicin, a compound in white willow bark whose
name comes from the herb's genus, *Salix.*

White willow grew on the banks of the Nile.
Ancient Egyptians considered it a symbol of joy.
The Hebrews adopted the beautiful tree. In
Leviticus 23:40, God commands them to cele-
brate the autumn harvest festival by setting up
temporary shelters covered with willow boughs:
"Take . . . boughs of willow . . . and rejoice
7 days."

But the willow became a Jewish symbol of
sorrow after the destruction of the first Temple
in Jerusalem (586 BC), which resulted in the
Babylonian exile. Consider the willow's transformation in Psalm 137: "By the rivers of Babylon, where we sat down, and there we wept,
when we remembered Zion. Upon the willows,
we hanged up our harps, for they that led us
there captive asked of us . . . songs." Since that
time, the graceful tree has been known as
weeping willow.

Healing History

Since 500 BC, Chinese physicians have prescribed white willow bark to relieve pain and
fever. Those uses took five centuries to arrive in
Europe. The 1st-century Greek physician
Dioscorides was the first Westerner to recommend willow bark for pain and inflammation,
but his prescription did not catch on. A century
later, the Roman doctor Galen recommended the
herb only for the vague purpose of "drying up
humors."

As the centuries passed, herbalists prescribed
white willow bark for many ailments, including
suppressing sexual desire. Seventeenth-century
English herbalist Nicholas Culpeper noted, "The
leaves, bark, and seed are used to stanch bleeding . . . stay vomiting . . . provoke urine . . . take
away warts . . . and clear the face and skin from
spots and discolourings. . . . The leaves bruised
and boiled in wine stays the heat of lust in man
or woman, and quite extinguishes it if it be long
used."

At the time, white willow was not commonly
used to treat pain, but Culpeper touted the work
of one Mr. Stone, who demonstrated its "great

efficacy . . . in intermittent fever [malaria]." Culpeper concluded that white willow bark "is likely to become an object worthy of . . . attention."

He referred to the research of Rev. Edmund Stone, a physician-minister in Chipping-Norton in Oxfordshire, England. Stone hoped to find a less expensive substitute for cinchona bark, the first effective treatment for malaria, which had been a scourge throughout Europe since ancient times.

In 1757, Stone collected some white willow bark for the medicinal uses that Culpeper had described and happened to taste it. He was surprised at its bitterness, which reminded him of cinchona. Stone wondered if willow bark might be a poor person's cinchona for fever and chills.

From the perspective of the Doctrine of Signatures, the medieval belief that a plant's physical appearance pointed to its medicinal uses, the signs looked promising. Willows grow along cool, damp riverbanks and in swampy lowlands, exactly the environments that physicians of Stone's era (wrongly) believed produced malaria and other illnesses marked by fever, or "ague."

For 6 years, Stone pulverized white willow bark, brewed a bitter tea with the powder, and gave his experimental medicine to 50 people with fevers. According to Stone, most of his patients' agues and chills disappeared shortly after drinking his concoction.

Stone wrote a report touting white willow bark as a cheap substitute for cinchona: "As this tree delights in a moist or wet soil where agues chiefly abound, the general maxim that many natural maladies carry their cures along with them, or that their remedies lie not far from the cause was so very [appropriate] to this particular case that I could not help applying it."

On April 25, 1763, Stone sent his report to the Royal Society, England's most prestigious scientific organization. Its publication in the society's journal, *Philosophical Transactions*, later that year finally popularized white willow bark in the West as a treatment for fever—more than 2,000 years after the Chinese had first used it for that purpose.

Alas, white willow was no cinchona. It contains no quinine, the drug that treats malaria. Nonetheless, it brought down other fevers and quickly became Europe's drug of choice for fever, pain, and inflammation.

Colonists introduced the tree into North America and found many Native American tribes using the bark of native willows to treat pain, chills, and fever.

Around 1828, French and German chemists extracted white willow bark's active compound, salicin. Ten years later, an Italian chemist isolated salicin's precursor, salicylic acid, which is very similar to aspirin. However, chemists made the first aspirin from another herb that contains salicin, meadowsweet (page 319).

During the mid-19th century, researchers showed that both salicin and salicylic acid reduce fever and relieve pain and inflammation. Unfortunately, they also have unpleasant—and potentially hazardous—side effects: nausea, diarrhea, bleeding, stomach ulceration, ringing in the ears (tinnitus), and at high doses, respiratory paralysis and death.

Chemists tinkered with salicylic acid, hoping to preserve its benefits while minimizing its side effects. In 1853, German chemists added a molecular acetyl group to an extract of meadowsweet to create acetylsalicylic acid. The new compound was as effective as salicylic acid. It still caused salicylic acid's side effects, but they were less debilitating.

"Acetylsalicylic acid" was quite a mouthful, so the synthesizers took the "a" from acetyl and "spirin" from meadowsweet's genus name, *Spirea*, to create "aspirin." News of aspirin's synthesis was published in an obscure German medical journal—and forgotten for 50 years.

In the 1890s, a German drug chemist, Felix Hoffman, got upset that his father's rheumatoid arthritis medications brought him so little relief. Hoffman was an employee of Fredrich Bayer and Company. He began looking for a better pain reliever. He delved into the journals and found the old reports of aspirin. Hoffman prepared the drug, and his father's condition improved significantly.

At first, Hoffman's superiors at Bayer were not interested in aspirin, but eventually, they changed their minds. In 1899, Bayer released it in Europe and North America under the brand name Aspirin.

Aspirin quickly became the household drug of choice for a broad range of everyday ailments. Then, in a landmark trademark-protection battle, Bayer lost its trademark on Aspirin. The court ruled that the term had passed into general usage.

Contemporary herbalists recommend white willow bark for headache, fever, arthritis, and other pain and inflammation, plus prevention of heart attack.

Therapeutic Uses

Aspirin may have been created from meadowsweet, but white willow bark contains more salicylates, making it the more potent pain reliever.

PAIN, INFLAMMATION, FEVER. Try white willow any time that you think you need an over-the-counter pain reliever. The herb is not as potent as pharmaceutical aspirin, but, compared with the little white pills, willow bark causes fewer side effects.

Commission E, the expert panel that evaluates herbal medicines for the German counterpart of the FDA, approves white willow bark for the treatment of fever, headaches, and muscle and joint pain.

OSTEOARTHRITIS. German researchers gave 59 people with osteoarthritis of the hip and/or knee either a standard pharmaceutica (diclofenac) or white willow bark (180 milligrams salacin/day). The drug worked better, but the herb worked almost as well. Using standard tests of arthritis, 48 percent of the diclofenac users reported significant improvement, for the white willow group, 40 percent.

LOW BACK PAIN. German scientists gave 210 people with back pain either a placebo or white willow bark (120 milligrams or 240 milligrams salacin). In the placebo group, 6 percent reported significant pain relief. But in the herb groups, the figures were 15 percent (low dose) and 3 percent (high dose).

European researchers reviewed 80 studies of white willow bark for low back pain. Their conclusion: It works.

HEART ATTACK AND STROKE. Low-dose aspirin has become a standard preventive and first-aid for heart attack. Aspirin helps prevent and dissolve the blood clots that trigger heart attack and most strokes. A cup of willow bark tea contains a similar low dose of aspirin-like salicin.

There have been no studies on willow bark as an aspirin substitute for heart attack prevention, but biochemically, the herb should be expected to have similar value. If you've been advised to take low-dose aspirin regularly, ask your physician about including willow bark in your regimen.

MENSTRUAL CRAMPS. Like aspirin, white willow contains enough salicylate to suppress the action of compounds called prostaglandins that are involved in menstrual cramps. If you have mild cramps, the herb may help.

Intriguing Possibilities

A laboratory study suggests that white willow may reduce blood sugar (glucose) levels. The herb's effect on diabetes in humans, if any, remains unclear.

Regular aspirin use has also been associated with reduced risk of colo-rectal cancer. White willow bark may provide similar preventive benefits.

Rx Recommendations

For a decoction to relieve pain, fever, and inflammation, use 1 teaspoon of powdered bark per cup of cold water and soak for 8 hours, then strain if you wish. Drink up to 3 cups a day. White willow tastes bitter and astringent. You can add honey and lemon or mix the herb with an herbal beverage tea.

To help prevent heart attack and stroke, drink 1 cup a day.

When using commercial preparations, follow package directions.

Safety

Pregnant women should not use white willow. In animal studies, aspirin is associated with an increased risk of birth defects. The herb is not as powerful, but better safe than sorry.

Do not give white willow bark to children under age 16 with fevers related to colds, flu, or chickenpox. It may cause Reye's syndrome, a rare but potentially fatal condition. Aspirin clearly causes Reye's. White willow has never been directly linked to Reye's, but it's similar. Do not give this herb to children with colds, flu, or chickenpox.

Aspirin upsets some people's stomachs. White willow bark is less potent and rarely causes this problem, but stomach upset is still possible in those particularly sensitive to aspirin. If stomach upset, nausea, or tinnitus develops, reduce your dose or stop using the herb.

People with chronic gastrointestinal conditions, such as ulcers and gastritis, should not use the herb.

Aspirin also triggers asthma attacks in some people. If you are aspirin-sensitive, do not use white willow bark.

Pregnant and nursing women should not use white willow bark.

Do not give white willow to children under 2. In older children who do no have colds, flu, or chickenpox, adjust the recommended dose based on the child's weight. Give a 50-pound child one-third of the dose a 150-pound adult would take.

If you're over 65, start with a low dose, and increase only if necessary.

Inform health professionals of the herbs you use. Problematic herb-drug interactions are possible.

White willow may cause allergic reactions or other unexpected side effects. If any develop, reduce your dose or stop taking it. For more on herb safety, see Chapter 2.

If symptoms get worse or persist longer than 2 weeks, consult a health professional promptly.

Gardening

White willow is a beautiful tree that reaches 75 feet. It has rough, grayish brown bark and long, thin leaves on flexible branches.

White willows grow in almost any moist garden soil under full sun. Buy saplings at nurseries or propagate them from first-year branches several feet in length rooted in water or from foot-long hardwood cuttings taken in spring or fall and rooted the same way.

Willows grow quickly and must be pruned regularly. Harvest the bark from older branches during pruning and dry it in the sun or in an oven on low.

WITCH HAZEL
A Cooling, Soothing Astringent

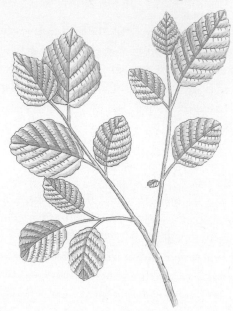

Family: Hamamelidaceae; no other members

Genus and species: *Hamamelis virginiana*

Also known as: Winterbloom, snapping hazelnut, and hamamelis

Parts used: Leaves and bark

The next time people pooh-pooh herbal healing, ask what they think of witch hazel. The clear, pungent liquid extract of this bushy herb is a standard home remedy for cuts, bruises, hemorrhoids, and other minor skin conditions. More than 1 million gallons of witch hazel are sold each year in the United States, making it one of the nation's most widely used healing herbs.

The "hazel" in this herb's name comes from its similarity to the common hazelnut. As for the "witch," some say that early colonists used the shrub to make brooms, witches' favorite form of transportation. Others trace it to witch hazel's winter flowering and the loud "pop" when it disperses its seeds, supposedly evidence of occult influence.

For the record, the herb's name has nothing to do with witchcraft. In medieval Middle English, "witch" was spelled "wych" and meant pliant or flexible. Witch hazel's branches are, indeed, flexible—so springy, in fact, that Native Americans used them to make bows.

Healing History

Witch hazel was highly valued in Native American medicine. Many tribes rubbed a decoction of the herb on cuts, bruises, insect bites, aching joints, sore muscles, and sore backs. They also drank witch hazel tea to stop internal bleeding, prevent miscarriage, and treat colds, fevers, sore throats, and menstrual pain.

Some colonists adopted witch hazel, but it did not become popular until the 1840s, when a medicine man of the Oneida tribe reportedly introduced the plant to Theron T. Pond of Utica, New York. Pond was impressed with the plant's astringent properties and its ability to treat skin conditions. In 1848, he began marketing witch hazel extract as Pond's Golden Treasure. Later, the name was changed to Pond's Extract, which became a commercial hit. Witch hazel water has been with us ever since.

Early witch hazel water was simply a strained decoction of the shrub's leaves and twigs that contained tannins, which made the extract highly astringent. By the late 19th century, manufacturers switched to steam distillation, a simpler process but one that left the resulting water with little if any of the plant's astringent tannins—and controversy erupted.

King's American Dispensatory (1898), the text used by Eclectic physicians, forerunners of today's naturopaths, asserted: "The decoction is very useful in hemorrhage, diarrhea, dysentery, swellings, inflammations, tumors, hemorrhoids, epistaxis [nosebleed], and uterine hemorrhage following delivery. . . . [However] since the introduction of the distilled extract [witch hazel] has been largely abandoned. . . . The fluid extract has little to recommend it."

Nonetheless, witch hazel was listed as an anti-inflammatory astringent in the *U.S. Pharmacopoeia*, a standard drug reference, from 1862 through 1916 and in the *National Formulary*, the pharmacists' reference, from 1916 to 1955. The *National Formulary* finally dropped it because in 1947, the 24th edition of *The Dispensatory of the United States* stated that witch hazel "is so nearly destitute of medicinal virtues, it scarcely deserves official recognition. . . . [Its continued use serves only to fill] the need in American families for an embrocation [liniment] which appeals to the psychic influence of faith."

Yet today, witch hazel can be found on the shelves of every pharmacy. Contemporary herbalists sidestep the controversy by recommending only the decoction of witch hazel bark, which contains astringent tannins. They are unanimous in their praise of the herb's cooling, astringent action when used externally for cuts, burns, scalds, bruises, inflammation, and hemorrhoids. They also recommend it as a gargle for sore throat and sores in the mouth and internally to treat diarrhea.

Therapeutic Uses

While it's true that steam-distilled witch hazel water contains no astringent tannins, several studies show that it still retains astringent action, presumably from other compounds in the plant.

HEMORRHOIDS AND SKIN PROBLEMS. Commercial witch hazel water may lack tannins, but it contains other compounds with reported antiseptic, anesthetic, astringent, and anti-inflammatory action. Witch hazel water is an ingredient in Fleet Medicated Wipes for hemorrhoids, Tucks pads, and several over-the-counter treatments for poison ivy, oak, and sumac.

Commission E, the expert panel that evaluates herbal medicines for the German counterpart of the FDA, approves witch hazel for hemorrhoids and skin inflammations.

SUNBURN. German researchers gave 30 people with sunburn one of three treatments: a medically inactive placebo cream, a skin cream containing aloe gel and vitamin E (both recommended for skin problems), or a lotion containing 10 percent witch hazel distillate. Participants applied their treatments three times over 48 hours. Although differences in redness were not clearly visible to the naked eye, they were to an instrument called a chromameter—and the witch hazel lotion reduced redness best.

Another German study compared witch hazel with a chamomile preparation and hydrocortisone, an over-the-counter anti-inflammatory drug, in 24 people with sunburn. The hydrocortisone worked best, but witch hazel was almost as effective and "clearly superior" to the chamomile lotion.

Rx Recommendations

It's most convenient to use commercial witch hazel water, which is available in pharmacies.

If you'd like to make an extra-astringent decoction, boil 1 teaspoon of powdered leaves or twigs per cup of water for 10 minutes. Strain and cool. Apply the liquid directly or mix it into a skin lotion.

For a bitter, astringent gargle, use 1 teaspoon of bark per cup of boiling water. Steep for 10 minutes, then strain.

Safety

The medical literature contains no reports of harm from using witch hazel externally or as a gargle, but most experts advise against ingesting this herb.

You may use witch hazel externally on anyone, but dilute it for use on children under age 2.

Witch hazel may cause allergic reactions or other unexpected side effects. If any develop, reduce your dose or stop taking it. For more on herb safety, see Chapter 2.

If symptoms get worse or persist longer than 2 weeks, consult a health professional promptly.

Gardening

Witch hazel's Latin name refers to Virginia, but the shrub grows all over the eastern United States. Most commercial witch hazel is grown in the Carolinas and Tennessee.

Witch hazel is a perennial that drops its leaves each autumn. Its single root sends up several twisting stems that fork into many flexible, hairy branches. It blooms long after most other flowers have disappeared-—from September to December, depending on location. That's how it got one of its common names, winterbloom. As a late bloomer, it makes a colorful addition to gardens.

The shrub's spidery yellow flowers appear at

the same time that the previous year's fruits mature. Its woody seed pods burst open with an audible pop and propel their two hard black seeds up to 25 feet. The seeds are edible and have been compared with hazelnuts, hence the name snapping hazelnut.

Witch hazel grows from seeds or twig cuttings. Refrigerate seeds at around 40°F for several months before planting to encourage germination. Cuttings generally produce roots in about 10 weeks.

Witch hazel grows best in moist, rich, sandy or peaty soil under partial shade, but it tolerates poorer soil and full sun. Harvest the leaves and twigs at any time and dry them in the sun or in a oven on low.

YARROW
The Herbal Bandage

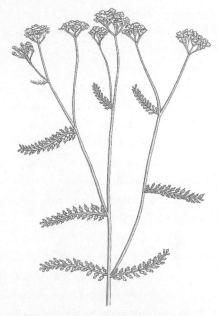

Family: Compositae; other members include daisy, dandelion, and marigold

Genus and species: *Achillea millefolium*

Also known as: Thousand weed, milfoil, soldier's woundwort, *herbe militaire*, nosebleed wort, bloodwort, and bad man's plaything

Parts used: Leaves, stems, and flowers

Legend has it that during the Trojan War, Achilles stopped the bleeding of his fellow soldiers' wounds by applying yarrow's fernlike leaves. Scientists have discovered that the mythological hero may have been onto something.

Yarrow contains substances that help stop bleeding and have pain-relieving and anti-inflammatory properties helpful in wound treatment, among other uses.

Healing History

Achilles defined yarrow's use in herbal healing for more than 2,500 years. Dioscorides, a 1st-century physician attached to Roman legions, recommended rubbing the crushed plant on wounds.

The herb's many popular names—*herbe militaire*, nosebleed wort, soldier's woundwort, and bloodwort—attest to its use as a blood stopper during the Middle Ages. (The word "wort" is Old English for plant.) Perhaps from an association with brawling, yarrow also became linked to ruffians, earning the name bad man's plaything.

Around Achilles' time, ancient Chinese physicians were prescribing Asian yarrow to treat inflammations, bleeding, heavy menstrual flow, and dog- and snakebites. The Chinese also used yarrow in the ritual of the *I Ching*, the oracle consulted to predict the future. Today, people use coins, but the traditional way to cast the *I Ching* involved dried yarrow stems. India's Ayurvedic physicians recommended yarrow to treat fevers.

Sixteenth-century British herbalist John Gerard suggested yarrow for "swellings . . . of the privie parts." In the 17th century, John Parkinson advised, "If it be put into the nose, assuredly it will stop the bleeding of it." And his contemporary Nicholas Culpeper wrote, "An ointment of the leaves cures wounds . . . restrains violent bleedings . . . is good for inflammations and ulcers . . . and is excellent for the piles [hemorrhoids]."

Colonists introduced yarrow into North America. Native Americans adopted it enthusiastically as an external treatment for wounds and burns and as an internal treatment for colds, sore throats, arthritis, toothaches, insomnia, and indigestion.

America's 19th-century Eclectic physicians, forerunners of today's naturopaths, considered yarrow a "tonic upon the venous system" but downplayed its age-old role in wound treatment. Their text, *King's American Dispensatory* (1898), recommended the herb for bloody urine, incontinence, hemorrhoids, menstrual cramps, diarrhea, dysentery, and "hemorrhage where the bleeding is small in amount."

Contemporary herbalists recommend yarrow as an "herbal Band-Aid." They also prescribe it for fevers and urinary tract infections and as a digestive aid.

Therapeutic Uses

If Achilles had had some yarrow on hand when his vulnerable heel was wounded, he might have survived the Trojan War.

WOUNDS. Yarrow contains many compounds that support its traditional use as a wound treatment. Two of them, achilletin and achilleine, spur blood coagulation. Several more—azulene, camphor, chamazulene, eugenol, menthol, quercetin, rutin, and salicylic acid—have anti-inflammatory and pain-relieving action. Several others—tannins, terpeniol, and cineol—are antiseptic.

DIGESTIVE UPSETS. Chamazulene, one of the compounds in yarrow (and chamomile), helps relax the smooth muscle tissue of the digestive tract. This makes the herb a stomach-soothing antispasmodic. Commission E, the expert panel that evaluates herbal medicines for the German counterpart of the FDA, endorses yarrow as a digestive aid.

MENSTRUAL CRAMPS. Antispasmodics

relax not only the digestive tract but also other smooth muscles, such as the uterus. This lends some credence to yarrow's use in treating menstrual cramps.

STRESS, ANXIETY, AND INSOMNIA. Yarrow contains a small amount of a hypnotic chemical called thujone, the effects of which have been compared to marijuana. The thujone in yarrow may account for the herb's traditional use as a sedative. In large amounts, thujone is poisonous, but the recommended amounts of yarrow do not cause harm.

Intriguing Possibility

Two animal studies have shown that yarrow protects the liver from toxic chemical damage, and Indian researchers have found that yarrow helps treat hepatitis. So, it may be useful in liver disorders.

Rx Recommendations

To treat wounds, press fresh leaves and flowers into cuts and scrapes until you can wash and bandage them. To help promote healing, apply the herb as a poultice on clean wounds and inflamed skin.

For an infusion to soothe indigestion, use 1 to 2 teaspoons of dried herb per cup of boiling water. Steep for 10 to 15 minutes, then strain. Drink up to 3 cups a day. Yarrow tastes tangy and bitter, with some astringency. To improve the flavor, add honey, sugar, or lemon or mix the herb with an herbal beverage blend.

As a homemade tincture, use ½ to 1 teaspoon up to three times a day.

When using commercial preparations, follow package directions.

Safety

Anyone may use yarrow externally, but it may cause allergic reactions or other unexpected side effects. If any develop, reduce your dose or stop taking it.

High doses of yarrow may turn urine dark brown. This is harmless and no cause for alarm.

Pregnant and nursing women should not ingest this herb.

The medical literature contains no reports of toxicity from yarrow, but people who are allergic to ragweed may develop a rash from contact with the plant. For more on herb safety, see Chapter 2.

If symptoms get worse or persist longer than 2 weeks, consult a health professional promptly.

Gardening

Yarrow is an attractive 3-foot perennial covered with delicate hairs. Its feathery leaves are divided into what seem like thousands of tiny leaflets—hence its names thousand weed and milfoil (a corruption of *mille feuille*, the French term for 1,000 leaves). Yarrow's numerous tiny white flowers develop in dense clusters on flat-topped, umbrella-like stalks in summer.

Yarrow grows easily from seeds or root divisions planted in spring or fall. Sow seeds just under the surface of fine soil and keep them moist until they germinate, usually within 2 weeks. Thin seedlings to 12-inch spacing. Yarrow adapts to many soil types but needs good drainage and does best in moderately rich soil under full sun. Divide plants every few years to keep them growing vigorously.

Harvest yarrow when the plants are in bloom and hang them to dry.

YOHIMBE

This Age-Old African Aphrodisiac Treats Erectile Dysfunction

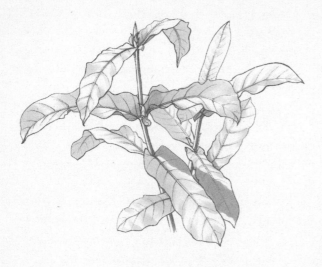

Family: Rubiaceae; other members include coffee, gardenia, and madder

Genus and species: *Pausinystalia yohimbe*

Also known as: No other common names

Parts used: Bark extract

Yohimbe is a prime example of the disdain Western science has shown toward traditional approaches to sex problems. Granted, many traditional aphrodisiacs—oysters, rhino tusk, tiger testicles—are worthless. But for 80 years after a compound in yohimbe bark, yohimbine, was first shown to have erection-boosting effects, Western researchers dismissed it. More than a decade before Viagra took the world by storm, the news that the Food and Drug Administration (FDA) had approved yohimbine for erection difficulties was greeted by thundering silence. Yohimbine still gets little respect. But for erectile dysfunction (ED), it works about as well as pharmaceutical erection medications. It also shows promise for problems they can't treat.

Healing History

For centuries, Africans used yohimbe bark as an aphrodisiac that restored faltering erections. Scientists scoffed. Then in 1896, a compound isolated from the bark, yohimbine, was shown to stimulate erection in both animals and humans. Scientists ignored this report.

Fast forward to the 1980s, when several studies showed that yohimbine, increases blood flow into the penis and helps treat ED. A dozen years before Viagra, the FDA approved yohimbine for ED treatment. It was—and still is—marketed by prescription under three brand names: Yohimbine, Yocon, and Aphrodyne. But few people know of the natural, herbal alternative to Viagra.

Therapeutic Uses

ERECTILE DYSFUNCTION. First, let's define the term "aphrodisiac." It refers to herbs, foods, and drugs that stimulate sexual arousal. Traditionally, a man with an erection was assumed to be sexually aroused, so the term was also applied to anything that enhanced erection. However, today we know that men can have erections without feeling sexually aroused and visa versa. As a result, modern sex researchers draw a distinction between things that stimulate sexual desire and arousal on the one hand, and things that stimulate erection on the other. Yohimbine (and Viagra and the other erection medications) improve erection, but they do not enhance libido.

Since the 1980s, more than a dozen studies have shown that yohimbine treats ED. In 1997, British researchers analyzed seven studies and concluded that compared with placebo treatment, yohimbine users were almost four times more likely to raise erections. Since then, several other studies have confirmed this effect. German researchers gave 85 men with ED either a placebo or yohimbine (10 milligrams three times/day). After 8 weeks, 45 percent of the placebo group reported erection improvement, but in the yohimbine group, 71 percent.

Intriguing Possibilities

Some men can raise erections, but can't ejaculate. British researchers gave yohimbine (20 milligrams) to 29 men with ejaculatory dysfunction. With the herb's help, 16 (55 percent) were able to ejaculate.

University of Texas researchers gave 25 women complaining of arousal difficulties either a placebo or a combination of yohimbine and L-arginine, an amino acid precursor to nitric oxide, a compound crucial to sexual arousal. The women then viewed erotic videos. Compared with those taking the placebo, the women who took the herb-amino acid product reported greater sexual arousal.

Yale researchers gave 50 depression sufferers either Prozac plus a placebo or the drug plus yohimbine. The drug/herb group reported significantly greater mood elevation.

Rx Recommendations

Most studies have used 15 to 30 milligrams/day. Yohimbe products are widely available over the counter (OTC) at health food stores and supplement shops. Unfortunately, according to an analysis by FDA chemists, many OTC products contain only trace amounts of yohimbine. If you're interested in using this herb to treat ED, ask your doctor for a prescription and follow the label directions.

Safety

Possible side effects include increased heart rate and blood pressure, nervousness, irritability, headache, dizziness, tremor, and flushing. Very large doses may cause paralysis and psychosis. Do not exceed the recommended dose.

Do not mix yohimbine-based drugs with Viagra or other erection medications.

Children should not use yohimbe. If you're over 65, start with a low dose, and increase only if necessary.

Pregnant and nursing women should not use this herb.

Inform health professionals of the herbs you use. Problematic herb-drug interactions are possible.

Yohimbe may cause allergic reactions or other unexpected side effects. If any develop, reduce your dose or stop taking it. For more on herb safety, see Chapter 2.

If symptoms get worse, consult a health professional promptly.

Gardening

Yohimbe is an evergreen tree native to Cameroon, Gabon, and the Republic of the Congo. It is not grown in the United States.

Chapter 6

USING THE HEALING HERBS: QUICK REFERENCE GUIDES

When you have a cold, which herbs should you reach for? How about when you have a headache? Anxiety? Indigestion?

This quick reference guide can help you make the right choice. It organizes the herbs discussed throughout the book into three categories: (1) conditions; (2) healing actions, such as antibiotic, decongestant, and so on; and (3) other uses, such as insect repellent and weight control.

Consumer Precautions

Before using any herb medicinally, read its profile in Chapter 5, especially the information on safety and side effects. Also read Chapter 2, which contains general safe-use guidelines. Follow all of the recommendations in both chapters.

The charts on the following pages list only the most potentially hazardous herb side effects. Other side effects are possible. In addition, any herb may cause allergic reactions.

Healing herbs are best used in consultation with a physician. This is especially true if you have a chronic condition such as asthma, arthri-

tis, cancer, diabetes, heart disease, or high blood pressure.

Herbal oils are highly concentrated and should not be ingested unless you're under the care of a naturopath or professional herbalist. Even a small amount—a teaspoon—can be toxic, even fatal. Keep herbal oils away from children and pets, and never allow children or pets to ingest herbal oils.

A Special Note to Women

With few exceptions, pregnant and nursing women should not ingest medicinal amounts of healing herbs because of the possibility of harming the fetus or infant.

Most herbal digestive aids have antispasmodic action, that is, they help to relax the smooth muscle lining the digestive tract. The uterus is also a smooth muscle, so it, too, may be affected by antispasmodic herbs. However, many herbal digestive aids have traditionally been used to stimulate the uterus and promote menstruation, so it's possible that taking large amounts may, over time, increase the risk of miscarriage.

This contradiction appears to be dose-related. Made with a dose of 1 to 2 teaspoons of freshly grated root, ginger tea is a safe, effective treatment for the morning sickness of pregnancy. In extremely large doses, however—20 to 40 teaspoons of root—it may induce uterine contractions.

The antispasmodic herbs are popular ingredients in cooking. Pregnant and nursing women may feel free to use culinary amounts of these herbs.

It's by no means clear from the research to date if all herbal digestive aids stimulate the uterus when taken in large doses, but given the traditional uses of antispasmodic herbs, pregnant women—and women who are trying to conceive—are best advised not to use medicinal amounts.

Conditions and Their Herbal Remedies

CONDITION	HERB(S)	SPECIAL PRECAUTIONS
Acne	Aloe	
	Tea tree oil	For external use only: As little as a teaspoon of tea tree oil can be toxic. Do not ingest it. Keep it away from children.
AIDS	Garlic	Garlic is anticoagulant and may cause bruising and/or delay blood clotting.
	St. John's wort	If you take an antidepressant or a protease inhibitor, consult a physician before using St. John's wort.
Alzheimer's disease	Coffee	Coffee contains caffeine, which may cause jitters, irritability, insomnia, and addiction.
	Ginkgo	Ginkgo is anticoagulant and may cause bruising and/or delay blood clotting.
	Saffron	
Antidepressant-induced sex problems	Ginkgo	Ginkgo is anticoagulant and may cause bruising and/or delay blood clotting.
Anxiety	Ashwagandha	
	Bacopa	
	Cannabis	In states that have not legalized medical marijuana, use of cannabis may lead to arrest and imprisonment.
	Catnip	
	Celery	Long-term use of celery seed may deplete potassium stores.
	Chamomile	

CONDITION	HERB(S)	SPECIAL PRECAUTIONS
Anxiety (cont.)	Ginkgo	
	Gotu kola	
	Hop	
	Kava	
	Lavender	
	Lemon balm	Lemon balm interferes with thyroid-stimulating hormone. If you have an underactive thyroid (hypothyroidism), consult a physician before using it.
	Motherwort	
	Passionflower	
	Rhodiola	
	Scullcap	
	Yarrow	
Aphrodisiac	Maca	
	Muira puama	
Arthritis (Osteoarthritis)	Angelica	Angelica may cause a rash on exposure to sunlight.
	Arnica	
	Black haw	
	Boneset	
	Boswellia	
	Cat's claw	
	Chamomile	
	Chaparral	
	Comfrey	Comfrey should not be ingested.
	Devil's claw	
	Echinacea	
	Evening primrose	
	Fenugreek	Fenugreek has estrogenic action. People with a history of abnormal blood clots (thromboembolism), inflammation of the blood vessels (thrombophlebitis), heart disease, or stroke should consult their physicians before using it.
	Gentian	

CONDITION	HERB(S)	SPECIAL PRECAUTIONS
	Ginger	
	Horsetail	Long-term use of horsetail, juniper, nettle, and vervain may deplete potassium stores.
	Juniper	
	Licorice	Long-term use of licorice may cause water retention, elevated blood pressure, and a hormone imbalance (pseudoaldosteronism).
	Meadowsweet	Meadowsweet and white willow contain aspirin-like compounds. If you are aspirin-sensitive, consult a physician before using it. Do not give meadowsweet to children under 16 with fever. It may cause Reye's syndrome.
	Nettle	
	Red pepper	
	Rose	
	St. John's wort	If you take an antidepressant, consult a physician before using St. John's wort.
	Turmeric	
	Vervain	Vervain may depress heart rate and constrict bronchial passages. If you have heart disease, high blood pressure, diabetes, or asthma, consult a physician before using it.
	While willow	
Asthma	Angelica	Angelica may cause a rash on exposure to sunlight.
	Borage	
	Boswellia	
	Cocoa (dark chocolate)	Cocoa (dark chocolate), coffee, kola, maté, and tea all contain caffeine, which may cause jitters, irritability, insomnia, and addiction.
	Coffee	
	Cordyceps	
	Ephedra	Ephedra may raise blood pressure and cause jitters, irritability, and insomnia. People with high blood pressure, heart or kidney disease, or a history of stroke should not use it. In very large doses, ephedra may cause potentially fatal heart problems.

CONDITION	HERB(S)	SPECIAL PRECAUTIONS
Asthma (cont.)	Kola	
	Maté	
	Tea	
Athlete's foot	*For external use:*	
	Tea tree	As little as a teaspoon of tea tree oil may be toxic. Do not ingest it and keep it away from children and pets.
Attention deficit/ hyperactivity disorder (ADHD)	Bacopa	
	Lemon balm	Lemon balm interferes with thyroid-stimulating hormone. If you have an underactive thyroid (hypothyroidism), consult a physician before ingesting it.
	Passionflower	
Bad breath	Alfalfa	
	Parsley	Long-term use of large amounts of parsley may deplete potassium stores.
Benign prostate enlargement	Nettle	Long-term use of large amounts of nettle may deplete potassium stores.
	Pumpkin seed	
	Pygeum	
	Saw palmetto	
Bleeding	Blackberry	
	Shepherd's purse	Shepherd's purse may cause powerful uterine contractions.
	Witch hazel	
	Yarrow	
Bronchitis (see also Cough)	Angelica	
	Barberry	
	Cordyceps	
	Echinacea	
	Garlic	Garlic is an anticoagulant and may cause bruising and/or delay blood clotting.
	Marshmallow	
	Pelargonium	

CONDITION	HERB(S)	SPECIAL PRECAUTIONS
Burns (see also Pain)	*For external use:*	Wash burns before applying herbal medicines. Extensive burns that raise blisters require professional care.
	Aloe	
	Chamomile	
	Comfrey	
	Echinacea	
	Gotu kola	
	Marshmallow	
	Passionflower	
	St. John's wort	
	Witch hazel	
	Yarrow	
Cancer prevention	Alfalfa	
	Apple	
	Ashwagandha	
	Bilberry	
	Blackberry	
	Black cohosh	
	Cat's claw	
	Cocoa (dark chocolate)	Cocoa (dark chocolate) and tea contains caffeine, which may cause jitters, irritability, insomnia, and addiction.
	Cranberry	
	Dandelion	
	Flax	
	Garlic	Garlic is an anticoagulant and may cause bruising and/or delay blood clotting.
	Ginseng	
	Maitake	
	Pomegranate	
	Raspberry	
	Reishi	
	Rhodiola	

CONDITION	HERB(S)	SPECIAL PRECAUTIONS
Cancer prevention (cont.)	Rooibos	
	Shiitake	
	Soybean	Soybean may reduce sperm count. Soybean is estrogenic. Women with hormonal conditions who have been advised to avoid birth control pills should consult their physicians before ingesting soy in amounts greater than a few servings of tofu per week.
	Stevia	
	Tea (green)	
	Turmeric	
Cancer treatment	Boarge	
	Echinacea	
	Maitake	
	Mistletoe	Mistletoe may slow heart rate and affect blood pressure. If you have heart disease, diabetes, high blood pressure, or a history of stroke, consult your physician before using it.
	Reishi	
	Rhodiola	
	Shiitake	
	Tea (green)	Tea contains caffeine, which may cause jitters, irritability, insomnia, and addiction.
Canker sores	Licorice	Long-term use of licorice may cause water retention, elevated blood pressure, and a hormone imbalance (pseudoaldosteronism).
Cataracts	Bilberry	
	Blackberry	
	Cranberry	
	Raspberry	
	Turmeric	
Childbirth recovery	Lavender	
Cholera	Barberry	Cholera is potentially fatal. Use herbs in conjunction with professional care.
	Goldenseal	

CONDITION	HERB(S)	SPECIAL PRECAUTIONS
Cirrhosis	Ginseng	
	Licorice	Long-term use of licorice may cause water retention, elevated blood pressure, and a hormone imbalance (pseudoaldosteronism).
	Milk thistle	
Cluster headache	Red pepper	
Colds and flu (see also Cough)	Angelica	
	Boneset	
	Cocoa (dark chocolate)	Cocoa (dark chocolate), coffee, and tea contain caffeine, which may cause jitters, irritability, insomnia, and addiction.
	Coffee	
	Echinacea	
	Elderberry	
	Eleutherococcus	
	Ephedra	Ephedra may raise blood pressure and cause jitters, irritability, and insomnia. People with high blood pressure, heart or kidney disease, or a history of stroke should not use it. In very large doses, ephedra may cause potentially fatal heart problems.
	Eucalyptus	
	Garlic	
	Ginger	
	Ginseng	
	Hyssop	
	Licorice	Long-term use of licorice may cause water retention, elevated blood pressure, and a hormone imbalance (pseudoaldosteronism).
	Marshmallow	
	Meadowsweet	Meadowsweet contains aspirin-like compounds. If you are aspirin-sensitive, consult a physician before using it. Do not give meadowsweet to children under 16 with fever. It may cause Reye's syndrome.
	Mullein	
	Pelargonium	

CONDITION	HERB(S)	SPECIAL PRECAUTIONS
Colds and flu (see also Cough) (cont.)	Peppermint	
	Rose	
	Slippery elm	
	Tea	
Cold sores (see Herpes and cold sores)		
Colic	Dill	
	Fennel	
	Slippery elm	
Congestive heart failure (see also Diuretics in "Healing Actions" chart	Buchu	All these herbs are diuretic and may cause potassium depletion.
	Celery	
	Dandelion	
	Hawthorn	
	Juniper	
	Nettle	
	Parsley	
	Sarsaparilla	
	Uva-ursi	
Conjunctivitis	Barberry	
Constipation	Apple	
	Buckthorn	Buckthorn, cascara sagrada, rhubarb, and senna may cause abdominal distress.
	Cascara sagrada	
	Psyllium	
	Rhubarb	
	Senna	
Cough	Angelica	Angelica may cause a rash on exposure to sun light.
	Cocoa (dark chocolate)	Cocoa (dark chocolate), coffee, kola, maté, and tea all contain caffeine, which may cause jitters, irritability, insomnia, and addiction.
	Coffee	

CONDITION	HERB(S)	SPECIAL PRECAUTIONS
	Ephedra	Ephedra may raise blood pressure and cause jitters, irritability, and insomnia. People with high blood pressure, heart or kidney disease, or a history of stroke should not use it. In very large doses, ephedra may cause potentially fatal heart problems.
	Eucalyptus	
	Fenugreek	Fenugreek has estrogenic action. People with a history of abnormal blood clots (thromboembolism), inflammation of the blood vessels (thrombophlebitis), heart disease, or stroke should consult their physicians before using it.
	Horehound	
	Hyssop	
	Kola	
	Licorice	Long-term use of licorice may cause water retention, elevated blood pressure, and a hormone imbalance (pseudoaldosteronism).
	Marshmallow	
	Maté	
	Mullein	
	Pennyroyal	
	Peppermint	
	Slippery elm	
	Tea	
	Thyme	
Depression	Chamomile	
	Coffee	Coffee and tea contain caffeine, which may cause jitters, irritability, insomnia, and addiction.
	Rhodiola	
	Saffron	
	St. John's wort	If you take any antidepressants, consult your physician before using St. John's wort.
	Tea	
	Turmeric	

CONDITION	HERB(S)	SPECIAL PRECAUTIONS
Diabetes	Aloe	
	Apple	
	Ashwagandha	
	Barberry	
	Bitter melon	
	Celery	Long-term use of celery may deplete potassium.
	Cinnamon	
	Eleutherococcus	
	Evening primrose	
	Fenugreek	Fenugreek has estrogenic action. People with a history of abnormal blood clots (thromboembolism), inflammation of the blood vessels (thrombophlebitis), heart disease, or stroke should consult their physicians before using it.
	Flax	
	Garlic	Garlic is an anticoagulant and may cause bruising or delay clotting.
	Ginger	
	Ginseng	
	Gotu kola	
	Milk thistle	
	Pomegranate	
	Red pepper	
	Reishi	
	Sage	
	Stevia	
	Tea	Tea contains caffeine and may cause jitters, irritability, insomnia, and addiction.
	Turmeric	
Diabetic neuropathy	Red pepper	
Diabetic retinopathy	Bilberry	
	Blackberry	
	Cranberry	
	Ginkgo	
	Raspberry	

CONDITION	HERB(S)	SPECIAL PRECAUTIONS
Diarrhea	Apple	
	Barberry	
	Bayberry	Bayberry may change the body's sodium-potassium balance. If you have high blood pressure, heart disease, diabetes, kidney disease, or a history of stroke, consult a physician before using it.
	Bilberry	
	Blackberry	
	Chamomile	
	Dill	
	Goldenseal	
	Meadowsweet	Meadowsweet contains aspirin-like compounds. If you are aspirin-sensitive, consult a physician before using it.
	Mullein	
	Psyllium	
	Purslane	
	Raspberry	
	Red pepper	
	Rhubarb	Large doses of rhubarb have laxative action and may cause abdominal distress.
	Slippery elm	
	Tea	Tea contains caffeine and may cause jitters, irritability, insomnia, and addiction.
	Uva-ursi	Long-term use of uva-ursi may deplete potassium stores.
Dizziness	Ginger	
	Ginkgo	
Dry skin	Borage	
Ear infection	Echinacea	
	Garlic	Garlic is an anticoagulant and may cause bruising or delay blood clotting.
Eczema	Borage	
	Evening primrose	
	Tea	Tea contains caffeine and may cause jitters, irritability, insomnia, and addiction.

CONDITION	HERB(S)	SPECIAL PRECAUTIONS
Emphysema	Eucalyptus	
	Ginseng	
	Peppermint	
Erectile dysfunction (due to poor blood flow)	Ginkgo	
	Ginseng	
	Saffron	
	Yohimbe	
Fatigue	Ashwagandha	
	Cocoa (dark chocolate)	Cocoa (dark chocolate), coffee, kola, maté, and tea all contain caffeine and may cause jitters, irritability, insomnia, and addiction.
	Coffee	
	Eleutherococcus	
	Ephedra	Ephedra may raise blood pressure and cause jitters, irritability, and insomnia. People with high blood pressure, heart or kidney disease, or a history of stroke should not use it. In very large doses, ephedra may cause potentially fatal heart problems.
	Ginseng	
	Kola	
	Maté	
	Rhodiola	
	Tea	
Fever	Andrographis	Andrographis is an anticoagulant and may cause bruising or delay blood clotting.
	Bayberry	Bayberry may change the body's sodium-potassium balance. If you have high blood pressure, heart disease, diabetes, kidney disease, or a history of stroke, consult a physician before using it.
	Black haw	
	Meadowsweet	Meadowsweet and white willow contain aspirin-like compounds. If you are aspirin-sensitive, consult a physician before using these herbs.
	White willow	

CONDITION	HERB(S)	SPECIAL PRECAUTIONS
Fibroids	Black cohosh	
Fibromyalgia	Cannabis	In states that have not legalized medical marijuana, use of cannabis may lead to arrest and imprisonment.
	Red pepper	
Flu (see Colds and flu)		
Food poisoning prevention	Echinacea	
	Rosemary	
	Sage	
	Thyme	
	Turmeric	
Food poisoning treatment	Angelica	Angelica may cause a rash in sensitive people exposed to direct sunlight.
	Apple	
	Barberry	
	Bayberry	Bayberry may change the body's sodium-potassium balance. If you have high blood pressure, heart disease, diabetes, kidney disease, or a history of stroke, consult a physician before using it.
	Burdock	
	Catnip	
	Chamomile	
	Cinnamon	
	Clove	
	Dill	
	Echinacea	
	Garlic	Garlic is an anticoagulant and may cause bruising or delay blood clotting.
	Ginseng	
	Goldenseal	
	Meadowsweet	Meadowsweet contains aspirin-like compounds. If you are aspirin-sensitive, consult a physician before using it.
	Mullein	
	Peppermint	

CONDITION	HERB(S)	SPECIAL PRECAUTIONS
Gallstone prevention	Coffee	Coffee contains caffeine and may cause jitters, irritability, insomnia, and addiction.
	Dandelion	Long-term use of dandelion may deplete potassium stores.
Gas (flatulence)	Dill	
Genital warts	Shiitake	
Giardiasis	Barberry	
	Elecampane	
	Goldenseal	
Glaucoma	Bilberry	
	Blackberry	
	Cannabis	In states that have not legalized medical marijuana, use of cannabis may lead to arrest and imprisonment.
	Cranberry	
	Raspberry	
Gout (see also Pain)	Celery	Long-term use of celery and nettle may deplete potassium stores.
	Coffee	Coffee contains caffeine and may cause jitters, irritability, insomnia, and addiction.
	Nettle	Long-term use of nettle may deplete potassium stores.
Gum disease prevention	Aloe	
	Chaparral	
	Cinnamon	
	Elderberry	
	Eucalyptus	
	Goldenseal	
	Myrrh	
	Neem	Small amounts of neem oil are toxic. Use it only in commercial toothpastes.
Hay fever	Astragalus	
	Butterbur	
	Clove	
	Nettle	Long-term use of nettle and parsley may deplete potassium stores.
	Parsley	

CONDITION	HERB(S)	SPECIAL PRECAUTIONS
Headache	Black haw	
	Eucalyptus	
	Feverfew (migraine)	
	Meadowsweet	Meadowsweet and white willow contain aspirin-like compounds. If you are aspirin-sensitive, consult a physician before using these herbs.
	Peppermint	
	Red pepper (cluster headache)	
	White willow	
Hearing loss	Ginkgo	
Heart disease (see also High blood pressure and High cholesterol)	Alfalfa	
	Angelica	
	Apple	
	Artichoke	
	Ashwagandha	
	Astragalus	
	Barberry	
	Bilberry	
	Blackberry	
	Cat's claw	
	Celery	
	Cocoa (dark chocolate)	Cocoa (dark chocolate) and tea (green) contains caffeine and may cause jitters, irritability, insomnia, and addiction.
	Cordyceps	
	Cranberry	
	Elderberry	
	Eleutherococcus	
	Evening primrose	
	Flax	
	Garlic	Garlic and shepherd's purse are anticoagulants and may cause bruising or delay blood clotting.

CONDITION	HERB(S)	SPECIAL PRECAUTIONS
Heart disease (see also High blood pressure and High cholesterol) (cont.)	Ginger	
	Ginkgo	
	Ginseng	
	Hawthorn	
	Meadowsweet	Meadowsweet and white willow contain aspirin-like compounds. If you are aspirin-sensitive, consult a physician before using these herbs.
	Motherwort	
	Pomegranate	
	Purslane	
	Raspberry	
	Red clover	
	Reishi	
	Rhodiola	
	Rooibos	
	Rose	
	Sage	
	Shepherd's purse	
	Soybean	Soybean may suppress sperm count. It also has estrogenic action. Women with hormonal conditions who have been advised to avoid birth control pills should consult their physicians before take soy in amounts greater than a few servings of tofu per week.
	Stevia	
	Tea (green)	
	Turmeric	
	White willow	
Heart rhythm normalization	Rhodiola	
Hemorrhoids	*For external use:*	
	Blackberry	
	Mullein	
	Psyllium	

CONDITION	HERB(S)	SPECIAL PRECAUTIONS
	Shepherd's purse	Shepherd's purse may cause powerful uterine contractions.
	Slippery elm	
	Tarragon	
	Witch hazel	
	For internal use:	
	Butcher's broom	
	Horse chestnut	
Hepatitis	Licorice	Long-term use of licorice may cause water retention, elevated blood pressure, and a hormone imbalance (pseudoaldosteronism).
	Maitake	
	Milk thistle	
	Shiitake	
Herpes and cold sores	*For external use:*	
	Comfrey	
	Hyssop	
	Lemon balm	Lemon balm interferes with thyroid-stimulating hormone. If you have an underactive thyroid (hypothyroidism), consult a physician before ingesting it.
	Licorice	Long-term use of licorice may cause water retention, elevated blood pressure, and a hormone imbalance (pseudoaldosteronism).
	Peppermint	
	Uva-ursi	Long-term use of uva-ursi may deplete potassium stores.
	For internal use:	
	Echinacea	
	Garlic	Garlic is an anticoagulant and may cause bruising or delay blood clotting.
	Lemon balm	
	Reishi	

CONDITION	HERB(S)	SPECIAL PRECAUTIONS
High blood pressure (see also Diuretics in Healing Actions)	Barberry	
	Black cohosh	Black cohosh is estrogenic. Women with a history of blood clots (thromboembolism) or inflammation of the blood vessels (thrombophlebitis), heart disease, or stroke should consult their physicians before using it.
	Buchu	
	Cat's claw	
	Celery	Long-term use of celery may deplete potassium stores.
	Cocoa (dark chocolate)	Cocoa (dark chocolate) contains caffeine and may cause jitters, irritability, insomnia, and addiction.
	Dandelion	
	Evening primrose	
	Garlic	Garlic is an anticoagulant and may cause bruising or delay blood clotting.
	Ginger	
	Ginseng	
	Gotu kola	
	Hawthorn	
	Hibiscus	
	Juniper	
	Mistletoe	Mistletoe may slow heart rate and affect blood pressure. If you have heart disease, diabetes, high blood pressure, or a history of stroke, consult a physician before using it.
	Motherwort	
	Nettle	Long-term use of nettle and parsley may deplete potassium stores.
	Parsley	
	Pomegranate	
	Purslane	
	Rhodiola	
	Sarsaparilla	
	Soybean	Soybean may suppress sperm count. It also has estrogenic action. Women with hormonal conditions who have been advised to avoid birth control pills should consult their physicians before take soy in amounts greater than a few servings of tofu per week.

CONDITION	HERB(S)	SPECIAL PRECAUTIONS
	Stevia	
	Uva-ursi	
	Valerian	
High cholesterol	Alfalfa	
	Apple	
	Artichoke	
	Ashwagandha	
	Bacopa	
	Cat's claw	
	Celery	Long-term use of celery may deplete potassium stores.
	Cinnamon	
	Cocoa (dark chocolate)	Cocoa (dark chocolate) and tea contains caffeine and may cause jitters, irritability, insomnia, and addiction.
	Evening primrose	
	Fenugreek	Fenugreek and soybean have estrogenic action. Soybean may suppress sperm count. People with a history of blood clots (thromboembolism) or blood vessel inflammation (thrombophlebitis), heart disease, or stroke should consult a physician before using fenugreek or soybean in quantities greater than a few servings of tofu per week.
	Flax	
	Garlic	Garlic is an anticoagulant and may cause bruising or delay blood clotting.
	Ginger	
	Ginseng	
	Hawthorn	
	Purslane	
	Psyllium	
	Red pepper	
	Scullcap	
	Shiitake	

CONDITION	HERB(S)	SPECIAL PRECAUTIONS
High cholesterol (cont.)	Soybean	Women with hormonal conditions who have been advised to avoid birth control pills should consult their physicians before ingesting soybean in amounts greater than a few servings of tofu per week.
	Tea	
	Turmeric	
HIV/AIDS	Shiitake	
Hives	Nettle	Long-term use of nettle and parsley may deplete potassium stores.
	Parsley	
Hypothyroidism	Bacopa	
Infertility (male)	Ashwagandha	
	Ginseng	
	Tea	Tea contains caffeine and may cause jitters, irritability, insomnia, and addiction.
Infertility (female)	Tea	Tea contains caffeine and may cause jitters, irritability, insomnia, and addiction.
Insomnia	Cannabis	In states that have not legalized medical marijuana, use of cannabis may lead to arrest and imprisonment.
	Catnip	
	Celery	Long-term use of celery may deplete potassium stores.
	Chamomile	
	Hop	
	Lavender	
	Lemon balm	Lemon balm interferes with thyroid-stimulating hormone. Those with underactive thyroid (hypothyroidism) should consult a physician before using it.
	Motherwort	
	Passionflower	
	Rhodiola	
	Scullcap	
	Valerian	
	Yarrow	

CONDITION	HERB(S)	SPECIAL PRECAUTIONS
Intermittent claudication	Ginkgo	
Irritable bowel syndrome	Artichoke	
	Cannabis	In states that have not legalized medical marijuana, use of cannabis may lead to arrest and imprisonment.
	Caraway	
	Peppermint	
	Turmeric	
Jet lag	Cocoa (dark chocolate)	Cocoa (dark chocolate), coffee, kola, mate, and tea all contain caffeine and may cause jitters, irritability, insomnia, and addiction.
	Coffee	
	Ephedra	Ephedra may raise blood pressure and cause jitters, irritability, and insomnia. People with high blood pressure, heart or kidney disease, or a history of stroke should not use it. In very large doses, ephedra may cause potentially fatal heart problems.
	Ginseng	
	Kola	
	Maté	
	Tea	
Kidney disease	Cordyceps	
Kidney stone prevention	Coffee	Coffee and tea contain caffeine, which may cause jitters, irritability, insomnia, and addiction.
	Horsetail	
	Pumpkin seed	
	Tea	
Lead poisoning	Apple	
	Garlic	Garlic is an anticoagulant and may cause bruising or delay blood clotting.
Leprosy (Hansen's disease)	Garlic	Garlic is an anticoagulant and may cause bruising or delay blood clotting.
	Gotu kola	
Lice (head lice)	*For eternal use:*	
	Tea tree	

CONDITION	HERB(S)	SPECIAL PRECAUTIONS
Lymphedema	Butcher's broom	
Macular degeneration	Bilberry	
	Blackberry	
	Cranberry	
	Ginkgo	
	Raspberry	
	Saffron	
Menopausal discomforts	Angelica	All these herbs have estrogenic action. Women who have been advised not to use birth control pills should consult their physicians before using them.
	Black cohosh	
	Fennel	
	Flax	
	Ginseng	
	Hop	
	Kava	
	Licorice	Long-term use of licorice may cause water retention, elevated blood pressure, and a hormonal imbalance (pseudoaldosteronism).
	Maca	
	Red clover	
	Rhubarb	Large doses of rhubarb have laxative action and may cause abdominal distress.
	Sage	
	St. John's wort	
	Soybean	
Menstrual cramps (see also Pain)	Black cohosh	
	Black haw	
	Chaste tree	
	Fennel	Fennel, fenugreek, and red clover have estrogenic action. Women who have been advised not to use birth control pills should consult their physicians before using them.
	Fenugreek	

CONDITION	HERB(S)	SPECIAL PRECAUTIONS
	Feverfew	
	Ginger	
	Lavender	
	Red clover	
	Yarrow	
Menstrual flow, heavy	Goldenseal	
Menstruation, delayed	Celery	Long-term use of celery may deplete potassium stores.
	Chaste tree	
	Fenugreek	Fenugreek has estrogenic action. Women who have been advised not to use birth control pills should consult their physicians before using them.
	Motherwort	
	Parsley	
	Pennyroyal	
	Rhubarb	Large doses of rhubarb have laxative action and may cause abdominal distress.
	Shepherd's purse	Shepherd's purse may cause powerful utterine contractions.
Menstruation, heavy	Chaste tree	
	Coffee	Coffee contains caffeine and may cause jitters, irritability, insomnia, and addiction.
	Shepherd's purse	Shepherd's purse may cause powerful utterine contractions.
Migraine	Butterbur	
	Feverfew	
Morning sickness	Ginger	
	Raspberry	
Motion sickness	Ginger	
Mouth sores	Blackberry	
Multiple sclerosis	Cannabis	In states that have not legalized medical marijuana, use of cannabis may lead to arrest and imprisonment.

CONDITION	HERB(S)	SPECIAL PRECAUTIONS
Muscle soreness and cramping	Arnica	Arnica is toxic. Ingest only homeopathic microdoses.
	Cinnamon	
	Purslane	
Muscle strength improvement	Ashwagandha	
Mushroom poisoning	Milk thistle	
Nausea	Cannabis	In states that have not legalized medical marijuana, use of cannabis may lead to arrest and imprisonment.
	Ginger	
	Peppermint	
Neuropathy (nerve pain)	Cannabis	In states that have not legalized medical marijuana, use of cannabis may lead to arrest and imprisonment.
Obesity	Bitter melon	
	Coffee	Coffee and tea contain caffeine and may cause jitters, irritability, insomnia, and addiction.
	Ephedra	Ephedra may raise blood pressure and cause jitters, irritability, and insomnia. People with high blood pressure, heart or kidney disease, or a history of stroke should not use it. In very large doses, ephedra may cause potentially fatal heart problems. Coffee and other herbs containing caffeine increase ephedra's effects and side effects. Ephedra and coffee should be used for weight control only under medical supervision.
	Maitake	
	Purslane	
	Tea	
Osteoarthritis (see Arthritis)		
Osteoporosis prevention	Eleutherococcus	
	Soybean	Soybean may suppress sperm count. It also has estrogenic action. Women with hormonal conditions who have been advised to avoid birth control pills should consult a physician before ingesting soy in amounts greater than a few servings of tofu per week.
	Tea	Tea contains caffeine, which may cause jitters, irritability, insomnia, and addiction.

CONDITION	HERB(S)	SPECIAL PRECAUTIONS
Parkinson's disease	Coffee	Coffee contains caffeine, which may cause jitters, irritability, insomnia, and addiction.
Pain (see also Anesthetic in "Healing Actions" table)	*For external use:*	
	Comfrey	
	For internal use:	
	Andrographis	
	Arnica	
	Black haw	
	Boswellia	
	Cannabis	In states that have not legalized medical marijuana, use of cannabis may lead to arrest and imprisonment.
	Coffee	Coffee, maté, and tea contain caffeine, which may cause jitters, irritability, insomnia, and addiction.
	Devil's claw	
	Maté	
	Meadowsweet	Meadowsweet and white willow contain aspirin-like compounds. If you are aspirin-sensitive, consult physician before using these herbs.
	Passionflower	
	Peppermint	
	Red pepper	
	Tea	
	Vervain	Vervain may depress heart rate and construct bronchial passages. If you have heart disease, high blood pressure, diabetes, or athma, consult a physician before using it.
	White willow	
Pinkeye	Barberry	
Poison ivy, oak, and sumac	Aloe	
Postpartum hemorrhage	Shepherd's purse	Shepherd's purse may cause powerful uterine contractions.
Pre-eclampsia	Cocoa (dark chocolate)	Cocoa (dark chocolate) contains caffeine, which may cause jitters, irritability, insomnia, and addiction.

CONDITION	HERB(S)	SPECIAL PRECAUTIONS
Premenstrual syndrome (PMS)	Black cohosh	
	Buchu	Buchu, celery, dandelion, horsetail, juniper, nettle, parsley, sarsaparilla, and uva-ursi are diuretics and may deplete potassium stores.
	Celery	
	Chaste tree	
	Dandelion	
	Evening primrose	
	Fennel	Fennel has estrogenic action. Women with a history of blood clots (thromboembolism) or blood vessel inflammation (thrombophlebitis), heart disease, or stroke should consult a physician before using medicinal amounts.
	Horsetail	
	Juniper	
	Lavender	
	Nettle	
	Parsley	
	Sarsaparilla	
	Uva-ursi	
Prostate cancer	Fennel	
	Red clover	
	Saw palmetto	
Psoriasis	Aloe	
	Barberry	
	Gotu kola	
	Red pepper	
	Turmeric	
Radiation exposure	Eleutherococcus	
Reaction time improvement	Ashwagandha	

CONDITION	HERB(S)	SPECIAL PRECAUTIONS
Restless leg syndrome	St. John's wort	If you take an antidepressant, consult a physician before using St. John's wort.
	Valerian	
Rheumatoid arthritis	Borage	
	Boswellia	
	Cannabis	In states that have not legalized medical marijuana, use of cannabis may lead to arrest and imprisonment.
	Cat's claw	
	Evening primrose	
	Tea	Tea contains caffeine, which may cause jitters, irritability, insomnia, and addiction.
	Turmeric	
Scabies	For external use:	
	Tea tree	
	Turmeric	
Scalds (see Burns)		
Scurvy	Nettle	
Seasonal affective disorder (SAD)	St. John's wort	
Shingles	Red pepper	
Sinus infection	Andrographis	Andrographis is anticoagulant and may cause bruising and delay blood clotting.
	Pelargonium	
Sore throat	Fennel	Fennel has estrogenic action. Women with a history of blood clots (thromboembolism) or blood vessel inflammation (thrombophlebitis), heart disease, or stroke should consult a physician before using medicinal amounts.
	Licorice	Long-term use of licorice may cause water retention, elevated blood pressure, and a hormonal imbalance (pseudoaldosteronism).
	Marshmallow	
	Mullein	
	Sage	
	Slippery elm	

CONDITION	HERB(S)	SPECIAL PRECAUTIONS
Stress	Ashwagandha	
	Bacopa	
	Cannabis	In states that have not legalized medical marijuana, use of cannabis may lead to arrest and imprisonment.
	Catnip	
	Celery	Long-term use of celery may deplete potassium stores.
	Chamomile	
	Ginseng	
	Hop	
	Kava	
	Lavender	
	Lemon balm	Lemon balm interferes with thyroid-stimulating hormone. If you have an underactive thyroid (hypothyroidism), consult a physician before using it.
	Motherwort	
	Passionflower	
	Rhodiola	
	Scullcap	
	Yarrow	
Stretch marks	Gotu kola	
Stroke	Alfalfa	
	Angelica	
	Apple	
	Astragalus	
	Bilberry	
	Blackberry	
	Cat's claw	
	Celery	
	Cocoa (dark chocolate)	Cocoa (dark chocolate), coffee, and tea all contain caffeine, which may cause jitters, irritability, insomnia, and addiction.

CONDITION	HERB(S)	SPECIAL PRECAUTIONS
	Coffee	
	Cordyceps	
	Cranberry	
	Elderberry	
	Evening primrose	
	Garlic	Garlic is anticoagulant and may cause bruising or delay blood clotting.
	Ginger	
	Ginkgo	
	Ginseng	
	Hawthorn	
	Meadowsweet	Meadowsweet and white willow contain aspirin-like compounds. If you are aspirin-sensitive, consult a physician before using these herbs.
	Motherwort	
	Pomegranate	
	Raspberry	
	Reishi	
	Rhodiola	
	Rooibos	
	Rose	
	Soybean	Soybean may suppress sperm count. It also has estrogenic action. Women with hormonal conditions who have been advised to avoid birth control pills should consult a physician before ingesting soy in amounts greater than a few servings of tofu per week.
	Tea (green)	
	Turmeric	
	White willow	
Sunburn (see Burns)		
Tinnitus (ringing in the ears)	Horse chestnut	
Tonsilitis	Pelargonium	

CONDITION	HERB(S)	SPECIAL PRECAUTIONS
Toothache	*For external use only:*	Herbal oils are highly concentrated. If ingested, as little as a teaspoon may be toxic. Keep herbal oils away from children and pets.
	Clove oil	
	Tarragon oil	
Tooth decay preventions	*For topical application:*	
	Chaparral	
	Cinnamon	
	Neem	Neem oil is toxic if ingested. Use it only in commercial toothpastes.
	Peppermint	
	For ingestion:	
	Tea	Tea contains caffeine, which may cause jitters, irritability, insomnia, and addiction.
Ulcerative colitis	Boswellia	
	Turmeric	
Ulcers	Chamomile	
	Garlic	Garlic is an anticoagulant and may cause bruising or delay blood clotting.
	Ginger	
	Licorice	Long-term use of licorice may cause water retention, elevated blood pressure, and a hormone imbalance (pseudoaldosteroinism).
	Neem	Neem oil is toxic. Use it only under a physician's supervision.
	Turmeric	
Urinary incontinence	Cranberry	
Urinary tract infection prevention	Andrographis	Andrographis is an anticoagulant and may cause bruising or delay blood clotting.
	Cranberry	
	Dill	
	Horsetail	Long-term use of horsetail and nettle may deplete potassium stores.
	Nettle	

CONDITION	HERB(S)	SPECIAL PRECAUTIONS
Urinary tract infection treatment	Barberry	
	Garlic	Garlic is an anticoagulant and may cause bruising or delay blood clotting.
	Meadowsweet	Meadowsweet contains aspirin-like compounds. If you are aspirin-sensitive, consult a physician before using these herbs.
	Uva-ursi	Long-term use of uva-ursi may deplete potassium stores.
Varicose veins	Bilberry	
	Blackberry	
	Butcher's broom	
	Cranberry	
	Gotu kola	
	Horse chestnut	
	Hyssop	
	Raspberry	
	Tarragon	
Weight control (See Obesity)		
Wounds	For external use:	
	Aloe	
	Barberry	
	Blackberry	
	Burtdock	
	Chamomile	
	Comfrey	
	Echinacea	
	Eucalyptus	
	Fenugreek	
	Garlic	
	Gotu kola	
	Horsetail	
	Lavender	
	Lemon balm	

CONDITION	HERB(S)	SPECIAL PRECAUTIONS
Wounds (cont.)	Marshmallow	
	Passionflower	
	Rosemary	
	Sage	
	St. John's wort	
	Shepherd's purse	
	Slippery elm	
	Tarragon	
	Tea tree	
	Thyme	
	Uva-ursi	
	Witch hazel	
	Yarrow	
	For internal use:	
	Echinacea	
	Garlic	Garlic is an anticoagulant and may cause bruising or delay blood clotting.
Yeast infection (candidiasis)	Barberry	
	Chamomile	
	Cinnamon	
	Dandelion	
	Echinacea	
	Garlic	Garlic and pau d'arco are anticoagulants and may cause bruising and delay blood clotting.
	Pau d-arco	
	Tea tree	Do not ingest tea tree oil by mouth. As little as a teaspoon can be toxic. Keep away from children and pets.

Healing Actions of Herbs

ACTION	HERB(S)	SPECIAL PRECAUTIONS
Adaptogen	Ashwagandha	
	Eleutherococcus	
	Ginseng	
	Reishi	
	Rhodiola	
	Schisandra	
Anesthetic	*For external use:*	Do not ingest herbal oils. As little as a teaspoon may be toxic. Keep herbal oils away from children and pets.
	Cinnamon oil	
	Clove oil	
	Peppermint oil	
Antibiotic (antibacterial)	Apple	
	Artichoke	
	Barberry	
	Bayberry	
	Boneset	
	Burdock	
	Catnip	
	Chamomile	
	Cinnamon	
	Clove	
	Dill	
	Echinacea	
	Garlic	Garlic and pau d'arco are anticoagulants and may cause bruising and delay blood clotting.
	Ginseng	
	Goldenseal	
	Licorice	Long-term use of licorice may cause water retention, elevated blood pressure, and a hormone imbalance (pseudoaldosteroinism).
	Meadowsweet	Meadowsweet contains aspirin-like compounds. If you are aspirin-sensitive, consult a physician before using this herb.

ACTION	HERB(S)	SPECIAL PRECAUTIONS
Antibiotic (antibacterial) (cont.)	Myrrh	
	Pau d'arco	
	Peppermint	
	Reishi	
	St. John's wort	If you take antidepressant medication, consult a physician before using St. John's wort.
	Tea tree	Do not ingest tea tree oil by mouth. As little as a teaspoon can be toxic. Keep away from children and pets.
	Thyme	
Antibiotic (antifungal)	Aloe	
	Artichoke	
	Barberry	
	Burtdock	
	Chamomile	
	Clove	
	Dandelion	Long-term use of dandelion may deplete potassium stores.
	Echinacea	
	Garlic	Garlic is an anticoagulant and may cause bruising and delay blood clotting.
	Goldenseal	
	Licorice	Long-term use of licorice may cause water retention, elevated blood pressure, and a hormone imbalance (pseudoaldosteroinism).
	St. John's wort	If you take antidepressant medication, consult a physician before using St. John's wort.
	Tea tree	Do not ingest tea tree oil by mouth. As little as a teaspoon can be toxic. Keep away from children and pets.
Antibiotic (antiparasitic, antiprotozoan)	Barberry	
	Bayberry	Bayberry may change the body's sodium-potassium balance. If you have high blood pressure, heart disease, diabetes, kidney disease, or a history of stroke, consult a physician before using it.
	Clove	
	Elecampane	

ACTION	HERB(S)	SPECIAL PRECAUTIONS
	Garlic	Garlic is an anticoagulant and may cause bruising and delay blood clotting.
	Goldenseal	
	Myrrh	
	Turmeric	
Anticoagulant	Garlic	These herbs may cause bruising and delay blood clotting.
	Shepherd's purse	
Antidepressant	Coffee	Coffee contains caffeine, which may cause jitters, irritability, insomnia, and addiction.
	St. John's wort	If you take antidepressant medication, consult a physician before using St. John's wort.
Antihistamine	Clove	
	Nettle	Long-term use of nettle may deplete potassium stores.
Anti-inflammatory	Andrographis	Andrographis is an anticoagulant and may cause bruising and delay blood clotting.
	Angelica	Angelica may cause a rash in sensitive people exposed to direct sunlight.
	Bacopa	
	Black haw	
	Boneset	
	Cat's claw	
	Chamomile	
	Chaparral	
	Echinacea	
	Fenugreek	
	Gentian	
	Ginger	
	Horsetail	Long-term use of horsetail, juniper, and vervain may deplete potassium stores.
	Juniper	
	Licorice	Long-term use of licorice may cause water retention, elevated blood pressure, and a hormone imbalance (pseudoaldosteroinism).
	Meadowsweet	Meadowsweet and white willow contain aspirin-like compounds. If you are aspirin-sensitive, consult a physician before using these herbs.

ACTION	HERB(S)	SPECIAL PRECAUTIONS
Anti-inflammatory (cont.)	Purslane	
	St. John's wort	If you take antidepressant medication, consult a physician before using St. John's wort.
	Turmeric	
	Vervain	Vervain may depress heart rate and constrict bronchial passages. If you have heart disease, high blood pressure, diabetes, or asthma, consult a physician before using it.
	White willow	
Antioxidant	Ashwagandha	
	Bacopa	
	Bilberry	
	Blackberry	
	Cat's claw	
	Chaparral	
	Cocoa (dark chocolate)	Cocoa (dark chocolate), coffee, and tea contain caffeine, which may cause jitters, irritability, insomnia, and addiction.
	Coffee	
	Cordyceps	
	Cranberry	
	Elderberry	
	Eleutherococcus	
	Muira puama	
	Pomegranate	
	Raspberry	
	Reishi	
	Tea	
	Turmeric	
Antiperspirant	Sage	
Antiseptic	*For external use on minor burns and wounds:*	
	Aloe	
	Apple	

ACTION	HERB(S)	SPECIAL PRECAUTIONS
	Blackberry	
	Catnip	
	Chamomile	
	Chaparral	
	Cinnamon	
	Clove	
	Eucalyptus	
	Garlic	
	Hop	
	Lemon balm	
	Licorice	
	Myrrh	
	Passionflower	
	Peppermint	
	Rosemary	
	Sage	
	St. John's wort	
	Slippery elm	
	Tarragon	
	Tea tree	
	Thyme	
	Turmeric	
	Yarrow	
	For internal use:	
	Echinacea	
	Ginseng	
Antiviral	Boneset	
	Cat's claw	
	Chamomile	
	Cinnamon	
	Echinacea	

ACTION	HERB(S)	SPECIAL PRECAUTIONS
Antiviral (cont.)	Ginger	
	Ginseng	
	Lemon balm	Lemon balm interferes with thyroid-stimulating hormone. If you have an underactive thyroid (hypothyroidism), consult a physician before using it.
	Pau d'arco	Pau d'arco is anticoagulant and may cause bruising and delay blood clotting.
	St. John's wort	If you take antidepressant medication, consult a physician before using St. John's wort.
Colonoscopy preparation	Senna	Senna may cause abdominal distress.
Decongestant	Angelica	
	Cocoa (dark chocolate)	Cocoa (dark chocolate), coffee, kola, maté, and tea contain caffeine, which may cause jitters, irritability, insomnia, and addiction.
	Coffee	
	Ephedra	Ephedra may raise blood pressure and cause jitters, irritability, and insomnia. People with high blood pressure, heart or kidney disease, or a history of stroke should not use it. In very large doses, ephedra may cause potentially fatal heart problems.
	Eucalyptus	
	Kola	
	Maté	
	Pennyroyal	
	Peppermint	
	Rosemary	
	Tea	
Digestive support	Angelica	Angelica may cause a rash in sensitive people exposed to direct sunlight.
	Artichoke	
	Caraway	
	Catnip	
	Chamomile	
	Cinnamon	

ACTION	HERB(S)	SPECIAL PRECAUTIONS
	Clove	
	Cocoa (dark chocolate)	Cocoa (dark chocolate) contains caffeine, which may cause jitters, irritability, insomnia, and addiction.
	Dandelion	
	Dill	
	Fennel	Fennel has estrogenic action. Women with a history of blood clots (thromboembolism) or blood vessel inflammation (thrombophlebitis), heart disease, or stroke should consult a physician before using medicinal amounts.
	Feverfew	
	Gentian	
	Ginger	
	Goldenseal	
	Hop	
	Horehound	
	Lavender	
	Lemon balm	Lemon balm interferes with thyroid-stimulating hormone. If you have an underactive thyroid (hypothyroidism), consult a physician before using it.
	Marshmallow	
	Papaya	
	Passionflower	
	Pennyroyal	
	Peppermint	
	Purslane	
	Red pepper	
	Rosemary	
	Sage	
	Slippery elm	
	Thyme	
	Turmeric	
	Yarrow	

ACTION	HERB(S)	SPECIAL PRECAUTIONS
Diuretic	Buchu	Long-term use of diuretic herbs may deplete potassium stores. Do not use diuretics for weight loss.
	Celery	
	Dandelion	
	Fennel	
	Horsetail	
	Juniper	
	Nettle	
	Parsley	
	Sarsaparilla	
	Uva-ursi	
Immune stimulation	For external use:	
	Aloe	
	For internal use:	
	Andrographis	Andrographis and garlic are anticoagulants and may cause bruising and delay blood clotting.
	Ashwagandha	
	Astragalus	
	Barberry	
	Bittter melon	
	Boneset	
	Cat's claw	
	Chamomile	
	Cordyceps	
	Echinacea	
	Eleutherococcus	
	Garlic	
	Ginger	
	Goldenseal	
	Gotu kola	

ACTION	HERB(S)	SPECIAL PRECAUTIONS
	Licorice	Long-term use of licorice may cause water retention, elevated blood pressure, and a hormone imbalance (pseudoaldosteronism).
	Maitake	
	Mistletoe	Mistletoe may slow heart rate and affect blood pressure. If you have heart disease, diabetes, high blood pressure, or a history of stroke, consult your physician before using it.
	Reishi	
	St. John's wort	If you take antidepressant medication, consult a physician before using St. John's wort.
	Shiitake	
	Turmeric	
Kidney protection	Reishi	
Labor stimulation	Shepherd's purse	Using herbs to induce labor requires medical supervision.
Labor support	Raspberry	
Lactation support	Chaste tree	
	Peppermint	
Laxative	Apple	
	Buckthorn	Buckthorn, cascara sagrada, rhubarb, and senna may cause abdominal distress. If you find yourself using them more than twice a month, consult a physician.
	Cascara sagrada	
	Coffee	Coffee contains caffeine, which may cause jitters, irritability, insomnia, and addiction.
	Psyllium	
	Rhubarb	
	Senna	
Liver protection	Andrographis	Andrographis is an anticoagulant and may cause bruising and delay blood clotting.
	Artichoke	
	Astragalus	
	Bacopa	
	Barberry	
	Cordyceps	

ACTION	HERB(S)	SPECIAL PRECAUTIONS
Liver protection (cont.)	Licorice	Long-term use of licorice may cause water retention, elevated blood pressure, and a hormone imbalance (pseudoaldosteronism).
	Maitake	
	Milk thistle	
	Reishi	
	Rhodiola	
	Turmeric	
Pregnancy support	Raspberry	
Sedative	Celery	Long-term use of celery may deplete potassium stores.
	Hop	
	Lavender	
	Lemon balm	Lemon balm interferes with thyroid-stimulating hormone. If you have an underactive thyroid (hypothyroidism), consult a physician before using it.
	Motherwort	
	Passionflower	
	Scullcap	
	Valerian	
	Yarrow	
Stimulant	Cocoa (dark chocolate)	Cocoa (dark chocolate), coffee, kola, mate, and tea all contain caffeine, which may cause jitters, irritability, insomnia, and addiction.
	Coffee	
	Ephedra	Ephedra may raise blood pressure and cause jitters, irritability, and insomnia. People with high blood pressure, heart or kidney disease, or a history of stroke should not use it. In very large doses, ephedra may cause potentially fatal heart problems.
	Ginseng	
	Kola	
	Maté	
	Tea	
Surgery recovery	Lavender	

ACTION	HERB(S)	SPECIAL PRECAUTIONS
Tranquilizer	Ashwagandha	
	Cannabis	In states that have not legalized medical marijuana, use of cannabis may lead to arrest and imprisonment.
	Catnip	
	Celery	Long-term use of celery may deplete potassium stores.
	Chamomile	
	Hop	
	Lavender	
	Lemon balm	Lemon balm interferes with thyroid-stimulating hormone. If you have an underactive thyroid (hypothyroidism), consult a physician before using it.
	Motherwort	
	Passionflower	
	Scullcap	
	Yarrow	

Other Uses of Herbs

USE	HERB(S)	SPECIAL PRECAUTIONS
Appetite loss	Ginseng	
Athletic performance enhancement	Coffee	Coffee contains caffeine, which may cause jitters, irritability, insomnia, and addiction.
	Ginseng	
	Peppermint	
	Rhodiola	
Cognitive function	Bacopa	
	Cocoa (dark chocolate)	Cocoa (dark chocolate), coffee, and tea contain caffeine, which may cause jitters, irritability, insomnia, and addiction.
	Coffee	
	Ginkgo	
	Ginseng	
	Gotu kola	
	Rhodiola	

USE	HERB(S)	SPECIAL PRECAUTIONS
Cognitive function (cont.)	Rosemary	
	Sage	
	Tea	
	Turmeric	
Insect repellent	Eucalyptus	
	Lavender	
	Neem	Neem oil and pennyroyal oil are toxic. Do not ingest them. Keep them away from children and pets.
	Pennyroyal oil	
Memory improvement	Bacopa	
	Eleutherococcus	
	Ginkgo	
	Ginseng	
Self-defense	Red pepper	
Wrinkles	*For external use:*	
	Rooibos	
	Tea	

References

How to Find the Latest Research on Medicinal Herbs

It's never been easier. Just visit PubMed (pubmed.gov), the Web site that catalogs most of the world medical literature. In the search bar, enter either the herb's common name (e.g., garlic) or its scientific name (*Allium sativum*). Abstracts of most studies published in the peer-reviewed medical literature come up. Research abstracts tend to be dense, but once you get used to the format, it's not difficult to read them.

Bibliography

Because of space limitations, we are unable to list the more than 1,000 medical journal articles used as sources for *The New Healing Herbs*. Source books are listed here.

Editors of the Pharmacist's Letter. *Natural Medicines Comprehensive Database.* www.naturaldatabase.therapeuticresearch .com/home

American Pharmaceutical Association. *Handbook of Nonprescription Drugs.* Washington, D.C.: American Pharmaceutical Association, 1996.

Backes, M. *Cannabis Pharmacy: The Practical Guide to Medical Marijuana.* New York: Black Dog & Leventhal Publishers, 2014.

Bassman, L. *The Whole Mind: The Definitive Guide to Complementary Treatments for Mind, Mood, and Emotion.* Novato, CA: New World Library, 1998.

Beinfield, H., and E. Korngold. *Between Heaven and Earth: A Guide to Chinese Medicine.* New York: Ballantine, 1991.

Blumenthal, M. *The ABC Clinical Guide to Herbs.* Austin, TX: American Botanical Council. 2003.

Blumenthal, M., et al. *Herbal Medicine: Expanded Commission E Monographs.* Austin, TX: American Botanical Council, 2000.

Blumenthal, M., et al. *The Complete German Commission E Monographs: Therapeutic Guide to Herbal Medicines.* Austin, TX: American Botanical Council and Integrative Medicine Communications, 1998.

Boyle, W. *Herb Doctors: Pioneers in 19th-Century American Botanical Medicine.* East Palestine, OH: Buckeye Naturopathic Press, 1988.

Brinker, F. J. *The Toxicology of Botanical Medicines.* 2nd ed. Portland, OR: Eclectic Medical Institute, 1987.

Brown, D. *Herbal Prescriptions for Better Health.* Rocklin, CA: Prima Publishing, 1996.

Burton Goldberg Group. *Alternative Medicine: The Definitive Guide.* Fife, WA: Future Medicine, 1994.

Chin, W. Y., and H. Keng. *An Illustrated Dictionary of Chinese Medicinal Herbs.* Sebastopol, CA: CRCS Publications, 1992.

Collinge, W. *The American Holistic Health Association Complete Guide to Alternative Medicine.* New York: Warner Books, 1996.

Conrow, R., and A. Hecksel. *Herbal Pathfinders: Voices of the Herb Renaissance.* Santa Barbara, CA: Woodbridge Press, 1983.

Coulter, H. L. *Divided Legacy.* Berkeley, CA: Homeopathic Educational Services, 1982.

Crenshaw, T. *The Alchemy of Love and Lust.* New York: Putnam, 1996.

Culpeper, N. *Culpeper's Complete Herbal and English Physician. 1826 ed.* Avon, England: Pitman Press, 1981.

Cummings, S., and D. Ullman. *Everybody's Guide to Homeopathic Medicines.* New York: Tarcher-Putnam, 1997.

Cumston, C. G. *An Introduction to the History of Medicine.* New York: Dorset Press, 1987.

Der Marderosian, A., and L. Liberti. *Natural Product Medicine.* Philadelphia: George F. Stickley, 1988.

DeSmet, P. A., ed. *Adverse Effects of Herbal Drugs.* Berlin: Springer-Verlag, 1993.

De Waal, M. *Medicinal Herbs in the Bible.* York Beach, ME: Samuel Weiser, 1984.

Dobelis, I. N., ed. *Magic and Medicine of Plants.* Pleasantville, NY: Reader's Digest, 1986.

Duke, J. A. *Ginseng: A Concise Handbook.* Algonac, MI: Reference Publications, 1989.

———. *The Green Pharmacy.* Emmaus, PA: Rodale, 1997.

———. *Handbook of Medicinal Herbs.* Boca Raton, FL: CRC Press, 1985.

Ehrenreich, B., and D. English. *Witches, Midwives, and Nurses: A History of Women Healers.* Detroit: Black and Red, 1973.

Eskinazi, D., et al., eds. *Botanical Medicine: Efficacy, Quality Assurance, and Regulation.* Larchmont, NY: Mary Ann Liebert, 1999.

Facts and Comparisons. *Drug Facts and Comparisons, 1999 and 2000.* St. Louis, MO: Facts and Comparisons Publishing Group, 1999 and 2000.

Felter, H. W., and J. U. Lloyd. *King's American Dispensatory.* 18th ed., 1898. Portland, OR: Eclectic Medical Publications, 1983.

Foster, S. *Echinacea Exalted!* Brixley, MO: Ozark Beneficial Plant Project, 1985.

———. *Herbal Bounty.* Salt Lake City: Peregrine Smith Books, 1984.

Foster, S., and J. A. Duke. *A Field Guide to Medicinal Plants: Eastern and Central North America* (Peterson Field Guide #40). Boston: Houghton Mifflin, 1990.

Foster, S., and V. E. Tyler. *Tyler's Honest Herbal.* 4th ed. New York and London: Haworth Herbal Press, 1999.

Fratkin, J. *Chinese Herbal Patent Formulas.* Boulder, CO: Shya Publications, 1986.

Fugh-Berman, A. *Alternative Medicine: What Works.* Tucson: Odonian Press, 1996.

Fulder, S. *Ginseng: Magical Herb of the East.* Northamptonshire, England: Thorsons Publishing, 1988.

Funfgeld, E. W., ed. *Rokan (Ginkgo Biloba): Recent Results in Pharmacology and Clinic.* Berlin: Springer-Verlag, 1988.

Gilman, A. G., et al, eds. *Goodman and Gilman's The Pharmacological Basis of Therapeutics.* 7th ed. New York: Macmillan, 1985.

Graedon, J., and T. Graedon. *Graedon's Best Medicine: From Herbal Remedies to High-Tech Rx Breakthroughs.* New York: Bantam Books, 1991.

Grieve, M. *A Modern Herbal. Volumes I and II.* New York: Dover, 1971.

Griffith, H. W. *The Complete Guide to Vitamins, Minerals, Supplements, and Herbs.* Tucson: Fisher Books, 1988.

Hallowell, M. *Herbal Healing: A Practical Introduction.* Bath, England: Ashgrove Press, 1985.

Harris, B. C. *Comfrey: What You Need to Know.* New Canaan, CT: Keats Publishing, 1982.

Harris, L. J. *The Book of Garlic.* Berkeley, CA: Aris Books, 1979.

Herbrandson, D. *Shaker Herbs and Their Medicinal Uses.* New Gloucester, ME: Shaker Heritage Society, Sabbathday Lake, 1985.

Heyn, B. *Ayurvedic Medicine.* Northamptonshire, England: Thorsons Publishing, 1987.

Hobbs, C. *The Ginsengs: A Users Guide.* Santa Cruz, CA: Botanica Press, 1996.

———. *Herbal Remedies for Dummies.* Foster City, CA: IDG Books, 1998.

Hoffman, D. *The Holistic Herbal.* Dorset, England: Element Books, 1983.

Hou, J. P. *Ginseng: The Myth and the Truth.* North Hollywood, CA: Wilshire Book Co., 1978.

Keville, K., and M. Green. *Aromatherapy: A Complete Guide to the Healing Art.* Freedom, CA: Crossing Press, 1995.

Kiangsu Institute of Modern Medicine. *Encyclopedia of Chinese Drugs,* vol. 2. Shanghai: Shanghai Scientific and Technical Publications, 1977.

Kloss, J. *Back to Eden.* Loma Linda, CA: Back to Eden Books, 1988.

Koch, H. P., and L. D. Lawson, eds. *Garlic: The Science and Therapeutic Application of Allium Sativum and Related Species.* Baltimore: Williams and Wilkins, 1996.

Kowalchik, C., and W. H. Hylton, eds. *Rodale's Illustrated Encyclopedia of Herbs.* Emmaus, PA: Rodale, 1987.

Kreig, M. B. *Green Medicine: The Search for Plants That Heal.* Chicago: Rand McNally, 1964.

Lad, V., and D. Frawley. *The Yoga of Herbs.* Santa Fe: Lotus Press, 1986.

Law, D. *The Concise Herbal Encyclopedia.* New York: St. Martin's Press, 1973.

Leung, A. Y. *Encyclopedia of Common Natural Ingredients Used in Food, Drugs, and Cosmetics.* New York: John Wiley & Sons, 1980.

Lewis, W., and M. P. F. Elvin-Lewis. *Medical Botany.* New York: John Wiley & Sons, 1974.

Lust, J. *The Herb Book.* New York: Bantam, 1974.

Marti-Ibaez, F. *The Epic of Medicine.* New York: Bramhall House, 1962.

McCaleb, R., et al. *The Herb Research Foundation's Encyclopedia of Popular Herbs.* Roseville, CA: Prima Publishing, 2000.

McGuffin, M., et al., eds. *American Herbal Products Association Botanical Safety Handbook.* Boca Raton, FL: CRC Press, 1997.

McIntyre, M. *Herbal Medicine for Everyone.* London: Penguin, 1988.

Medical Economics. *PDR for Herbal Medicines.* Montvale, NJ: Medical Economics, 1998.

Micozzi, M. S. *Fundamentals of Complementary and Alternative Medicine.* New York: Churchill Livingstone, 1996.

Millspaugh, C. F. *American Medicinal Plants.* 1892 ed. New York: Dover, 1974.

Morse, F. *The Story of the Shakers.* Woodstock, VT: Countryman Press, 1986.

Mowrey, D. B. *Next Generation Herbal Medicine.* Lehi, UT: Cormorant Books, 1988.

————. *The Scientific Validation of Herbal Medicine.* Lehi, UT: Cormorant Books, 1986.

Murray, M. *Natural Alternatives to Over-the-Counter and Prescription Drugs.* New York: William Morrow, 1994.

————. *The 21st Century Herbal.* Bellevue, WA: Vita-Line, 1987.

Murray, M., and J. Pizzorno. *Encyclopedia of Natural Medicine.* Rocklin, CA: Prima Publishing, 1991.

Olsen, C. *Australian Teatree Oil Guide.* Pagosa Springs, CO: Kali Press, 1997.

Pendergrast, M. *Uncommon Grounds: The History of Coffee and How It Transformed Our World.* New York: Basic Books, 1999.

Pizzorno, J., and M. Murray. *A Textbook of Natural Medicine.* Kenmore, WA: Bastyr University Publications, 1996.

Reid, D. P. *Chinese Herbal Medicine.* Boston: Shambhala, 1987.

Riddle, J. M. *Eve's Herbs: A History of Contraception and Abortion in the West.* Cambridge, MA: Harvard University Press, 1997.

Schechter, S. *Fighting Radiation with Foods, Herbs, and Vitamins.* Brookline, MA: East West Health Books, 1988.

Simon, J. E., and L. Grant, eds. *Proceedings of the First National Herb Growing and Marketing Conference.* West Lafayette, IN: Purdue University Cooperative Extension Service, 1986.

————. *Proceedings of the Second National Herb Growing and Marketing Conference.* West Lafayette, IN: Purdue University Cooperative Extension Service, 1987.

Simon, J. E., et al. *Proceedings of the Fourth National Herb Growing and Marketing Conference.* Silver Spring, PA: International Herb Growers and Marketers Association, 1989.

Spencer, J. W., and J. J. Jacobs. *Complementary/Alternative Medicine: An Evidence-Based Approach.* St. Louis: Mosby, 1999.

Spinella, M. *The Psychopharmacology of Herbal Medicine.* Cambridge, MA: MIT Press, 2001.

Spoerke, D. *Herbal Medications.* Santa Barbara, CA: Woodbridge Press, 1980.

Starr, P. *The Social Transformation of American Medicine.* New York: Basic Books, 1982.

Stuart, M., ed. *The Encyclopedia of Herbs and Herbalism.* New York: Grosset & Dunlap, 1979.

Strehlow, W., and G. Hertzka. *Hildegard of Bingen's Medicine.* Santa Fe: Bear, 1988.

Tannahill, R. *Food in History.* New York: Stein & Day, 1973.

Tierra, M. *The Way of Herbs.* New York: Pocket Books, 1983.

Tyler, V. *Herbs of Choice: The Therapeutic Use of Phytomedicinals.* New York: Hawthorn Press, 1994.

Tyler, V. E., et al. *Pharmacognosy.* 9th ed. Philadelphia: Lea and Febiger, 1988.

Ullman, D. *The Consumer's Guide to Homeopathy.* New York: G. P. Putnam's Sons, 1995.

Weed, S. S. *Wise Woman Herbal for the Childbearing Years.* Woodstock, NY: Ash Tree Publishing, 1985.

Weil, A. *Natural Health, Natural Medicine.* Boston: Houghton Mifflin, 1990.

Weiner, M., and J. A. Weiner. *Herbs That Heal.* Mill Valley, CA: Quantum Books, 1994.

Weiner, M. A. *Earth Medicine, Earth Food.* New York: Macmillan, 1980.

————. *The People's Herbal.* New York: Perigee/Putnam, 1984.

————. *Weiner's Herbal.* New York: Stein & Day, 1980.

Weiss, G., and S. Weiss. *Growing and Using the Healing Herbs.* Emmaus, PA: Rodale, 1985.

Weiss, R. F. *Herbal Medicine.* Beaconsfield, England: Beaconsfield Publishers, 1988.

Werbach, M., and M. Murray. *Botanical Influences on Illness.* Tarzana, CA: Third Line Press, 1994.

Wheelwright, E. G. *Medicinal Plants and Their History.* New York: Dover, 1974.

White, L., and S. Foster. *The Herbal Drugstore: The Best Natural Alternatives to Over-the-Counter and Prescription Medicines.* Emmaus, PA: Rodale, 2000.

White, L., and S. Mavor. *Kids, Herbs, and Health.* Loveland, CO: Interweave Press, 1998.

Willard, T. *Textbook of Modern Herbology.* Calgary, Alberta, Canada: Progressive Publishing, 1988.

Wren, R. C. *Potter's New Cyclopaedia of Botanical Drugs and Preparations.* Essex, England: C. W. Daniel, 1988.

Zhu, C-H. *Clinical Handbook of Chinese Prepared Medicines.* Brookline, MA: Paradigm Publications, 1989.

Index

Underscored page references indicate sidebars and tables. **Boldface** references indicate illustrations.

About the Author

*L*ibrary Journal has called Michael Castleman "one of the nation's top health writers." He has been the herbal medicine columnist for *Herb Quarterly* magazine since 1988. His articles on herbal medicine have appeared in many publications and online, including *Prevention, Reader's Digest, Redbook, Family Circle, AARP Magazine, Natural Health, Herb Companion*, Salon.com, WebMD.com, and PsychologyToday.com.

Castleman is the author of 13 consumer medical books with a total of more than 2 million copies in print. They include: *Blended Medicine*, a home medical guide that combines the best of mainstream and alternative medicine for 100 common conditions; *Nature's Cures*, an exploration of the science behind 30 alternative therapies; *Before You Call the Doctor* (coauthored with Anne Simons, M.D., and Bobbie Hasselbring) a self-care home medical guide; and *Building Bone Vitality* (coauthored with Amy Lanou, Ph.D.), a guide to osteoporosis prevention and treatment that argues against calcium supplements. Castleman has also written three mystery novels.

A former adjunct professor at the University of California, Berkeley, Graduate School of Journalism, where he taught medical writing, Castleman has won several awards for excellence in journalism.

He lives in San Francisco.